360° Around Shoulder Instability

Roman Brzóska • Giuseppe Milano
Pietro S. Randelli • Ladislav Kovačič
Editors

360° Around Shoulder Instability

Springer

European Society of Sports Traumatology, Knee Surgery & Arthroscopy
ESSKA

Editors
Roman Brzóska
Shoulder and Upper Limb Department
St. Luke's Hospital
Bielsko-Biała
Poland

Pietro S. Randelli
Istituto Ortopedico Gaetano Pini
Prima Clinica Ortopedica
Milan
Italy

Giuseppe Milano
Department of Medical and Surgical Specialties, Radiological Sciences, and Public Health
University of Brescia
Brescia
Italy

Department of Bone and Joint Surgery
Spedali Civili
Brescia
Italy

Ladislav Kovačič
Department of Traumatology
University Medical Centre Ljubljana
Ljubljana
Slovenia

ISBN 978-3-662-61073-2 ISBN 978-3-662-61074-9 (eBook)
https://doi.org/10.1007/978-3-662-61074-9

This Springer imprint is published by the registered company Springer-Verlag GmbH, DE part of Springer Nature.
The registered company address is: Heidelberger Platz 3, 14197 Berlin, Germany

To Mariangela. Don't look back in anger. There is always a good chance to take. Someday, somehow…

GM

To Krištof, Klemen and Jernej - amazing boys. Being with you is pleasure and happiness. The future is all in front of you. Go ahead with brave and decisive steps. You can realize your dreams.

Ladislav Kovačič

Preface

As a continuation of the tradition, initiated during the first ESA Biennale Meeting in Rome, we share with you another monograph, which is a collection of speeches that were presented during the ESA second meeting. The title of this book is uniform with the title of the last meeting "360 degrees around shoulder instability" which took place on 5–7 October 2017 in Kraków/Bielsko-Biała, Poland.

The book you are holding is a compendium which includes summaries of scientific reports on the treatment of shoulder instability, but also original studies, made available by many experienced and widely recognized shoulder surgeons.

In this book, as the title says, we started a discussion on the diagnosis and treatment of anterior instability in all its aspects. Then we tried to discuss the problems in the treatment of posterior, multidirectional instability and those less common forms of instability whose recognition and effective treatment still pose many problems in daily practice even for the most experienced surgeons. Scientific reports indicate that we still lack clear and transparent guidelines in the treatment of shoulder instability and we are still looking for new solutions to expand the portfolio of modern treatment methods, giving new tools and solutions to shoulder surgeons.

The dynamic development of shoulder surgery enables continuous progress in this field, bringing new methods, especially in arthroscopic techniques. We know that the effectiveness of instability treatment is best judged by time. Many methods, especially at the beginning of the arthroscopic era, did not withstand the test of time.

Enriched by these experiences, we are still looking for better surgical solutions; furthermore our knowledge about indications is also maturing. Learning from experience, we also know more and more about the irreplaceable role of rehabilitation and physiotherapy in the treatment of shoulder instability. Contemporary treatment, especially of posterior and multidirectional instability, practically would not exist without the correct cooperation of orthopedic surgeons, physiotherapists, and sometimes doctors of other specialties.

This book is composed according to the program of the ESA meeting in Krakow/Bielsko-Biała, presenting the problem of shoulder instability in all its aspects. You will find in it explanation of the underlying causes of these pathologies, a multidisciplinary approach facilitating understanding of etiology, diagnostics, and finally treatment methods.

The involvement of scientists representing basic sciences gives a broad perspective to the issues raised and sets out some new directions for cooperation between various fields of medicine and medical science.

We have long stopped treating the problem of instability as a mechanical issue—consisting only in the treatment of organic damage. We have an increasing knowledge of the pathophysiology of these phenomena. We are able to determine the probability of recurrence of instability with much greater precision, combining facts from the interview, constitutional conditions of the patient and his activity. The defining feature of this monograph is numerous algorithms that are useful in making decision when planning the treatment.

Almost all lecturers who participated in the ESA meeting in Krakow/Bielsko-Biała agreed to participate in the creation of this book and share their experiences. We also invited our American, Canadian, and Indian colleagues to share with us their perspective on the current approach to anterior instability.

Thanks to the support of ESSKA management and Springer's professional help, this monograph could be created in such high quality. We hope that readers will receive answers to many bothering questions and help in making daily decisions in effective treatment of patients suffering from various forms of shoulder instability.

Bielsko-Biała, Poland Roman Brzóska
Brescia, Italy Giuseppe Milano
Milan, Italy Pietro S. Randelli
Ljubljana, Slovenia Ladislav Kovačič

Contents

Part II Posterior Shoulder Instability

Part I

Anterior Shoulder Instability

1 Historical Outline of Anterior Shoulder Instability Treatment

Radovan Mihelic and Tomislav Prpic

The history of shoulder instability goes far back into the ancient era. It was on Egyptian papyrus dated some 2000 years. BC that a shoulder reduction was drawn (Fig. 1.1). This is the first known document on the subject. Next description comes from Hippocrates 400 BC showing a shoulder traction to reduce a dislocation (Fig. 1.2). This same method was later reintroduced by Kocher in 1870 [1]. It was even documented in *Hippocratic Corpus*, and some doctors use it still today [2].

The middle age has a lack of medical texts and methods, the Inquisition has occupied the attention of the unbelievers, and it was not popular to mess around with anatomy. Therefore, the work of Jean-François Malgaigne in 1855 is important; he described a bony lesion of the humeral head after anterior dislocation, which we now call the Hill-Sachs lesion [3]. Harold A. Hill and Maurice D. Sachs were two radiologists who have described a humeral defect as a result of repeated dislocations in 1940 [4].

The nineteenth century brings us some interesting papers explaining surgical methods to address the anterior instability. In 1819 Weinhold has published about a surgical reduction to the dislocated shoulder [5, 6]. The Czech surgeon named Eduard Albert made the first fusion of the shoulder in 1878 after serious condition due to recurrent instability, and he named it the arthrodesis [7]. Today it might seem a little exaggerated, but in 1882, Cramer in Germany used a humeral head resection for the chronically unstable shoulder [8].

Auguste Broca and Henri Albert Charles Antoine Hartmann in a paper published in 1890 in French have explained the anatomy of anterior capsular complex in unstable shoulder. They emphasized the role of the glenoid labrum for the joint stability [9].

At the turn to the twentieth century, two important papers appeared thus starting the modern era of shoulder treatment. The first was published in Germany by B. Perthes in 1906 about the surgery of the unstable shoulder [10]. In his paper he has explained the type of anterior capsular detachment that we today call "the Perthes lesion." The second, a paper that we consider a historic turn in shoulder understanding, was published in 1923 by Arthur Sidney Blundell Bankart [11]. He has explained that the detachment of the anterior capsule causes the anterior instability and it is necessary to reattach it in order to stabilize the joint. This short publication on two pages with no images has caused an impact so important that we consider this paper as a basic science in shoulder instability.

Almost at the same time, Vittorio Putti and Harry Platt (1923–1925) have published their surgical method for capsulolabral plication

R. Mihelic (✉)
Special Hospital Medico, Rijeka, Croatia

T. Prpic
University Orthopedic Clinic Lovran, Lovran, Croatia

R. Brzóska et al. (eds.), *360° Around Shoulder Instability*,
https://doi.org/10.1007/978-3-662-61074-9_1

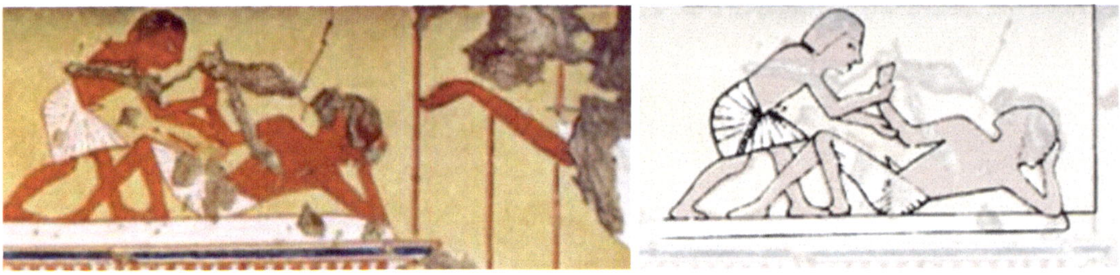

Fig. 1.1 Egyptian papyrus showing a shoulder reduction. (Reproduced from Davies, N. de Garis. Two Ramesside Tombs at Thebes. Robb de Peyster Tytus Memorial Series, Vol 5 1927. New York the Metropolitan museum of Art)

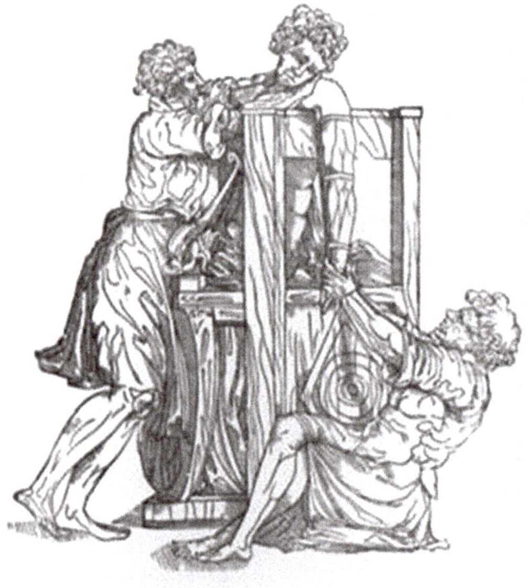

Fig. 1.2 "Inquisition type" of reduction on the Hippocratic device. (An Illustrated history by Ira M Rutkow pub 1993. A woodcut probably after a drawing by Francesco Salviati)

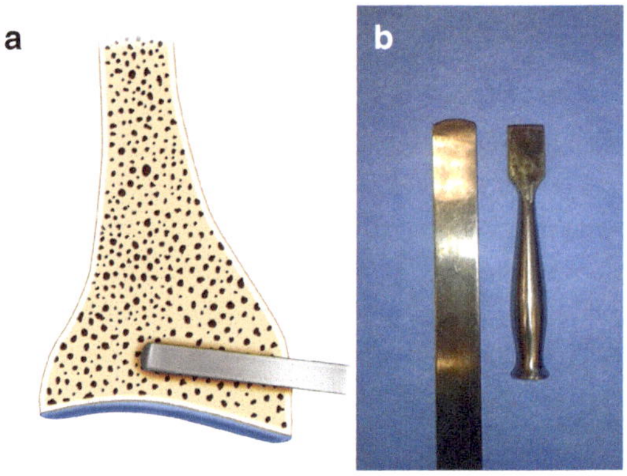

Fig. 1.3 (**a**) Schematic image of the bone block by Eden. (Drawing by the author). (**b**) Special chisels for Eden-Hybinette procedure used in our clinic in the 1980s

including the subscapularis muscle. There were two groups of surgical techniques: the first group have performed various variations of soft tissue tensioning, while the other group introduced a bone block to be used as an anterior plug that will prevent the humeral head to dislocate. So, let us go back to 1917. Then the first paper about the bone block procedure appeared by Eden (Fig. 1.3a, b). He used a cortical tibia graft and introduced it into the anterior glenoid rim [12]. In 1932 the similar procedure was published by Hybinette, only he used an iliac bone block [13]. At that time with no Internet, it was possible that two surgeons invented the same method and publish it in their country without knowing for each other. Around the year 1980 when I discovered the orthopedic world in the late 1970s of the twentieth century, this method was widely used in my country, so in my clinic we still preserve (in the museum) special chisels for this purpose.

Magnuson-Stack method in 1943 described transferring the subscapularis under the coracoid and over the biceps tendon to stabilize the joint [14]. Next similar soft tissue procedure was the one by Russian surgeon Boicev (1951) who has also transferred the subscapularis but over the conjoined tendon and fixed it more laterally [15].

The next important method was again the bone block stabilization. It was published in 1954 by Latarjet [16]. Four years later Helfet has published a similar method invented by Bristow who died before publishing it [17]. Therefore, it is now known as "Bristow-Latarjet" procedure which consisted of the coracoid transfer to the anterior glenoid rim. This method was so successful that nowadays it is wary popular, especially as a difficult arthroscopic procedure, just to show what we can achieve with mini invasive techniques. This technique has two effects: the first is a bone block limitation, and the second is a sling effect of the attached conjoint tendon which brings more tension to the anterior aspect of the joint.

It is a fact that hip and knee surgery developed much faster than shoulder. We can speculate about the reasons, but it is a fact. So, the 1st Symposium on Surgery of the Shoulder Region was held in Montreal in 1963. The first International Conference on Surgery of the Shoulder was organized in London in 1980.

1.1 Arthroscopy: The Modern Era

Lanny Johnson in London has performed the first arthroscopic stabilization of the shoulder in 1980, the same year of the London Conference [18]. He used staples and had recurrence in 15–25%, but it was only the beginning. In fact, arthroscopic techniques had the same aim as Bankart, that is, to refix the labrum to the glenoid. For this purpose, some implants were necessary. Seven years later, two Americans Morgan and Caspari have introduced transglenoid sutures with no implants (Fig. 1.4) [19, 20]. The 1990s was the era of huge development of arthroscopic techniques and solutions. All kinds of implants were invented including wires, staples, screws, and anchors. Still the recurrent rate was between 4 and 35% long after that. Arthroscopy enabled a precise visualization of the entire shoulder joint, and new precise classification of several types of capsulolabral tear was introduced.

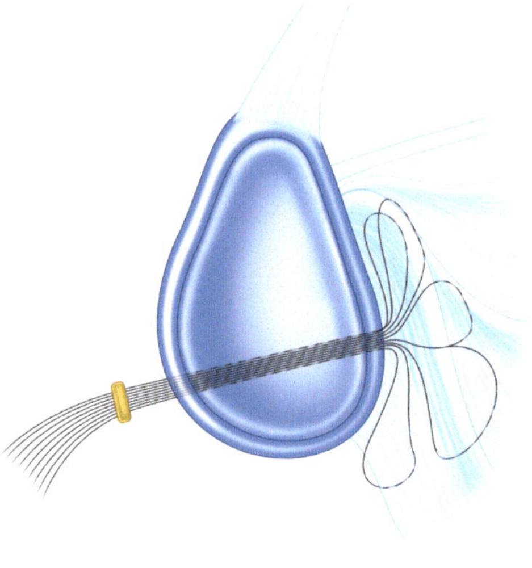

Fig. 1.4 Transglenoid sutures by Caspari. (Caspari RB (1988) Arthroscopic reconstruction for anterior shoulder instability. Tech Orthop 3:1)

The evolution of arthroscopic techniques enables complex and demanding extraarticular surgeries where almost everything is possible. The technology and industry encourage the surgeons to it. New generations of arthroscopic equipment and young and courageous surgeons send us the message: "only the sky is our limit"!

References

1. Kocher ET. Eine neue Reduktionsmethode für Schulterverrenkung. Berliner Klin Wochenschrift. 1870;7:101–5.
2. Hippocrates Corpus Hippocraticum—De articulis. Corpus Hippocrat. p. 201.
3. Malgaigne J-F. Traité des fractures et des luxations. Paris: Baillière; 1855. p. 454–570.
4. Hill HA, Sachs MD. The grooved defect of the humeral head. Radiology. 1940;35:690–700.
5. Randelli P, Cucchi D, Butt U. History of shoulder instability surgery. Knee Surg Sports Traumatol Arthrosc. 2016;24:305–29.
6. Osmond-Clarke H. Habitual dislocation of the shoulder; the Putti–Platt operation. J Bone Joint Surg Br. 1948;30B:19–25.
7. Albert E. Die chirurgischen Krankheiten der Wirbelsäule,der Brust, des Schultergürtels und der oberen Gliedmassen. Lehrbuch der Chirurgie und Operationslehre: Vorlesungen für praktische Ärzte und Studirende, Band 2. Wien: Urban & Schwarzenberg; 1878.
8. Cramer F. Resektion des Oberarmkopfes wegen habitueller Luxation. Berl Klin Wochenschr. 1882;2:21–5.
9. Broca A, Hartmann AHAC. Contribution à l'étude des luxations de l'épaule (luxations dites incomplètes, décollements périostiques, luxations directes et luxations indirectes). Bull Société Anat Paris, Juin. 1890;1:312–36.
10. Perthes G. Ueber Operationen beihabitueller Schulterluxation. Dtsch Z Chir. 1906;85:199–227.
11. Bankart ASB. Recurrent or habitual dislocation of the shoulder joint. BMJ. 1923;2:1132–3. [PMC free article] [PubMed].
12. Eden RT. Zur Operation der habituellen Schulterluxation unter Mitteilung eines neuen ver-

fahrens bei Abriß am inneren Pfannenrande. Dtsch Z Chir. 1918;144:269–80.
13. Hybinette S. De la transplantationd'un fragment osseux pour remedier aux luxations recidivantes de l'épaule; constations et resultats operatoires. Acta Chir Scand. 1932;569:411–45.
14. Magnuson PB, Stack JK. Recurrent dislocation of the shoulder. J Am Med Assoc. 1943;123:889–92.
15. Boicev B. Sulla lussazione abituale della spalla. Chir Organi Mov. 1938;23:354–70.
16. Latarjet M. Traitement de la luxation récidivante de l'épaule. Lyon Chir. 1954;49:994–7. [PubMed].
17. Helfet AF. Coracoid transplantation for recurring dislocation of the shoulder. J Bone Joint Surg. 1958;4:198–202. [PubMed].
18. Johnson LL. Arthroscopy of the shoulder. Orthop Clin North Am. 1980;11:197–204.
19. Caspari RB. Arthroscopic reconstruction for anterior shoulder instability. Tech Orthop. 1988;3(1):59–66.
20. Morgan CD, Bodenstab AB. Arthroscopic Bankart suture repair: technique and early results. Arthroscopy. 1987;3:111–22.

The Anatomy in Shoulder Instability

2

Ángel Calvo Díaz, Pablo Carnero Martín de Soto, and Néstor Zurita Uroz

2.1 Introduction

The glenohumeral joint is the most commonly dislocated joint of the body [1], with an incidence of 24 per 100,000 cases per year [2]. The bony anatomy of the articular surfaces of the humeral head and the glenoid allows a great arc of mobility but leads to a relatively unstable joint. The glenoid fossa is a shallow articular surface that covers a small portion of the humeral head. Thus, the surrounding soft tissues, such as the labrum, capsular attachment, and glenohumeral ligaments, have a key role on maintaining articular congruency. The mechanisms responsible for compensating the bony instability of the joint are varied and complex. In general, they can be divided into static and dynamic stabilizers (Fig. 2.1). Static stabilizers are the most important, as their isolated injury can develop recurrent instability. This group comprises the labrum, the articular capsule, and the glenohumeral ligaments. These last are often visualized as reinforcements of the capsule, so the term capsuloligamentous complex is frequently used to describe its anatomy and combined function. The main goal of the static stabilizers is to maintain congruency during the last degrees of movement [3] and to provide passive stability to the joint. The dynamic stabilizers are the musculotendinous structures whose contractions maintain the humeral head centered during joint movement [4, 5] and include the rotator cuff, the scapular muscles, and the neuromuscular control that allows coordinated contraction of all these structures.

Understanding the anatomy of the bony and soft-tissue components of the glenohumeral joint is crucial to identify the pathological changes that occur in shoulder instability to optimize treatment procedures. Moreover, it is mandatory to recognize the normal variants, which are not infrequent, to avoid overtreating our patients, which can lead to suboptimal outcomes.

2.2 Anatomy

2.2.1 Bone Anatomy

The glenohumeral joint is a ball-and-socket joint formed by the rounded head of the humerus and the cup-like depression of the scapula called the glenoid fossa. The glenoid articular surface covers about 25–33% of the surface of the humeral head, leaving a relatively unstable joint (Fig. 2.2).

The glenoid cavity is pear- or oval shaped (in 88% and 12% of cases, respectively [6]) and retroverted 5° to 7°, whereas the humeral head is retroverted 30°. The angle between the humeral head and the diaphysis is about 130°–150° [7].

Á. Calvo Díaz · P. Carnero Martín de Soto (✉)
Arthrosport Zaragoza, Zaragoza, Spain

N. Zurita Uroz
IMED Elche Hospital, Alicante, Spain

R. Brzóska et al. (eds.), *360° Around Shoulder Instability*,
https://doi.org/10.1007/978-3-662-61074-9_2

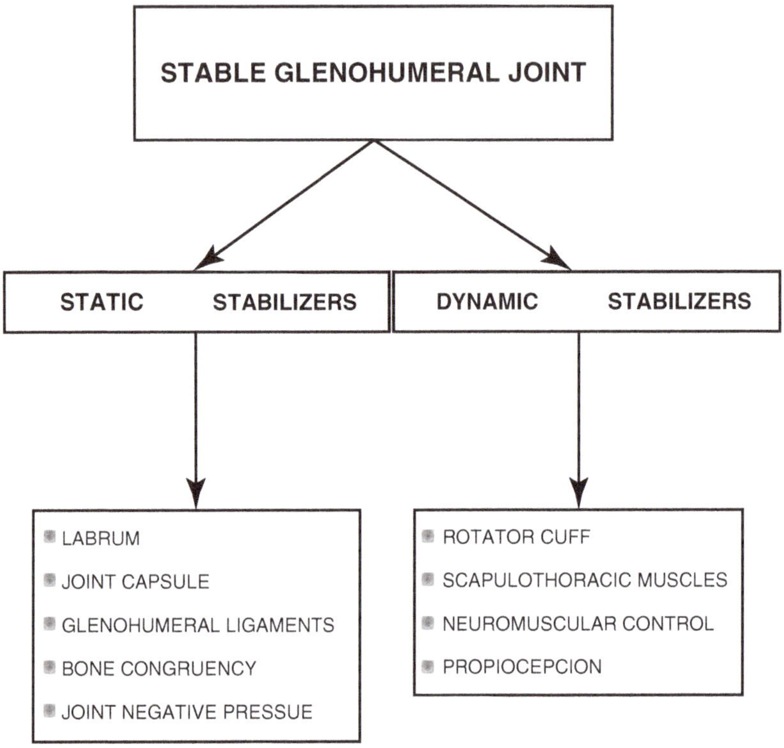

Fig. 2.1 Stabilizers of the shoulder

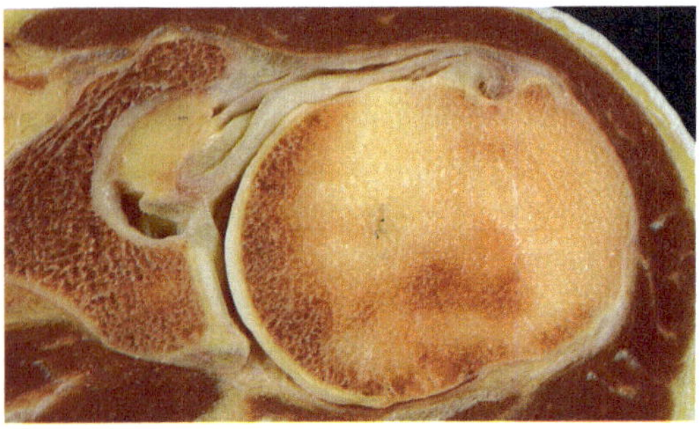

Fig. 2.2 Axial cut of the shoulder in cadaveric specimen. A large mismatch between articular surfaces of the humeral head and the glenoid fossa is visible

The humeral head cartilage is thicker centrally and thinner peripherally, in contrast to the glenoid articular cartilage, which is thinner centrally and thicker peripherally. The central area of the glenoid, also called the "bare area" or "bare spot," has a recognizable depression of the cartilage and should not be mistaken for a cartilage defect. This area has double function in providing osseous stability to the joint. First, it deepens the concave shape of the glenoid to increase the contact with the humeral head. Second, this greater contact between articular surfaces creates a negative pressure environment in the joint in which the glenoid fossa "suctions" the humeral head, impeding its migration during movement [8]. The labrum, the capsule, and the synovial fluid are also important in this mechanism [9].

An analogous bare area can be found on the posterolateral zone of the humeral head, between the cartilage and the insertion of the infraspinatus. A Hill–Sachs lesion should not be confounded with this physiological finding (Fig. 2.3).

2.2.2 Soft-Tissue Anatomy

2.2.2.1 Labrum

The labrum is a fibrous and fibrocartilagenous ring attached around the margin of the glenoid cavity. Peripherically, it is composed of collagen fibers disposed circularly and radially and has close relationships with the attachment of the long head of the biceps tendon, the joint capsule, and the glenohumeral ligaments. Medially, the transitional zone provides firm attachment to the glenoid.

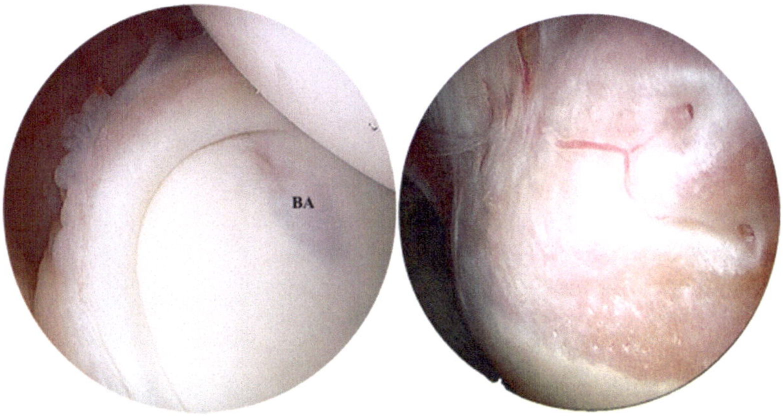

Fig. 2.3 Glenoid and humeral head cartilage: bare areas (BA)

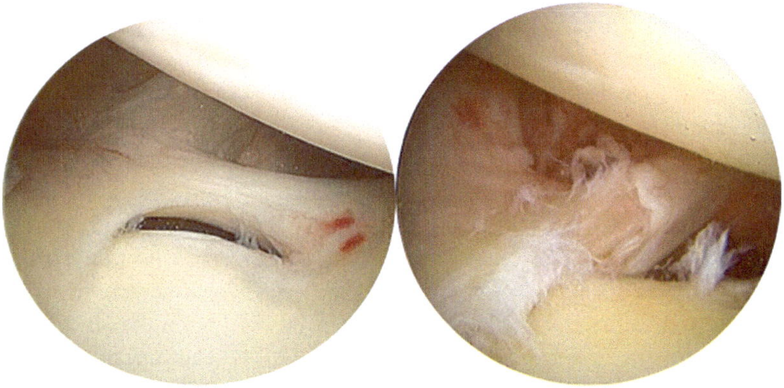

Fig. 2.4 Left: Sublabral foramen. Right: Buford complex, in which a cord-like thick middle glenohumeral ligament and absent anterosuperior labrum are visible

The main function of the labrum is increasing the contact area between the glenoid fossa and the humeral head by about 30–50% [10], which favors a greater articular congruency. In addition, it restrains the anterior or posterior displacement of the humeral head and "seals" the space between the articular surfaces, helping to maintain the negative pressure in the joint.

Different anatomical variants have been described in labrum insertion and should not be confounded with pathological changes (Fig. 2.4). The *sublabral recess* may be found superiorly in the glenoid. It is a variation of the insertion of the bíceps–labral complex at the 11 to 1 o'clock positions. It is frequently seen as an incomplete detachment of the labrum that partially shows the superior border of the glenoid neck. It is formed by a reflexion of the synovial layer that covers the articular margin of the glenoid and the labrum, and does not generate instability of the labrum or the long head of biceps tendon insertion, so it should not be addressed as a superior labrum anterior-posterior (SLAP) tear. The *sublabral foramen* is a complete detachment of the antero-superior labrum that does not extend inferiorly to the 9 o'clock position in the left shoulder or the 3 o'clock position in the right shoulder. This finding is not involved in the development of shoulder instability, as the remaining inferior labrum, which is the most important in providing stability, remains intact. The sublabral foramen is visible in less than 20% of patients [11]. The *Buford complex* was described as a "cord-like" middle glenohumeral ligament that originated directly from the superior labrum at the base of the biceps tendon associated with no anterior-superior labral tissue present between this attachment and the mid-glenoid notch [12]. Its incidence ranges from 1.5 to 6% [11–13], and there is common agreement in considering it a normal variant, as its surgical fixation to the glenoid rim could cause important restriction to external rotation and elevation [12]. Indeed, the presence of a cord-like middle glenohumeral ligament has been identified as a protective factor against instability [11, 14]. However, few case reports have been published about patients with recurrent shoulder instability associated with the Buford complex [15, 16]. In addition, the abnormalities of the anterosuperior labrum, including the Buford complex and sublabral hole, may influence shoulder biomechanics as patients usually present an increased internal rotation and variations at the superior glenohumeral ligament and the rotator interval [17]. However, the clinical implications of these findings are uncertain. Although a relationship between variants of the anterosuperior labrum and SLAP lesions has been documented [11, 17, 18], it has not been established with shoulder instability.

2.2.2.2 Capsuloligamentous Complex

The joint capsule inserts into the glenoid margin of the scapula and the anatomic neck of the humerus. It is made of collagen fibers disposed circularly and radially and support the tensile forces when the joint abducts and rotates. It is reinforced by the glenohumeral ligaments that, together with the capsule, tighten when the shoulder reaches the last degrees of movement.

There are two recesses located between the reinforcements of the glenohumeral ligaments and the rotator cuff muscles. The subscapular recess, or *Weitbrecht foramen*, is an opening of the anterior capsule located between the superior glenohumeral ligament and the superior border of the subscapularis tendon and communicates the joint with the subtendinous bursa of the subscapularis. The *axillary recess* or *axillary pouch* is located between the anterior and the posterior bundles of the inferior glenohumeral ligament.

The anterior capsular insertion can be divided into three types depending on the location on the glenoid margin. In type I, capsular attachment reaches the glenoid and labrum. In type II, the capsule attaches on the glenoid within 1 cm of the labrum. In type III, the capsule attaches more than 1 cm medial to the labrum [19]. As the capsule attachment becomes farther away from the labrum, it becomes thinner, the recesses are larger, and the capsuloligamentous complex is less resistant [19, 20].

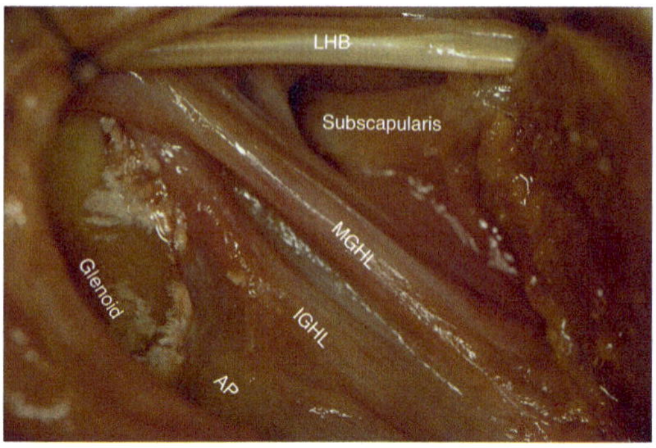

Fig. 2.5 Anterior structures of the shoulder seen from posterior on a cadaveric specimen. *LHB* long head of the biceps tendon, *MGHL* middle glenohumeral ligament, *IGHL* inferior glenohumeral ligament, *AP* axillary pouch

The glenohumeral ligaments are fibrous reinforcements of the joint capsule that restrain the humeral head translation when the range of motion reaches its maximum. Different ligaments have been described with diverse functions (Fig. 2.5).

- The superior glenohumeral ligament (SGHL) originates from the supraglenoid tubercle, anterior to the insertion of the long head of the biceps tendon, and inserts on the cephalic side of the lesser tuberosity, medial to the bicipital groove. Its location and thickness are very variable, as it can be not visible in 59% of cases [11]. It acts stabilizing the shoulder in adduction, limiting the inferior and posterior translation. The SGHL also forms the "*bicipital pulley*" together with the coracohumeral ligament, which prevents dislocation of the biceps tendon intraarticularly.
- The middle glenohumeral ligament (MGHL) originates from the anterosuperior glenoid rim, close to the origin of the SGHL, and inserts onto the anatomic neck of the humerus, adjacent to the lesser tuberosity. It is often seen as a thin layer anterior to the subscapularis tendon, but can be visualized as a thick cord-like structure, as in the Buford complex. It prevents anterior translation of the humeral head when the shoulder is in mid-abduction of 45° and external rotation.

- The inferior glenohumeral ligament (IGHL) has three distinct parts: the anterior bundle, the axillary pouch, and the posterior bundle. The anterior bundle of the IGHL originates from the anteroinferior labrum and glenoid neck, the posterior bundle of the IGHL from the posterior labrum and the glenoid neck, and the axillary pouch from the inferior labrum. The common insertion is at the inferior and medial part of the anatomic neck. The IGHL has the least variability of the glenohumeral ligaments and is the main stabilizer of the shoulder. When it is in adduction, it remains lax and folded, but when the shoulder is at 90° of abduction and external rotation, the axillary pouch unfolds and the anterior bundle tightens to limit anterior translation of the head. At abduction and internal rotation, the posterior bundle tightens and limits posterior translation and excessive internal rotation. This selective function of its parts has been described as a "*hammock effect*" that allows great range of motion while maintaining stability of the joint.

2.2.2.3 Rotator Interval

The rotator interval is a triangular space marked by the anterior border of the supraspinatus tendon, the superior border of the subscapularis tendón, and the base of the coracoid process. It contains several structures such as the SGHL, the coracohumeral ligament, the long head of the biceps tendon, and the anterosuperior capsule. It has been reported that it has a role in glenohumeral stability. Its functions are limiting inferior translation of the humeral head with the arm adducted; limiting external rotation; and controlling anterior and posterior translation during adduction and flexion–extension. Therefore, a wide rotator interval leads to an increased anterior, posterior, and inferior humeral head translation [21]. However, during shoulder arthroscopy it is difficult to assess whether a rotator interval is widened as there are no measurement methods described, so the indication of performing a rotator interval closure as an associated procedure to treat shoulder instability is debated [22].

2.3 Dynamic Stabilizers

The musculotendinous structures of the rotator cuff reinforce the whole capsular area except in the axillary recess and the rotator interval. Their contraction keeps the humeral head centered during joint movement in the mid-range of motion. Thus, the action of the stabilizers of the shoulder can be explained as a continuum, in which at the beginning and the mid-phase of the movement the static stabilizers remain lax and the contraction of the rotator cuff tendons provide congruity. When the extreme range of motion is reached, stability depends on the static elements.

Proprioception of the shoulder is crucial in its dynamic stabilization. The glenohumeral capsule is richly innervated by mechanoreceptors [4] that send information to the cerebral cortex to establish a pathway that finishes with a coupled contraction of the muscles of the rotator cuff and the scapulothoracic space to provide stability of the joint during movement [5]. A torn or stretched capsule can cause disturbance of the mechanoreceptors and delay of the proprioceptive signal, slowing the feedback response of the musculotendinous units, so that injury of the static stabilizers can also cause disruption of the dynamic stabilizers.

2.4 Pathology

Shoulder instability is a complex pathological entity with different clinical presentations. Several classifications have been described according to its etiology (traumatic versus atraumatic instability), direction of instability (anterior, posterior, multidirectional), timing (acute, locked, recurrent), associated injuries (with versus without bone loss), or a combination of these factors (TUBS versus AMBRII). This variety of classifications shows that the clinical spectrum of shoulder instability is wide. Therefore, the anatomical lesions present depend on the clinical setting of the patient. Thus, injuries found during surgery will be different in patients with recurrent anterior traumatic instability than in those with atraumatic multidirectional instability with associated hyperlaxity, and, consequently, the surgical approach should be different in each case.

It is accepted that the origin of the dysfunction in most cases is the combined injury of the static stabilizers. The labrum avulsion secondary to the dislocation or subluxation of the humeral head is often associated with pathological capsular redundancy, whether congenital or acquired. In addition, the mechanoreceptors of the capsule can become damaged in capsular injury, which promotes an impaired response of the dynamic stabilizers as well. However, in some cases the isolated capsular redundancy can cause shoulder instability without labrum detachment.

In other cases, the origin of the instability can be found in an abnormal pattern of contraction of the musculotendinous units around the shoulder. Neuromuscular pathology, such as muscular dystrophy, cause a weakness of the rotator cuff muscles that impedes keeping the humeral head centered during shoulder motion. In these cases, a certain capsular laxity is needed to develop the instability, so the static stabilizers are not disconnected from these infrequent types of instability.

2.5 Labrum Injury

Our understanding of labrum injuries has increased in recent years thanks to the development of arthroscopy, and different lesions have been described in both acute dislocations and chronic instabilities.

After an anterior traumatic shoulder dislocation, the most common sequel is a complete avulsion of the anteroinferior labrum of the glenoid rim and the periosteum, known as the *Bankart lesion*. This finding is almost constant in cases of recurrent instability [23], as it is a major cause of the instability [24]. When the injury comprises a marginal fracture of the anteroinferior portion of the glenoid neck instead of labrum detachment, it is known as a Bony-Bankart.

The *anterior labroligamentous periosteal sleeve avulsion* (ALPSA lesion) is often visualized in patients with multiple dislocations [23, 25]. It consists of a complete detachment of the labrum and the glenohumeral ligaments from the glenoid rim but maintaining a bundle of the glenoid neck periosteum, so the detached structures retract medially and are scarred to the medial glenoid neck, being unable to limit the anterior translation of the humeral head (Fig. 2.6).

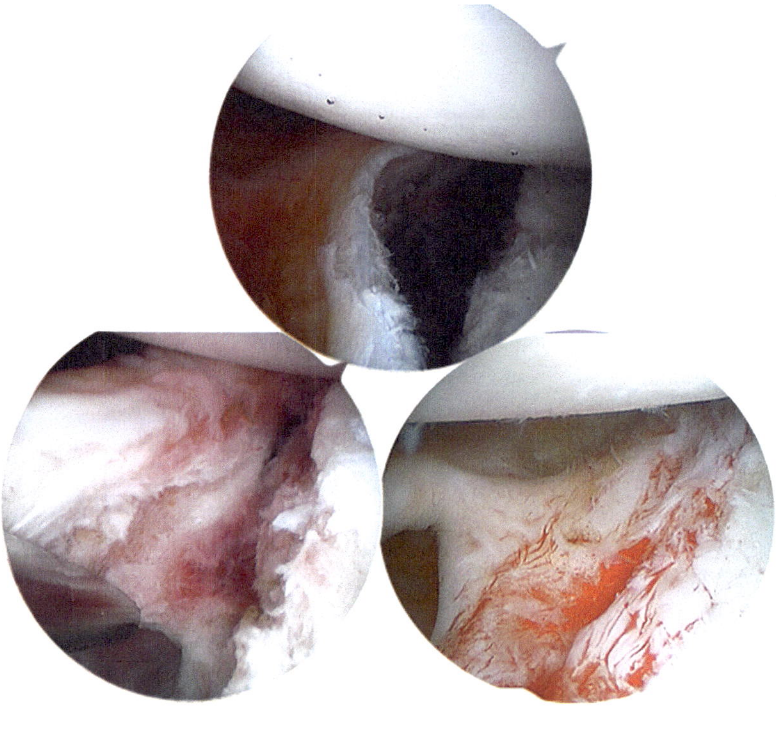

Fig. 2.6 Up: Anterior Bankart lesion; down left: anterior Bony-Bankart; down right: ALPSA lesion

A *Perthes lesion* is an incomplete avulsion without displacement of the anteroinferior labrum with a medially striped but intact periosteum [26]. It is an uncommon lesion that rarely causes gross instability, but should be suspected in patients with subluxation of the joint and recurrent pain.

The *glenoid labral articular disruption* (GLAD) *lesion* was first described by Neviaser in 1993. This lesion occurs when there is a defect in the articular cartilage of the anteroinferior glenoid in addition to the labral tear, which is not fully detached [27]. Similar to the Perthes lesion, the predominant symptom is these cases is not instability, but pain.

All these injuries just described are not exclusive to the anteroinferior labrum. In cases of posterior shoulder instability, analogous lesions can be found on the posteroinferior labrum, added to incomplete detachments of the superficial portion of the posterior labrum, which are known as *Kim's lesions*. These incomplete tears usually appear as a consequence of repetitive movements of flexion, adduction, and internal rotation, so athletes such as throwers or weightlifters are prone to these disruptions. They do not cause gross instability symptoms, but instead origin pain and shoulder dysfunction.

2.6 Capsular Injury

A plastic irreversible elongation of the anteroinferior capsule is frequently seen in patients with anterior recurrent instability [23]. Global capsular redundancy is a usual feature in hyperlaxity and multidirectional instability, whereas in unidirectional instability stretching of the anteroinferior portion of the capsule is paramount [28]. It is difficult to determine when an increased capsular volume is congenital or acquired, but it seems logical that perhaps the most frequent origin combines an inherent predisposition and a traumatic component [29]. However, capsular insertions below the labrum (i.e., type III) predispose to glenohumeral hypermobility or even instability without traumatic antecedent.

The humeral avulsion of the glenohumeral ligaments (*HAGL lesion*) is a variant of capsular injury after an acute dislocation. Reported in 2–9% of patients with shoulder instability [30, 31], this injury usually happens when the arm is placed in maximal abduction and external rotation. Anterior HAGL represents 93% of the cases, whereas posterior accounts for only 7% [30]. These lesions can be easily missed during shoulder arthroscopy if they are not suspected, especially in cases without a concomitant Bankart lesion. Consequently, placing the scope on the anterosuperior and anterior portals while abducting and externally rotating the arm must be routinely performed to visualize the humeral insertion of the capsuloligamentous complex.

2.7 Bone Injury

2.7.1 Glenoid

Several glenoid bony configurations can predispose to recurrent instability. Glenoid bone loss is the most common and has received more attention than other matters, as it is considered an important contributor to recurrent shoulder instability. Previous reports show that recurrence rates after arthroscopic soft-tissue procedures for anterior instability are 4–6% [29, 32], but when there is significant bone loss, either at the glenoid rim or at the posterolateral aspect of the humeral head, the rate is as high as 89% [32] even after lower-energy traumas.

Following an initial shoulder dislocation, an osseous defect on the anteroinferior margin of the glenoid is present in up to 22% of patients and in up to 88% of patients with recurrent instability [33, 34]. This defect predisposes to instability during the middle range of motion as the concavity of the rim is lost, so the humeral head finds no stop to anterior translation. Moreover, the suction effect of the glenoid is missed as it loses its cup shape.

The loss of the normal shape of the glenoid can be assessed radiographically or arthroscopically. Computed tomography scans permit obtaining tridimensional reconstructions of the glenohumeral joint that allow quantifying the bone defect. On the other hand, arthroscopic

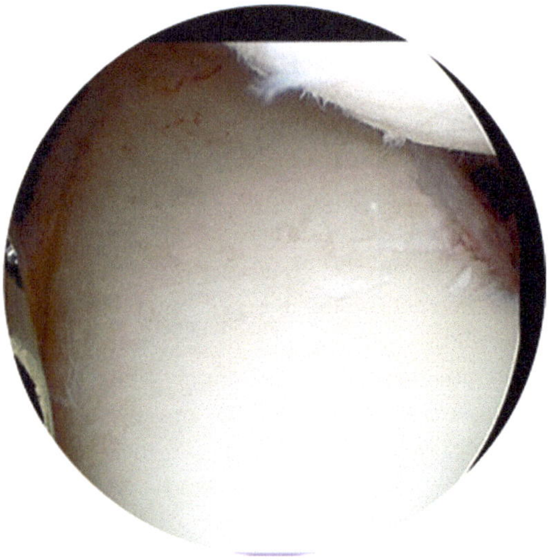

Fig. 2.7 Anteroinferior significant glenoid bone loss causing an "inverted pear" morphology of the glenoid

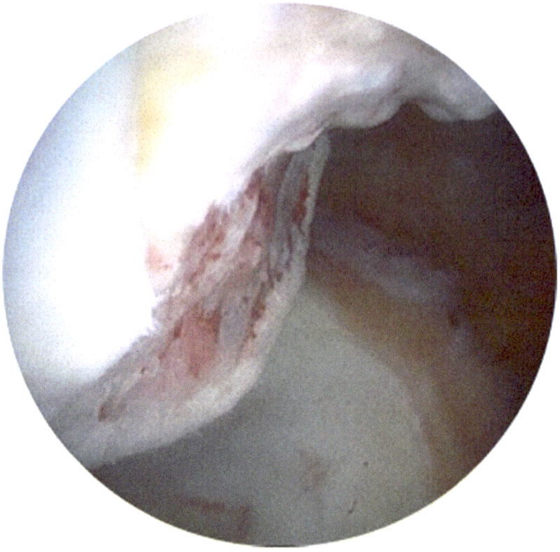

Fig. 2.8 Hill–Sachs lesion

examination provides direct visualization of the glenoid, as it would appear as an "inverted pear" shape in cases of significant bone loss (Fig. 2.7). Furthermore, anteroinferior bone defects can be measured with a calibrated probe inserted through the posterior portal. Using the bare area of the glenoid as the landmark, the posteroinferior and anteroinferior radii of the glenoid can be measured and compared.

There is common agreement on considering 25% of anteroinferior glenoid bone loss as the critical point at which arthroscopic soft-tissue procedures are not sufficient for correcting instability, so a glenoid grafting technique should be performed. This limit was determined after biomechanics studies reported that a defect measuring 30% of the diameter of the inferior glenoid causes a decrease in the contact area across the entire glenoid of 40%, whereas the mean contact pressure for the entire glenoid increased by nearly 100% and mean contact pressures in the anteroinferior quadrant increased by 300–400% [35]. If an isolated soft-tissue repair were to be performed in a patient with this glenoid bone loss, it would have to resist this overload at the repair interface, dramatically increasing the likelihood of failure.

Abnormalities of glenoid anatomy and version have been studied in the setting of multidirectional and posterior instability. It has been shown that glenoid retroversion is higher in patients with posterior instability compared to control subjects or patients with anterior instability [36]. Interestingly, when shoulder retroversion reaches 16°, the incidence of contralateral injuries is increased [37]. However, it is unknown whether osseous changes precede the development of instability or whether instability itself causes the bony changes. Furthermore, although the exact amount of glenoid retroversion necessary to affect shoulder joint stability is unclear, the connection between retroversion and posterior instability exists, so future research about this issue will aid us to obtain clear conclusions.

2.7.2 Humeral Head

A posterolateral bone defect is frequently seen after initial shoulder dislocation. This finding, called the *Hill–Sachs lesion*, is present in up to 51–65% of cases after the first episode of dislocation, and the rate is higher in chronic instability [23, 29] (Fig. 2.8). As previously stated, there is a bare area between the insertion of the rotator cuff and the humeral head cartilage that should not be confused with an injury.

The presence of a Hill–Sachs lesion predisposes to recurrent instability, even after an arthroscopic soft-tissue procedure stabilization [32, 38]. Therefore, correct identification and quantification of the deformity is mandatory during shoulder arthroscopy. Complete visualization of the injury can be obtained by placing the scope in the antero-superior portal and rotating the shoulder.

The orientation of the lesion is important in the development of recurrent instability. If the medial border of the Hill–Sachs defect passes the medial border of the glenoid during external rotation, it will "engage" and facilitate dislocation, so it will be considered an "engaging" injury. If the medial border of the Hill–Sachs lesion does not overpass the glenoid, rather if it is not large enough or the orientation of the injury does not fit with the medial border of the glenoid, the complete arc of motion of the shoulder can be achieved and there will be a small likelihood of dislocation, so it will be considered as a "non-engaging" lesion. In case of an engaging lesion, additional surgical procedures such as infraspinatus tendon tenodesis may be required.

2.8 Conclusions

Shoulder anatomy is particularly complex and requires a thorough knowledge by the orthopedic surgeon. Anatomical variants should not be confounded with pathological findings. Moreover, different anatomical lesions can be found depending on the type of instability and the functional requirements of the patient, so the surgical procedures must be carefully chosen to achieve optimal outcomes when treating shoulder instability.

References

1. Nabian MH, Zadegan SA, Zanjani LO, Mehrpour SR. Epidemiology of joint dislocations and ligamentous/tendinous injuries among 2,700 patients: five-year trend of a tertiary center in Iran. Arch Bone Jt Surg. 2017;5(6):426–34.
2. Krøner K, Lind T, Jensen J. The epidemiology of shoulder dislocations. Arch Orthop Trauma Surg. 1989;108(5):288–90.
3. Turkel SJ, Panio MW, Marshall JL, Girgis FG. Stabilizing mechanisms preventing anterior dislocation of the glenohumeral joint. J Bone Joint Surg Am. 1981;63(8):1208–17.
4. Jerosch J, Castro WH, Halm H, Drescher H. Does the glenohumeral joint capsule have proprioceptive capability? Knee Surg Sports Traumatol Arthrosc. 1993;1(2):80–4.
5. Tibone JE, Fechter J, Kao JT. Evaluation of a proprioception pathway in patients with stable and unstable shoulders with somatosensory cortical evoked potentials. J Shoulder Elb Surg. 1997;6(5):440–3.
6. Anetzberger H, Putz R. The scapula: principles of construction and stress. Acta Anat (Basel). 1996;156(1):70–80.
7. Cyprien JM, Vasey HM, Burdet A, Bonvin JC, Kritsikis N, Vuagnat P. Humeral retrotorsion and glenohumeral relationship in the normal shoulder and in recurrent anterior dislocation (scapulometry). Clin Orthop Relat Res. 1983;175:8–17.
8. Itoi E. Pathophysiology and treatment of atraumatic instability of the shoulder. J Orthop Sci. 2004;9(2):208–13.
9. Habermeyer P, Schuller U, Wiedemann E. The intra-articular pressure of the shoulder: an experimental study on the role of the glenoid labrum in stabilizing the joint. Arthroscopy. 1992;8(2):166–72.
10. Huber WP, Putz RV. Periarticular fiber system of the shoulder joint. Arthroscopy. 1997;13(6):680–91.
11. Ilahi OA, Labbe MR, Cosculluela P. Variants of the anterosuperior glenoid labrum and associated pathology. Arthroscopy. 2002;18(8):882–6.
12. Williams MM, Snyder SJ, Buford D Jr. The Buford complex—the "cord-like" middle glenohumeral ligament and absent anterosuperior labrum complex: a normal anatomic capsulolabral variant. Arthroscopy. 1994;10(3):241–7.
13. Ide J, Maeda S, Takagi K. Normal variations of the glenohumeral ligament complex: an anatomic study for arthroscopic Bankart repair. Arthroscopy. 2004;20(2):164–8.
14. Morgan CD, Rames RD, Snyder SJ. Arthroscopic assessment of anatomic variations of the glenohumeral ligaments associated with recurrent anterior shoulder instability. Orthop Trans. 1992;16:727–8.
15. del Rey FC, Vázquez DG, López DN. Glenohumeral instability associated with Buford complex. Knee Surg Sports Traumatol Arthrosc. 2009;17(12):1489–92.
16. Nishinaka N, Uehara T, Tsutsui H. Recurrent posterior dislocation of the shoulder associated with the Buford complex. J Clin Orthop Trauma. 2016;7(1):55–60.
17. Rao AG, Kim TK, Chronopoulos E, McFarland EG. Anatomical variants in the anterosuperior aspect of the glenoid labrum: a statistical analysis of seventy-three cases. J Bone Joint Surg Am. 2003;85A(4):653–9.
18. Kanatli U, Ozturk BY, Bolukbasi S. Anatomical variations of the anterosuperior labrum: prevalence and association with type II superior labrum anterior-posterior (SLAP) lesions. J Shoulder Elb Surg. 2010;19(8):1199–203.

19. Pouliart N, Boulet C, Maeseneer MD, Shahabpour M. Advanced imaging of the glenohumeral ligaments. Semin Musculoskelet Radiol. 2014;18(4):374–97.
20. Eberly VC, McMahon PJ, Lee TQ. Variation in the glenoid origin of the anteroinferior glenohumeral capsulolabrum. Clin Orthop Relat Res. 2002;400:26–31.
21. Provencher MT, Dewing CB, Bell SJ, McCormick F, Solomon DJ, Rooney TB, Stanley M. An analysis of the rotator interval in patients with anterior, posterior, and multidirectional shoulder instability. Arthroscopy. 2008;24(8):921–9.
22. Itoigawa Y, Itoi E. Anatomy of the capsulolabral complex and rotator interval related to glenohumeral instability. Knee Surg Sports Traumatol Arthrosc. 2016;24(2):343–9.
23. Yiannakopoulos CK, Mataragas E, Antonogiannakis E. A comparison of the spectrum of intra-articular lesions in acute and chronic anterior shoulder instability. Arthroscopy. 2007;23(9):985–90.
24. Hantes M, Raoulis V. Arthroscopic findings in anterior shoulder instability. Open Orthop J. 2017;11:119–32.
25. Spatschil A, Landsiedl F, Anderl W, Imhoff A, Seiler H, Vassilev I, Klein W, Boszotta H, Hoffmann F, Rupp S. Posttraumatic anterior-inferior instability of the shoulder: arthroscopic findings and clinical correlations. Arch Orthop Trauma Surg. 2006;126(4):217–22.
26. Wischer TK, Bredella MA, Genant HK, Stoller DW, Bost FW, Tirman PF. Perthes lesion (a variant of the Bankart lesion): MR imaging and MR arthrographic findings with surgical correlation. AJR Am J Roentgenol. 2002;178(1):233–7.
27. Neviaser TJ. The GLAD lesion: another cause of anterior shoulder pain. Arthroscopy. 1993;9(1):22–3.
28. McMahon PJ, Dettling JR, Sandusky MD, Lee TQ. Deformation and strain characteristics along the length of the anterior band of the inferior glenohumeral ligament. J Shoulder Elb Surg. 2001;10(5):482–8.
29. Cuéllar R, Ruiz-Ibán MA, Cuéllar A. Anatomy and biomechanics of the unstable shoulder. Open Orthop J. 2017;11:919–33.
30. Marco SM, Lafuente JLÁ, Ibán MAR, Heredia JD. Controversies in the surgical management of shoulder instability: associated soft tissue procedures. Open Orthop J. 2017;11:989–1000.
31. Bui-Mansfield LT, Banks KP, Taylor DC. Humeral avulsion of the glenohumeral ligaments: the HAGL lesion. Am J Sports Med. 2007;35(11):1960–6.
32. Burkhart SS, De Beer JF. Traumatic glenohumeral bone defects and their relationship to failure of arthroscopic Bankart repairs: significance of the inverted-pear glenoid and the humeral engaging Hill–Sachs lesion. Arthroscopy. 2000;16(7):677–94.
33. Edwards TB, Boulahia A, Walch G. Radiographic analysis of bone defects in chronic anterior shoulder instability. Arthroscopy. 2003;19(7):732–9.
34. Taylor DC, Arciero RA. Pathologic changes associated with shoulder dislocations. Arthroscopic and physical examination findings in first-time, traumatic anterior dislocations. Am J Sports Med. 1997;25(3):306–11.
35. Greis PE, Scuderi MG, Mohr A, Bachus KN, Burks RT. Glenohumeral articular contact areas and pressures following labral and osseous injury to the anteroinferior quadrant of the glenoid. J Shoulder Elb Surg. 2002;11(5):442–51.
36. Owens BD, Campbell SE, Cameron KL. Risk factors for posterior shoulder instability in young athletes. Am J Sports Med. 2013;41(11):2645–9.
37. Gottschalk MB, Ghasem A, Todd D, Daruwalla J, Xerogeanes J, Karas S. Posterior shoulder instability: does glenoid retroversion predict recurrence and contralateral instability? Arthroscopy. 2015;31(3):488–93.
38. Balg F, Boileau P. The instability severity index score. A simple pre-operative score to select patients for arthroscopic or open shoulder stabilisation. J Bone Joint Surg Br. 2007;89(11):1470–7.

Predictor Factors in Anterior Shoulder Instability

3

Boris Poberaj

3.1 Age

The age is one of the key risk factors for primary and recurrent instability. The epidemiologic study [1] using cohort of patients aged 10–16 years has shown that among 10- to 13-year-old patients, there was considerably lower rate of primary and recurrent dislocations. The reason for lower recurrence rate in younger adolescents seems to be more elastic capsule resilient to structural damage and more lateral attachment of the anterior capsule to the glenoid. The statistics among 14- to 16-year-old individuals for primary and recurrent dislocations is comparable to high-risk adults 17–20 years old. Recurrent dislocation in adolescents after a primary anterior dislocation usually occurs within 2 years with incidence of 76.7% [2]. The patients in this study were treated after first dislocation with sling immobilization in internal rotation for 1 week; then early movement was allowed as pain allows with physiotherapy for 8 weeks. Another systematic review and meta-analysis [3] that included 1324 patients have shown 51% of recurrence after first dislocation in the age group of 15–20 years, 49% in the age group of 15–30 years, and 36% in the group of 21–40 years.

B. Poberaj (✉)
Aspetar Orthopaedic and Sports Medicine Hospital, Doha, Qatar

3.2 Gender and Race

In general males have greater risk of shoulder dislocation than females because they participate more commonly in higher-risk contact sports. Also many traditional collision sports have modified rules in the women's version. Kardouni et al. [4] reported 15,426 incident shoulder dislocations in US soldiers with greater risk in male population. At the same time, male soldiers had a 20% decreased odds of chronic or recurrent injury than female soldiers. This is in line with other reports of no significant difference in recurrence rates based on sex. Incidence on recurrent dislocation is similar in both genders during the adolescence [2]. In the study of Kardouni, results indicate that white people may have a greater risk for sustaining shoulder dislocations than other races.

3.3 Associated Fractures and Axillary Nerve Lesions

Bony fracture of anterior glenoid and Hill-Sachs deformity importantly increase the risk of recurrence.

The presence of a greater tubercle fracture of the humerus decreased the risk of recurrence rate for 4–7 times. This was postulated due to decreased range of motion in external rotation and abduction, which is usual sequel after such traumas.

R. Brzóska et al. (eds.), *360° Around Shoulder Instability*,
https://doi.org/10.1007/978-3-662-61074-9_3

An axillary nerve palsy does not affect the structural integrity of the joint but results in decreased movement of the limb for a significant period of time.

3.4 Other Factors

Hyperlaxity increases recurrence for up to three times following a first-time dislocation.

Immobilization in external or internal position has no influence on recurrence rate, as well as duration of immobilization.

Overhead athletes, collision sports, and overhead manual workers have increased risk of recurrence.

3.5 Diagnostic Value of Clinical Tests

There are numerous clinical tests for anterior shoulder instability. The most commonly used are apprehension, relocation, and release tests.

The apprehension test is done with the patient supine with the arm in 90° abduction, the elbow in 90° of flexion, and progressive external rotation. The test is positive in case of an apprehensive feeling and negative if only pain is present.

The relocation test is literarily continuation of apprehension test with depression of the humeral head by posterior-directed force to the humerus. It is considered positive if it provides relief of the apprehensive feeling. At the same time, external rotation can be proceeded to its maximal range.

The anterior release test is continuation of relocation test with sudden release of posterior-directed force to the humerus. The test is positive in case of recurrent apprehensive feeling.

Kampen et al. [5] confirmed good diagnostic accuracy of individual tests with overall accuracy more than 80% with highest score for release test with 86.4%.

The assessment of anterior apprehension test was further studied by Milgrom et al. [6] in cohort of patients with first-time shoulder dislocations and minimum follow-up of 75 months. The mean age of the patients was 20 years, and the tests were performed 6 weeks after first traumatic dislocation, followed by rehabilitation. Those with a positive test result have had a 79% rate of recurrent dislocation, and those with a negative test result had a 53% rate. Also those with a positive test sustained redislocation earlier than those with a negative test result.

Finally, shoulder apprehension is more complex than a pure mechanical problem as it reflects the scar at the brain level that prevents the performance of specific movements [7]. Brain activity changes can predict the successful postsurgical outcome. Decreased activity in premotor and orbitofrontal cortex is a key factor for a successful surgical outcome.

3.6 Predictors of Dislocation After Shoulder Stabilization

Younger patient's age and increased numbers of documented preoperative dislocations increase the likelihood of stabilization failures [8]. It seems also that shoulder dislocations that require physician relocation are more likely to have significant pathological lesions like bigger bone defects, which potentially increase risk of failure of operative stabilization. The number of dislocations and age at first dislocation are the most significant predictors of glenoid bone loss [9]. Patients with three or more preoperative dislocations required physician relocation had postoperative recurrent dislocation rate of 24.4% compared with 2.4% for patients who had none in the cohort of 73 patients. These data support the promoters of surgical intervention for the first-time dislocation [10].

3.7 Surgery for the First-Time Dislocation

Main reasons to support surgery for the first-time dislocation are:

- At age of 16–27 years, the redislocation rate is up to 80%.
- Young patients with three or more dislocations before surgery have up to 25% recurrence rate after surgery.

- Glenohumeral osteoarthritis in chronic instability is 10–20 times greater.

The reasons to not support the first-time dislocation are:

- Approx. 20% of surgeries among young athletes would be unnecessary.
- Additional 14% of the surgeries would be unsuccessful.

3.8 Summary

Young age 16–27 years, male gender, and collision sports are predictors for primary glenohumeral (GH) dislocation.

The supine apprehension test 6 weeks [11] after first GH dislocation can help in predicting risk of recurrent instability.

Age 20 years or less with more than three preoperative dislocations predicts significant risk of revision surgery.

Any shoulder stabilization study with only 2-year follow-up should be interpreted with caution.

References

1. Leroux T, Ogilvie-Harris D, Veillette C, Chahal J, Dwyer T, Khoshbin A, Henry P, Mahomed N, Wasserstein D. The epidemiology of primary anterior shoulder dislocations in patients aged 10 to 16 years. Am J Sports Med. 2015;43:2111–7.
2. Roberts SB, Beattie N, McNiven ND, Robinson CM. The natural history of primary anterior dislocation of the glenohumeral joint in adolescence. Bone Joint J. 2015;97-B:520–6.
3. Olds M, Ellis R, Donaldson K, Parmar P, Kersten P. Risk factors which predispose first-time traumatic anterior shoulder dislocations to recurrent instability in adults: a systematic review and meta-analysis. Br J Sports Med. 2015;49:913–23.
4. Kardouni JR, McKinnon CJ, Seitz AL. Incidence of shoulder dislocations and the rate of recurrent instability in soldiers. Med Sci Sports Exerc. 2016;48-11:2150–6.
5. Kampen DA, Berg T, Woude HJ, Castelein RM, Terwee CB, Willems WJ. Diagnostic value of patient characteristics, history, and six clinical tests for traumatic anterior shoulder instability. J Shoulder Elb Surg. 2013;22:1310–9.
6. Milgrom C, Milgrom Y, Petrova DR, Jaber S, Beyth S, Finestone AS. The supine apprehension test helps predict the risk of recurrent instability after a first-time anterior shoulder dislocation. J Shoulder Elb Surg. 2014;23:1838–42.
7. Zanchy D, Cunningham G, Lädermann A, Ozturk M, Hoffmeyer P, Haller S. Brain activity in the right-frontal pole and lateral occipital cortex predicts successful post-operatory outcome after surgery for anterior glenohumeral instability. Sci Rep. 2017;7(1):498.
8. Wasserstein D, Dwyer T, Veillette C, Gandhi R, Chahal J, Mahomed N, Harris DO. Predictors of dislocation and revision after shoulder stabilization in Ontario, Canada, from 2003 to 2008. Am J Sports Med. 2013;41(9):2034–40.
9. Milano G, Grasso A, Russo A, Magarelli N, Santagada DA, Deriu L, Baudi P, Bonomo L, Fabbriciani C. Analysis of risk factors for glenoid bone defect in anterior shoulder instability. Am J Sports Med. 2011;39(9):1870–6.
10. Gasparini G, Benedetto M, Cundari A, Gori M, Orlando N, McFarland EG, Galasso O, Castricini R. Predictors of functional outcomes and recurrent shoulder instability after arthroscopic anterior stabilization. Knee Surg Sports Traumatol Arthrosc. 2016;24(2):406–13.
11. Safran O, Milgrom C, Petrova DR, Jaber S, Finestone A. Accuracy of the anterior apprehension test as a predictor of risk for redislocation after a first traumatic shoulder dislocation. Am J Sports Med. 2010;38-5:972–5.

Basic Science on Shoulder Instability

4

Tim Kraal, William D. Regan,
and Christiaan J. A. van Bergen

4.1 Introduction

The shoulder has an impressive wide range of motion in three dimensions, but sometimes, this comes at a price. The glenohumeral joint is the most commonly dislocated joint in the human body. Basic science research on shoulder instability is of paramount importance to understand the biomechanics of the shoulder, including static and dynamic constraints that control stability. Several studies have investigated joint contact pressures and contact areas in various arm positions, as well as the way they are affected by bone loss caused by instability [1–3]. Furthermore, other biomechanical studies have investigated the effects of surgical stabilizing procedures on joint biomechanics.

Glenohumeral stability is a complex issue, reliant on a multitude of static and dynamic factors, which cannot be simulated in a biomechanical study. There is intrinsic stability from the glenoid concavity and the congruency of the glenoid and labrum with the humeral head. Although the articular surface of the humeral head is about three times larger than the articular surface of the glenoid, the radius of curvature of the humeral head and the glenoid is within 2 mm of each other in most cases [4]. Furthermore the capsuloligamentous structures are a (patient-specific) static restraint, mainly important in the end range of motion [5, 6]. In the apprehension position, i.e., combined abduction and external rotation, the labrum and the inferior glenohumeral ligament (IGHL) resist antero-inferior translation [7]. The labrum itself is a fibrocartilaginous structure attached to the glenoid rim, and it increases the depth of the glenoid. Its collagen fibres are oriented in a circumferential manner, and are densely packed at the core layer. The antero-inferior part of the labrum has the highest elastic modulus and yield stress; it is the thickest and strongest part of the labrum, providing maximal resistance to translational forces of the humeral head [8]. In addition to these intrinsic and static restraints, there is dynamic muscle control. The prime movers of the shoulder include the rotator cuff and the deltoid. These, and other muscles to a lesser degree, create a joint reaction force, compressing the humeral head in the concave glenoid fossa. Muscle activation is directed by proprioception, mediated by mechanoreceptors in tendons. Although in a cadaveric specimen the individual muscles can be dissected, the tendons can be clamped and loaded individually with computer-controlled actuators; these models are still a simplification of reality [9, 10].

T. Kraal
Spaarne Gasthuis, Hoofddorp, The Netherlands

W. D. Regan
Division of Arthroscopic, Reconstructive Surgery and Joint Preservation, University of British Columbia, Vancouver, BC, Canada

C. J. A. van Bergen (✉)
Amphia, Breda, The Netherlands
e-mail: cvanbergen@amphia.nl

R. Brzóska et al. (eds.), *360° Around Shoulder Instability*,
https://doi.org/10.1007/978-3-662-61074-9_4

Another factor which is difficult to account for in basic science research is the negative intra-articular pressure. In vivo, this is a physiological contributing factor to shoulder stability, but in most cadaveric specimens the joint is vented with dissection before testing. Most researchers believe that the effect of venting is relatively small during muscle contraction (active range of motion), and that negative intra-articular pressure is more important when the arm is in a resting position [6, 9]. Other limitations to basic science studies are that most of the cadaveric specimens used in these studies are usually from elderly donors, and this does not match the target population of instability surgery. In addition, the dynamic coupled motion of scapulo-thoracic and glenohumeral joint is not tested. This remains an unsolved limitation. Taking the above into account, the aim of this chapter is to increase the understanding of basic science as it pertains to the shoulder biomechanics of shoulder stability.

4.2 Biomechanical Testing Models in Shoulder Instability

Measuring shoulder stability can be done in various ways, but there are a couple of accepted general principles in the way shoulder models are tested. Contact area and contact pressures can be measured with pressure sensors or pressure sensitive films from approximately 0.1 mm thickness. The contact area is important because it is inversely related to the contact pressure. The test model ideally allows for six degrees of freedom for glenohumeral motion, internal/external rotation, abduction/adduction, flexion/extension, antero-posterior translation, supero-inferior translation, and compression/distraction. To define the neutral position of humeral rotation, the bicipital groove is placed directly anteriorly, and the humerus is then externally rotated 10° [6]. Furthermore, the test model needs to take into account the combined scapulothoracic motion. For example, a rhythm of 2:1 means that a composite of 90° of abduction consists of 60° of glenohumeral and 30° of scapulothoracic abduction [10]. The shoulder needs to be loaded, but it is arguable which compressive force (in Newtons) is required. The term "non-weight bearing" is somewhat inappropriate because maximum joint pressures can exceed a subject's own bodyweight [11]. A compressive load of around 50N can be used to centralize the humeral head in the glenoid socket, and thus to define the neutral position. During testing, a compressive load of up to 440N is used to simulate the in vivo glenohumeral joint reaction force, as this is the estimated maximal compressive load during the range of motion of daily life activities [12, 13]. Stability can be measured as the required translational force until dislocation, but more frequently, the required force to reach a normalized distance anteriorly (e.g., 10 mm of anterior translation of the humeral head) is defined as the outcome parameter for stability [14]. Translation can be measured by lasers, or with a linear potentiometer, accurately measuring displacement in millimeters. For strength testing of surgical procedures like a Bankart repair or Latarjet reconstruction, cyclic loading until failure is used. The term joint biomechanics can be considered as an umbrella to express parameters such as stability, contact area, contact pressures, and the direction of the force couples.

4.2.1 Pathophysiology of Shoulder Instability

An anterior shoulder dislocation can cause damage to several structures in the joint. The Bankart lesion, an avulsion of the anteroinferior labrum with the attachment site of the IGHL is frequently called the "essential lesion" [15]. Over the last two decades, arthroscopic Bankart repair has become the mainstay of treatment in shoulder instability. However, clinical studies have shown that bone loss is a crucial factor for the success rate of arthroscopic Bankart repair [16, 17]. To appreciate why bone loss is so important, basic science studies can improve our understanding of the biomechanical consequences of bone loss on the glenohumeral joint.

4.2.2 Prevalence of Bone Loss

The prevalence of bone loss in shoulder instability is high. Griffit et al. reported 41% of glenoid bone loss after a primary dislocation and 86% after recurrent dislocations [18]. This is in line with the study of Piasecki, who found 49–89% of glenoid bone loss and 70–100% of humeral side bone loss in patients with recurrent instability [19]. Likewise, Widjaja found combined defects in 54% of patients after traumatic anterior shoulder dislocations [20]. On the glenoid side, bone loss can occur as a fragment type, the so-called bony Bankart, or as the erosion type, which is seen more often in chronic instability. On the humeral side, the Hill-Sachs lesion is a compression fracture of the posterior humeral head caused by the anterior glenoid rim when the shoulder dislocates. These combined defects of the glenoid and humeral head are called bipolar bone loss. Both are important risk factors for recurrence of instability.

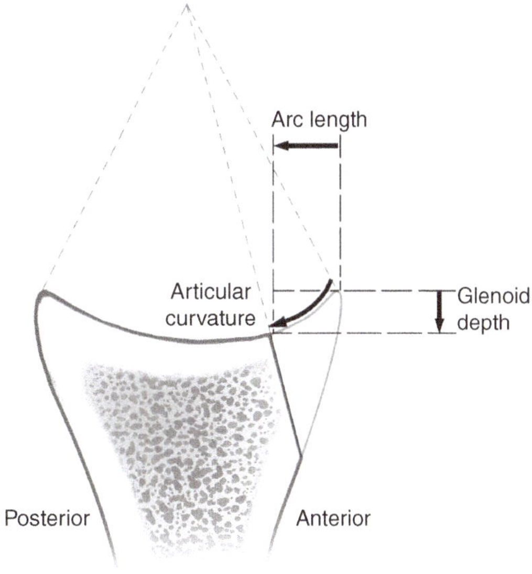

Fig. 4.1 Schematic drawing of the three factors that alter the intrinsic stability associated with anterior glenoid bone loss: depth, articular surface, and arc length. (Reprinted from: Yamamoto N et al. Stabilizing Mechanism in Bone-Grafting of a Large Glenoid Defect. Journal of Bone and Joint Surgery—Series A. 2010;92(11):2059–66. With permission from Wolters Kluwer Health, Inc.)

4.2.3 How Joint Biomechanics Are Altered by Labral Detachment and Bone Loss

The physiological maximum joint contact pressure occurs with combined abduction and external rotation [21]. Anterior labrum detachment and bone loss of the anterior glenoid rim alter the intrinsic stability in several ways. The glenoid depth is reduced, the arc length and articular curvature are decreased, and the contact area that articulates with the humeral head is decreased (Fig. 4.1) [22]. The average antero-posterior width of the glenoid is approximately 23–27 mm and the depth is 5–6 mm [2, 6, 13]. With this relatively small concavity, it is understandable that small amounts of bone loss on the anterior glenoid can have important consequences on the stability of the glenohumeral joint.

Removal of the antero-inferior labrum decreases the contact area by 10% (SD 7–15%) and increases the contact pressure by 12% (SD 8–20%), compared to the intact situation [12]. A decreased force required to dislocate the shoulder was confirmed in many biomechanical studies after creation of a Bankart lesion [3, 23]. Yamamoto et al. showed that joint stability can be restored with a Bankart repair if there is no bone loss, or only a small amount of bone loss [23]. Joint biomechanics are changed to a more marked extent in case of associated anterior glenoid bone loss compared to a Bankart lesion. Increasing glenoid bone loss progressively increases the mean contact pressures in the glenohumeral joint. This effect is most pronounced at the antero-inferior quadrant. A shift of the contact pressures can be seen, with reduced forces in the postero-superior quadrant and increased forces in the antero-inferior quadrant [23]. Greis et al. showed that a glenoid defect of 20% resulted in an increase in the mean contact pressure over 40% across the entire glenoid, and over 200% of normal in the anteroinferior quadrant (Fig. 4.2) [12]. Subsequently, a glenoid defect of 30% resulted in an increase of the contact pressure on the antero-inferior cartilage of 300–400% compared to the intact state. Furthermore, the required maximum

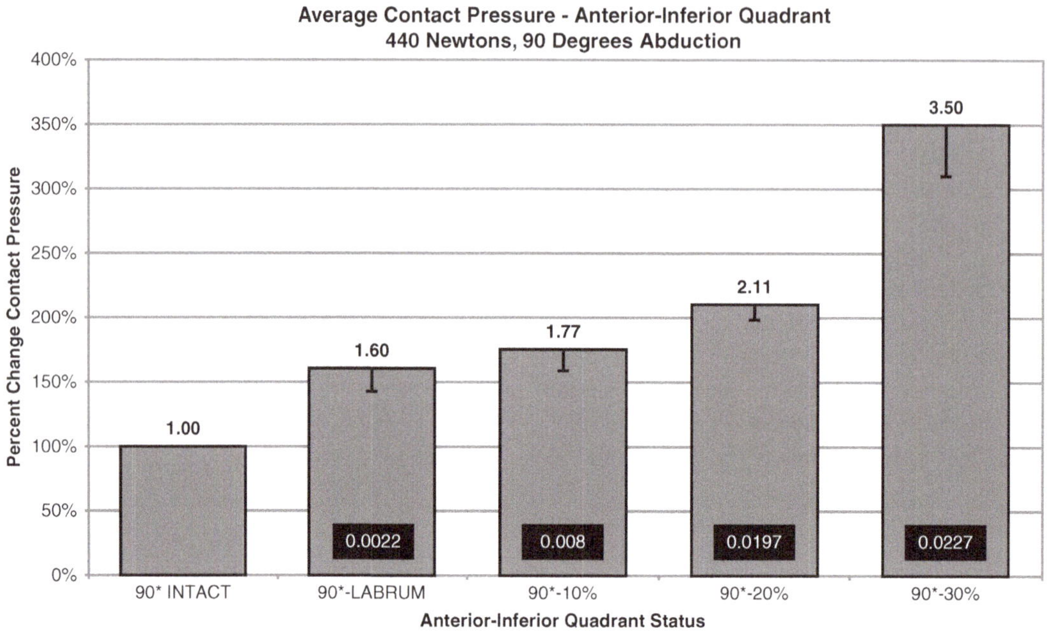

Fig. 4.2 Mean contact pressures in the antero-inferior quadrant at 90° of abduction under 440N compressive load. Contact pressure is shown in percentages relative to the intact situation for labral detachment and bone loss (10, 20, and 30%). *p* values are shown within each bar. (Reprinted from: Greis P et al. Glenohumeral articular contact areas and pressures following labral and osseous injury to the anteroinferior quadrant of the glenoid. J Shoulder Elb Surg. 2002;11(5):442–51. With permission from Elsevier)

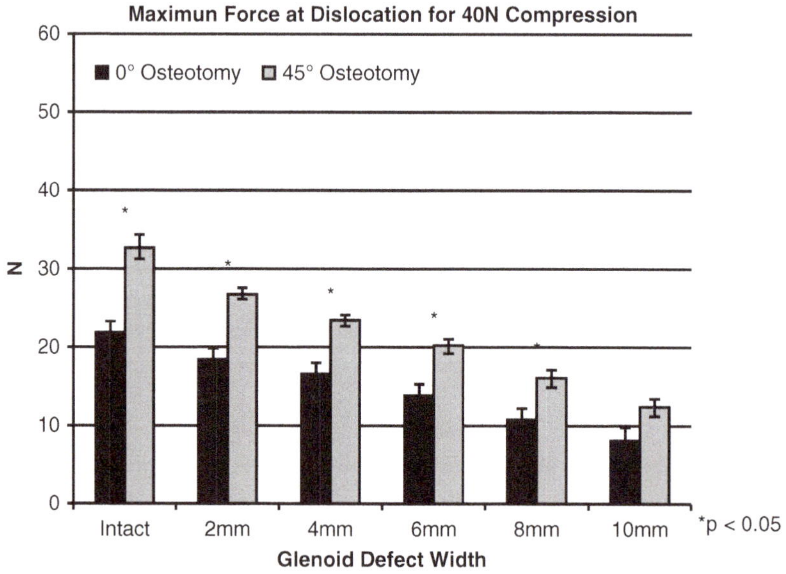

Fig. 4.3 Maximum force required to dislocate the shoulder (in N) was given for the intact state and for increasing glenoid defects. Data are shown for bone loss parallel to the long axis of the glenoid at an angle of 45°. (Reprinted from: Shin SJ et al. The effect of defect orientation and size on glenohumeral instability: a biomechanical analysis. Knee Surgery, Sport Traumatol Arthrosc. 2016;24(2):533–9. With permission from Springer Nature)

force to dislocate the shoulder decreased proportionally with an increase in the glenoid defect size [2]. Shin et al. concluded that bony stability was decreased significantly with any size defect larger than 2 mm, equivalent to 7.5% of the glenoid width (Fig. 4.3) [2].

These studies have clearly shown how joint biomechanics are altered in case of a Bankart lesion and bone loss in shoulder instability. It is hypothesized that these alterations could possibly play a role in the degenerative changes that are seen in natural history studies on shoulder instability [24].

4.2.4 The "Critical Size Defect" in Bankart Repair Procedures

Because bone loss is considered the primary reason for failure after arthroscopic Bankart repair, authors have tried to establish the "critical size" defect [16, 25]. This is an attempt to define the amount of bone loss in which joint stability can still be restored with an arthroscopic Bankart procedure. If bone loss exceeds the "critical size," a bone graft procedure to augment the anterior glenoid, such as a Latarjet procedure, should be performed. The "critical size" of bone defects has decreased over the years. In 1990, Matsen considered a defect as large as one third of the glenoid as the threshold for a bone graft procedure [26]. Bigliani and Itoi both mentioned 25% in 1998 and 2000 [27, 28]. Shin et al. in 2016 concluded that 15% is the maximum amount of bone loss in which stability can be restored with an arthroscopic Bankart procedure [29].

4.2.5 How to Quantify Bone Loss, and to Simulate It in Biomechanical Research

There are several ways to quantify the amount of bone loss. One of the most widely used methods is the "perfect circle" method [30]. In this method, the defect size is expressed as a percentage of the antero-posterior diameter of the glenoid. The inferior two thirds of the glenoid is the shape of a true circle [31]. On a 3D CT scan with subtraction of the humeral head, a perfect circle can be drawn on the en face view of the glenoid. The diameter of the best-fit circle is measured, and bone loss can be measured as the distance from the circle to the anterior glenoid rim (Fig. 4.4) [32]. Nonetheless, the creation of a simulated glenoid defect in biomechanical studies is sometimes slightly different. First of all, the orientation of glenoid bone loss was first believed to occur in a 45-degree angle of the superior-inferior axis of the glenoid, and simulated in this orientation in biomechanical studies [12, 33]. However, cohort studies with CT analysis of Griffith and Saito [18, 34] have shown that bone loss occurs most often parallel to the long axis of the glenoid. Therefore, the orientation of simulated glenoid defects was parallel to the superior–inferior axis, or long axis, of the glenoid in more recent studies (Fig. 4.5) [2, 3, 35].

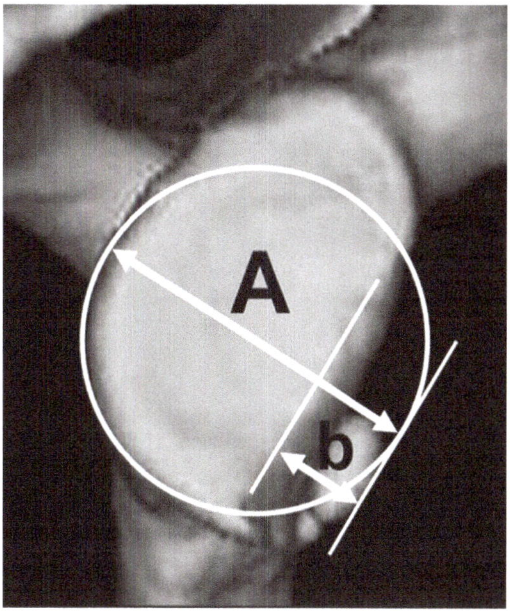

Fig. 4.4 A method to quantify glenoid bone loss. The defect width (b) as a ratio against the diameter of the inferior glenoid circle (A). (Reprinted from: Sugaya H. Techniques to evaluate glenoid bone loss. Curr Rev Musculoskelet Med. 2014;7(1):1–5. With permission from Springer Nature)

4.2.6 Hallmark Studies on "Critical Size Defect"

In 2000, Itoi et al. created glenoid defects oriented 45° to the long axis of the glenoid. The force needed to move the humeral head a normalized distance anteriorly was measured. It was found that stability was not restored after a Bankart repair with a defect of 25% of the glenoid

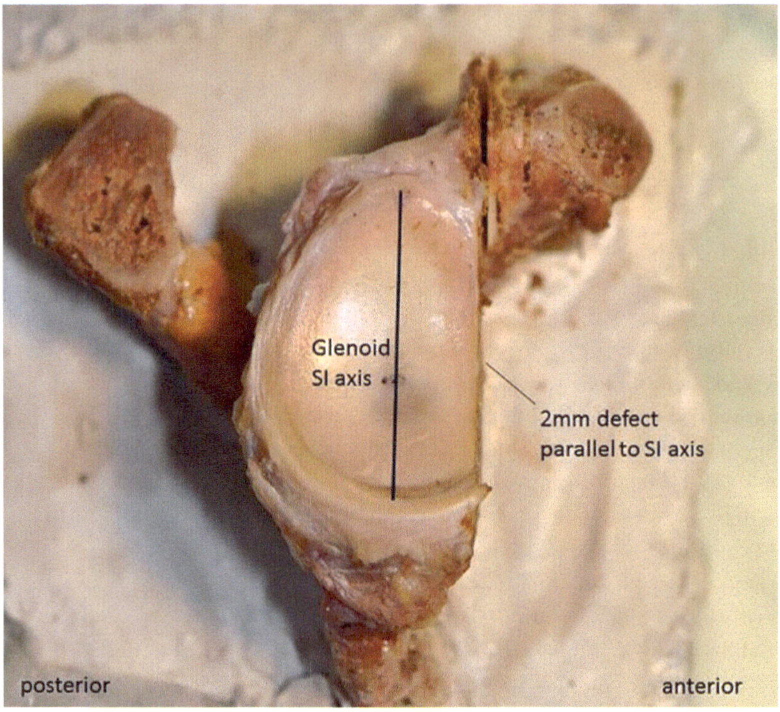

Fig. 4.5 Example of a 2 mm defect from the anterior edge of the glenoid rim, parallel to the superior-inferior axis. (Reprinted from: Shin SJ et al. The effect of defect orientation and size on glenohumeral instability: a biomechanical analysis. Knee Surgery, Sport Traumatol Arthrosc. 2016;24(2):533–9. With permission from Springer Nature)

width, which corresponds to 6–7 mm. Furthermore, external rotation was affected if the glenoid defect was 25% or more of the glenoid width, because the capsule was tensioned by closing the gap over the glenoid defect [27].

In 2010, Yamamoto et al. created glenoid defects in 2 mm stepwise increments parallel to the long axis of the glenoid [22]. The peak translational force required to move the humeral head 10 mm anteriorly was measured as the outcome for stability. With a 6 mm anterior glenoid defect (equivalent to 25% of the glenoid width) and a Bankart repair, the peak translational force was significantly lower than the intact state. Therefore, 6 mm of anterior glenoid bone loss was considered the critical size in which a Bankart repair could not restore the stability.

In a study of Yamamoto et al. in 2014, joint contact pressures were measured in an intact situation, with a labral detachment, with progressive anterior glenoid bone, and after a Bankart repair. Bone defects were created along the superior–inferior glenoid axis, with the percentages corresponding to the widest glenoid diameter in the anterior–posterior direction. In the situation of a 30% bone defect, the glenohumeral contact area was not restored, and the mean contact pressures remained elevated after a Bankart repair. In addition, the peak contact pressure shifted anteriorly in this situation. Glenohumeral contact mechanics were restored to baseline values after Bankart repair in 10 and 20% bone defects [23].

In the study of Shin et al. (2016), 10, 15, 20, and 25% defects were created parallel to the superior–inferior axis of the glenoid. Bankart repair was performed with three 2.4 mm metal suture anchors (SutureTak Arthrex) at the 3, 4 and 5.30 o'clock positions. The amount of humeral head translation with an externally applied antero-inferior load was the outcome parameter representing stability. The antero inferior humeral head translation was increased for all translational loads after a Bankart repair for defects of 15% or more. This was significantly increased compared to the intact condition and the Bankart repair condition without glenoid bone defect. Furthermore, there was significantly less external rotation after a Bankart repair in the 15% defect situation compared with the Bankart repair in the intact condition. Therefore, Shin et al. concluded that 15% or more anterior glenoid bone loss is the critical value for which bone graft procedures should be considered [29].

4.2.7 Bipolar Bone Loss

Although the above-mentioned studies about "critical size" defect are very relevant for our understanding of shoulder instability, these studies only take into account the glenoid side of the osseous defects. This is an oversimplification of reality because shoulder instability is often based on combined glenoid and humeral bony defects, i.e., bipolar bone loss. Far less biomechanical studies have been conducted to investigate the role of bipolar bone loss. But it is understandable that the size of a Hill-Sachs lesion influences the "critical degree" of the glenoid defect. Gottschalk et al. have showed this in a biomechanical study with a variety of combined defects [36]. Glenoid defects were created parallel to the superior–inferior axis, and humeral head defects were made in the posterior superolateral portion. A progressive decrease in stability was found with increase in combined defects, and the decrease in stability was greater for combined lesions than for isolated defects. The decrease in stability (required translational force) reached significance for the combination of a 19% humeral head defect with a 20% glenoid defect. The translation distance to dislocation decreased significantly for the combination of a 19% humeral head defect with a 10% glenoid defect. Based on these results, the authors suggested a bone graft procedure for combined defects with glenoid defects of 10–20%.

In a comparable study, Arciero et al. tried to accurately reproduce Hill-Sachs defects in a biomechanical cadaveric study. 3D CT scans were used from a cohort of 142 instability patients to re-create small (0.87 cm^3, 25th percentile) and medium (1.47 cm^3, 50th percentile) Hill-Sachs lesions with respect to their volumetric size. Glenoid defects were created parallel to the long axis of the glenoid in 2 mm increments. Bankart repair was done with a transosseous technique using No. 2 fiberwire. The peak translational force required to move the humeral head 10 mm anteriorly was the primary outcome measure for stability. It was found that after a Bankart repair, the peak translational force decreased significantly for a 4 mm glenoid defect in combination with a small sized Hill-Sachs defect, and for a 2 mm glenoid defect in combination with a medium sized Hill-Sachs defect (Fig. 4.6) [3]. The authors therefore concluded that even small combined defects may require surgical strategies other than an arthroscopic Bankart procedure alone. However, the clinical relevancy of this work is limited by the fact that currently there is no consensus on how to determine the width and depth of Hill-Sachs defects in an accurate and reproducible way.

4.2.8 Alternatives to a Bone Graft Procedure in Bipolar Bone Loss

An alternative to a Latarjet procedure in the case of combined bone loss is an arthroscopic Bankart repair plus a remplissage procedure, in which the humeral head defect is filled with the posterior capsule and infraspinatus. Grimberg et al. conducted a biomechanical study to compare a Bankart repair only versus a Bankart repair with a remplissage. Bankart lesions were created from 3 to 6 o'clock and humeral head defects were 2 × 2 × 0.5 cm (length × width × depth). A load was applied to the humeral head in the anterior direction and the displacement was measured. The most significant finding of this study was that a Bankart repair alone could not restore the stability to the intact state in the case of a Bankart lesion combined with a humeral head defect. Stability was restored to the intact state by the Bankart repair with remplissage [37]. However, external rotation was significantly limited (from 62° to 51°) in the latter situation, although it is arguable if this has any clinical consequences. Besides this study, there is very limited biomechanical data available on Bankart repairs in combination with a remplissage procedure.

Another alternative, especially if there is a large Hill-Sachs defect, is a Weber derotational osteotomy. With this procedure, popularized in Germany in the 70s and 80s, the humeral head with its Hill-Sachs defect is rotated posterolaterally with respect to the humeral shaft [38]. Excellent stability can be

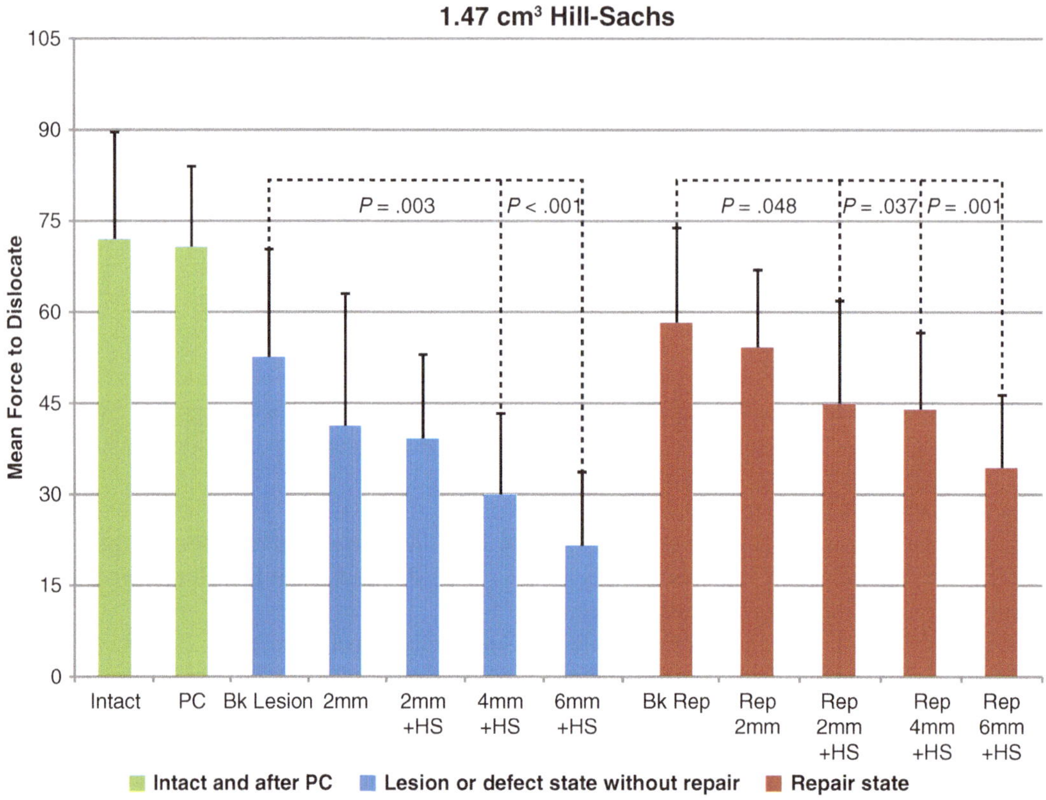

Fig. 4.6 Mean force required to dislocate the shoulder in shoulders with a 1.47 cm^3 (medium size) Hill-Sachs (HS) defect and increasing (2, 4, and 6 mm) glenoid bone loss. Data are shown for the intact situation, after posterior capsulotomy (PC), after creation of a Bankart lesion (Bk), and after the Bankart repair (Rep). (Reprinted from Arciero R et al. The Effect of a Combined Glenoid and Hill-Sachs Defect on Glenohumeral Stability: A Biomechanical Cadaveric Study Using 3-Dimensional Modeling of 142 Patients. Am J Sports Med. 2015;43(6):1422–9. With permission from SAGE Publications Inc.)

achieved, but the complication rate of this procedure is high, reported to be 100% in one study (including plate removal) [39]. Other options to treat instability with large Hill-Sachs defects are to fill the defect with an osteoarticular allograft or with a partial resurfacing metal implant. To our knowledge, the biomechanical consequences of these procedures have not been studied.

4.2.9 Restoration of Joint Biomechanics with the Latarjet Procedure

The alternative to an arthroscopic Bankart procedure is a bone graft procedure to augment the anterior glenoid. The most commonly used technique is the Latarjet procedure, in which the coracoid is used as an autograft to restore the anterior glenoid [40]. The goal of the Latarjet procedure is not only to stabilize the shoulder joint, but also to recreate a stable surface for the humeral head, increasing the effective contact area and decreasing the joint contact pressure. Furthermore, the anterior shift of peak loads associated with glenoid bone loss is restored to normal, without limiting external rotation, theoretically decreasing the chance of development of early osteoarthritis that can be seen with chronic instability. It has been shown that the mean radius of the inferior coracoid is the best match to re-establish the native radius of curvature of the glenoid [41]. Since the conjoined tendon of the coracobrachialis and the short head of the biceps remain attached to the coracoid, a concomitant stabilizing sling effect

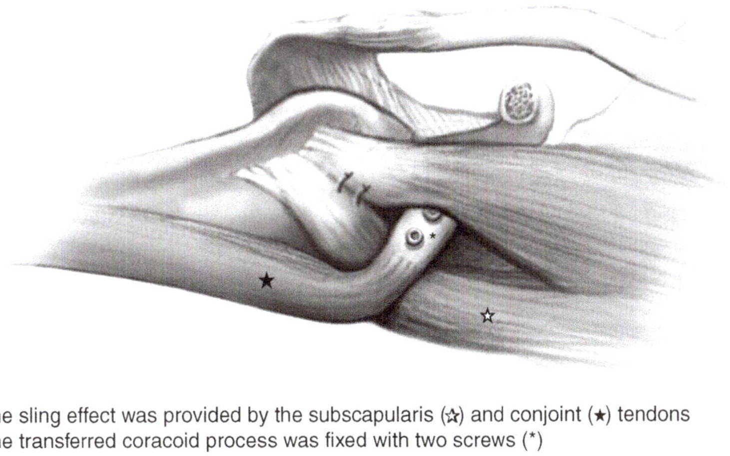

Fig. 4.7 Schematic illustration of the sling effect at the end range of motion. The sling effect is provided by the subscapularis (dark star) and the conjoined tendon (light star). The coracoid transfer is fixed with two screws (∗). The split subscapularis muscle works as a barrier, and the transferred conjoined tendon adds tension to the inferior portion of the subscapularis. (Reprinted from: Yamamoto N et al. Stabilizing mechanism of the Latarjet procedure—A cadaveric study. J Bone Jt Surg Am. 2013;95(15):1390–1397. With permission from Wolter Kluwer Health, Inc.)

is provided together with the subscapularis muscle that is split to facilitate exposure. It is assumed that the sling effect acts mainly in the end range of motion, and that the recreation of the glenoid concavity is more important in mid-range [24]. Alternatives to the coracoid as a bone graft are the distal clavicle, a J-graft of the iliac crest or allografts from the distal tibia or the scaphoid, but these techniques are beyond the scope of this chapter.

4.2.10 The Sling Effect

Biomechanical studies have tried to quantify the contribution of the sling effect in the shoulder following a Latarjet procedure. The peak translational force required to move the humeral head a normalized distance anteriorly was studied by Yamamoto et al. after a Latarjet procedure and after removal of the conjoined tendons from the coracoid graft. The created glenoid defect was 6 mm, parallel to the superior–inferior axis of the glenoid. The subscapularis and conjoined tendon were loaded with pulleys and weights. It was found that the required force to translate the humeral head decreased by 76–77% at the end range of motion and 51–52% in the mid-range position when the conjoined tendons were removed from the coracoid, compared to the standard Latarjet procedure (Fig. 4.7) [14]. Although the applied loads in their experiment were relatively low (30N at maximum), the authors concluded that the sling effect is the main stabilizing mechanism of the Latarjet procedure. Payne et al conducted a different biomechanical cadaveric study to investigate the sling effect, wherein they compared the Latarjet (classic technique) with a "conjoined tendon only" transfer after creation of a 20% glenoid defect. In the latter situation, the conjoined tendon was transferred through a split in the subscapularis and fixated with suture anchors to the anterior glenoid, and loaded in the physiologic line of pull. An anteroinferior translational force was applied through a pulley attached to the proximal humerus. The conjoined tendon only transfer did decrease the anterior translation, and the apex of the humeral head shifted even more posteriorly with the increasing abduction and external rotation compared to the intact specimen, because the conjoined tendon tightened in the apprehensive position. However, the authors emphasized the importance of the bone block itself, because the conjoined tendon alone was insufficient to resist anterior translation and preserve normal joint biomechanics at higher loads of 40N [42].

4.2.11 The Position of the Bone Graft

The position of the bone graft in relation to the articular surface can be recessed (medially), flush, or proud (laterally). It has been clearly shown that the flush position is the most optimal position to restore joint biomechanics [13]. No differences in contact pressure compared to the defect state, i.e., before reconstruction with a bone graft, were found if the bone graft was placed 2 mm recessed. In other words, increased mean contact pressures and high edge loading in the anteroinferior quadrant were not solved with a recessed graft. With placement of the graft 2 mm proud, the contact area was reduced, and there was edge loading in the anteroinferior quadrant with peak contact pressures of up to 250% compared to the intact state. Furthermore, in combined abduction and external rotation, a shift in the contact pressure to the posterosuperior quadrant was seen. The authors stated that their results indicate that the risk of development of osteoarthritis is the highest in the proud position. After restoration of a 30% glenoid defect with a flush bone graft, the mean contact pressure could almost be restored to normal, i.e., 120% compared to the intact state.

4.2.12 The Orientation of the Bone Graft

The effect of bone graft orientation has also been studied. In the classic technique, the inferior surface of the coracoid is fixed to the anterior glenoid and the lateral aspect of the coracoid is used as the articular surface (Fig. 4.8a). In the congruent arc technique, the coracoid is rotated 90° and the medial aspect is fixed to the anterior glenoid and the inferior

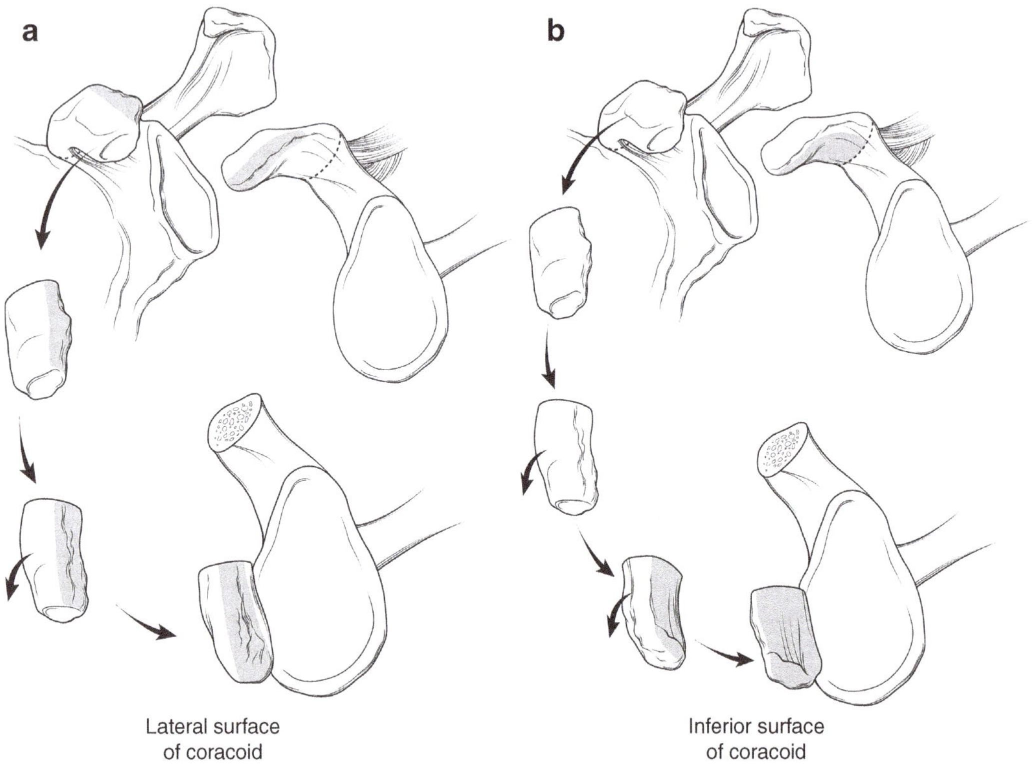

Fig. 4.8 Illustration of the (**a**) classic latarjet technique and (**b**) the congruent arc technique in which the coracoid is rotated 90°, so that the wider inferior surface becomes congruent with the articular surface. (Reprinted from: Ghodadra N et al. Normalization of glenohumeral articular contact pressures after Latarjet or iliac crest bone-grafting. J Bone Jt Surg-Ser A. 2010;92(6):1478–89. With permission from Wolters Kluwer Health, Inc.)

aspect now becomes congruent with the articular surface of the glenoid (Fig. 4.8b) [10]. The lateral aspect of the coracoid is about 24% smaller than the inferior surface, or in other words, the coracoid is wider than being thick. Therefore, the additional benefit of a congruent arc technique is a larger articular surface to augment the anterior glenoid bone loss, which can lead to decreased contact pressures [13]. Indeed, Ghodadra et al. showed that with the congruent arc technique the articular surface area (measured as the glenoid diameter) can be restored completely from a 30% defect state, whereas with the classic technique the surface area could not be restored completely, but can be restored up to within 5% of the intact state. Furthermore, at 60° and 90° of abduction, the mean contact pressure was significantly lower for the congruent arc technique compared to the classic technique. Similarly, Montgomery et al. found a larger articular surface width in the congruent arc technique (13 ± 2 mm), compared to the classic technique (10 ± 2 mm). With the congruent arc technique, glenoid defects of up to 50% of the glenoid width could be restored, whereas defects of up to 35% could be restored in the classic technique [1]. This is in line with the findings in the sophisticated biomechanical study of Boons et al., which shows that a wider glenoid articular surface can be constructed with the congruent arc technique. As a result, the congruent arc technique allowed a significantly greater anterior humeral head translation on the glenoid before an endpoint was reached [43]. However, the downside of the congruent arc technique is twofold. The fixation strength, tested by cyclic loading of the conjoined tendon to the first visible motion and load to failure, is significantly lower in the congruent arc technique compared to the classic technique [1]. There is also a greater risk of coracoid fracture, as the area for screw fixation is smaller in the congruent arc technique. In addition, there is a potentially greater risk of nonunion, because the congruent arc technique has a smaller graft surface to consolidate with the anterior glenoid.

4.2.13 Is There a Maximum to the Stabilizing Effect of the Latarjet?

The stabilizing effect of the Latarjet procedure has been studied in the presence of associated humeral head defects. In theory, a large humeral head defect can still pass the anterior glenoid, even after a Latarjet procedure. Patel et al. created glenoid defects parallel to the long axis of the glenoid. The conjoined tendon was removed from the coracoid and the coracoid was placed against the glenoid in the classic orientation. Humeral head defects were created representing 6, 19, 31, and 44% of the humeral head diameter (Fig. 4.9) [44]. After the coracoid bone graft in the 20% glenoid defect state, the authors found a significant decrease in stability, measured as a distance to dislocation, for humeral head defects of 31% (5/8 of the diameter) or greater. These findings suggest that there is a limit in the stabilizing effect of the Latarjet in relatively large

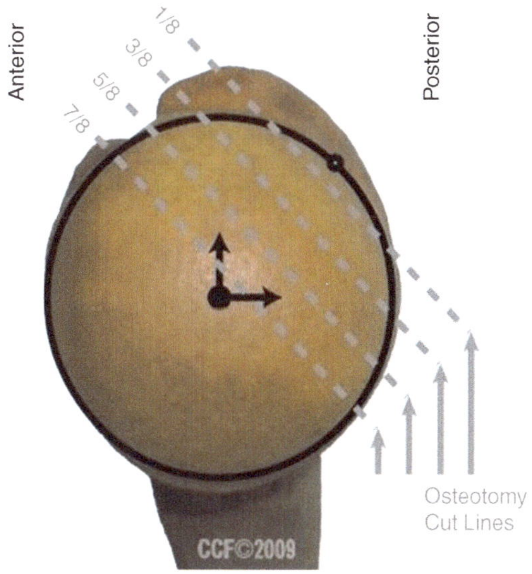

Fig. 4.9 Illustration demonstrating the progressive series of the osteotomy cuts used to simulate humeral head defects. Osteotomy cuts were made at 6%, 9%, 31%, and 44% of the projected diameter of the humeral head, respectively. (Reprinted from: Patel RM et al. The Effects of Latarjet Reconstruction on Glenohumeral Kinematics in the Presence of Combined Bony Defects. Am J Sports Med. 2016;44(7):1818–24. With permission from SAGE publications Inc.)

combined defects, and perhaps additional humeral sided surgery (such as a remplissage) may be needed.

4.3 Conclusions

In summary, the following lessons can be learned from basic science studies on shoulder instability and stabilization:

- Shoulder instability is a complex issue involving static and dynamic components, and not all contributing factors can be simulated in biomechanical studies, especially dynamic muscle control.
- The physiological maximum joint contact pressures occur with combined abduction and external rotation.
- A Bankart lesion results in a decreased contact area, increased contact pressures across the joint, and decreased force required to dislocate the shoulder. These can be restored with a Bankart repair if there is no glenoid bone loss.
- Anterior glenoid bone loss progressively increases the mean contact pressures in the glenohumeral joint, with an antero-inferior shift of peak contact pressures toward the antero-inferior quadrant. A 30% glenoid defect results in a fourfold (or 390%) increase in the contact pressure in the antero-inferior quadrant.
- The changes in joint biomechanics are a possible cause of both recurrent instability and the development of degenerative changes of the shoulder.
- The "critical size" of bony glenoid defects which justifies a bone graft procedure is difficult to define, but can be as small as 15% of the glenoid diameter, or even less (10%, or 2–4 mm) in the case of humeral head defects, i.e., bipolar bone loss.
- Joint biomechanics can be restored to normal with a Latarjet procedure, provided that the bone graft is placed flush with the glenoid articular surface.
- The congruent arc technique allows restoration of larger glenoid defects compared to the classic technique, but the fixation surface and the fixation strength is decreased.

References

1. Montgomery SR, Katthagen JC, Mikula JD, Marchetti DC, Tahal DS, Dornan GJ, et al. Anatomic and biomechanical comparison of the classic and congruent-arc techniques of the Latarjet procedure. Am J Sports Med. 2017;45(6):1252–60.
2. Shin SJ, Ko YW, Scott J, McGarry MH, Lee TQ. The effect of defect orientation and size on glenohumeral instability: a biomechanical analysis. Knee Surg Sports Traumatol Arthrosc. 2016;24(2):533–9.
3. Arciero R, Parrino A, Bernhardson AS, Diaz-Doran V, Obopilwe E, Cote MP, et al. The effect of a combined glenoid and Hill-Sachs defect on glenohumeral stability: a biomechanical cadaveric study using 3-dimensional modeling of 142 patients. Am J Sports Med. 2015;43(6):1422–9.
4. Soslowsky LJ, Flatow EL, Bigliani LU, Mow VC. Articular geometry of the glenohumeral joint. Clin Orthop Relat Res. 1992;285:181–90. https://doi.org/10.1097/00003086-199212000-00023.
5. Lazarus MD, Sidles JA, Harryman DT, Matsen FA. Effect of a chondral-labral defect on glenoid concavity and glenohumeral stability. A cadaveric model. J Bone Joint Surg Am [Internet]. 1996;78(1):94–102.
6. Lippitt SB, Vanderhooft JE, Harris SL, Sidles JA, Harryman DT, Matsen FA. Glenohumeral stability from concavity-compression: a quantitative analysis. J Shoulder Elb Surg. 1993;2(1):27–35.
7. O'Brien SJ. Capsular restraints to anterior-posterior motion of the abducted shoulder. J Shoulder Elb Surg. 1995;4:298–308.
8. Smith CD, Masouros SD, Hill AM, Wallace AL, Amis AA, Bull AMJ. Tensile properties of the human glenoid labrum. J Anat. 2008;212(1):49–54.
9. McMahon PJ, Chow S, Sciaroni L, Yang BY, Lee TQ. A novel cadaveric model for anterior-inferior shoulder dislocation using forcible apprehension positioning. J Rehabil Res Dev. 2003;40(4):349–59.
10. de Beer JF, Roberts C. Glenoid bone defects-open Latarjet with congruent arc modification. Orthop Clin North Am. 2010;41(3):407–15.
11. Westerhoff P, Graichen F, Bender A, Halder A, Beier A, Rohlmann A, et al. In vivo measurement of shoulder joint loads during activities of daily living. J Biomech. 2009;42(12):1840–9.
12. Greis PE, Scuderi MG, Mohr A, Bachus KN, Burks RT. Glenohumeral articular contact areas and pressures following labral and osseous injury to the anteroinferior quadrant of the glenoid. J Shoulder Elb Surg. 2002;11(5):442–51.
13. Ghodadra N, Gupta A, Romeo AA, Bach BR, Verma N, Shewman E, et al. Normalization of glenohumeral articular contact pressures after Latarjet or iliac crest bone-grafting. J Bone Joint Surg Am. 2010;92(6):1478–89.

14. Yamamoto N, Muraki T, An K, Sperling J. The stabilizing mechanism of the Latarjet procedure: part II. J Bone Joint Surg Am. 2013;95-A(15):1390–7.
15. Bankart AS, Cantab MC. Recurrent or habitual dislocation of the shoulder-joint. Clin Orthop Relat Res. 1993;(291):3–6.
16. Burkhart SS, De Beer JF. Traumatic glenohumeral bone defects and their relationship to failure of arthroscopic Bankart repairs: significance of the inverted-pear glenoid and the humeral engaging Hill-Sachs lesion. Arthroscopy. 2000;16(7):677–94.
17. Porcellini G, Campi F, Pegreffi F, Castagna A, Paladini P. Predisposing factors for recurrent shoulder dislocation after arthroscopic treatment. J Bone Joint Surg Am. 2009;91(11):2537–42.
18. Griffith JF, Antonio GE, Yung PSH, Wong EMC, Yu AB, Ahuja AT, et al. Prevalence, pattern, and spectrum of glenoid bone loss in anterior shoulder dislocation: CT analysis of 218 patients. AJR Am J Roentgenol. 2008;190(5):1247–54.
19. Piasecki DP, Verma NN, Romeo AA, Levine WN, Bach BR, Provencher MT. Glenoid bone deficiency in recurrent anterior shoulder instability: diagnosis and management. J Am Acad Orthop Surg. 2009;17(8):482–93.
20. Widjaja AB, Tran A, Bailey M, Proper S. Correlation between Bankart and Hill-Sachs lesions in anterior shoulder dislocation. ANZ J Surg. 2006;76(6):436–8.
21. Conzen A, Eckstein F. Quantitative determination of articular pressure in the human shoulder joint. J Shoulder Elb Surg. 2000;9(3):196–204.
22. Yamamoto N, Muraki T, Sperling JW, Steinmann SP, Cofield RH, Itoi E, et al. Stabilizing mechanism in bone-grafting of a large glenoid defect. J Bone Joint Surg Am. 2010;92(11):2059–66.
23. Yamamoto A, Massimini DF, Distefano J, Higgins LD. Glenohumeral contact pressure with simulated anterior labral and osseous defects in cadaveric shoulders before and after soft tissue repair. Am J Sports Med. 2014;42(8):1947–54.
24. Pauzenberger L, Dyrna F, Obopilwe E, Heuberer PR, Arciero RA, Anderl W, et al. Biomechanical evaluation of glenoid reconstruction with an implant-free J-bone graft for anterior glenoid bone loss. Am J Sports Med. 2017;45(12):2849–57.
25. Balg F, Boileau P. The instability severity index score. A simple pre-operative score to select patients for arthroscopic or open shoulder stabilisation. J Bone Joint Surg Br [Internet]. 2007;89(11):1470–7.
26. Matsen FA III and Thomas SC: Glenohumeral Instability. In Surgery of the Musculoskeletal System. Evart CMC (ed.). Churchill Livingstone New York 1990;3:1439–69.
27. Itoi E. The effect of a glenoid defect on anteroinferior stability of the shoulder. J Bone Joint Surg Am. 2000;82-A(1):35–46.
28. Bigliani LU, Newton PM, Steinmann SP, Connor PM, McIlveen SJ. Glenoid rim lesions associated with recurrent anterior dislocation of the shoulder. Am J Sports Med [Internet]. 1998;26(1):41–5.
29. Shin SJ, Koh YW, Bui C, Jeong WK, Akeda M, Cho NS, et al. What is the critical value of glenoid bone loss at which soft tissue Bankart repair does not restore glenohumeral translation, restricts range of motion, and leads to abnormal humeral head position? Am J Sports Med. 2016;44(11):2784–91.
30. Sugaya H, Moriishi J, Dohi M, Kon Y, Tsuchiya A. Glenoid rim morphology in recurrent anterior glenohumeral instability. J Bone Joint Surg Am. 2003;85(5):878–84.
31. Huysmans PE, Haen PS, Kidd M, Dhert WJ, Willems JW. The shape of the inferior part of the glenoid: a cadaveric study. J Shoulder Elb Surg. 2006;15(6):759–63.
32. Sugaya H. Techniques to evaluate glenoid bone loss. Curr Rev Musculoskelet Med. 2014;7(1):1–5.
33. Yamamoto N, Itoi E, Abe H, Kikuchi K, Seki N, Minagawa H, et al. Effect of an anterior glenoid defect on anterior shoulder stability: a cadaveric study. Am J Sports Med. 2009;37(5):949–54.
34. Saito H, Itoi E, Sugaya H, Minagawa H, Yamamoto N, Tuoheti Y. Location of the glenoid defect in shoulders with recurrent anterior dislocation. Am J Sports Med. 2005;33(6):889–93.
35. Kaar SG, Fening SD, Jones MH, Colbrunn RW. Stability: a cadaveric study of simulated Hill-Sachs. J Bone Joint Surg Am Vol. 2011;38(3):594–9.
36. Gottschalk LJ, Walia P, Patel RM, Kuklis M, Jones MH, Fening SD, et al. Stability of the glenohumeral joint with combined humeral head and glenoid defects. Am J Sports Med. 2015;44(4):933–40.
37. Grimberg J, Diop A, Ghosn RB, Lanari D, Canonne A, Maurel N. Bankart repair versus Bankart repair plus remplissage: an in vitro biomechanical comparative study. Knee Surg Sports Traumatol Arthrosc. 2016;24(2):374–80.
38. Weber BG, Simpson LA, Hardegger F. Rotational humeral osteotomy for recurrent anterior dislocation of the shoulder associated with a large Hill-Sachs lesion. J Bone Joint Surg Am. 1984;66(9):1443–50.
39. Brooks-Hill AL, Forster BB, van Wyngaarden C, Hawkins R, Regan WD. Weber osteotomy for large Hill-Sachs defects: clinical and CT assessments. Clin Orthop Relat Res. 2013;471(8):2548–55.
40. Latarjet M. Treatment of recurrent dislocation of the shoulder. Lyon Chir. 1954;49(8):994–7.
41. DeHaan A, Munch J, Durkan M, Yoo J, Crawford D. Reconstruction of a bony Bankart lesion: best fit based on radius of curvature. Am J Sports Med. 2013;41(5):1140–5.
42. Payne WB, Kleiner MT, McGarry MH, Tibone JE, Lee TQ. Biomechanical comparison of the Latarjet procedure with and without capsular repair. Clin Orthop Surg. 2016;8(1):84–91.
43. Boons HW, Giles JW, Elkinson I, Johnson JA, Athwal GS. Classic versus congruent coracoid positioning during the Latarjet procedure: an in vitro biomechanical comparison. Arthroscopy. 2013;29(2):309–16.
44. Patel RM, Walia P, Gottschalk L, Kuklis M, Jones MH, Fening SD, et al. The effects of Latarjet reconstruction on glenohumeral kinematics in the presence of combined bony defects. Am J Sports Med. 2016;44(7):1818–24.

Benign Joint Hypermobility Syndrome (BJHS)

5

Adrian Błasiak

5.1 Introduction

The laxity of connective tissue and mobility of joints ranges from normal, in cases of the established literature range of motion (majority of the population), and abnormal in patients with connective tissue disorders [Marfan syndrome, Ehlers–Danlos syndrome (EDS), osteogenesis imperfecta]. Generalized joint laxity is commonly seen in healthy people with no complaints; hence, it has no association with arthralgia [1]. When the range of motion of multiple joints exceeds a scope adequate to age, sex, and ethnic origin, it can be considered to be a normal variant. Laxity without complaints, in some situations, can be an advantage, for example, in sports such as gymnastics or in ballet and artistic dance [2].

5.2 Definition

The first mention in the literature, as hypermobility syndrome, was by Kirk et al. [3] for the situation in which this joint laxity was associated with musculoskeletal complaints. Benign joint hypermobility syndrome (BJHS) is defined as the presence of musculoskeletal symptoms in individuals with hypermobility in the absence of systemic rheumatic disease. The prefix "benign" is used to distinguish it from systemic diseases (Marfan syndrome, osteogenesis imperfecta, etc.). This syndrome is considered to be a benign form of congenital connective tissue defect, as a result of improper protein synthesis. Some researchers indicate that BJHS is clinically identical to the former type III of EDS [4].

5.3 Epidemiology

About 10–20% of individuals present with joint hypermobility, especially children, adolescents, and females [5]. According to other authors, the prevalence of BJHS is established at 5% [6], increases to 10% in the European population, and reaches as much as 25–30% in particular ethnic groups (Asians, West Africans) [7–9]. Hypermobility in children decreases with age [10]. Although generalized joint hypermobility is a common finding, symptoms of BJHS such as chronic pain and fatigue can be seen in approximately 3% of the general population [11].

5.4 Pathogenesis

Many genetic and environmental factors contribute to the development of this syndrome. The underlying issues of BJHS are factors such as

A. Błasiak (✉)
Shoulder and Upper Limb Department, St. Luke's Hospital, Bielsko-Biała, Poland
e-mail: blasiak@lukasza.pl

R. Brzóska et al. (eds.), *360° Around Shoulder Instability*,
https://doi.org/10.1007/978-3-662-61074-9_5

protein synthesis defect, resulting in imbalance of the proportion of type I and III collagen, synthesis of type V collagen, and fibrillin, which is essential for the formation of elastic fibers.

The genetic background is deficient or incomplete and controversial. There is a lack of clear correlation between gens mutations and joint hypermobility syndrome [12]. In less than 10% of patients, a single mutation in the gene TNXB, coding for the extracellular matrix glycoprotein Tenascin X, can be observed. These patients are more likely to present dermatological signs such as skin hyperextensibility, velvety skin, and easy bruising [13, 14]. The second important factor responsible for development of symptoms is localized biomechanical overloading, resulting in chronic soft tissue injury caused by joint laxity and either minor or major joint instability. Repetitive microtrauma leads to altered kinematics, followed by overload on other joints and further soft tissue injuries, causing joint and diffuse musculoskeletal pain. It is proven that patients with joint hypermobility syndrome have deficits of proprioceptive acuity [15]. The typical signs of classic inflammatory arthritis such as prolonged morning stiffness (lasting >30 min), edema, and swelling are absent. The symptoms appear either after intense physical activity or repetitive microtrauma, and the pain usually starts later in the day [11].

5.5 Diagnosis

The diagnosis of BJHS is made when the patient presents with pain associated with hypermobility of multiple joints and systemic rheumatic diseases have been excluded. The patient's history and the clinical examination are crucial. The goals are (1) to identify individuals with generalized hyperlaxity, (2) to either confirm or exclude systemic connective tissue diseases, and (3) to assess the condition of affected joints [16]. Not all patients who have generalized joint hypermobility are at risk of developing joint hypermobility syndrome. About 3.3% of women and 0.6% of men will suffer chronic pain, fatigue, or other complaints [17]. BJHS can be suspected when taking a history by using a simple five-point questionnaire described by Hakim et al. [18] for the screening of joint hypermobility (Table 5.1).

When assessed, the degree of hypermobility should be scored and documented.

The first scoring system was devised by Carter and Wilkinson [19]. Subsequently, Beighton et al. modified the system for use in bone and joint disorders. They gave one point for each side of the body for the paired tests and one for forward bend. The range of scoring is thus between 0 and 9, with high scores denoting greater joint laxity [20] (Table 5.2).

See Figs. 5.1, 5.2, 5.3, 5.4, 5.5, 5.6, 5.7, 5.8, and 5.9.

However, certain individuals, particularly in different ethnic groups, would demonstrate such hypermobility according to a scoring system

Table 5.1 Questions to ask patients with suspected joint hypermobility

1. Do you consider yourself double-jointed?
2. Can you now (or could you ever) place your hands flat on the floor without bending your knees?
3. Can you now (or could you ever) bend your thumb to touch your forearm?
4. As a child, did you amuse your friends by contorting your body into strange shapes or could you do the splits?
5. As a child or teenager, did your shoulder or kneecap dislocate on more than one occasion?

Positive responses to 2 of 5 questions have a sensitivity of 84% and specificity of 85% for BJHS
Source: Adapted from Hakim AJ, Cherkas LF, Grahame R, et al. The genetic epidemiology of joint hypermobility: a population study of female twins. Arthritis Rheum 2004;50(8):2640–2644 [18]

Table 5.2 Beighton scoring system for joint hypermobility (adapted from Junge et al. [21])

Passive dorsiflexion of the fifth metacarpophalangeal joint to >90°	Scoring 1 point for each side (max 2)
Passive apposition of thumb to the flexor aspect of forearm	Scoring 1 point for each side (max 2)
Hyperextension of the elbow >10°	Scoring 1 point for each side (max 2)
Hyperextension of the knee >10°	Scoring 1 point for each side (max 2)
Flexion of the trunk with knees straight and both palms resting easily on floor	Scoring 1 point

When obtaining at least 4 points (of 9) in adults, generalized hypermobility can be stated

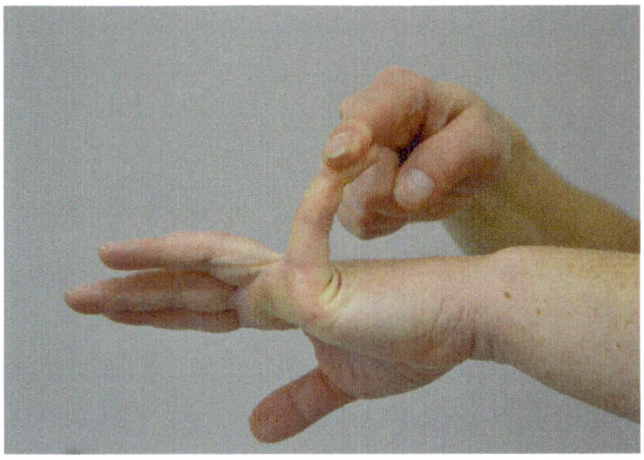

Fig. 5.1 Passive dorsiflexion of fifth metacarpophalangeal joint to 90°: left side

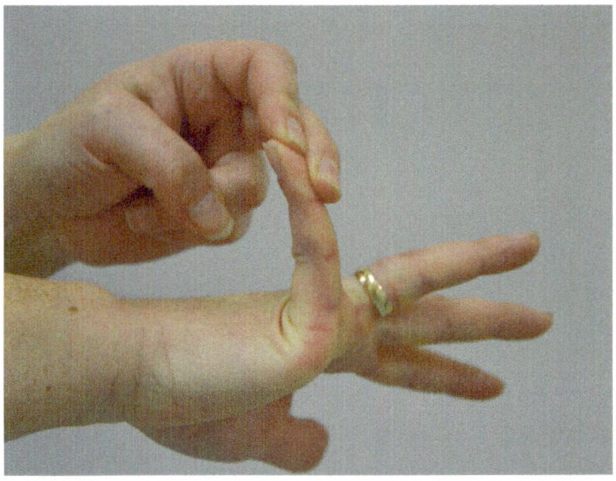

Fig. 5.2 Passive dorsiflexion of fifth metacarpophalangeal joint to 90°: right side

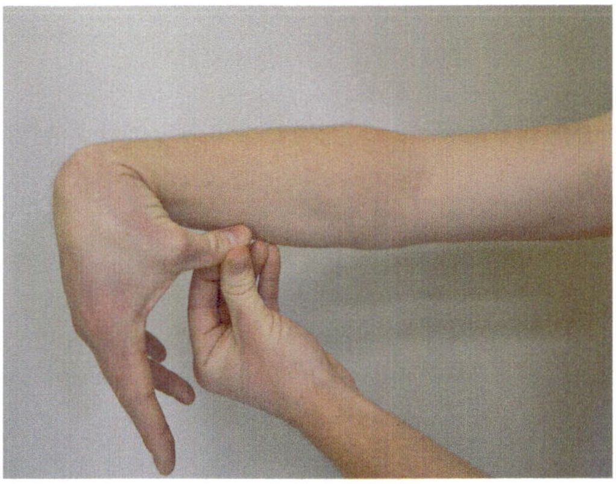

Fig. 5.3 Passive apposition of thumb to flexor aspect of forearm: right side

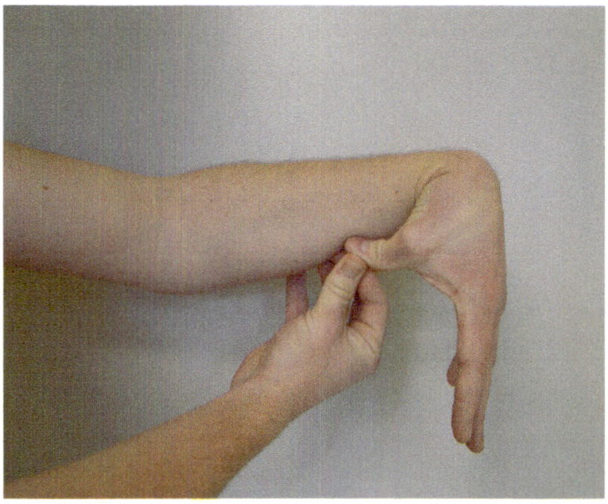

Fig. 5.4 Passive apposition of thumb to flexor aspect of forearm: left side

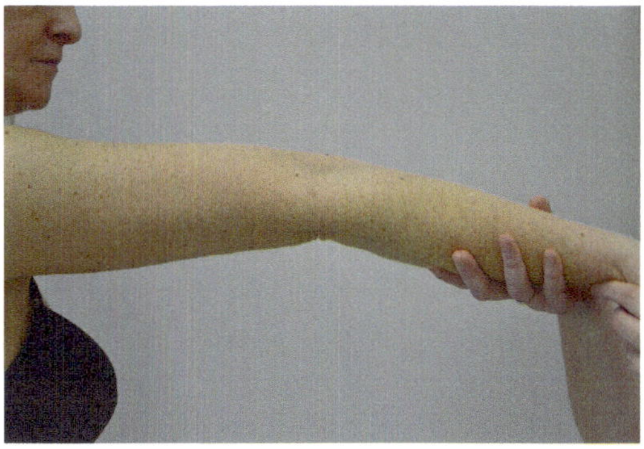

Fig. 5.5 Hyperextension of elbow 10°: right side

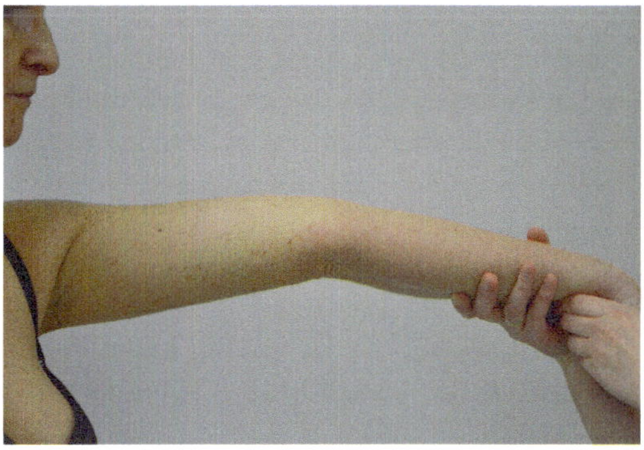

Fig. 5.6 Hyperextension of elbow 10°: left side

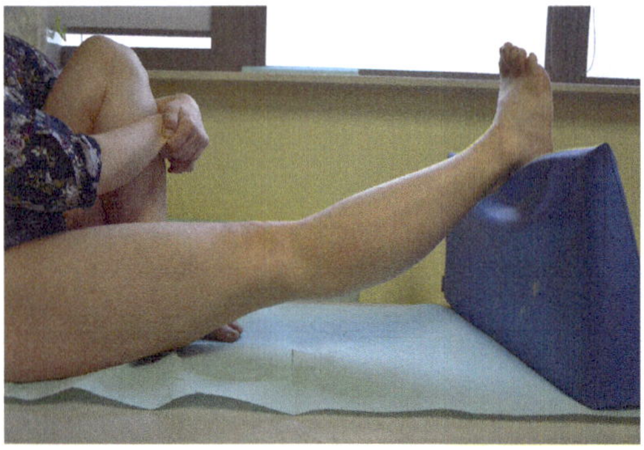

Fig. 5.7 Hyperextension of knee 10°: right side

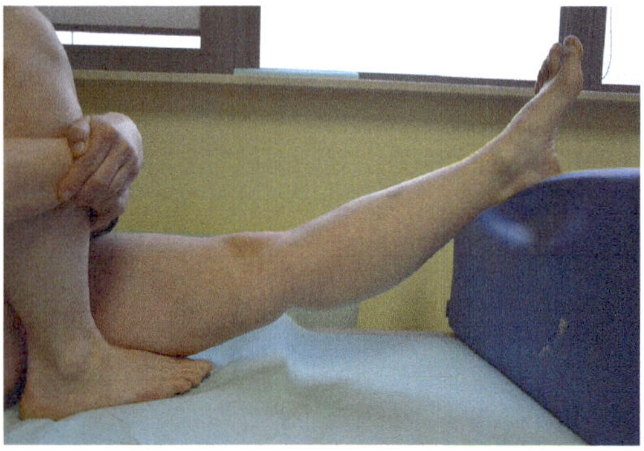

Fig. 5.8 Hyperextension of knee 10°: left side

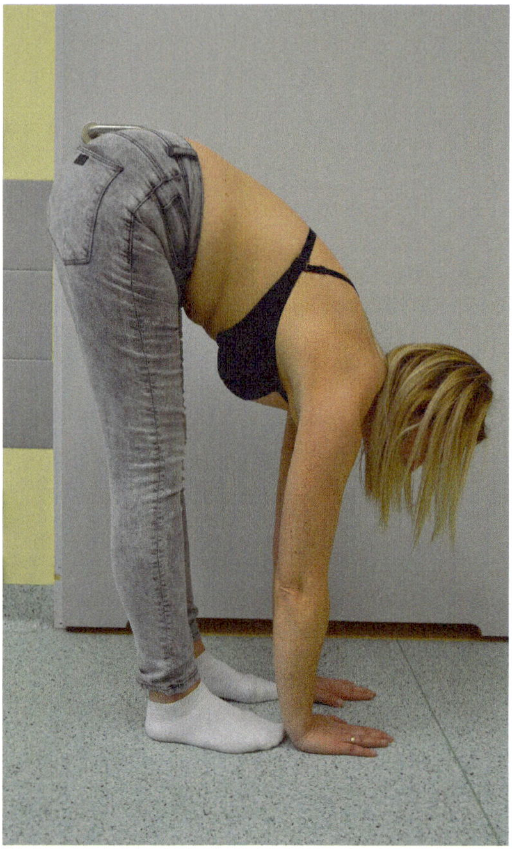

Fig. 5.9 Flexion of trunk with knees straight and both palms resting easily on floor

but still remain asymptomatic. Consequently, a working group of the British Society for Rheumatology addressed this issue. As a result, criteria were proposed in Brighton in 1999 and were published the following year [22]. Table 5.3 presents the revised Brighton criteria.

Brighton criteria are most commonly used for diagnosing of BJHS, although Bulbena et al. proposed their own criteria to determine hypermobility syndrome [23]. Joint-related problems including scoliosis, lordosis, genu valgum, pes planus, and patellar instability move to the forefront of all complaints. However, other extraarticular signs [24] such as bruising, hernias, muscle dystonia, skin hyperextensibility, arrhythmia, headaches, anxiety, orthostasis, and abdominal pain may be mentioned [24–26]. Typically, pain is described as dull and can be either constant or self-limited. Commonly, weight-bearing joints of the lower extremity such as the knee and ankle are involved [11]. The musculoskeletal pain is usually diffuse and very often associated with fatigue, as seen in up to 84% of patients [27].

5.6 Differential Diagnosis

BJHS is a diagnosis of exclusion. Thus, the most important issue is to identify other symptoms of potential systemic connective tissue disease. Joint hypermobility could be congenital in nature, although when affecting a single joint it might be a result of long-time stretch-training, inflammatory diseases of joints or connective tissue, and posttraumatic. Establishment of diagnosis in professional athletes such as gymnasts and in professional ballet and other dancers is a challenge because they have increased range of motion acquired in long-lasting stretching exercises. In these cases, all individuals should be screened for

Table 5.3 Brighton criteria

Major criteria
• Beighton score of at least 4 (Table 5.2)
• Arthralgia for longer than 3 months in four or more joints
Minor criteria
• Beighton score of 1, 2, or 3 (Table 5.2)
• Arthralgia (3-month duration) in one to three joints or back pain (3-month duration) or spondylosis, spondylolysis, spondylolisthesis
• Dislocation or subluxation in more than one joint, or in one joint on more than one occasion
• Three or more soft-tissue lesions (e.g., epicondylitis, tenosynovitis, bursitis)
• Marfanoid habitus [tall, slim, span greater than height (1.03 ratio), upper segment less than lower segment (<0.89 ratio), arachnodactyly]
• Skin striae, hyperextensibility, thin skin, or abnormal scarring
• Ocular signs: drooping eyelids, myopia, antimongoloid slant
• Varicose veins, hernia, or uterine or rectal prolapse
• Mitral valve prolapse
Requirement for diagnosis: any one of the following:
• Two major criteria
• One major plus two minor criteria
• Four minor criteria
• Two minor criteria and unequivocally affected first-degree relative in family history

extraarticular signs such as skin hypextensibility, hyperelasticity of auricular cartilage, or abdominal disorders. Examining the range of motion in joints that have not undergone stretch training is very useful to distinguish BJHS from generalized hyperlaxity. Hereditary defects of connective tissue are excluded in genetic testing, and traumatic reasons are detectable while taking the history. It is very important to exclude other causes of chronic musculoskeletal pain, because BJHS is a nonprogressive and noninflammatory condition and joint laxity decreases with age.

5.7 Management

There is no specific treatment of BJHS. One of the most important issues is modification of lifestyle by education of patients to avoid excessive joint movements and exercises that may aggravate symptoms and lead to joint injury such as meniscal, cartilage, and ligament lesions. Regular moderate exercises are indicated. Overtraining, especially focused on increasing joint flexibility, may lead to injuries and is contraindicated. Physiotherapy, including proprioceptive and neuromuscular training, taping, and bracing, could prevent injuries and improve gait [28–30]. Nonsteroidal antiinflammatory drugs administered periodically or before physical activity are helpful in reducing pain during daily activities or athletic competition. Cooperation with physiotherapists and personalizing of training and exercises may be useful and relieve symptoms [31, 32]. Stabilization of the joint could be achieved indirectly through strengthening programs of periarticular musculature. Some authors indicate supplementation of vitamin C in addressing some cutaneous features and vitamin D for increasing bone mineral density [33].

5.8 Conclusion

BJHS is a quite common finding in the general population, affecting the quality of life. In fact, the term joint hypermobility is misleading, because the problem affects not only joints but the connective tissue overall; therefore, it is a systemic disorder. Diagnosis of BJHS is crucial for improvement of daily living and more appropriate management and care in cases of extraarticular symptoms. However, the diagnosis requires a high level of clinical suspicion. Therefore, in every case of joint pain without other supporting symptoms, BJHS should be taken into account.

A specific physical examination should be performed. Education and explanation to the patients about the issues of their disease will provide protection of their joints and lifestyle modification to prevent further damage.

5.9 Clinical Implications

The crucial clinical implication for orthopedic surgeons regarding the presence of BJHS is that diagnosing instability in one of the joints obliges them to exclude the presence or lack of instability in other joints.

Furthermore, one must have in mind that potential surgical treatment of an unstable joint in the presence of BJHS is related to a higher risk of recurrence.

Some individuals find advantages in increased laxity, especially athletes in sports such as gymnastics, swimming, and ballet.

References

1. de Inocencio Arocena J, Ocaña Casas I, Benito Ortiz LB. Laxitud articular: prevalencia y relación con dolor musculosquelético. Joint hypermobility: prevalence and relationship with musculoskeletal pain. An Pediatr (Barc). 2004;61:162–6.
2. Scheper MC, de Vries JE, de Vos R, Verbunt J, Nollet F, Engelbert RH. Generalized joint hypermobility in professional dancers: a sign of talent or vulnerability? Rheumatology. 2013;52(4):651–8.
3. Kirk JA, Ansell BM, Bywaters EL. The hypermobility syndrome. Ann Rheum Dis. 1967;26:419.
4. Tinkle BT, Bird HA, Grahame R, Lavallee M, Levy HP, Sillence D. The lack of clinical distinction between the hypermobility type of Ehlers–Danlos syndrome and the joint hypermobility syndrome (a.k.a. hypermobility syndrome). Am J Med Genet A. 2009;149A:2368.
5. Hakim AJ, Grahame R. Joint hypermobility. Best Pract Res Clin Rheumatol. 2003;17:989–1004.
6. Jessee EF, Owen DS, Sagar KB. The benign hypermobile joint syndrome. Arthritis Rheum. 1980;23:1053.
7. Birrell F, Adebajo A, Hazleman BL, Silman A. High prevalence of joint laxity in West Africans. Br J Rheumatol. 1994;33:56–9.
8. Remvig L, Jensen DV, Ward RC. Epidemiology of general joint hypermobility and basis for the proposed criteria for benign joint hypermobility syndrome: review of the literature. J Rheumatol. 2007;34:804.
9. Clark CJ, Simmonds JV. An exploration of the prevalence of hypermobility and joint hypermobility syndrome in Omani women attending a hospital physiotherapy service. Musculoskeletal Care. 2011;9:1.
10. Silverman S, Constine L, Harvey W, Grahame R. Survey of joint mobility and in vivo skin elasticity in London schoolchildren. Ann Rheum Dis. 1975;34:177–80.
11. Scheper MC, de Vries JE, Verbunt J, Engelbert RH. Chronic pain in hypermobility syndrome and Ehlers–Danlos syndrome (hypermobility type): it is a challenge. J Pain Res. 2015;8:591–601.
12. Malfait F, Hakim AJ, De Paepe A, Grahame R. The genetic basis of the joint hypermobility syndromes. Rheumatology. 2006;45:502.
13. Bristow J, Carey W, Egging D, et al. Tenascin-X, collagen, elastin, and the Ehlers–Danlos syndrome. Am J Med Genet C Semin Med Genet. 2005;139C(1):24–30.
14. Chiarelli N, Carini G, Zoppi N, et al. Transcriptome-wide expression profiling in skin fibroblasts of patients with joint hypermobility syndrome/Ehlers–Danlos syndrome hypermobility type. PLoS One. 2016;11(8):e0161347.
15. Bates AV, Alexander CM. Kinematics and kinetics of people who are hypermobile. A systematic review. Gait Posture. 2015;41(2):361–9.
16. Kumar B, Lenert P. Joint hypermobility syndrome: recognizing a commonly overlooked cause of chronic pain. Am J Med. 2017;130:640–7.
17. Scheper MC, Engelbert RH, Rameckers EA, Verbunt J, Remvig L, Juul-Kristensen B. Children with generalised joint hypermobility and musculoskeletal complaints: state of the art on diagnostics, clinical characteristics, and treatment. Biomed Res Int. 2013;2013:121054.
18. Hakim AJ, Cherkas LF, Grahame R, et al. The genetic epidemiology of joint hypermobility: a population study of female twins. Arthritis Rheum. 2004;50(8):2640–4.
19. Carter C, Wilkinson J. Persistent joint laxity and congenital dislocation of the hip. J Bone Joint Surg Br. 1964;46B:40–5.
20. Beighton P, Solomon L, Soskolne CL. Articular mobility in an African population. Ann Rheum Dis. 1973;32:413–8.
21. Junge T, Jespersen E, Wedderkopp N, Juul-Kristensen B. Inter-tester reproducibility and inter-method agreement of two variations of the Beighton test for determining generalized joint hypermobility in primary school children. BMC Pediatr. 2013;13:214.
22. Grahame R, Bird HA, Child A, et al. The revised (Brighton 1998) criteria for the diagnosis of benign joint hypermobility syndrome (BJHS). J Rheumatol. 2000;27:1777–9.
23. Bulbena A, Duro J, Porta M, Faus S, Vallescar R, Martin-Santos R. Clinical assessment of hypermobile joints: assembly criteria. J Rheumatol. 1992;19:115–22.
24. Mishra MB, Ryan P, Atkinson P, Taylor H, Bell J, Calver D, et al. Extraarticular features of benign joint hypermobility syndrome. Br J Rheumatol. 1996;35:861–6.
25. Bendik EM, Tinkle BT, Al-shuik E, et al. Joint hypermobility syndrome: a common clinical disorder associated with migraine in women. Cephalalgia. 2011;31(5):603–13.
26. Zarate N, Farmer AD, Grahame R, et al. Unexplained gastrointestinal symptoms and joint hypermobility: is connective tissue the missing link? Neurogastroenterol Motil. 2010;22(3):252–78.
27. Voermans NC, Knoop H, van de Kamp N, Hamel BC, Bleijenberg G, van Engelen BG. Fatigue is a frequent and clinically relevant problem in Ehlers–Danlos syndrome. Semin Arthritis Rheum. 2010;40(3):267–74.
28. Camerota F, Galli M, Cimolin V, et al. The effects of neuromuscular taping on gait walking strategy in a patient with joint hypermobility syndrome/Ehlers–Danlos syndrome hypermobility type. Ther Adv Musculoskelet Dis. 2015;7(1):3–10.

29. Simmonds JV, Keer RJ. Hypermobility and the hypermobility syndrome. Man Ther. 2007;12(4):298–309.
30. Ferrel WR, Tennant N, Sturrock RD, Ashton L, Creed G. Amelioration of symptoms by enhancement of proprioception in patients with joint hypermobility syndrome. Arthritis Rheum. 2004;50:3323–8.
31. Russek LN. Examination and treatment of a patient with hypermobility syndrome. Phys Ther. 2000;80:386–98.
32. McCormack M, Briggs J, Hakim A, Grahame R. Joint laxity and the benign joint hypermobility syndrome in student and professional ballet dancers. J Rheumatol. 2004;31:173–8.
33. Castori M, Morlino S, Pascolini G, Blundo C, Grammatico P. Gastrointestinal and nutritional issues in joint hypermobility syndrome/Ehlers–Danlos syndrome, hypermobility type. Am J Med Genet C Semin Med Genet. 2015;169C(1):54–75.

Anterior Shoulder Instability Diagnosis: Clinical Examination

6

Sanjay Desai

6.1 History

Age and the level of activity are the some of the most important factors in diagnosis and management of shoulder instability. The mechanism of injury, position of the arm, and the type of symptoms at the time of injury can provide useful information. Injury with the arm in abducted and externally rotated position typically leads to anterior shoulder instability. Whether it was reduced under sedation or relocated spontaneously, this gives useful information about shoulder laxity. The number of dislocations and activities when it happens is important in predicting the extent of soft-tissue damage as well as damage to the glenoid bone. Similarly, the location of the Hill–Sachs lesion can be determined by knowing the degree of abduction when the arm went into forceful external rotation. The severity of the force and the constitutional quality of the soft tissue or collagen are important factors that determine whether the shoulder subluxes or frankly dislocates. Lastly, a history of epilepsy or a family history of connective tissue disorders such as Ehlers–Danlos syndrome and Marfans syndrome can be of great relevance.

6.2 General Clinical Examination

It is mandatory to expose both the shoulders and look for wasting of muscles, asymmetry, and abnormal scapular position. Assessment for neurovascular injury is an essential part of basic examination of any shoulder injury. One may need to feel for the deltoid contraction to rule out axillary nerve injury, as active movement can be difficult to elicit in an acutely injured shoulder. Both active and passive evaluation of range of movement, including external rotation with the arm on the side and with arms abducted 90°, will immediately raise suspicion of conditions such as locked posterior dislocation or persistent unreduced anterior dislocation. Strength testing, particularly of the rotator cuff muscles, must be performed. The supraspinatus can be tested by applying resistance to forward elevation of the arm in 90°, infraspinatus power is tested by applying resistance to external rotation with arms on the side and subscapularis by the lift-off and belly-press sign [1]. One must ask if the patient can subluxate the shoulder at will, which would help identify "voluntary" or "habitual" instability. Lastly, thorough evaluation for generalized ligament laxity will give clues not only about the quality of the collagen/capsule but also help in selecting the appropriate stabilization procedure, if required.

S. Desai (✉)
Breach Candy Hospital and Research Centre, Bhatia General Hospital, Mumbai, India

R. Brzóska et al. (eds.), *360° Around Shoulder Instability*,
https://doi.org/10.1007/978-3-662-61074-9_6

6.3 Shoulder Examination: Provocative Test

6.3.1 Apprehension Test

The most time tested "anterior apprehension" sign was first described by Rowe et al. [2, 3]. The test is done either in standing or supine position, with the arm abducted 90°; the shoulder is externally rotated until the patient is apprehensive of it coming out. Rowe stated that all their patients tested positive when examined in this fashion; however, the test could be positive in other conditions with pain and weakness in the shoulder [3]. The author prefers to examine in standing position with one hand holding the forearm, keeping the shoulder in 90° of abduction and gradually increasing external rotation, while the fingers of the other hand of the examiner on the coracoid anteriorly and the thumb posteriorly gently push the humeral head in the anterior direction (Fig. 6.1). The test is considered positive when the patient experiences the same feeling of 'humeral head coming out, however, pain by itself may not be a reliable sign of instability [4, 5]. The apprehension test has a specificity of 95.7–100% and a sensitivity of 50–55.6% [6, 7]. It has many variations, but all of them essentially aim to provoke the humeral head to go over the anterior edge of the glenoid. The augmentation test, crank test, and fulcrum test are examples of variations of what is principally the apprehension test [8, 9].

6.3.2 The Relocation Test

Described by Frank Jobe, the test is performed with the patient supine and the shoulder over the edge of the examination table [10]. The arm is pushed into maximum abduction and external rotation until the patient complains of pain. The examiner then places the other hand on the humeral head and pushes it posteriorly to 'relocate' the head and the pain is relieved, which means the test is positive (Fig. 6.2). Jobe described that the pain is caused by rotator impingement secondary to instability. This test has been studied by Lo and Speer [4, 11], who concluded that the test is useful if done for instability rather than secondary impingement. The test has a high specificity when evaluated for apprehension, which is relieved by relocation [11]. However, it is not useful for the diagnosis of instability if only pain is used as a criterion instead of apprehension.

6.3.3 Surprise Test

After relocating the humeral head, if you suddenly release the pressure and the patient is apprehensive again, this is called the Surprise test, described by Silliman and Hawkins [12]. Similar to the other test for instability, the test is not reliable if only pain is used as the criterion. Also, patients are often uncomfortable when undergoing this test because there is a risk of subluxation or even dislocation when the test is being done.

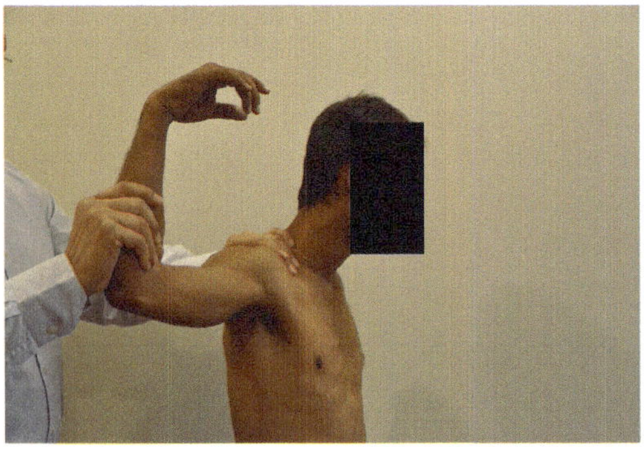

Fig. 6.1 Apprehension test

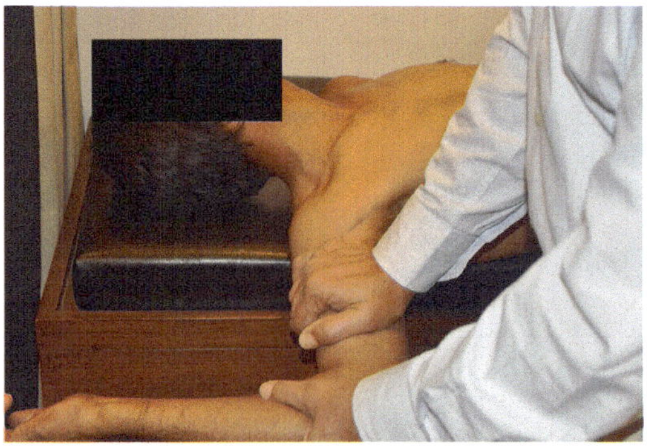

Fig. 6.2 Relocation test

6.3.4 Posterior Instability Test

In this test as described by Kessel, the examiner applies a posteriorly directed force along the axis of the humerus, with the arm flexed 90° and in adduction, with internal rotation (Fig. 6.3) [13]. However, the position of subluxation is not the same in every patient. Hence, the test has low sensitivity, besides the test has not been validated.

6.3.5 Jerk Test

Described by Matsen et al., an axial force is applied to the arm, which is adducted, internally rotated, and in 90° of flexion [14]. A jerk may be felt as the humeral head subluxates posteriorly. The examiner then extends the arm away from the body, and another clunk is felt as the humeral head relocates. In our experience it is difficult to reproduce this test in all patients with posterior instability, although it may be specific, because the exact position of posterior instability is variable among patients.

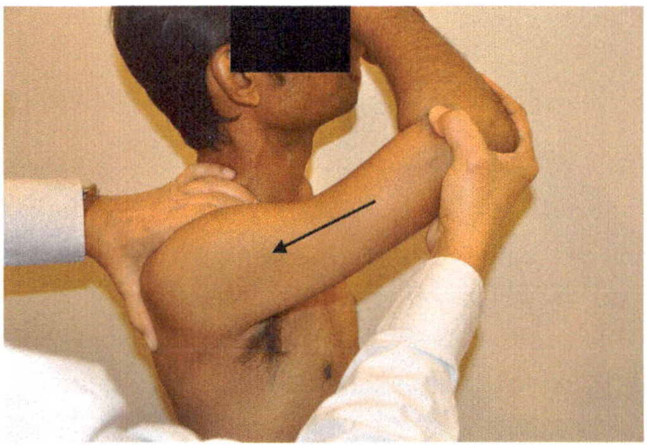

Fig. 6.3 Posterior instability test

6.4 Shoulder Examination: Laxity Testing

6.4.1 Beighton Hypermobility Score

The clinician should be able to differentiate between laxity and instability. Laxity is the extent of normal, symptom-free translation of the humeral head over the glenoid. Laxity is determined by the looseness of the passive stabilizers. Excessive laxity could be localized to only the shoulder or may be generalized. The Beighton hypermobility score is a relatively simple method of quantifying generalized ligament laxity [15]. One point is awarded for each, for dorsiflexion of fifth finger and thumb, hyperextension of the knees and elbows, and ability to forward flex with palms touching the floor (Fig. 6.4). Of a total score of 9, more than 4 would be significant laxity. Patients with significant laxity are more likely to develop instability and are at a higher risk of failure of the stabilization procedure.

6.4.2 Shoulder Laxity: Passive Humeral Head Translation

The drawers test and load-shift test are two common methods of assessing shoulder laxity. The

Fig. 6.4 Beighton score

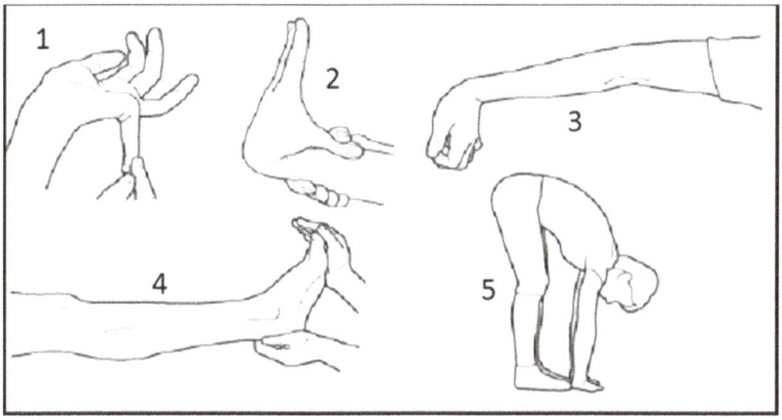

translation of the humeral head can be assessed in millimeters or as a percentage of the humeral head shifting over the edge of the glenoid. However, one must bear in mind that there is a wide range of normal laxity that allows asymptomatic translation of the humeral head over the glenoid rim. This normal translation could be more pronounced when performed under anesthesia.

The *anterior drawer test* described by Gerber is one method of assessing the laxity of the shoulder [16]. This test is performed with the patient in supine position and the shoulder beyond the edge of the table, with the arm in about 80°–100° of abduction, 0°–20° of flexion, and external rotation, while the elbow remains flexed. With one hand, the examiner stabilizes the scapula by holding the scapular spine and coracoid while the other hand holds the proximal humerus and translates the head anteriorly to feel if it glides over the anterior edge of the glenoid (Fig. 6.5). However, it can be difficult to maintain the arm in the described position as well as stabilize the scapula. We prefer to hold the patient's forearm or hand and hold the humerus with the other hand, applying anterior or posterior force (Fig. 6.6). The second method of testing laxity is the *load-shift test* described by Hawkins [12]. The test is performed with the patient in sitting position, with the arm in about 20° of abduction, 20° of flexion, and neutral rotation. One hand of the examiner is over the shoulder to stabilize the scapula, and the humeral head is held by the other hand to apply an anterior or posterior force to translate the head over the glenoid rim (Fig. 6.7). The load-shift test has not been validated by any biomechanical evaluation. Tzannes and Murrell evaluated the load-shift test and found 100% specificity but only 50% sensitivity [17]. In agreement with Hawkins, they emphasized the importance of loading the humeral head onto the glenoid when executing the test. My personal experience is that it is easier to examine the patient for shoulder laxity in supine position. Not only is the patient more relaxed, it is also easier to keep the arm in 40°–50° of abduction, which is the position for the greatest laxity.

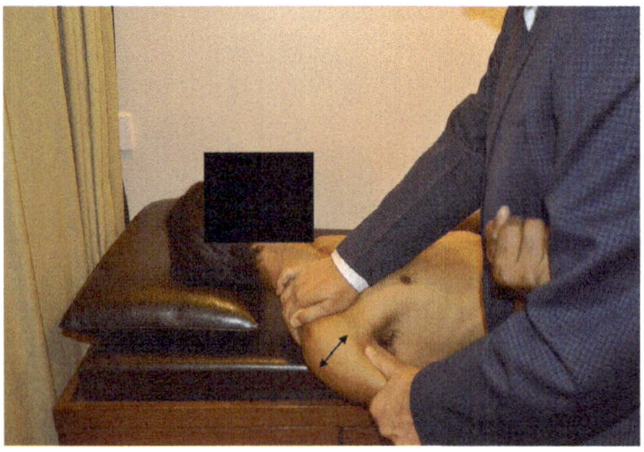

Fig. 6.5 Gerber and Ganz drawer test

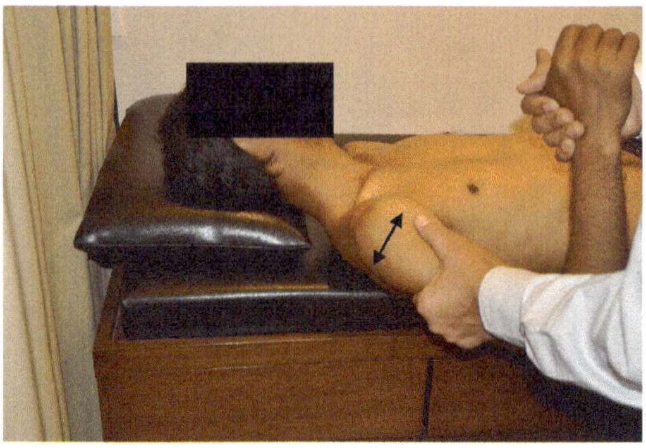

Fig. 6.6 Modified anterior-posterior drawer test

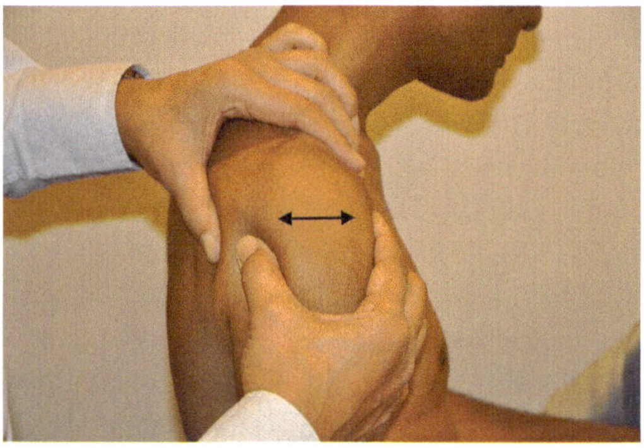

Fig. 6.7 Load-shift test

6.4.3 Sulcus Test

Described by Neer and Foster in 1980 [18] as a measure of inferior laxity, with reference to multidirectional instability, this test is performed with the patient in sitting position with the arms by the side in neutral rotation and elbows flexed 90°. The elbow is held by the examiner and a downward pull is applied along the axis of humerus, translat-

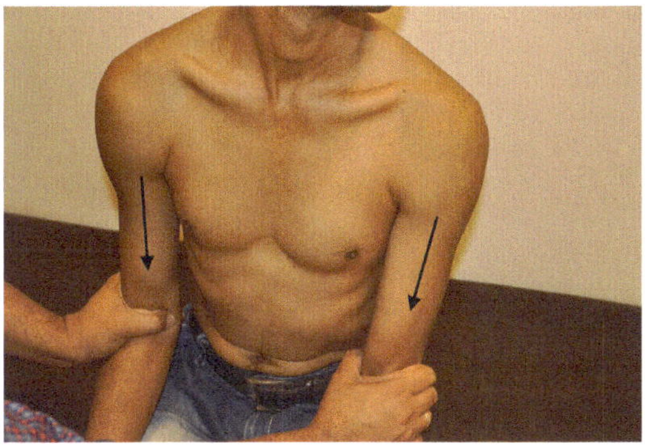

Fig. 6.8 Sulcus test

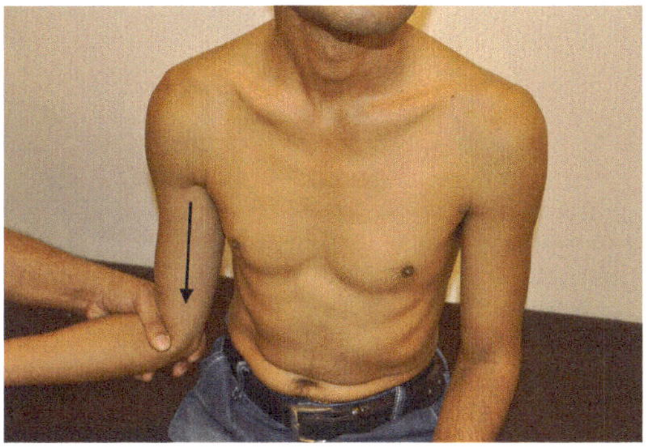

Fig. 6.9 Sulcus test in external rotation

ing the humeral head inferiorly, thereby creating a sulcus or gap in the subacromial region (Fig. 6.8). The test is repeated with the arm in external rotation (Fig. 6.9). If the sulcus increases in comparison to neutral rotation, then a rotator interval lesion is suspected. The sulcus sign can be graded: more than 2 cm is grade 3, 1.5–2 cm is grade 2, and less than 1.5 cm is grade 1. There are several issues with the sulcus test: one, it has not been validated, and two, asymptomatic individuals can have inferior translation. Also, there is no absolute translation that defines inferior instability.

6.4.4 Gagey's Hyperabduction Test

This test was described by O. Gagey and N. Gagey to assess the laxity of the inferior glenohumeral ligament complex [19]. With one hand the examiner holds the elbow of the patient and the other hand stabilizes the scapula. The arm is gradually abducted until the scapula starts moving. It is considered positive if the passive abduction is more than 105° (Fig. 6.10). The test is more valuable when it produces pain and the passive abduction is greater in comparison to the opposite side.

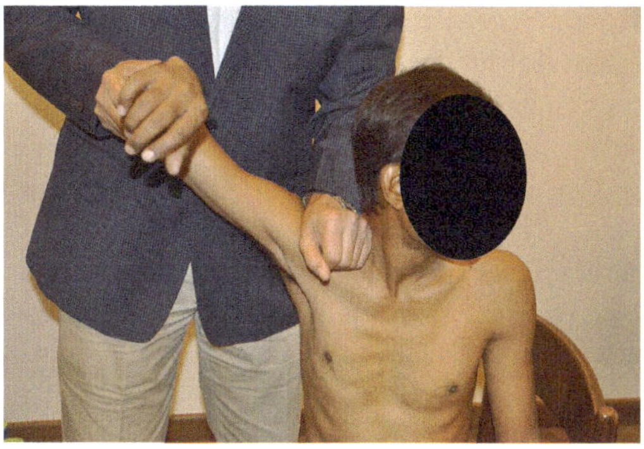

Fig. 6.10 Gagey test

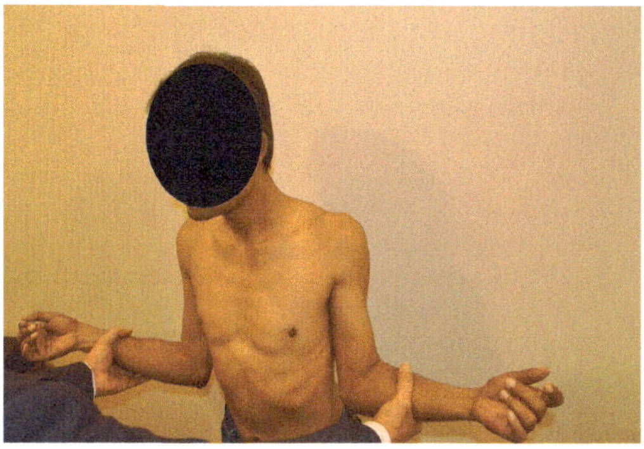

Fig. 6.11 Walch test

6.4.5 Walch Test

The patient is examined in a sitting position, arms adducted by the side of the body and elbows flexed 90° with examiner standing behind the patient [20]. The Walch test is considered positive when there is passive external rotation greater than 90° (Fig. 6.11). The test helps in identifying constitutional anterior hyperlaxity of the shoulder.

6.5 Conclusion

A thorough history and examination of both well exposed shoulders, is mandatory. Laxity assessment is critical and must not be confused with instability.

In my experience, both the drawers and load-shift test are difficult to execute accurately, with consistency, and therefore are not easy to interpret. The various laxity tests and the Beighton criteria can give a reasonable idea of the condition of the soft tissues. The apprehension test and relocation test can be specific for anterior glenohumeral instability. However, it is the comprehensive correlation of history, clinical findings, and imaging that helps in making the final accurate diagnosis.

References

1. Gerber C, Hersche O, Farron A. Isolated rupture of subscapularis tendon. J Bone Joint Surg Am. 1996;78(7):1015–23.
2. Rowe CR, Zarins B. Recurrent transient subluxation of the shoulder. J Bone Joint Surg Am. 1981;63(6):863–72.
3. Rowe CR, Zarins B, Ciullo JV. Recurrent anterior dislocation of the shoulder after surgical repair. Apparent causes of failure and treatment. J Bone Joint Surg Am. 1984;66(2):159–68.
4. Lo IK, Nonweiler B, Woolfrey M, Litchfield R, Kirkley A. An evaluation of the apprehension, relocation and surprise tests for anterior shoulder instability. Am J Sports Med. 2004;32(2):301–7.
5. Tzannes A, Paxinos A, Callanan M, Murrell GA. An assessment of the interexaminer reliability of test for shoulder instability. J Shoulder Elb Surg. 2004;13(1):18–23.
6. Jobe FW, Kvitne RS, Giangarra CE. Shoulder pain in the overhand or throwing athlete. The relationship of anterior instability and rotator cuff impingement. Orthop Rev. 1989;18(9):963–75.
7. Farber AJ, Castillo R, Clough M, Bahk M, McFarland EG. Clinical assessment of three common test for traumatic anterior shoulder instability. J Bone Joint Surg Am. 2006;88(7):1467–74.
8. Silliman JF, Hawkins RJ. Current concepts and recent advance in the athlete's shoulder. Clin Sports Med. 1991;10(4):693–705.
9. Matsen FA, Kirby RM. Office evaluation and management of shoulder pain. Orthop Clin N Am. 1982;13(3):453–75.
10. Jobe FW, Gingarra CE, Kvitne RS, Glousman RE. Anterior capsulolabral reconstruction of the shoulder in athletes in overhand sports. Am J Sports Med. 1991;19(5):428–34.
11. Speer KP, Hannafin JA, Altchek DW, Warren RF. An evaluation of shoulder relocation test. Am J Sports Med. 1994;22(2):177–83.
12. Silliman JF, Hawkins RJ. Classification and physical diagnosis of instability of the shoulder. Clin Orthop. 1993;291:7–19.
13. Kessel L. Clinical disorders of the shoulder, vol. 1. Edinburgh: Churchill Livingstone; 1982.
14. Matsen FA, Thomas SC, Rockwood CA, Wirth MA. Glenohumeral instability, in the shoulder. Philadelphia: Saunders; 1990. p. 611–755.
15. Beighton P, Horan F. Orthopaedic aspects of the Ehlers-Danlos syndrome. J Bone Joint Surg Br. 1969;51(3):444–53.
16. Gerber C, Ganz R. Clinical assessment of instability of the shoulder. With special reference to anterior and posterior drawer tests. J Bone Joint Surg Br. 1984;66(4):551–6.
17. Tzannes A, Murrell GA. Clinical examination of the unstable shoulder. Sports Med. 2002;32(7):447–57.
18. Neer CS, Foster CR. Inferior capsular shift for involuntary inferior and multidirectional instability of the shoulder. A preliminary report. J Bone Joint Surg Am. 1980;62(6):897–908.
19. Gagey OJ, Gagey N. The hyperabduction test. J Bone Joint Surg Br. 2001;83(1):69–74.
20. Walch G, Agostini J, Levigne C, Nove-Josserand L. Recurrent anterior and multidirectional instability of the shoulder. Rev Chir Orthop Reparatrice Appar Mot. 1995;81:682–90.

Scapulothoracic Dyskinesis and Anterior Shoulder Instability

7

Shahbaz S. Malik, Benjamin Jong, Lionel Neyton, and Peter B. MacDonald

7.1 Introduction

Shoulder motion is dependent on couple motion between scapula and humerus also known as scapulohumeral (SH) rhythm [1] whilst shoulder stability is dependent on static and dynamic restraints. Static restraints include glenoid labrum [2, 3], the articular surfaces [4], capsulo-ligamentous structures [5–9] and a negative intra-capsular pressure [10–12]. Dynamic restraints are the rotator cuff muscles that maintain the head of the humerus concentric on the glenoid [3, 13, 14]. In order for the shoulder to function efficiently, both the humerus and the scapula movement must be coordinated and coherent [15]. The scapula's anatomy is unique in that it forms part of both the acromioclavicular (AC) joint and the gleno-humeral (GH) joint and is linked to the axial skeleton via the clavicle. This makes the scapula mobile in many directions. Hence the motion, stability, performance and motor control of shoulder is linked with scapular performance [1]. There is an increasing interest in biomechanics of the scapula and its role in the pathology of shoulder which will be covered in this chapter.

S. S. Malik (✉) · B. Jong · P. B. MacDonald
Pan Am Clinic, University of Manitoba, Winnipeg, MB, Canada

L. Neyton
Centre Orthopédique Santy, Lyon, France

7.2 Scapular Dyskinesis

The term scapular dyskinesia or scapular winging is routinely used to describe the altered motion of scapula [15]. Winging refers to a visual description of the scapula without differentiating the abnormality being static or dynamic or indeed both [15]; dyskinesia, however, represents abnormal active movements mediated by neurologically controlled factors [1]. Given that the motion and position can be affected by a number of factors (Fig. 7.1), detachment of muscles or ACJ instability, the term *dyskinesis* is more inclusive and preferred [16] as it is neither an injury nor a musculoskeletal diagnosis [17]. Although the examination finding of dyskinesis may be a consequence of an injury, it is not always the case [18]. Dyskinesis can also be caused by muscle imbalance and proximal kinetic chain weakness [19]. According to the consensus statement of the second scapular summit, scapular dyskinesis is (1) medial border prominence as a result of either atypical inactive position of scapula and/or during active scapular kinesis (2) inferior angle prominence and/or premature elevation of scapula or shrugging on raising the arm and/or (3) accelerated inferior scapula rotation while lowering the arm [16, 20].

Scapular dyskinesis is a result of general reaction usually to pain arising from the shoulder and not a specific response to GH joint disorder. It is difficult to determine, however, if scapular dyskinesis is the

R. Brzóska et al. (eds.), *360° Around Shoulder Instability*,
https://doi.org/10.1007/978-3-662-61074-9_7

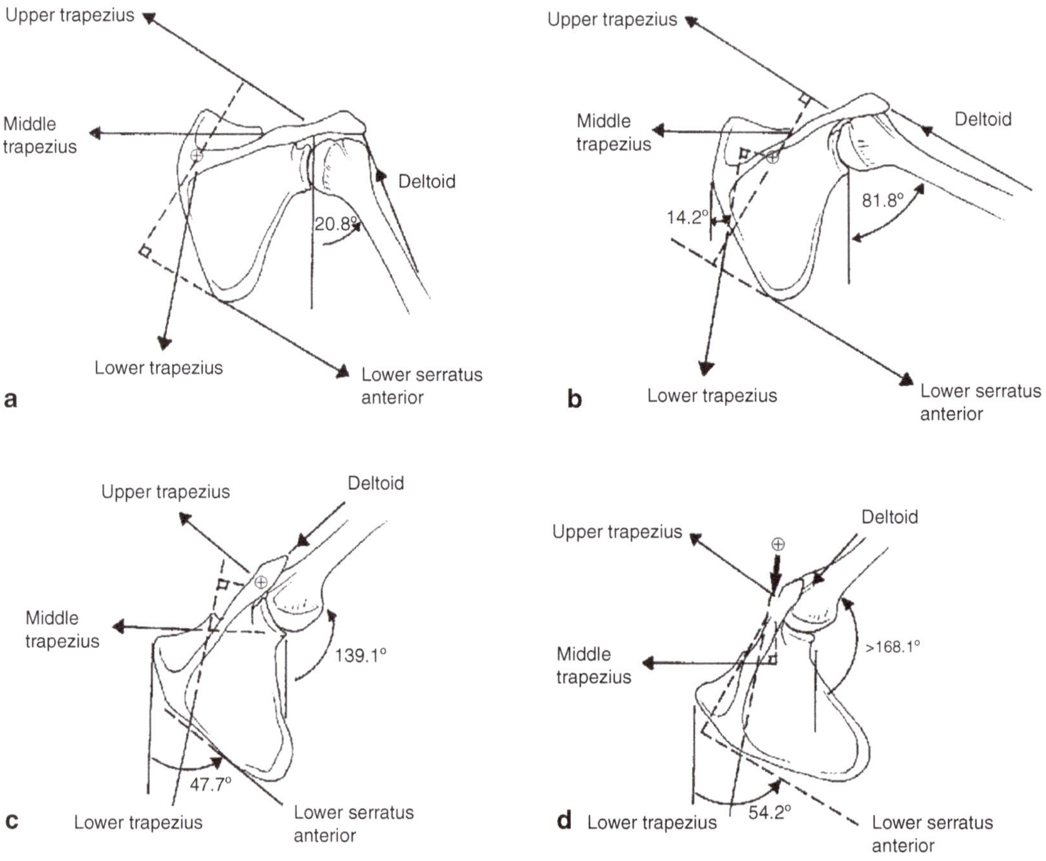

Fig. 7.1 A biomechanical model of scapular rotation. (**a** and **b**). In early phases of arm abduction, serratus anterior and upper & lower trapezius act as rotators and stabilisers with their long lever arms. (**c**) as the arm continues to abduct, the scapula rotates further with long serratus anterior and lower trapezius moment arms and short upper trapezius moment arm. (**d**) shows arm in maximum elevation. In this position, the lower trapezius continues to pull along its long axis while the scapular instant centre of rotation (shown as ⊕) migrates from the root of scapular spine towards the acromioclavicular joint. (Adapted with permission from Bagg SD, Forrest WJ [78])

cause of or a result of shoulder pain [21]. Dyskinesis has multiple causes and includes shoulder disorders such as shoulder impingement syndrome [22–26], rotator cuff pathology [27, 28], adhesive capsulitis [28, 29], labrum injuries [15, 18, 30] and shoulder instability [25, 28, 31]. It refers to causes as a result of bone pahtology such as clavicular fractures, non-union or mal-union with shortening angulation or rotation as well as excessive thoracic kyphosis [1, 18]. There can also be neurological causes such as cervical radiculopathy, spinal accessory nerve or long thoracic nerve palsies [1, 15, 18, 32].

Prevalence of shoulder dyskinesis is reported to be 61% in overhead athletes and 33% in non-overhead athletes [33]. Previous studies have shown that 33–100% of patients with various shoulder pathologies have scapular dyskinesis [34–37]. In order to restore the shoulder function in those with shoulder pathology, it is essential to evaluate scapulothoracic joint and more so for overhead athletes [38].

The typical mechanisms of dyskinesis have alterations of muscular activation or coordination, and soft tissue stiffness [1]. The scapular muscles, upper and lower trapezius and serratus anterior control the movement of scapula by coordinating as a force couple in task-specific movements [39]. The scapular stability has the most contribution from

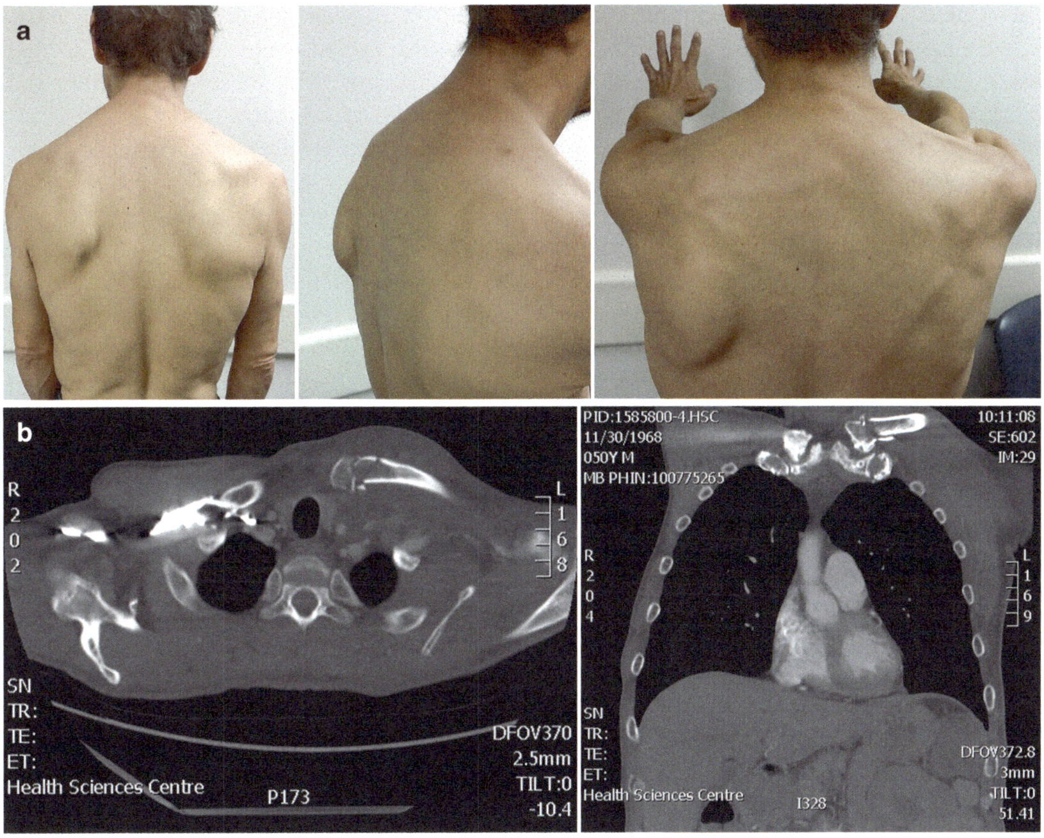

Fig. 7.2 (**a**) A 50-year-old patient with scapular dyskinesis following a left medial clavicle fracture. The left inferomedial border is prominent (SICK position) with arm at side (left), in 45° of forward elevation (middle) and at 90° of elevation (right). (**b**) CT scan of patient in (**a**) showing axial (left) and coronal (right) views which show a medial clavicle fracture causing scapular dyskinesis

these muscles [40, 41]; therefore, abnormal scapular kinematics can result from uncoordinated force coupling (Fig. 7.2). Patients with shoulder impingement have been found to have an overactive upper trapezius and underactive lower trapezius and serratus anterior [22, 23]. Scapular kinematics are also subject to change as a result of muscle or ligament tightness, such as decreased flexibility of either the pectoralis minor or the short head of biceps muscle. This creates excessive anterior tilt and protraction of scapula due to pull on the coracoid [42, 43].

There is further risk of excessive scapular anterior tilt and internal rotation by posterior capsule or shoulder muscles [44]. Whatever may be the cause of dyskinesis, the endpoint is scapula protraction irrespective of the arm position i.e., whether at rest or moving. As scapula protraction is the least favourable position for an ideal shoulder function, and it therefore exacerbates symptoms of impingement and rotator cuff compression by reducing the subacromial space and thus potentially decreasing the RC strength [41, 45]. Protraction can also lead to an increase in strain of the anterior gleno-humeral ligaments as occurs during the late cocking phase of throwing and can be critical for internal impingement [46].

7.3 Clinical Evaluation of Glenohumeral Instability

According to Kibler et al. [1] scapular dyskinesis should primarily be evaluated through visual observation, symptom alteration testing and examination of the surrounding structures. However, there are numerous physical examinations for the assessment of scapular dyskinesis described in the literature [47]. Nonetheless, scapula examination should be part of shoulder examination.

Observation: The assessment of scapula starts with a clinical examination of the shoulder from the posterior aspect. Both shoulders should be assessed for resting posture and symmetry. In some overhead athletes, the dominant shoulder can appear to be in a somewhat lower position in comparison to the contralateral side [48]. It can be helpful to mark superior and inferior medial borders of scapula. The evidence of the altered position of scapula at rest should be sought (Fig. 7.1) which is termed SICK position (Scapular malposition, Inferior medial border prominence, Coracoid pain and malposition and dysKinesis of scapular movement) [49]. This is illustrated by apparent inferior drooping and is due to anterior scapular tilting [50].

Palpation: This should include palpation of the upper and lower trapezius to assess for tender spots as well as pectoralis minor and latissimus dorsi. It is important to identify if there is muscle stiffness and inhibition or hyperactivity secondary to pain as it may need to be treated as part of the clinical issue [50]. The clavicle should be assessed for shortening, malrotation, or angulation and AC and SC joints evaluated for instability.

Mobilisation: Assessment of scapular dyskinesis includes visual observation [51–53] and as such focus should be on the scapula medial border motion as the arm raises and when it comes down [54]. Patients are required to carry out the test with 3–5 lb weights in each hand raising and lowering the arm in forward flexion from maximal elevation down to the starting position and repeat it 3–5 times [52, 53]. It is important for muscles to maintain the closed chain mechanism and therefore requires coordinated sequenced muscle activation [50]. There is increased scapular internal rotation if there is failure to maintain this, resulting in medial border prominence [51, 55]. When seen on the symptomatic side, this is noted as an 'yes' (prominence detected) or 'no' (prominence not detected). There is correlation between biomechanically demonstrated dyskinesis and the medial border projection in those patients that exhibit symptoms [56]. This scoring system has proven interobserver reliability and clinical utility [52, 56].

Special tests: To fully evaluate scapular dyskinesis during an assessment of injured shoulder, there are two commonly employed tests: the scapular assistance test (SAT) and scapular retraction test (SRT). The corrective movements using these two tests can modify the symptoms the patients elicit with the method of correction and therefore offer information on the role of scapular dyskinesis in overall shoulder dysfunction presented in patients with instability and how it can be resolved [57, 58]. While both these tests are useful for evaluation of rotator cuff strength in relation to scapula, SAT is more specific for scapular involvement in impingement and SRT for labral symptoms. To carry out SAT, examiner aids in upward rotation and posterior tilt by application of gentle force as the patient lifts the arm upwards (Fig. 7.3) [57, 58]. The positive result is concluded if the (1) impingement

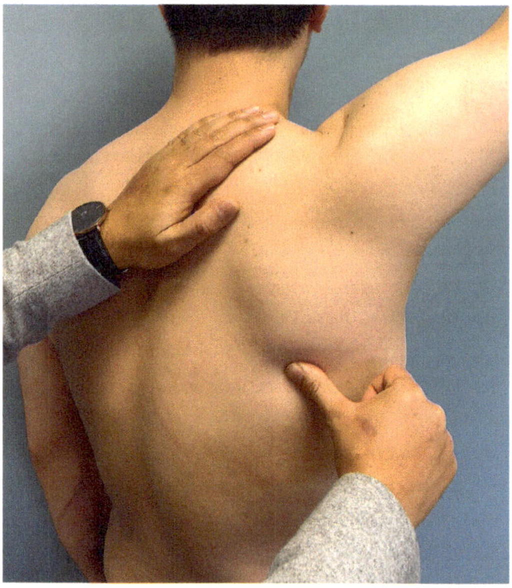

Fig. 7.3 Scapular assistance test (SAT): As the arm is elevated, the examiner assists serratus anterior and lower trapezius muscle activity by pushing the scapula in upward rotation. The positive result is concluded if the (1) impingement symptoms of painful arc are alleviated and (2) the range of movement is increased with assistance of the examiner

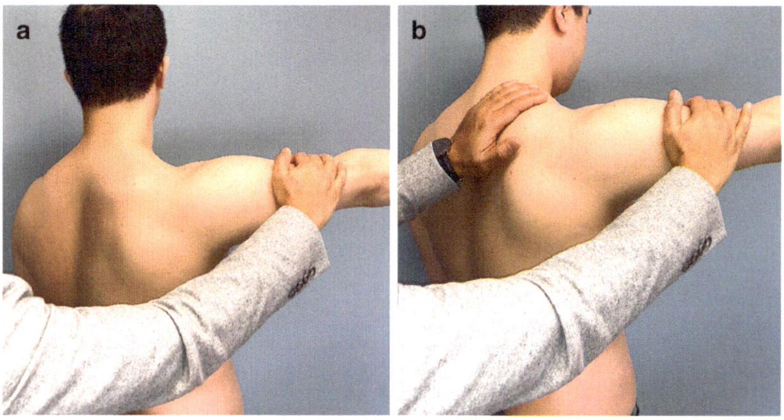

Fig. 7.4 Scapular retraction test (SRT). (**a**) An empty can test is performed first to assess the supraspinatus. (**b**) Stabilise the medial scapular border and reapply the muscle test. The result is positive if stabilisation of the scapular border results in a decrease in symptoms

symptoms of painful arc are alleviated and (2) the range of movement is increased. For SRT, the examiner needs to grade the strength of supraspinatus as per usual rotator cuff muscle tests. It is also valuable in assessment of labral injury in association with dynamic labral shear (DLS) [45, 59] and is performed by physically stabilising the scapula in a retracted position while the test is repeated to grade muscle strength or DLS (Fig. 7.4). The test is considered positive either upon lessening the internal impingement symptoms in the retracted position, usually caused by labral pathology or if the strength of supraspinatus grade is higher than before [50, 54]. It is important to establish here that a positive test can only establish scapular dyskinesis involvement in creating symptoms and not in diagnosis of an underlying shoulder injury. This should prompt the physician to enrol the patient for scapular rehabilitation at an early stage in order to improve scapular dyskinesis [50].

According to Kibler et al. [51] scapular dyskinesis can be divided into four categories depending on abnormal movement patterns of scapula in three planes: medial scapular border prominence, superior scapular border prominence, inferior scapular border prominence and the symmetric pattern (Table 7.1). This system is based on visual inspection [51] and is widely used in clinical setting [51, 60–62].

Although the scapula is the focus of assessment, it goes without saying again that examining for shoulder pathology should always be in the forefront. This is because a shoulder injury can cause or be aggravated by concomitant scapula dyskinesis [18].

Table 7.1 Shows detailed description of scapular dyskinesis

Pattern	Description
Type I	Abnormal sagittal plane movements with anterior and posterior tilt—inferior scapular border prominence
Type II	Abnormal transverse plane movements with internal and external rotations—medial scapular border prominence
Type III	Scapula elevation and abnormal coronal plane movement with upward and downward rotations—superior scapular border prominence
Type IV	Bilateral symmetrical scapula

7.3.1 Alternative Methods of Assessment

In addition to subjective assessment of scapula as above, there are objective measurements such as scapula displacement [63, 64] from the torso. This is a plain yet an objective method. In the lateral scapular slide test (LSST), the scapula lifts up and readings are taken of the scapular distance from the inferior angle of scapula to thoracic spinous process in the same horizontal line at 0°, 40° and 90° of shoulder abduction in the coronal plane (Fig. 7.5). The measurements are taken

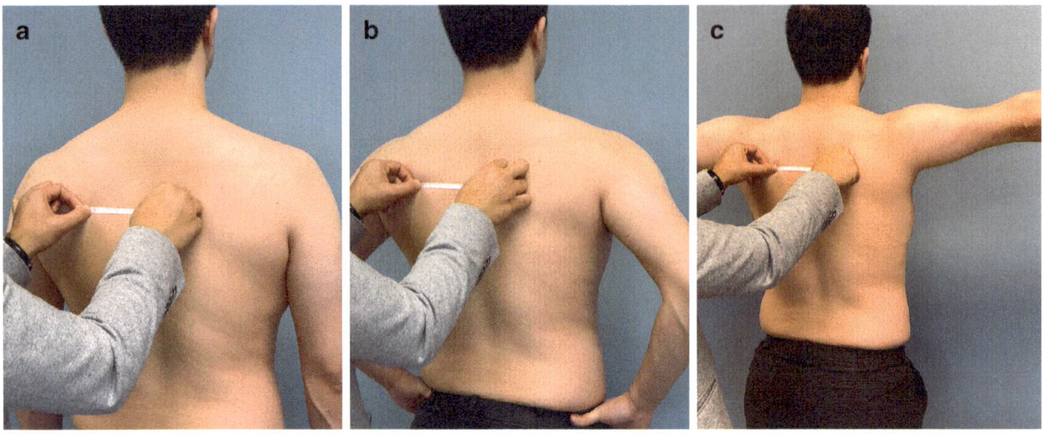

Fig. 7.5 Lateral scapular slide test (LSST). The scapula lifts up and readings are taken of the scapular distance from the inferior angle of scapula to the thoracic spinous process in the same horizontal line at 0° (**a**), 40° (**b**) and 90° (**c**) of shoulder abduction in the coronal plane. Measurements are taken bilaterally; a positive test is indicated by a bilateral difference of greater than 1.5 cm

bilaterally—a positive test is indicated by a bilateral difference of greater than 1.5 cm [63]. The downside of this technique is that it only provides static assessment of the scapula [60]. Another objective way to assess the scapula is with motion analysis systems [23, 53] or optoelectronic tracking systems which can quantify scapular kinematics in a complex three dimension [29, 65–68] and provide more quantitative data on scapular movements. Despite these alternatives offering an objective way to assess the scapula for dyskinesis, in practical terms they have limited use in the clinical setting.

7.4 Scapular Movements

7.4.1 At Rest Position

Scapular angles at *rest* are variable in different studies. The ST angle with the arm by side and relaxed ranges from −5.3° to +5.4° (negative values denote downward scapular rotation) [69–73]. Interestingly, rest angles varied significantly in population according to age demographics with older population recording a higher scapular angle compared to the younger cohort (mean age, 70 vs. 35 years; angle, +4.6° vs −9.4° respectively) [74]. As a result, glenoid is upward facing in the older population and downwardly facing in the younger population. A further analysis of healthy overhead athletes showed 3.46° scapular upward rotation in the dominant shoulder and 2° scapular upward rotation in non-dominant shoulder [75].

7.4.2 Elevation

During shoulder elevation in the sagittal plane, the scapula has little contribution to the total shoulder elevation, a period known as an initial setting phase [72, 76, 77]. Although there is no consensus on the duration of the setting phase, there are also no fixed values on the range. The range has been reported to be from 0 to 30°, 60° or 90° [72, 76, 77]. There is disagreement on how much the scapula rotates [71, 73, 78, 79] but a majority of academics agree that it rotates upwards in a linear manner while externally rotating and tilting posteriorly in a non-linear fashion [72, 73, 76, 77, 79].

The scapular movement pattern varies according to different anatomic planes. Thus in elevation, the scapula is more rotated upwardly at 60° in the frontal plane than the other two planes [72, 73] and also in the frontal plane at 90° and 120° of elevation, in comparison to sagittal and scapular plane elevation [73]. Although scapula internal rotation (IR) reduces throughout elevation in all three planes, it is more internally rotated in the sagittal plane than the frontal plane when compared to abduction and scapular plane [72, 73]. Similarly, scapula posteriorly tilts the most in the sagittal plane compared to the other two planes [77].

7.5 Anterior Glenohumeral Instability and Scapular Dyskinesis

As discussed above, scapular dyskinesis can be seen in a variety of shoulder pathologies with the increasing number of literature to support this [26, 28, 54, 80]. Anterior GH instability is one of the most frequent shoulder pathologies. This section will cover scapular dyskinesis in relation to instability.

Scapular dyskinesis and unstable GH joint are often associated with each other as alteration in the static and dynamic scapular movements present in the setting of GH instability [81]. Dyskinesis can be seen in micro-traumatic type of instability such as multidirectional instability as well as in traumatic recurrent instability [15]. It is reportedly present in up to 80% of instability patients [34, 35, 49]. When the shoulder is in apprehension position i.e., shoulder abduction, horizontal abduction and excessive external rotation, it is the inferior glenohumeral ligament (anterior band) that acts as the primary static restraint to anterior GH translation [82]. Scapular posturing leading to pathologic anterior tensile loads and shear forces according to biomechanical studies include excessive anterior tilting (type I) and internal rotation and protraction (type II) [51, 81]. This leads the GH angle beyond the 'safe zone' [50]. Excessive upper medial border prominence (type III) is clinically seen as a shrug manoeuvre due to activity of the upper trapezius [15]. The position created by the lack of acromial elevation results in impingement as the arm elevates establishing 'impingement/instability' connection [83].

When shoulders of asymptomatic subjects are compared to those with anterior shoulder instability, the scapula is rotated downwardly at *rest* position in asymptomatic patients [34]. During *elevation* of the shoulder in the scapular plane, there is a greater SH ratio from 0 to 90° of elevation in patients with anterior shoulder instability when compared to unimpaired control subjects [35, 84] and further still when SH ratio from 90° to maximum shoulder elevation was significantly lower in instability group compared to control group [35]. This suggests that ST movement increases from 90° to maximal shoulder elevation [80]. The effect of any altered scapular posturing is generation of excessive tensile loads and shear forces experienced by the anterior band of the inferior GH ligament [81]. It is also clear that scapular IR seems to be the most common and defining alteration during clinical examination of injured patients [56].

7.6 Management of Scapular Dyskinesis

7.6.1 Investigations

Initial investigation should be aimed to establish if there is any underlying cause of dyskinesis. Plain radiographs are simple, quick and feasible to obtain and are useful for assessment of bony morphology such as the clavicle, AC joint and GH joint. Plain film radiography has been suggested to have excellent reliability in evaluation of type I and II scapula dyskinesis [85]. Nerve conduction studies can be useful in trauma cases where there is concern of injury to nerves such as the spinal accessory nerve, long thoracic nerve or dorsal scapular nerve. Magnetic resonance imaging with or without arthrogram aids in diagnosis of labral pathology. Case reports have suggested that in some instances MRI can assist in diagnosing the aetiology of symptomatic scapular dyskinesis [86].

Three-dimensional MRI and wing computed tomography (CT) have been explored for evaluation of scapular dyskinesis [62, 87, 88]. As both CT and MRI are done in the decubitus position, it therefore alleviates the scapula of gravity and the resulting motion. What is unknown is whether decubitus or erect position has an effect on scapular kinematics [85].

7.6.2 Treatment

The mainstay of treatment for scapular dyskinesis is non-operative in the form of rehabilitation which can also be employed pre-operatively or post-operatively [89, 90]. The goal of treatment is to ease the symptoms attributed to muscular stiffness or trigger points in order to regain the muscle strength and activation patterns [57, 91]. The aim of pre-operative rehabilitation is to reestablish kinetic chain activation patterns in order to maximise scapular stabiliser activation and control the ability of scapula to retract. The sequence of scapular rehabilitation should be from proximal to distal with the goal to attain the position of ideal scapular function which is posterior tilt, external rotation and upward elevation [18].

In the post-operative period, core stability exercises can be initiated whilst the shoulder is immobilised. Core stability and strengthening can help improve the three-dimensional control of scapular movement, accomplished through kinetic chain exercises for hip and torso strengthening and scapular retraction. Both scapular protraction and retraction are assisted by hip and trunk flexion and extension exercises [18]. After establishing core stability, the attention should shift to muscles controlling scapular movements, lower trapezius (LT) and serratus anterior (SA). Closed chain axial load and 'clock' exercises can strengthen the scapular stabilisers whilst keeping the load to minimum on repair site. The SA muscle acts as a powerful external rotator of the scapula, whereas the LT acts as a stabiliser of the acquired scapular position [18, 50]. If rotator cuff strength exercises need to be administered, combined exercises of scapular stability and humeral head depression restore the compressor cuff activation function off a stablised scapular [50].

The outcome of non-operative treatment with scapular rehabilitation for GH joint instability depends on the underlying pathology as discussed previously. Those with instability from traumatic causes frequently present with ligament injury with or without bony injury preventing normal ball and socket joint kinematics. However, those with micro-trauma may be able to regain the function by restoring the coupled SH rhythm to maximise concavity/compression and ball and socket kinematics. Any rehabilitation with effective scapular control and resulting muscle activation in MDI patients frequently yields successful outcome as it is a very muscle-dependent problem [50].

7.7 Conclusion

Shoulder instability whether traumatic or multi-directional can be a cause of shoulder pain which is associated with scapular dyskinesis. When examining the shoulder joint for any pathology, scapula assessment should be an integral part of the evaluation. When there is an underlying anatomical injury, this must be remedied in order for scapular kinematics to be normal. Rehabilitation under physiotherapy supervision is still an optimum way to improve the functional outcome whether used as a non-operative, pre-operative or post-operative option.

References

1. Kibler WB, Ludewig PM, McClure PW, et al. Clinical implications of scapular dyskinesis in shoulder injury: the 2013 consensus statement from the 'scapular summit'. Br J Sports Med. 2013;47:877–85. https://doi.org/10.1136/bjsports-2013-092425.
2. Howell SM, Galinat BJ. The glenoid-labral socket. A constrained articular surface. Clin Orthop Relat Res. 1989;(243):122–5.
3. Lippitt SB, Vanderhooft JE, Harris SL, et al. Glenohumeral stability from concavity-compression: a quantitative analysis. J Shoulder Elb Surg. 1993;2:27–35. https://doi.org/10.1016/S1058-2746(09)80134-1.
4. Matsen FA, Fu FH, Hawkins RJ, Soslowsky L, Flatow E, Biglini L, et al. Stabilization of the glenohumeral joint by articular contact and by contact in the subacromial space. In: Matsen III F, Fu F, Hawkins R, editors. The shoulder: a balance of mobility and stability. Rosemont: American Academy of Orthopaedic Surgeons; 1993.
5. O'Connell PW, Nuber GW, Mileski RA, Lautenschlager E. The contribution of the glenohumeral ligaments to anterior stability of the shoulder joint. Am J Sports Med. 1990;18:579–84. https://doi.org/10.1177/036354659001800604.
6. Ovesen J, Nielsen S. Stability of the shoulder joint. Cadaver study of stabilizing structures.

Acta Orthop Scand. 1985;56:149–51. https://doi.org/10.3109/17453678508994342.
7. Terry GC, Hammon D, France P, Norwood LA. The stabilizing function of passive shoulder restraints. Am J Sports Med. 1991;19:26–34. https://doi.org/10.1177/036354659101900105.
8. Turkel SJ, Panio MW, Marshall JL, Girgis FG. Stabilizing mechanisms preventing anterior dislocation of the glenohumeral joint. J Bone Joint Surg Am. 1981;63:1208–17.
9. Jerosch J, Steinbeck J, Schröder M, Castro WHM. Arthroscopic resection of the acromioclavicular joint (ARAC). Knee Surg Sports Traumatol Arthrosc. 1993;1:209–15. https://doi.org/10.1007/BF01560209.
10. Kumar VP, Balasubramaniam P. The role of atmospheric pressure in stabilising the shoulder. An experimental study. J Bone Joint Surg Br. 1985;67:719–21.
11. Warner JJ, Deng X, Warren RF, et al. Superoinferior translation in the intact and vented glenohumeral joint. J Shoulder Elb Surg. 1993;2:99–105. https://doi.org/10.1016/1058-2746(93)90007-4.
12. Gibb TD, Sidles JA, Harryman DT, et al. The effect of capsular venting on glenohumeral laxity. Clin Orthop Relat Res. 1991;(268):120–7.
13. Blasier RB, Guldberg RE, Rothman ED. Anterior shoulder stability: contributions of rotator cuff forces and the capsular ligaments in a cadaver model. J Shoulder Elb Surg. 1992;1:140–50. https://doi.org/10.1016/1058-2746(92)90091-G.
14. Rockwood CA. Anterior glenohumeral instability. In: Rockwood Jr CA, Matsen III FA, editors. The shoulder. 4th ed. Philadelphia: Saunders/Elsevier; 2009.
15. Kibler WB, Sciascia A. Current concepts: scapular dyskinesis. Br J Sports Med. 2010;44:300–5. https://doi.org/10.1136/bjsm.2009.058834.
16. Kibler WB, Ludewig PM, McClure P, et al. Scapular Summit 2009: introduction. July 16, 2009, Lexington, Kentucky. J Orthop Sports Phys Ther. 2009;39:A1–A13. https://doi.org/10.2519/jospt.2009.0303.
17. Wright AA, Wassinger CA, Frank M, et al. Diagnostic accuracy of scapular physical examination tests for shoulder disorders: a systematic review. Br J Sports Med. 2013;47:886–92. https://doi.org/10.1136/bjsports-2012-091573.
18. Roche SJ, Funk L, Sciascia A, Kibler WB. Scapular dyskinesis: the surgeon's perspective. Shoulder Elbow. 2015;7:289–97. https://doi.org/10.1177/1758573215595949.
19. Kibler WB, Press J, Sciascia A. The role of core stability in athletic function. Sports Med. 2006;36:189–98. https://doi.org/10.2165/00007256-200636030-00001.
20. Second Scapula Summit. Unpublished consensus statement. Lexington, Kentucky; 2006.
21. Hickey D, Solvig V, Cavalheri V, et al. Scapular dyskinesis increases the risk of future shoulder pain by 43% in asymptomatic athletes: a systematic review and meta-analysis. Br J Sports Med. 2018;52:102–10. https://doi.org/10.1136/bjsports-2017-097559.
22. Cools AM, Witvrouw EE, Declercq GA, et al. Scapular muscle recruitment patterns: trapezius muscle latency with and without impingement symptoms. Am J Sports Med. 2003;31:542–9.
23. Ludewig PM, Cook TM. Alterations in shoulder kinematics and associated muscle activity in people with symptoms of shoulder impingement. Phys Ther. 2000;80:276–91.
24. McClure PW, Michener LA, Karduna AR. Shoulder function and 3-dimensional scapular kinematics in people with and without shoulder impingement syndrome. Phys Ther. 2006;86:1075–90.
25. Struyf F, Cagnie B, Cools A, et al. Scapulothoracic muscle activity and recruitment timing in patients with shoulder impingement symptoms and glenohumeral instability. J Electromyogr Kinesiol. 2014;24:277–84.
26. Timmons MK, Thigpen CA, Seitz AL, et al. Scapular kinematics and subacromial-impingement syndrome: a meta-analysis. J Sport Rehabil. 2012;21:354–70.
27. Mell AG, LaScalza S, Guffey P, et al. Effect of rotator cuff pathology on shoulder rhythm. J Shoulder Elb Surg. 2005;14:S58–64.
28. Ludewig PM, Reynolds JF. The association of scapular kinematics and glenohumeral joint pathologies. J Orthop Sports Phys Ther. 2009;39:90–104.
29. Fayad F, Roby-Brami A, Yazbeck C, et al. Three-dimensional scapular kinematics and scapulohumeral rhythm in patients with glenohumeral osteoarthritis or frozen shoulder. J Biomech. 2008;41:326–32.
30. Myers JB, Laudner KG, Pasquale MR, et al. Glenohumeral range of motion deficits and posterior shoulder tightness in throwers with pathologic internal impingement. Am J Sports Med. 2006;34:385–91.
31. Ogston JB, Ludewig PM. Differences in 3-dimensional shoulder kinematics between persons with multidirectional instability and asymptomatic controls. Am J Sports Med. 2007;35:1361–70.
32. Jayasinghe GS. Scapula dyskinesis: a review of current concepts and evaluation of assessment tools. Curr Sports Med Rep. 2018;17:338–46. https://doi.org/10.1249/JSR.0000000000000526.
33. Burn MB, McCulloch PC, Lintner DM, et al. Prevalence of scapular dyskinesis in overhead and nonoverhead athletes: a systematic review. Orthop J Sports Med. 2016;4:2325967115627608.
34. Warner JJ, Micheli LJ, Arslanian LE, et al. Scapulothoracic motion in normal shoulders and shoulders with glenohumeral instability and impingement syndrome. A study using Moiré topographic analysis. Clin Orthop Relat Res. 1992;(285):191–9.
35. Paletta GA, Warner JJ, Warren RF, et al. Shoulder kinematics with two-plane x-ray evaluation in patients with anterior instability or rotator cuff tearing. J Shoulder Elb Surg. 1997;6:516–27.
36. Kawasaki T, Yamakawa J, Kaketa T, et al. Does scapular dyskinesis affect top rugby players during a game season? J Shoulder Elb Surg. 2012;21:709–14. https://doi.org/10.1016/j.jse.2011.11.032.
37. Myers JB, Oyama S, Hibberd EE. Scapular dysfunction in high school baseball players sustaining

throwing-related upper extremity injury: a prospective study. J Shoulder Elb Surg. 2013;22:1154–9. https://doi.org/10.1016/j.jse.2012.12.029.
38. Huang T-S, Huang C, Ou H-L, Lin J-J. Scapular dyskinesis: patterns, functional disability and associated factors in people with shoulder disorders. Man Ther. 2016;26:165–71. https://doi.org/10.1016/j.math.2016.09.002.
39. Magarey ME, Jones MA. Dynamic evaluation and early management of altered motor control around the shoulder complex. Man Ther. 2003;8:195–206. https://doi.org/10.1016/S1356-689X(03)00094-8.
40. Kibler WB, Chandler TJ, Shapiro R, Conuel M. Muscle activation in coupled scapulohumeral motions in the high performance tennis serve. Br J Sports Med. 2007;41:745–9. https://doi.org/10.1136/bjsm.2007.037333.
41. Smith J, Dietrich CT, Kotajarvi BR, Kaufman KR. The effect of scapular protraction on isometric shoulder rotation strength in normal subjects. J Shoulder Elb Surg. 2006;15:339–43. https://doi.org/10.1016/j.jse.2005.08.023.
42. Borstad JD, Ludewig PM. The effect of long versus short pectoralis minor resting length on scapular kinematics in healthy individuals. J Orthop Sports Phys Ther. 2005;35:227–38. https://doi.org/10.2519/jospt.2005.35.4.227.
43. Ellenbecker TS, Cools A. Rehabilitation of shoulder impingement syndrome and rotator cuff injuries: an evidence-based review. Br J Sports Med. 2010;44:319–27. https://doi.org/10.1136/bjsm.2009.058875.
44. Laudner KG, Moline MT, Meister K. The relationship between forward scapular posture and posterior shoulder tightness among baseball players. Am J Sports Med. 2010;38:2106–12. https://doi.org/10.1177/0363546510370291.
45. Kibler WB, Sciascia A, Dome D. Evaluation of apparent and absolute supraspinatus strength in patients with shoulder injury using the scapular retraction test. Am J Sports Med. 2006;34:1643–7. https://doi.org/10.1177/0363546506288728.
46. Mihata T, McGarry MH, Kinoshita M, Lee TQ. Excessive glenohumeral horizontal abduction as occurs during the late cocking phase of the throwing motion can be critical for internal impingement. Am J Sports Med. 2010;38:369–74. https://doi.org/10.1177/0363546509346408.
47. Lange T, Struyf F, Schmitt J, et al. The reliability of physical examination tests for the clinical assessment of scapular dyskinesis in subjects with shoulder complaints: a systematic review. Phys Ther Sport. 2017;26:64–89. https://doi.org/10.1016/j.ptsp.2016.10.006.
48. Warth RJ, Millett PJ. Physical examination of the shoulder: an evidence-based approach. New York: Springer; 2015.
49. Burkhart SS, Morgan CD, Kibler WB. The disabled throwing shoulder: spectrum of pathology Part III: the SICK scapula, scapular dyskinesis, the kinetic chain, and rehabilitation. Arthroscopy. 2003;19:641–61. https://doi.org/10.1016/s0749-8063(03)00389-x.
50. Kibler WB, Sciascia AD. Disorders of the scapula and their role in shoulder injury: a clinical guide to evaluation and management. Cham: Springer; 2017.
51. Kibler WB, Uhl TL, Maddux JWQ, et al. Qualitative clinical evaluation of scapular dysfunction: a reliability study. J Shoulder Elb Surg. 2002;11:550–6. https://doi.org/10.1067/mse.2002.126766.
52. McClure P, Tate AR, Kareha S, et al. A clinical method for identifying scapular dyskinesis, part 1: reliability. J Athl Train. 2009;44:160–4. https://doi.org/10.4085/1062-6050-44.2.160.
53. Tate AR, McClure P, Kareha S, et al. A clinical method for identifying scapular dyskinesis, part 2: validity. J Athl Train. 2009;44:165–73. https://doi.org/10.4085/1062-6050-44.2.165.
54. Kibler WB, Sciascia A, Wilkes T. Scapular dyskinesis and its relation to shoulder injury. J Am Acad Orthop Surg. 2012;20:364–72. https://doi.org/10.5435/JAAOS-20-06-364.
55. Ludewig PM, Cook TM, Nawoczenski DA. Three-dimensional scapular orientation and muscle activity at selected positions of humeral elevation. J Orthop Sports Phys Ther. 1996;24:57–65. https://doi.org/10.2519/jospt.1996.24.2.57.
56. Uhl TL, Kibler WB, Gecewich B, Tripp BL. Evaluation of clinical assessment methods for scapular dyskinesis. Arthroscopy. 2009;25:1240–8. https://doi.org/10.1016/j.arthro.2009.06.007.
57. Kibler WB. The role of the scapula in athletic shoulder function. Am J Sports Med. 1998;26:325–37. https://doi.org/10.1177/03635465980260022801.
58. Rabin A, Irrgang JJ, Fitzgerald GK, Eubanks A. The intertester reliability of the Scapular Assistance Test. J Orthop Sports Phys Ther. 2006;36:653–60. https://doi.org/10.2519/jospt.2006.2234.
59. Ben Kibler W, Sciascia AD, Hester P, et al. Clinical utility of traditional and new tests in the diagnosis of biceps tendon injuries and superior labrum anterior and posterior lesions in the shoulder. Am J Sports Med. 2009;37:1840–7. https://doi.org/10.1177/0363546509332505.
60. Huang T-S, Huang H-Y, Wang T-G, et al. Comprehensive classification test of scapular dyskinesis: a reliability study. Man Ther. 2015;20:427–32. https://doi.org/10.1016/j.math.2014.10.017.
61. Huang T-S, Ou H-L, Huang C-Y, Lin J-J. Specific kinematics and associated muscle activation in individuals with scapular dyskinesis. J Shoulder Elb Surg. 2015;24:1227–34. https://doi.org/10.1016/j.jse.2014.12.022.
62. Park J-Y, Hwang J-T, Kim K-M, et al. How to assess scapular dyskinesis precisely: 3-dimensional wing computer tomography—a new diagnostic modality. J Shoulder Elb Surg. 2013;22:1084–91. https://doi.org/10.1016/j.jse.2012.10.046.
63. Odom CJ, Taylor AB, Hurd CE, Denegar CR. Measurement of scapular asymmetry and assessment of shoulder dysfunction using the lateral scapular slide test: a reliability and validity study. Phys

Ther. 2001;81:799–809. https://doi.org/10.1093/ptj/81.2.799.
64. Hong J, Barnes MJ, Leddon CE, et al. Reliability of the sitting hand press-up test for identifying and quantifying the level of scapular medial border posterior displacement in overhead athletes. Int J Sports Phys Ther. 2011;6:306–11.
65. Chu Y, Akins J, Lovalekar M, et al. Validation of a video-based motion analysis technique in 3-D dynamic scapular kinematic measurements. J Biomech. 2012;45:2462–6. https://doi.org/10.1016/j.jbiomech.2012.06.025.
66. Forthomme B, Crielaard J-M, Croisier J-L. Scapular positioning in Athlete's shoulder: particularities, clinical measurements and implications. Sports Med. 2008;38:369–86. https://doi.org/10.2165/00007256-200838050-00002.
67. Shakeri H, Keshavarz R, Arab AM, et al. Scapular position and orientation during abduction, flexion and scapular plane elevation phase. Iran Rehabil J. 2014;12:22–30.
68. van den Noort JC, Wiertsema SH, Hekman KMC, et al. Reliability and precision of 3D wireless measurement of scapular kinematics. Med Biol Eng Comput. 2014;52:921–31. https://doi.org/10.1007/s11517-014-1186-2.
69. Freedman L, Munro RR. Abduction of the arm in the scapular plane: scapular and glenohumeral movements. A roentgenographic study. J Bone Joint Surg Am. 1966;48:1503–10.
70. Poppen NK, Walker PS. Normal and abnormal motion of the shoulder. J Bone Joint Surg Am. 1976;58:195–201.
71. Mandalidis DG, Mc Glone BS, Quigley RF, et al. Digital fluoroscopic assessment of the scapulohumeral rhythm. Surg Radiol Anat. 1999;21:241–6.
72. Fung M, Kato S, Barrance PJ, et al. Scapular and clavicular kinematics during humeral elevation: a study with cadavers. J Shoulder Elb Surg. 2001;10:278–85. https://doi.org/10.1067/mse.2001.114496.
73. Ludewig PM, Phadke V, Braman JP, et al. Motion of the shoulder complex during multiplanar humeral elevation. J Bone Joint Surg Am. 2009;91:378–89. https://doi.org/10.2106/JBJS.G.01483.
74. Talkhani IS, Kelly CP. Scapulothoracic rhythm in normal male volunteers. Biomed Sci Instrum. 1997;34:327–31.
75. Oyama S, Myers JB, Wassinger CA, et al. Asymmetric resting scapular posture in healthy overhead athletes. J Athl Train. 2008;43:565–70. https://doi.org/10.4085/1062-6050-43.6.565.
76. Inman VT, Saunders JB, Abbott LC. Observations of the function of the shoulder joint. 1944. Clin Orthop Relat Res. 1996;(330):3–12. https://doi.org/10.1097/00003086-199609000-00002.
77. McClure PW, Michener LA, Sennett BJ, Karduna AR. Direct 3-dimensional measurement of scapular kinematics during dynamic movements in vivo. J Shoulder Elb Surg. 2001;10:269–77. https://doi.org/10.1067/mse.2001.112954.
78. Bagg SD, Forrest WJ. A biomechanical analysis of scapular rotation during arm abduction in the scapular plane. Am J Phys Med Rehabil. 1988;67:238–45.
79. van der Helm FC, Pronk GM. Three-dimensional recording and description of motions of the shoulder mechanism. J Biomech Eng. 1995;117:27–40. https://doi.org/10.1115/1.2792267.
80. Struyf F, Nijs J, Baeyens J-P, et al. Scapular positioning and movement in unimpaired shoulders, shoulder impingement syndrome, and glenohumeral instability. Scand J Med Sci Sports. 2011;21:352–8. https://doi.org/10.1111/j.1600-0838.2010.01274.x.
81. Varacallo M, Mair SD. Anterior shoulder instability. In: StatPearls. Treasure Island: StatPearls Publishing; 2019.
82. Weiser WM, Lee TQ, McMaster WC, McMahon PJ. Effects of simulated scapular protraction on anterior glenohumeral stability. Am J Sports Med. 1999;27:801–5. https://doi.org/10.1177/03635465990270061901.
83. Jobe FW, Kvitne RS, Giangarra CE. Shoulder pain in the overhand or throwing athlete. The relationship of anterior instability and rotator cuff impingement. Orthop Rev. 1989;18:963–75.
84. von Eisenhart-Rothe R, Matsen FA, Eckstein F, et al. Pathomechanics in atraumatic shoulder instability: scapular positioning correlates with humeral head centering. Clin Orthop Relat Res. 2005;(433):82–9. https://doi.org/10.1097/01.blo.0000150338.27113.14.
85. Chen K, Deng S, Ma Y, et al. A preliminary exploration of plain-film radiography in scapular dyskinesis evaluation. J Shoulder Elb Surg. 2018;27:e210–8. https://doi.org/10.1016/j.jse.2017.12.032.
86. Morita W, Nozaki T, Tasaki A. MRI for the diagnosis of scapular dyskinesis: a report of two cases. Skelet Radiol. 2017;46:249–52. https://doi.org/10.1007/s00256-016-2528-y.
87. Sahara W, Sugamoto K, Murai M, Yoshikawa H. Three dimensional clavicular and acromioclavic ular rotations during arm abduction using vertically open MRI. J Orthop Res. 2007;25:1243–9. https://doi.org/10.1002/jor.20407.
88. Park J-Y, Hwang J-T, Oh K-S, et al. Revisit to scapular dyskinesis: three-dimensional wing computed tomography in prone position. J Shoulder Elb Surg. 2014;23:821–8. https://doi.org/10.1016/j.jse.2013.08.016.
89. Sciascia A, Cromwell R. Kinetic chain rehabilitation: a theoretical framework. Rehabil Res Pract. 2012;2012:1–9. https://doi.org/10.1155/2012/853037.
90. McMullen J, Uhl TL. A kinetic chain approach for shoulder rehabilitation. J Athl Train. 2000;35:329–37.
91. Kibler WB, McMullen J. Scapular dyskinesis and its relation to shoulder pain. J Am Acad Orthop Surg. 2003;11:142–51.

First Anterior Dislocation: Conservative Treatment

8

Robert Pełka and Wojciech Marek

8.1 Epidemiology

Anterior shoulder dislocation occurs relatively often. The prevalence of dislocation episodes is 11–56 per 100,000 persons per year; for the first episode of a shoulder dislocation, the prevalence is 8–26 per 100,000 persons per year. Therefore, this pathology is considered to be a serious problem [1–8].

Relying on the data recorded by emergency departments in the United States, we can confirm that the highest rate of dislocation incidents occurs between 10 and 30 years of age. Males have a much higher rate of dislocation episodes than females. Occurrences in adolescents are the most common [7].

Evaluating the age at first dislocation, we can state that the primary episode usually happens to children and young persons [9] (Fig. 8.1).

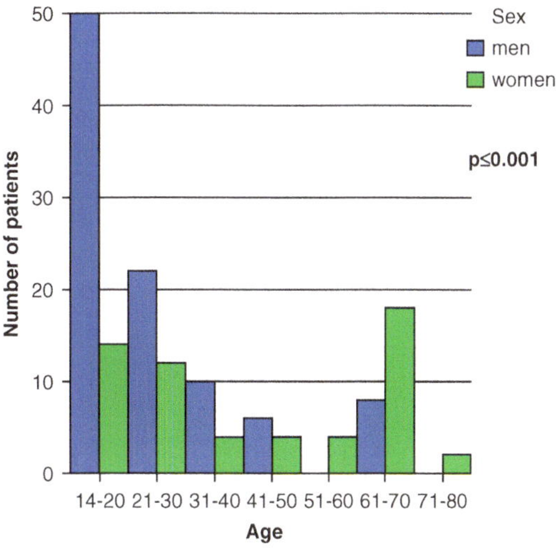

Fig. 8.1 Relationship of sex to age in years at first dislocation

8.2 Structural Lesions in the Shoulder

Although we can provide conservative treatment after the first shoulder dislocation, this first dislocation always causes intraarticular pathology, most often Hill–Sachs (Fig. 8.2) and Bankart lesions (Fig. 8.3). Conservative treatment helps to reduce pain after the injury, and rehabilitation supports recovery and faster return to sport activities [10].

8.3 Recurrence of Shoulder Instability and Its Factors

The most common problem after every kind of treatment, whether we choose conservative or surgical, is recurrence of the instability.

In predictors of recurrent instability, we can include age less than 25 years, contact or collision sports (handball, MMA, football, etc.), the

R. Pełka (✉) · W. Marek
NZOZ Ortopedia Opole/Głuchołazy, Opole, Poland

R. Brzóska et al. (eds.), *360° Around Shoulder Instability*,
https://doi.org/10.1007/978-3-662-61074-9_8

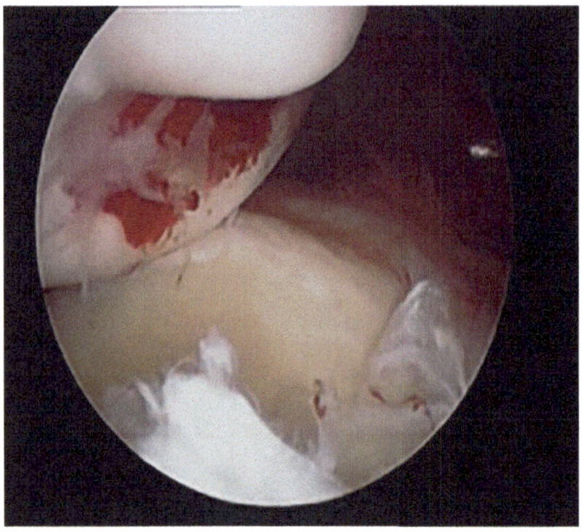

Fig. 8.2 Hill- Sachs Lesion

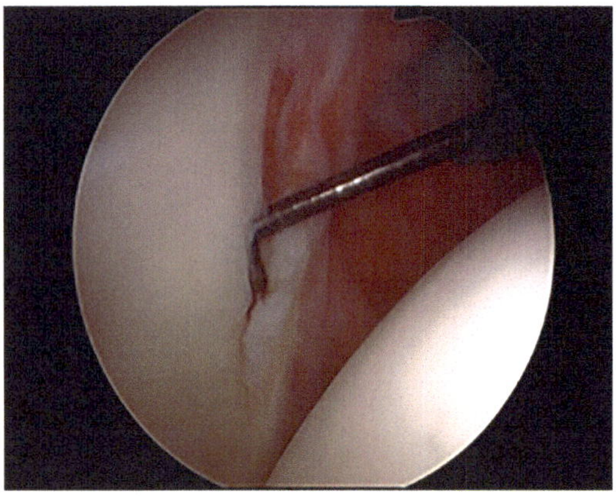

Fig. 8.3 Bankart lesion

character of the patient's occupation, such as using the arms above chest level, and the poorer quality of life among patients with instability. For estimating quality of life, we can use scales such as ASES, CMS, and WOSI [11].

The recurrence of instability essentially increases structural and functional abnormalities, including progressive labro-ligamentous injury and degeneration, loss of the anterior hinge, which is correlated to damage to the labrum and inferior glenohumeral ligament (IGHL), irreversible ligament and capsule elongation with plastic deformation and degeneration of anterior passive stabilizers. Habermeyer stated a third type of dislocation—the point of no return! [12] (Table 8.1). All these reasons make the

Table 8.1 Percentage of joint lesions in first and recurrent dislocations

	Single dislocation	Recurrent dislocations
Glenoid bone loss	41%	86% (10.8% bone loss)
Arthropathy	18%	40%

decision to operate or to apply conservative treatment very difficult, because a poor decision may lead to all the injuries just mentioned.

As far as is known, a recurrent instability demands surgical treatment, a rather doubt-free solution. In primary dislocations, however, we still have no established recommendations about the best actions [13, 14].

Conservative treatment and the decision to apply such treatments should be made according to the age of the patient at the first dislocation and with consideration of comorbidities such as hyperlaxity or quality of life. When valuating recurrence rate in relation to age, we can confirm that the highest prevalence of occurrence is also among young persons under 20 years of age and essentially decreases in adult groups: it is an age-related factor.

8.4 Treatment Recommendations Correlated with Age of Patient

Many orthopedic surgeons apply conservative treatment after the first anterior dislocation. The decision-making cycle is mostly correlated to the history of the first dislocation (traumatic, atraumatic) and what is shown by diagnostic imaging, with magnetic resonance imaging (MRI) as the gold standard, X-ray as the bone lesion predictor, and computed tomography (CT) scan for bone abnormalities and other comorbidities such as hyperlaxity (MDI, MDL). In the X-ray examination we should use AP and Y projections. We can provide for additional projections: West Point or Bernageau.

As conservative treatment in a first shoulder dislocation, closed reposition is used as the first intervention. In the nonoperative approach to a first dislocation, one can use shoulder immobilization in external or internal rotation for some period of time. In 2003 and 2007, the Ito team published articles describing, on the basis of MRI examination, the lower recurrence rate of secondary dislocation among patients immobilized in external rotation, especially in a younger subgroup [15, 16]. Analyzing pros and cons, some authors recently concluded that ER immobilization did not reduce the risk of recurring dislocations. In 2011, Whelan proved that there is no evidence showing that immobilization in external rotation is significantly better than in internal rotation [17]. Nowadays a majority of orthopedic surgeons recommend using only a standard arm sling, which might be more comfortable for the patient [15–18].

No consensus was ever established as to how long immobilization should be applied, but from 2 to 6 weeks is most often recommended: for young patients, 1 to 4 weeks, and for older, 1 to 2 weeks (Patterson). Immobilization for 1 week or less can cause a recurrence rate as high as 41%; whereas when 3 weeks of immobilization was applied, recurrence was about 37%. As the difference was not relevant, there is no recommendation to extend the period of immobilization [15–18].

Return to a competitive sports activity after the first anterior dislocation was as high as 73%. Return occurred for the rest of season, or part of it, or the whole season, most often after 5 days. There is no consensus about return to amateur sport activity [19]. The period of time for rehabilitation should be strictly connected with the return of range of motion (ROM) and proper dynamic stabilization of the scapula, but there is no strict time frame.

Physical exercise under the supervision of a physiotherapist such as strengthening shoulder muscles and dynamic stabilization decreases the risk of recurrence after primary shoulder dislocation by 25% [20]. We have shown that our rehabilitative approach seems to be effective in the conservative management of shoulder instability among adults with the first episode of traumatic anterior shoulder dislocation who are not involved in sports activity, and who are not overhead workers. Other nonoperative approaches to treatment of anterior dislocation may be changing work/sports activities and changing life habits (Table 8.2).

Table 8.2 Recurrence rate correlated with age [21, 22]

Age	Recurrence rate (%)
Overall	14–100
Less than 20 years	72–95
From 20 to 30 years	70–82
More than 30 years	25–30
More than 50 years	14–22

8.4.1 Adolescents

In adolescents under 14 years of age, there is no difference in recurrence after conservative treatment with immobilization or without; rather, immobilization works as a pain relief method. It is also very important to carefully examine young patients by paying attention to hyperlaxity and other comorbidities that can lead to other dislocations.

Children aged 14–18 years were 2.4 times more likely to experience recurrent instability than children aged 13 years and less (93% versus 40%). Children with a closed physis are 14 times more likely to experience recurrent instability compared to those with an open physis [23–25].

Thus, in an adolescent population (15–18 years of age), conservative treatment after the first traumatic shoulder dislocation, including immobilization in internal rotation, leads to a significantly higher and unacceptably high failure rate compared with early arthroscopic stabilization.

8.4.2 Adults 18–25 Years of Age

We can summarize some publications concerning young adults with the following statements.

Recurrent instability and deficits of shoulder function are common after primary nonoperative treatment of an anterior shoulder dislocation. There is substantial variation in the risk of instability, with younger males having the highest risk whereas females have a much lower risk.

Arthroscopic anatomic stabilization of traumatic, first-time anterior shoulder dislocations can be an effective and safe treatment that significantly reduces the recurrence rate of shoulder dislocations among young athletes when compared with conventional, nonoperative treatment.

There is evidence to suggest treatment of young patients with a first-time shoulder dislocation with anatomic Bankart repair, with the goal of lowering the rate of recurrent instability over the long term and improving short-term quality of life.

There are no studies showing that conservative treatment should be applied in this age group. Methods of conservative treatment should be used as pain relief and rehabilitation preceding surgery [26–28].

8.4.3 Adults 25–35 or 40 Years of Age

It is recommended that immediate arthroscopic stabilization be the treatment of choice in a subset of patients who are younger than 30 years and are higher-level athletes, for whom the timing for surgery is good or their sport is risky, such as rugby, football, kayaking, and rock climbing.

Longo and coworkers, in a giant systematic review including 2813 patients, defined mean redislocation rate as 32.2% (much higher post conservative treatment and internal rotation immobilization), 9.6% after arthroscopic treatment, 27.8% after lavage, and 37.5% after conservative treatment. Their studies have shown that immobilization in external rotation may lead to a 25.5% recurrence rate and in internal rotation to as much as 50.2% [29]. However, this is in contradiction to studies by Liavaag et al. and by Whelan et al. [17, 19].

Thus, although limited, the available evidence from randomized controlled trials (RCTS) supports primary surgery among young adults engaged in highly demanding sports or job activities. There is a lack of evidence to determine whether surgical or nonsurgical treatment is better for other categories of injury [30].

8.4.4 Adults More Than 40 Years of Age

Problems correlated with age greater than 40 years are other common injuries: rotator cuff, subscapularis (SSCAP) tear, fracture of the greater tuberosity and other fractures, and glenoid arthritis. Patients older than 40 years presenting with a first-time anterior shoulder dislocation with an associated fracture of the greater tuberosity have a significant rate of iatrogenic humeral neck fracture during closed reduction under sedation. For this group some should reconsider open reduction and assessment of other injuries at the same time [29, 31–33].

8.5 Conclusion

Although it has been proven that recurrence after first anterior dislocation has a high prevalence, conservative treatment should be our first step. Repositioning should be performed as quickly as possible, and with care, especially in older patients. Immobilization should provide pain relief at the first occurrence, but it should be not considered as a treatment in recurrences. An intensive rehabilitation protocol is an excellent instrument for recovery and has great impact on decreasing the recurrence rate [20, 34].

Careful examination and diagnostic imaging should be performed to decide whether to choose surgical treatment because most dislocations cause structural damages in the shoulder joint. After recurrent dislocations, surgical treatment should be considered as the first step. We should not use conservative treatment in dislocated shoulders where closed reduction is not possible, where intraarticular injuries are significant, and when hyperlaxity or bone defects are seen after dislocation.

Acute glenoid rim defect caused by first-time dislocation was evaluated by Spiegl et al.: his algorithm includes conservative strategy for small defects, that is, less than 5%, and operative methods for larger defects of the rim [35]. Applying this treatment algorithm for acute osseous Bankart

Table 8.3 Treatment suggestions after first anterior dislocation by age group

5–25 years of age Early surgical repair	Recurrence rate reduction from 80–90% to 3–15% Improved overall quality of life
25–35 years of age: Initial attempt at nonoperative management	Risk of repeated dislocation is lower (20–30%) Examples: high level of sports; demanding job activity
Over 40 years of age: Nonoperative treatment	Low recurrence rate 10–15%; Address associated injuries such as RC tears, neurological injury

lesions, consisting of a conservative strategy for small defect sizes and a surgical approach for medium-sized and large defects, leads to encouraging mid-term results and a low rate of recurrent instability in active patients. However, we still need more convincing studies, and the following suggestions should be considered (Table 8.3).

In the combined first and second group of patients (children, youths, young adults), because of the high risk of recurrence after conservative treatment, surgical procedures should be suggested.

For adults between 25 and 40 years of age, an initial attempt of nonoperative treatment is suggested, with the exception of people engaged in highly demanding sports or job activities.

For adults more than 40 years of age, the suggestion is nonoperative treatment, keeping any associated injuries in mind!

References

1. Liavaag S, Svenningsen S, Reikerås O, Enger M, Fjalestad T, Pripp AH, Brox JI. The epidemiology of shoulder dislocations in Oslo. Scand J Med Sci Sports. 2011;21(6):e334–40.
2. Kroner K, Lind T, Jensen J. The epidemiology of shoulder dislocations. Arch Orthop Trauma Surg. 1989;108(5):288–90.
3. Nordqvist A, Petersson CJ. Incidence and causes of shoulder girdle injuries in an urban population. J Shoulder Elb Surg. 1995;4(2):107–12.
4. Simonet WT, Melton LJ III, Cofield RH, Ilstrup DM. Incidence of anterior shoulder dislocation in Olmsted County, Minnesota. Clin Orthop Relat Res. 1984;186:186–91.
5. Owens BD, Agel J, Mountcastle SB, Cameron KL, Nelson BJ. Incidence of glenohumeral instability in collegiate athletics. Am J Sports Med. 2009;37(9):1750–4.
6. Owens BD, Dawson L, Burks R, Cameron KL. Incidence of shoulder dislocation in the United States military: demographic considerations from a high-risk population. J Bone Joint Surg Am. 2009;91(4):791–6.
7. Zacchilli MA, Owens BD. Epidemiology of shoulder dislocations presenting to emergency departments in the United States. J Bone Joint Surg Am. 2010;92(3):542–9.
8. Hovelius L. Incidence of shoulder dislocation in Sweden. Clin Orthop Relat Res. 1982;166:127–31.
9. Chalidis B, et al. Has the management of shoulder dislocation changed over time? Int Orthop (SICOT). 2007;31:385–9.
10. Baker CL. Intraarticular pathology in acute, first-time anterior shoulder dislocation: an arthroscopic study. Arthroscopy. 1994;10(4):478–9.
11. Sachs RA, Lin D, Stone ML, et al. Can the need for future surgery for acute traumatic anterior shoulder dislocation be predicted? J Bone Joint Surg Am. 2007;89:1665–74.
12. Habermeyer P, Gleyze P, Rickert M. Evolution of lesions of the labrum-ligament complex in posttraumatic anterior shoulder instability: a prospective study. J Shoulder Elb Surg. 1999;8:66–74.
13. Buscayret F, Edwards TB, Szabo I, et al. Glenohumeral arthrosis in anterior instability before and after surgical treatment: incidence and contributing factors. Am J Sports Med. 2004;32:1165–72.
14. Griffith JF, Antonio GE, Yung PS, et al. Prevalence, pattern, and spectrum of glenoid bone loss in anterior shoulder dislocation: CT analysis of 218 patients. AJR Am J Roentgenol. 2008;190:1247–54.
15. Itoi E, Hatakeyama Y, Kido T, Sato T, Minagawa M, Wakabayashi I, Kobayashi M. A new method of immobilization after traumatic anterior dislocation of the shoulder: a preliminary study. J Shoulder Elb Surg. 2003;12(5):413–5.
16. Itoi E, et al. Immobilization in external rotation after shoulder dislocation reduces the risk of recurrence. A randomized controlled trial. J Bone Joint Surg Am. 2007;89:2124–31.
17. Whelan DB, Lichtfeld R, Wambolt E, Dainty KN. External rotation immobilization for primary shoulder dislocation: a randomized controlled trial. Clin Orthop Relat Res. 2014;472(8):2380–6.
18. Liavaag S, Brox JI, Pripp AH, Enger M, Soldal LA, Svenningsen S. Immobilization in external rotation after primary shoulder dislocation did not reduce the risk of recurrence: a randomized controlled trial. J Bone Joint Surg Am. 2011;93(10):897–904. Epub 2011 Apr 15
19. Dickens JF, Owens BD, Cameron KL, Kilcoyne K, Allred CD, Svoboda SJ, Sullivan R, Tokish JM, Peck KY, Rue JP. Return to play and recurrent instability after in-season anterior shoulder

instability: a prospective multicenter study. Am J Sports Med. 2014;42(12):2842–50. https://doi.org/10.1177/0363546514553181. Epub 2014 Nov 5
20. Aronen JG, Regan K. Decreasing the incidence of recurrence of first time anterior shoulder dislocations with rehabilitation. Am J Sports Med. 1984;12:283–91.
21. Robinson CM, Howes J, Murdoch H, et al. Functional outcome and risk of recurrent instability after primary traumatic anterior shoulder dislocation in young patients. J Bone Joint Surg Am. 2006;88:2326–36.
22. Hovelius L, Olofsson A, Sandström B, et al. Nonoperative treatment of primary anterior shoulder dislocation in patients forty years of age and younger. A prospective twenty-five-year follow-up. J Bone Joint Surg Am. 2008;90:945–52.
23. Olds M, Donaldson K, Ellis R, Kersten P. Among children of 18 years old and under, what promotes recurrent shoulder instability after traumatic anterior shoulder dislocation? A systematic review and meta-analysis of risk factors. Br J Sports Med. 2016;50(18):1135–41. https://doi.org/10.1136/bjsports-2015-095149.
24. Shymon SJ, Roocroft J, Edmonds EW. Traumatic anterior instability of the pediatric shoulder: a comparison of arthroscopic and open Bankart repairs. J Pediatr Orthop. 2015;35(1):1–6.
25. Gigis I, Heikenfeld R, Kapinas A, Listringhaus R, Godolias G. Arthroscopic versus conservative treatment of first anterior dislocation of the shoulder in adolescents. J Pediatr Orthop. 2014;34(4):421–5. https://doi.org/10.1097/BPO.0000000000000108.
26. Robinson CM, Howes J, Murdoch H, Will E, Graham C. Functional outcome and risk of recurrent instability after primary traumatic anterior shoulder dislocation in young patients. Bone Joint Surg Am. 2006;88(11):2326–36.
27. Brophy RH, Marx RG. The treatment of traumatic anterior instability of the shoulder: nonoperative and surgical treatment. Arthroscopy. 2009;25(3):298–304.
28. Chahal J, Marks P, MacDonald P, Shah P, Theodoropoulos J, Ravi B, Whelan D. Anatomic Bankart repair compared with nonoperative treatment and/or arthroscopic lavage for first-time traumatic shoulder dislocation. Arthroscopy. 2012;28(4):565–75.
29. Longo UG, Loppini M, Rizzello G, Ciuffreda M, Maffulli N, Denaro V. Management of primary acute anterior shoulder dislocation: systematic review and quantitative synthesis of the literature. Arthroscopy. 2014;30(4):506–22. Level IV
30. Kirkley A, Werstine R, Ratjek A, Griffin S. Prospective randomized clinical trial comparing the effectiveness of immediate arthroscopic stabilization versus immobilization and rehabilitation in first traumatic anterior dislocations of the shoulder: long-term evaluation. Arthroscopy. 2005;21(1):55–63.
31. Atoun E, Narvani A, Even T, Dabasia H, Van Tongel A, Sforza G, Levy O. Management of first-time dislocations of the shoulder in patients older than 40 years: the prevalence of iatrogenic fracture. J Orthop Trauma. 2013;27(4):190–3. https://doi.org/10.1097/BOT.0b013e31826576f8.
32. Pevny T, Hunter RE, Freeman JR. Primary traumatic anterior shoulder dislocation among patients 40 years of age and older. Arthroscopy. 1998;14(3):289–94.
33. Wenner SM. Anterior dislocation of the shoulder in patients over 50 years of age. Orthopedics. 1985;8(9):1155–7.
34. Riccio I, de Sire A, Latte C, Pascarella F, Gimigliano F. Conservative treatment of traumatic shoulder instability: a case series study. Musculoskelet Surg. 2015;99(2):133–7. https://doi.org/10.1007/s12306-015-0373-0. Epub 2015 May 16
35. Spiegl UJ, Ryf C, Hepp P, Rillmann P. Evaluation of a treatment algorithm for acute traumatic osseous Bankart lesions resulting from first time dislocation of the shoulder with a two year follow-up. BMC Musculoskelet Disord. 2013;14:305. https://doi.org/10.1186/1471-2474-14-305.

9 Is There a Place for Conservative Treatment in Recurrent Anterior Shoulder Instability?

Patryk Kłaptocz

9.1 Functional Deficits in Anterior Shoulder Instability

The stability of the shoulder depends on many structures: the shape of the glenoid, humeral head retrotorsion, and the condition of the labrum, ligaments, and joint capsule [1, 2]. Many muscles are also responsible for dynamic shoulder stability, in particular, the rotator cuff muscles, but also the deltoid, pectoralis major, latissimus dorsi, teres major, and long head of biceps [3]. To ensure appropriate function and stability, we need right movement patterns and cooperation between these muscles [4, 5]. Proprioception also has a very large role in joint stability. Proprioceptors, which are receptors that sense joint position, are located in muscles, tendons, and joint capsules. Mechanoreceptors are also located in different layers of the skin, such as Pacinian and Messner corpuscles, Ruffini endings, and Merkel discs, which make a large sensorimotor contribution to joint stability [6]. Proprioception depends on many factors, including age, training level, awareness, fatigue, and body mass [7].

Shoulder disorders have an influence on proprioception. Joint position sense and kinesthesia are altered in patients with glenohumeral instability [8]. When ligaments, labrum, or even the articular surface are damaged, there is less stimulation from mechanoreceptors localized in these structures, which impacts the stability of the joint [9] by changing neuromotor control and disturbing the balance between stabilizer and phase muscles [10]. Pain may accompany instability, and increased stimulation from nociceptors decreases proprioception; these actions can lead to muscle atrophy [11].

Sadeghifar et al. [12] found reduced internal and external rotation range of motion and decreased internal and external rotation strength in anterior shoulder instability (AI). Other authors observed decreased electromyographic activity in the serratus anterior and supraspinatus muscles in comparison with normal shoulders [13]. Jaggi and coworkers carried out a dynamic electromyography study in patients with different kinds of shoulder instability [14]. They noted the pectoralis major (PM) and latissimus dorsi (LD) to be inappropriately active in AI, by 60% and 81%, respectively. A cadaveric study [15, 16] showed these two muscles at the end of the abduction and external rotation of the arm can produce anterior translation forces, especially when the PM and LD are not in correct balance with the rotator cuff muscles. In the study by Anju Jaggi [14] the authors observed also increased activation of the anterior deltoid (AD) in 22% of cases, but these acted mainly when displacement occurred. It is difficult to say that activation has a destabilizing impact to the joint, because there were no data

P. Kłaptocz (✉)
Shoulder and Upper Limb Department,
St. Luke's Hospital, Bielsko-Biała, Poland

R. Brzóska et al. (eds.), *360° Around Shoulder Instability*,
https://doi.org/10.1007/978-3-662-61074-9_9

about other parts of the deltoid, but it is commonly known that AD is important as an anterior stabilizer of the glenohumeral joint (GHJ) [17].

Warner and coworkers [18] observed scapulothoracic motion asymmetry in 64% of patients with anteroinferior shoulder instability compared to 18% of subjects with normal shoulders. In 36% of these cases, it was a winging scapula. The discussion still persists: is this a symptom, or could it be also partly a reason for shoulder instability?

Palleta et al. [19] assessed shoulder kinematics during scapular plane abduction with two-plane X-ray in patients with anterior instability and rotator cuff tear. All patients in the rotator cuff tear group demonstrated superior translation of the humeral head (HH), whereas 78% of the instability group presented with abnormal anterior translation. Both groups had altered scapulothoracic rhythm. Two years after open anterior stabilization and open rotator cuff repair, the patients were restudied. All these patients had demonstrated abnormalities of HH translation before surgery. The researchers noted that all the patients from the instability group and 86% of the cuff tear (CT) group had restored normal glenohumeral kinematics in both planes, but what was really interesting was that in the CT group the scapulothoracic rhythm became normal whereas in the instability group the altered rhythm persisted. This result suggests that instability patients need much more attention during their rehabilitation process.

9.2 Conservative Treatment Options and Effectiveness in Anterior Shoulder Instability

Nonoperative treatment consists of immobilization and physiotherapy. Even though immobilization is used quite often, controversy remains if a time of immobilization is warranted or whether early motion improves patient outcomes and decreases redislocation rates [20]. There is also no consensus regarding the position of immobilization. In the traditional way, the patient was immobilized in adduction and internal rotation for 3 weeks [21], although Itoi et al. [22] have demonstrated that immobilization in external rotation reduces the torn labrum better than internal rotation and decreases redislocation [23].

Rehabilitation principally includes different kinds of exercises such as isometric, isotonic, plyometric, and proprioceptive in closed or open kinetic chains and specific sport exercises until the patient has progressed to their previous activity level. If instability is acute, the beginning phase includes antiinflammatory and analgesic therapy as well [24].

Reviewing the scientific literature, we did not find many good quality studies confirming the high effectiveness of rehabilitation in AI. All such studies are characterized by the lack of a control group, with no comparison to other rehabilitation interventions; usually these are case or case-series studies. Unfortunately, retrospective studies also dominate.

Riccio et al. [25] assessed 32 cases with primary AI after a rehabilitation protocol that lasted for 3 months and consisted of five phases. Each phase included different goals and slow progression. The researchers described only the kind of exercises without describing the manner of execution; that is, no details of numbers of sets and repetitions were included. Thus, the protocol is not repeatable and not comparable to other data; the amount of physiotherapy sessions needed throughout the 3 months was also not stated. The authors noted an improvement in Rowe score from 45 to 80 and no new episodes of dislocation having occurred after 2 years by using their exercise program, but of importance is that athletes who use overhead motions and physical workers were excluded from the study.

The only shoulder instability rehabilitation program sufficiently defined to be reproducible is the protocol by Burkhead and Rockwood [26], which contained specific resistance exercises with a Theraband for the rotator cuff and deltoid muscles. The first phase includes five exercises with resistive progression, performed two or three times a day, with five repetitions with a 5-s hold. If the patient had no complaints, every 2–3 weeks the resistance was increased by changing the Theraband color. In the second phase the same exercises were prescribed but on a pulley kit, with weight exercises with load progression if the exercises ceased to be demanding. Patients were supervised for 8 weeks. If there was no improvement after 4 months, surgery was recommended. Burkhead and Rockwood investigated 140 shoulders with different kinds of instability and assigned them to the following groups:

1. Traumatic subluxation
   - Type 1—without previous subluxation
   - Type 2—with previous subluxation
2. Atraumatic subluxation
   - Type 3A—voluntary subluxation and psychological problems
   - Type 3B—voluntary subluxation and no psychological problems
   - Type 4—involuntary subluxation

To evaluate the subjects, the authors used a grading system suggested by Rowe and Zarins. They obtained the following results in AI: in type 1, only 18% had a good or excellent result; in type 2, only two shoulders of 29 (9%) had a good or excellent result. These two shoulders presented only mild degenerative changes and no Hill–Sachs lesion on radiographs. In comparison, 27% of traumatic posterior dislocations presented good or excellent results after the exercise program. In atraumatic cases, results were much better: 88% had good or excellent results in posterior or multidirectional instability, but only 50% in AI (four shoulders).

Aronen and Regan [27] conducted an experiment on 20 midshipmen with traumatic AI. The rehabilitation protocol began with immobilization and then progressed first to isometric, later to isotonic, and in the end isokinetic exercises. Subjects used internal and external rotation, flexion, extension, and adduction motions with a Theraband. Patients had to avoid activities that could induce subluxation until the goals of rehabilitation program were achieved. Authors reported a 75% success rate, so they suggested a program of specific exercises can decrease the rate of recurrence. This study was limited by the lack of data about inclusion and exclusion criteria.

Two cited studies are case series [25, 27] and one is a retrospective cohort [26]. Except the Rockwood program, there are not enough well-defined protocols to replicate and compare different rehabilitation modes. Authors use various tools to determine their results, so it is not possible to compare between studies. Qualification to the research group is also a weak aspect; only Burkhead assessed the range of damage in joint structures. Thus, such articles provide a low level of evidence and do not provide sufficient knowledge regarding qualification and duration of rehabilitation in AI. Therefore, there is high need of further good-quality research to evaluate the effects of different protocols on recurrence rates.

Fortunately, Eshoj et al. [28] is conducting such a study in Denmark: this is a multicenter, randomized, blinded experiment on 80 patients with traumatic AI. The subjects will be allocated to groups with different rehabilitation treatments for 12 weeks. Patients will have either a standardized, individualized, or physiotherapist-supervised neuromuscular shoulder exercise program or a self-managed shoulder exercise program. Also, the subjects will be allocated to groups based on primary and recurrent anterior instability. This is the first study to compare different rehabilitation treatments in traumatic AI, but at the same time, the first to investigate non-operative treatment effects in patients with recurrent shoulder dislocations.

Warby and coworkers [29] have done the first randomized control trial, which compared the Rockwood Instability Program to a program by Watson in atraumatic multidirectional instability patients without significant lesions of joint structures. The Watson MDI Program precisely described a rehabilitation protocol that consists primarily of individual assessment and reeducation of scapula position and movement, and only then addresses strengthening shoulder muscles. Watson recommends more sets and repetitions than Rockwood, starting with motor relearning (3 sets, 20 repetitions, twice a day), followed by an endurance dosage (3 sets, 10–15 reps, twice a day), then a strength dosage in later stages (4 sets, 8–12 reps, every second day). For most exercises, repetitions are held for 3 s. Patients underwent 12 sessions of physiotherapy lasting 30 min. Results showed a statistically significant difference between the two groups, the effects favoring the Watson program for WOSI at 12 weeks and for MISS and pain at 24 weeks. This study revealed that this kind of rehabilitation, with an individual approach to motor control deficits and a program of exercises, can determine the final results.

9.3 Conservative Treatment Versus Surgical Treatment

There are many more good-quality studies regarding surgical treatment (ST) in comparison to conservative treatment (CT) for patients with AI. We can quote here, for instance, Brophy and Marx [30], who noted a 46% recurrence rate after CT compared with 7% after ST at 2 years of follow-up. Johannsen et al. [31] also found that 56% of patients had recurrence after CT versus 3% after ST at 2 years of follow-up. In 10 years of observations, they noted 75% of the CT group demonstrated unsatisfactory results compared to 72% with good or excellent results in the ST group. Kirkley and colleagues [32] observed a recurrence rate of 16% after arthroscopy compared to 47% in conservative treatment.

All the papers mentioned describe primary shoulder instability. We can find much more evidence showing the superiority of surgical treatment over conservative treatment, but in general, the risk of recurrence in the CT group is three to ten times greater than in the ST group. If we consider treatment options in recurrent anterior shoulder instability, we will find in the literature only scientific reports regarding the surgical treatment approach and comparison between them [33–35].

9.4 Discussion

Much controversy is presently being seen in the management of anterior shoulder dislocation. First, we know that time and position of immobilization really do not matter for recurrence rate [36]. Second, the recurrence rate for nonoperative treatment is about 50%, and surgical procedures significantly reduce the prevalence of recurrence [32, 33, 37]. In young active patients, the recurrence rate can be very high, as much as 92–96% [38]. Thus, in reviewing the latest literature we can get the impression there is a greater trend in the direction of surgical treatment, even more often in primary AI. Further arguments supporting operation are progressive degenerative changes in joint structures. Hovelius and Saeboe [39] have observed patients for 25 years since their first episode of dislocation. All of them had arthropathy, which was more advanced with more episodes of dislocation. Buscayret and coworkers [40] had similar findings; 9.2% of AI patients had accompanying arthritis, and risk factors were age of first dislocation, period of time from dislocation to surgery, and bony lesions of the glenoid. After surgery, 19.7% of subjects had arthritis, but it was probably correlated with age, a larger amount of dislocation, and long follow-up. Increased occurrence of arthritis exists with decreased external rotation range of motion, but it is not known whether this a source of or an effect in joint changes. Habermeyer and coworkers [13] examined arthroscopically 91 shoulders to carefully evaluate joint structures in patients after one, two, three to five, six, and more episodes of dislocation. Studies have shown marked gradual degeneration of the anteroinferior labrum and capsuloligamentous complex along with increasing instability. Some authors [31, 32, 41] strongly recommend early arthroscopic repair after primary dislocation, which achieves better results.

On the other hand, although it seems inevitable, still there is no evidence showing that early repair after the first episode means better results than surgery in the recurrent state. Robinson and colleagues [42] made an RCT, double-blinded study to compare arthroscopy and lavage to arthroscopic Bankart repair. They discovered a decreased rate of recurrence after structural repair, but perceived that early repair does not seem to have functional benefits in stable shoulders at 2 years after intervention.

Lädermann and coworkers [43] came to interesting conclusions when they checked humeral head (HH) translation during functional arm movement. Despite reducing the risk of recurrence, anterior HH translation was not significantly decreased after surgical stabilization compared to pre-operation values. This micro-instability in operated patients can explain persisting pain, apprehension, inability to return to sport, and subsequent arthropathy.

9.5 Conclusion

Implementation of conservative treatment seems justified and is supported by scientific evidence in atraumatic shoulder instability [24]. It is usually the case of multidirectional (MDI) and posterior instability, but anterior instability can occur as well.

The study designed by Jaggi et al. [44] is still not published. This randomized controlled clinical trial will provide information whether the addition of surgical intervention to physiotherapy improves outcomes for patients with atraumatic shoulder instability who have sustained soft-tissue damage at the joint. Although today rehabilitation is the treatment of choice for such patients [24], it is already known that the type of rehabilitation affects the results in MDI patients [29]. We will see how large an influence different kinds of rehabilitation programs have in traumatic anterior primary and recurrent cases [28]. Keeping in mind structural lesions, deepening pathology, proprioception, and neuromotor deficits partly resulting from impaired sensory functions in damaged tissue, it seems that the trend toward an earlier operation is reasonable. If for some reason the patient cannot or does not want to undergo an operation, rehabilitation should contain, in addition to exercises, very precise education regarding safe functioning and avoiding stressful activities. The Stanmore Triangle can help with clinical decision making, as presented by Lewis et al. [45], who distinguish three types of instability (Fig. 9.1):

1. Traumatic with structural pathology
2. Atraumatic with structural pathology
3. Atraumatic without structural pathology but with abnormal muscle patterns.

The first type is dedicated to surgery, and the third type to rehabilitation and avoiding an operation. The second type is controversial and depends on how much muscle patterns are involved. In these cases we should pay attention to the history and examination although the evidence for either surgery or therapy is lacking. Conservative treatment can be also a good treatment option in acute anterior shoulder instability, even with structural damage, but also in in-season professional athletes, when it is really important to come back quickly to the arena [46].

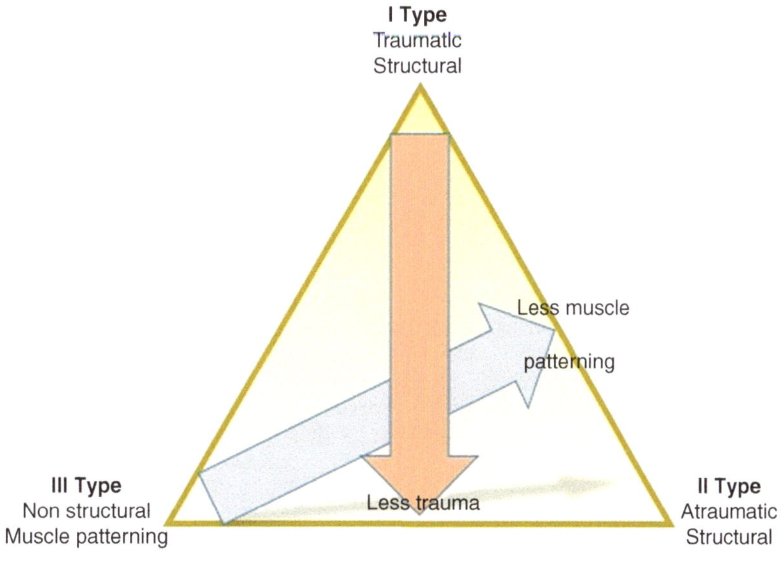

Fig. 9.1 The Stanmore Triangle

Surgical treatment, although it can significantly reduce the recurrence rate of instability, cannot restore scapulothoracic rhythm or totally correct HH translation. Thus, for complete treatment, appropriate rehabilitation is necessary. We know rehabilitation can be successful in many shoulder disorders. The question is whether rehabilitation should be applied first, as the less invasive treatment, or added after surgical treatment? Clinicians should not consider ST and CT as a competition, but as a common whole that merges to achieve the best possible result for the patient.

References

1. Tannenbaum E, Sekiya JK. Evaluation and management of posterior shoulder instability. Sports Health. 2011;3(3):e253–63.
2. Wang VM, Flatow EL. Pathomechanics of acquired shoulder instability: a basic science perspective. J Shoulder Elb Surg. 2005;14(1 Suppl S):2S–11S.
3. Debski RE, Sakone M, Woo SL, Wong EK, Fu FH, Warner JJ. Contribution of the passive properties of the rotator cuff to glenohumeral stability during anterior-posterior loading. J Shoulder Elb Surg. 1999;8(4):e324–9.
4. Herrington L, Horsley I, Rofl C. Evaluation of shoulder joint position sense in both asymptomatic and rehabilitated professional rugby players and matched controls. Phys Ther Sport. 2010;11(1):18–22.
5. Provencher MT, LeClere LE, King S, McDonald LS, Frank RM, Mologne TS. Posterior instability of the shoulder: diagnosis and management. Am J Sports Med. 2011;39(4):e874–86.
6. Grigg P. Peripheral neural mechanism in proprioception. J Sport Rehabil. 1994;3:2–17.
7. Goble DJ. Proprioceptive acuity assessment via joint position matching: from basic science to general practice. Phys Ther. 2010;90(8):1176–84.
8. Barden JM, Balyk R, Raso VJ. Dynamic upper limb proprioception in multidirectional shoulder instability. Clin Orthop Relat Res. 2004;420:181–9.
9. Lephart SM, Henry TJ. The physiological basis for open end and closed kinetic chain rehabilitation for upper extremity. J Sport Rehabil. 1996;5:71–87.
10. Myers JB, Ju YY, Hwang JH, McMahom PJ. Reflexive muscle activation alterations in shoulders with anterior glenohumeral instability. Am J Sports Med. 2004;32:1013–21.
11. Safran MR, Borsa PA, Lephart SM. Shoulder proprioception in baseball pitchers. J Shoulder Elb Surg. 2001;10:438–44.
12. Sadeghifar A, Ilka S, Dashtbani H, Sahebozamani M. A comparison of glenohumeral internal and external range of motion and rotation strength in healthy and individuals with recurrent anterior instability. Arch Bone Joint Surg. 2014;2(3):215–9.
13. Habermeyer P, Gleyze P, Rickert M. Evolution of lesions of the labrum–ligament complex in posttraumatic anterior shoulder instability: a prospective study. J Shoulder Elb Surg. 1999;8(1):66–74.
14. Jaggi A, Noorani A, Malone A, Cowan J, Lambert S, Bayley I. Muscle activation patterns in patients with recurrent shoulder instability. Int J Shoulder Surg. 2012;6(4):101–7.
15. Konrad GG, Jolly JT, Labriola JE, McMahon PJ, Debski RE. Thoracohumeral muscle activity alters glenohumeral joint biomechanics during active abduction. J Orthop Res. 2006;24:748–56.
16. Labriola JE, Lee TQ, Debski RE, McMahon PJ. Stability and instability of the glenohumeral joint: the role of shoulder muscles. J Shoulder Elb Surg. 2005;14:328.
17. Kido T, Itoi E, Lee SB, Neale PG, An KN. Dynamic stabilizing function of the deltoid muscle in shoulders with anterior instability. Am J Sports Med. 2003;31:399–403.
18. Warner JJ, Micheli LJ, Arslanian LE, Kennedy J, Kennedy R. Scapulothoracic motion in normal shoulders and shoulders with glenohumeral instability and impingement syndrome. A study using Moire topographic analysis. Clin Orthop. 1992;285:191–9.
19. Paletta GA Jr, Warner JJ, Warren RF, Deutsch A, Altchek DW. Kinematics with two-plane x-ray evaluation in patients with anterior instability or rotator cuff tearing. J Shoulder Elb Surg. 1997;6(6):516–27.
20. Hovelius L, Eriksson K, Fredin H. Recurrences after initial dislocation of the shoulder. Results of a prospective study of treatment. J Bone Joint Surg. 1983;65:343–9.
21. Kiviluoto O, Pasila M, Jaroma H, Sundholm A. Immobilization after primary dislocation of the shoulder. Acta Orthop Scand. 1980;51(6):915–9.
22. Itoi E, Sashi R, Minagawa H. Position of immobilization after dislocation of the glenohumeral joint. J Bone Joint Surg Am. 2001;83A:661–7.
23. Itoi E, Hatakeyama Y, Sato T. Immobilization in external rotation after shoulder dislocation reduces the risk of recurrence. A randomized controlled trial. J Bone Joint Surg. 2007;89:2124–31.
24. Wilk KE, Macrina LC, Michael M, Reinold MM. Non-operative rehabilitation for traumatic and atraumatic glenohumeral instability. N Am J Sports Phys Ther. 2006;1(1):16–31.
25. Riccio I, de Sire A, Latte C, Pascarella F, Gimigliano F. Conservative treatment of traumatic shoulder instability: a case series study. Musculoskelet Surg. 2015;99(2):133–7.
26. Burkhead WZ Jr, Rockwood CA Jr. Treatment of instability of the shoulder with an exercise program. J Bone Joint Surg Am. 1992;74:890–6.
27. Aronen JG, Regan K. Decreasing the incidence of recurrence of first time anterior shoulder dislocations with rehabilitation. Am J Sports Med. 1984;12:283–91.

28. Eshoj H, Rasmussen S, Frich LH, Hvass I, Christensen R, Jensen SL, Søndergaard J, Søgaard K, Juul-Kristensen B. A neuromuscular exercise programme versus standard care for patients with traumatic anterior shoulder instability: study protocol for a randomised controlled trial (the SINEX study). Trials. 2017;18:90.
29. Warby SA, Ford JJ, Hahne AJ, Watson L, Balster S, Lenssen R, Pizzari T. Comparison of 2 exercise rehabilitation programs for multidirectional instability of the glenohumeral joint. A randomized controlled trial. Am J Sports Med. 2018;46(1):87–97.
30. Brophy RH, Marx RG. The treatment of traumatic anterior instability of the shoulder: nonoperative and surgical treatment. Arthroscopy. 2009;25(3):298–304.
31. Jakobsen BW, Johannsen HV, Suder P, Søjbjerg JO. Primary repair versus conservative treatment of first-time traumatic anterior dislocation of the shoulder: a randomized study with 10-year follow-up. Arthroscopy. 2007;23(2):117.
32. Kirkley A, Griffin S, Richards C, Miniaci A, Mohtadi N. Prospective randomized clinical trial comparing the effectiveness of immediate arthroscopic stabilization versus shoulder. Arthroscopy. 1999;15(5):507–14.
33. Bottoni CR, Smith EL, Berkowitz MJ, Towle RB, Moore JH. Arthroscopic versus open shoulder stabilization for recurrent anterior instability: a prospective randomized clinical trial. Am J Sports Med. 2006;34(11):1730–7.
34. Freedman KB, Smith AP, Romeo AA, Cole BJ, Bach BR Jr. Open Bankart repair versus arthroscopic repair with transglenoid sutures or bioabsorbable tacks for recurrent anterior instability of the shoulder: a meta-analysis. Am J Sports Med. 2004;32(6):1520–15277.
35. Lenters TR, Franta AK, Wolf FM, Leopold SS, Matsen FA 3rd. Arthroscopic compared with open repairs for recurrent anterior shoulder instability. A systematic review and meta-analysis of the literature. J Bone Joint Surg Am. 2007;89(2):244–54.
36. Liavaag S, Brox JI, Pripp AH, Enger M, Soldal LA, Svenningsen S. Immobilization in external rotation after primary shoulder dislocation did not reduce the risk of recurrence: a randomized controlled trial. J Bone Joint Surg Am. 2011;93(10):897–904.
37. Hovelius L, Augustini BG, Fredin H. Primary anterior dislocation of the shoulder in young patients. J Bone Joint Surg. 1996;78A:1677–84.
38. te Slaa RL, Brand R, Marti RK. A prospective arthroscopic study of acute first-time anterior shoulder dislocation in the young: a five-year follow-up study. J Shoulder Elb Surg. 2003;12(6):529–34.
39. Hovelius L, Saeboe M. Neer Award 2008. Arthropathy after primary anterior shoulder dislocation: 223 shoulders prospectively followed up for twenty-five years. J Shoulder Elb Surg. 2009;18(3):339–47.
40. Buscayret F, Edwards TB, Szabo I, Adeleine P, Coudane H, Walch G. Glenohumeral arthrosis in anterior instability before and after surgical treatment: incidence and contributing factors. Am J Sports Med. 2004;32(5):1165–72.
41. Rugg CM, Hettrich CM, Ortiz S, Wolf BR, MOON Shoulder Instability Group, Zhang AL. Surgical stabilization for first-time shoulder dislocators: a multicenter analysis. J Shoulder Elb Surg. 2018;27(4):674–85.
42. Robinson CM, Jenkins PJ, White TO, Ker A, Will E. Primary arthroscopic stabilization for a first-time anterior dislocation of the shoulder. A randomized, double-blind trial. J Bone Joint Surg Am. 2008;90(4):708–21.
43. Lädermann A, Denard PJ, Tirefort J, Kolo FC, Chagué S, Cunningham G, Charbonnier C. Does surgery for instability of the shoulder truly stabilize the glenohumeral joint? A prospective comparative cohort study. Medicine (Baltimore). 2016;95:31.
44. Jaggi A, Alexander S, Herbert R, Funk L, Ginn KA. Does surgery followed by physiotherapy improve short and long term outcome for patients with atraumatic shoulder instability compared with physiotherapy alone? protocol for a randomized controlled clinical trial. BMC Musculoskelet Disord. 2014;15:439.
45. Lewis A, Kitamura T, Bayley JI. Mini symposium: shoulder instability. The classification of shoulder instability: new light through old windows. Curr Orthop. 2004;18:97–108.
46. Conti M, Garofalo R, Castagna A, Massazza G, Ceccarelli E. Dynamic brace is a good option to treat first anterior shoulder dislocation in season. Musculoskelet Surg. 2017;101(Suppl 2):169–73.

10 Soft-Tissue Procedures: Indications

Ladislav Kovačič

10.1 Introduction

Various open and arthroscopic surgical options are available to address anterior shoulder instability. The outcome is dependent on multiple intrinsic and extrinsic factors. The most important factor of instability and predictor of surgical treatment by far is the presence of bony injuries, including the bony Bankart lesion and Hill–Sachs lesion. In these specific conditions of bone deficiency in the glenohumeral joint, it is recognized that the recurrence after soft-tissue stabilization alone is unacceptably high [1–4]. When concerned, on the other hand, with patients with predominantly soft-tissue lesions, soft-tissue procedures and especially soft-tissue arthroscopic surgical repair for anterior shoulder stabilization can be as successful as other treatment options. To be able to perform an appropriate decision-making process before surgical treatment, adequate knowledge of the important risk factors for recurrence, and their influence on shoulder instability and prognosis of the surgical treatment, is necessary. Correct assessment of the lesions associated with anterior shoulder instability and appropriate patient selection regarding risk factors for recurrence are necessary for a successful surgical outcome [5, 6].

L. Kovačič (✉)
Department of Traumatology, University Medical Centre Ljubljana, Ljubljana, Slovenia
e-mail: ladislav.kovacic@kclj.si

R. Brzóska et al. (eds.), *360° Around Shoulder Instability*,
https://doi.org/10.1007/978-3-662-61074-9_10

10.2 The Diagnostic Process

Glenohumeral instability can be classified in many ways. Direction of the instability, its chronicity, and the etiology are probably the most important categories. To assess the risk of recurrence, it is necessary to understand the etiology and pathomechanics related to the glenohumeral instability. This understanding may aid in determining the patient's risk of recurrence and will also guide us to the appropriate choice of surgical procedure [7]. When assessing the patient with anterior shoulder instability, we should collect information not only regarding the underlying lesion but also regarding the specific condition of the shoulder joint and, furthermore, the patient's personality, level of activity, and expectations. The thorough history of the patient and clinical examination are of utmost importance. Diagnostic radiologic studies, which will further reveal the nature of the injury, are also essential [8, 9].

When the surgeon is deciding about further management and the surgical options for patients with anterior shoulder instability, we should ask ourselves: what are important data about the patient to know? In other words: what do I want to know about the patient? We should inquire about the age of the patient, age at time of the first dislocation, and the mode of injury at the first dislocation. Knowing the position of the arm during that dislocation event is useful.

Table 10.1 Important patient and injury characteristics that should be questioned during history, clinical examination, and diagnostic workup

What do I want to know about the patient?
Age of the patient and age at the time of the first dislocation
Gender
Mode of injury at first dislocation
Presence and quantity of instability events
Activities/sports participation
Shoulder laxity
Underlying lesion and concomitant lesions
Bone structure

Furthermore, it is important to understand the presence and quantity of the instability events. Patient characteristics are also important, including the patient's activity level and sports participation. We should determine shoulder laxity, underlying and concomitant lesions, and, probably the most important, the bone structure of the glenohumeral joint and the possibility of bony lesions (Table 10.1) [10].

10.3 Risk Factors That Predispose to Recurrence

Several authors have studied the risk factors for recurrence after shoulder instability treatment [11–13]. Some risk factors are more significant than others (Table 10.2). The instability severity score described and published by Balg and Boileau [11] and further validated by Rouleau [14] can help us to select the patient for soft-tissue or bony stabilization procedures [11, 14]. It was shown that important prognostic factors are age at the time of surgery, degree of sports participation, type of sport, shoulder hyperlaxity, visible Hill–Sachs lesion, and loss of glenoid contour on anteroposterior shoulder radiograph. Soft-tissue repair is advisable only if less than 5% of recurrence is estimated, which corresponds to less than 3 points in this scoring system.

The Presence and Quantity of Instability Events. According to some studies, presence and quantity of instability events are important risk factors. The number of shoulder dislocations may lead to plastic deformation or elongation of the joint capsule [15]. Furthermore, the number of

Table 10.2 Important risk factors for recurrence in anterior shoulder stabilization treatment

Significant	Less significant
Age at the time of first dislocation	Gender
Shoulder laxity	Mechanism of injury
Bone deficiency	Type of sports
Level of sport	Number of shoulder dislocations

Table 10.3 Recurrence rate in relationship to the number of preoperative dislocations [13, 16]

Number of dislocations	Recurrence rate (%)
1–2	11.1
3–4	17.8
6–10	43.3
11–20	43.4
>21	55.5

instability events has been associated with the presence of a bone defect on the glenoid and humeral side, the size of the bone defects, and the presence of a critical bone defect [12]. In fact, the glenoid bone defect is not a rare condition in anterior shoulder instability: it has been observed in 72% of the cases [12]. Another study reported on the recurrence rate in relationship to shoulder instability events (Table 10.3). The recurrence rate varies from 11.1% in the patients with 1 or 2 dislocation events to as high as 55.5% when the patients experience more than 21 shoulder dislocations [13, 16].

Shoulder Laxity. Shoulder laxity is included as a risk factor in almost all classifications of anterior shoulder instability. Recurrence tends to be threefold more likely in patients with shoulder laxity [6, 10, 11]. Shoulder laxity is not always easy to assess. The examiner should rely on the apprehension test, sulcus sign in neutral and external rotation position, load-shift test, amount of external rotation with the arm at the side, and Gagey's hyperabduction test (Fig. 10.1).

Underlying Lesion and Concomitant Lesions. Anteroinferior labro-ligamentous injury is the lesion most commonly found after an anterior shoulder luxation. The so-called Bankart lesion—the lesion of labro-ligamentous attachment on the anteroinferior part of the glenoid—can be found in 85–100% of young patients after anterior shoulder dislocation. The corresponding lesion

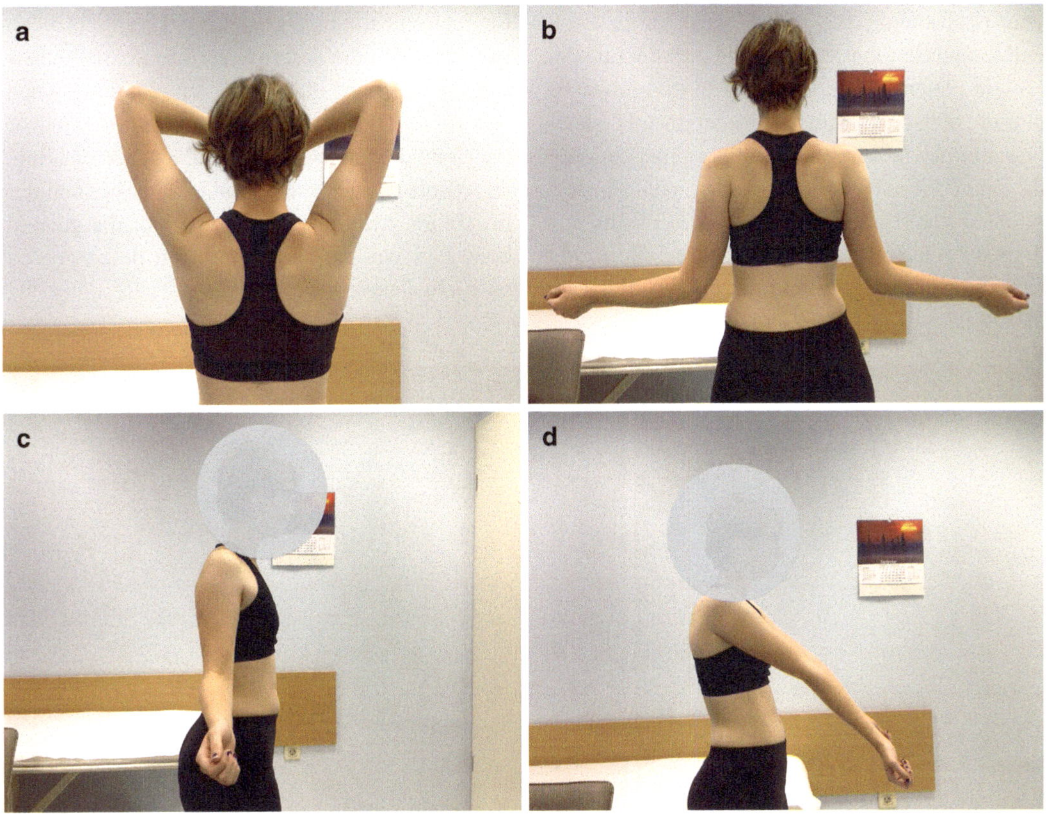

Fig. 10.1 Signs of shoulder laxity: excessive hyperabduction (**a**), external rotation with the arm at the side (**b**, **c**), and laxity of the joints (elbow hyperextension) (**d**)

on the humeral part, the Hill–Sachs lesion, can be found in 40–100% of young patients as well. Although being the most frequent lesions after anterior shoulder dislocation, these are not the only ones. Different pathological changes in soft tissue and bony structure can be detected as well: for example, the ALPSA lesion, SLAP lesion, HAGL lesion, capsular tear, capsular elongation, and rotator cuff tear. Of bone pathology, glenoid rim fracture and greater tuberosity fracture are the most common [17, 18]. Recognition of the underlying lesion is important to address the appropriate corresponding pathology as needed.

Bone Structure. Assessment of the bony structure is the most important factor when considering the possibility of a soft-tissue procedure for anterior shoulder instability stabilization. Burkhart and De Beer have found that the recurrence rate in patients with a significant bone defect was unacceptably high, as much as 67% in comparison to a 4% recurrence rate in patients with no bone defect [2]. This finding and the concept of engaging Hill–Sachs lesion has started to change the paradigm about anterior shoulder instability treatment. Surgeons began to study bone loss in the glenoid side first and later on the humeral side as well. Soft-tissue stabilization becomes appropriate only in the patient with a preserved effective glenoid arc. Although everyone recognizes bone loss as an important factor in the treatment decision algorithm, there are still some unanswered questions regarding this subject. How to measure bone loss? How much of the glenoid bone loss can be tolerated? What is the significant Hill–Sachs lesion? These are questions that are not fully answered at the moment. Although some scoring systems use a plain roentgenogram of the shoulder to assess bone loss, measurement on computed tomography (CT) scan or magnetic resonance imaging (MRI) is much more accurate (Fig. 10.2). The CT scan is absolutely recommended in cases where radiographs demonstrate glenoid or humeral bone loss, in patients with instability in mid-ranges of motion, in patients who have experienced dislocation after trivial trauma or a slight provocation at the initial episode, and in patients with a history of failed stabilization procedure, multiple dislocations, or bilateral dislocations, especially on the nondominant side. Several methods are available for quantification of glenoid and humeral bone loss [19, 20]. The description of those methods is beyond the scope of this chapter and is explained elsewhere. The important question is how much of the glenoid bone loss is acceptable when deciding about soft-tissue stabilization in anterior shoulder instability. At the beginning, 20% of the glenoid bone loss was set as a significant defect, based on some cadaveric studies [21, 22]. Recently, the

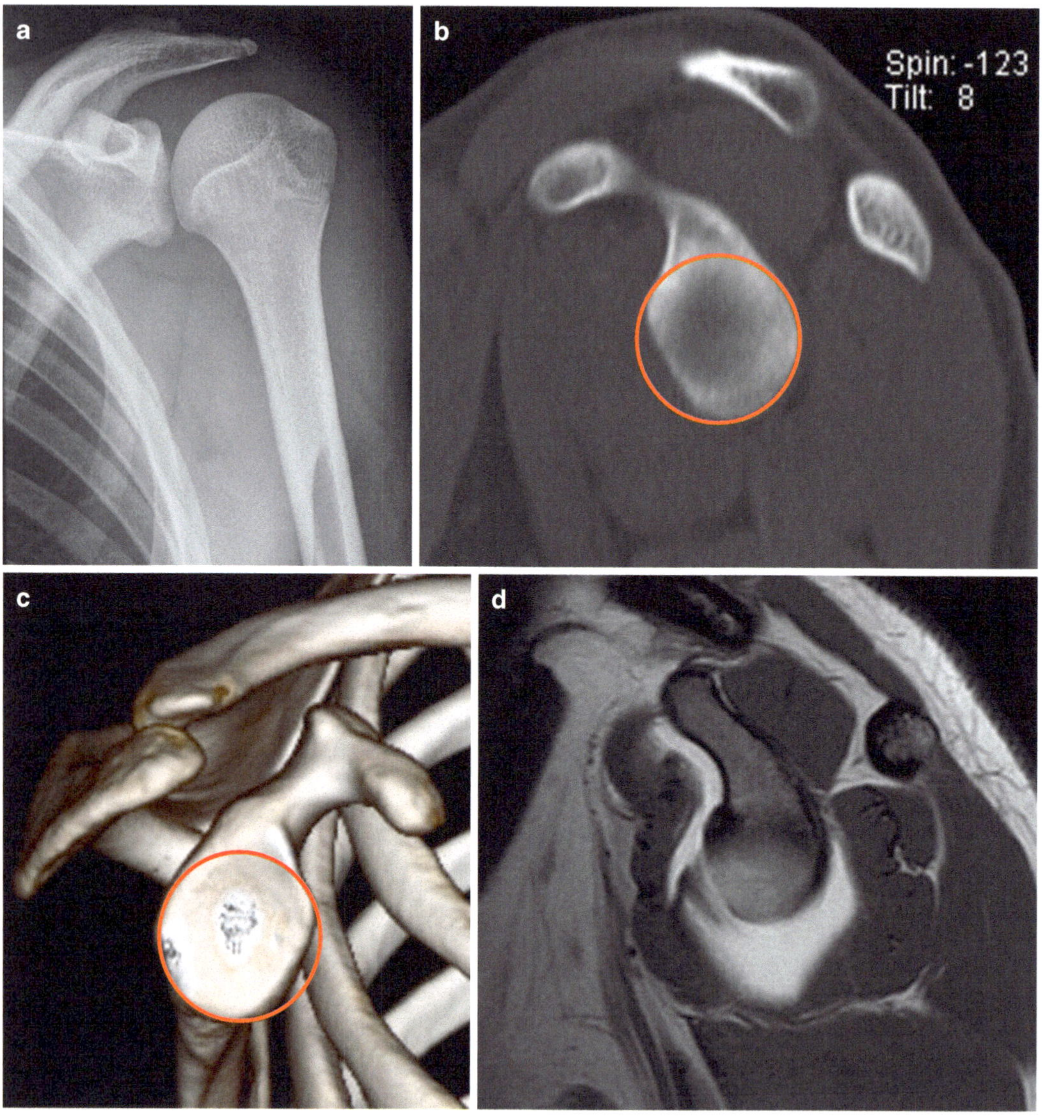

Fig. 10.2 Radiologic studies performed in patient with anterior shoulder instability reveal glenoid bone loss. Sclerotic contour loss on anterior glenoid rim (**a**). Best-fit circle shows anterior glenoid rim defect on sagittal plane (**b**) and 3-D reconstruction (**c**) on CT scan. The same method was applied on glenoid profile view on MRI in the sagittal plane (**d**)

threshold point was lowered significantly: only defects up to 15% of the glenoid surface might be ignored [23]. It is even more difficult to answer what is a significant Hill–Sachs lesion and how to measure it [11, 24, 25]. Nevertheless, the combination of both glenoid and humeral bony lesions seems to be the most relevant. Starting with the concept of engaging Hill–Sachs lesion and further development to the concept of the glenoid track by Itoi and Yamamoto [21, 22], we are closer to understanding shoulder instability on the basis of pathomechanics. The combined so-called bipolar lesions are responsible for the combined biomechanical effect. If a Hill–Sachs lesion extends medially over the glenoid tract (contact area of glenoid and humeral head in apprehension position), there is a risk of engagement [22]. And, as described in another study, when there is a glenoid bone loss of 2 mm, the medium-size Hill–Sachs lesion is significant. When there is a glenoid loss of 4 mm, the small-size Hill–Sachs lesion is already significant [26]. The role of the glenoid-sided and humeral-sided bone loss and the relationship between both has been additionally explained recently with the on-track/off-track concept, which gives us an improved understanding of this dynamic condition [27, 28]. Further studies are necessary to better understand the question of bone loss and especially to determine the limits of soft-tissue stabilization procedures.

10.4 Author's Preferred Treatment Scenarios

The combination of risk factors in a particular patient will influence our decision-making process, taking into account the factors of significant importance first, and second, the factors that are less important.

Scenario no. 1: A 17-year-old female basketball player with two dislocations in the past 6 months. On clinical examination, signs of hyperlaxity are present. Radiologic imaging reveals no glenoid bone lesion and a small Hill–Sachs lesion. ISIS score is 6.

Preferred treatment option: Arthroscopic Bankart repair, which will preserve the anatomy of the joint. Absence of important bone lesions and assumption of good-quality soft tissue allows us to predict a successful soft-tissue repair.

Scenario no. 2: A 24-year-old man who practices parachuting. He has had eight dislocations so far. No signs of hyperlaxity. He has no glenoid bone lesion and there is a small Hill–Sachs lesion seen on CT scan. ISIS score is 3.

Preferred treatment option: Bone block procedure; despite the absence of an important bone lesion, his activity is too risky to be exposed to danger.

Scenario no. 3: A 23-year-old man who practices kayaking. He has had more than 10 dislocations in 4 years. On clinical examination, he shows no signs of hyperlaxity. CT scan reveals small glenoid bone lesion of 10% and additional small Hill–Sachs lesion. ISIS score is 4.

Preferred treatment option: Bone block procedure. There is a borderline glenoid bone lesion with an additional lesion on the glenoid side. Number of dislocations is high, predisposing to low-quality soft tissue. Because of his activity level with arms working in apprehension position, a soft-tissue procedure is too risky.

Scenario no. 4: A 21-year-old man who performs sailing. He has had two dislocations and multiple episodes of subluxation. He has no signs of hyperlaxity. CT scan reveals small glenoid bone loss of 10% and a small Hill–Sachs lesion (width 8 mm, 2 mm deep). ISIS score is 4.

Preferred treatment option: Arthroscopic Bankart repair and remplissage. Despite the borderline glenoid bone deficiency, soft-tissue stabilization can give good results because of assumption of relatively good tissue quality. Additional remplissage will address an effective glenoid arc.

10.5 Summary

Arthroscopic soft-tissue stabilization procedures are generally safe and effective treatment options for patients suffering from anterior shoulder instability. However, meticulous attention should be given to individuals with risk factors for recurrence. Among these, bone deficiency, concomitant lesions, and quality of the anterior shoulder capsule are the

Table 10.4 Proposed algorithm for soft-tissue procedures

Bone structure	Procedure	Modifiers
Good capsule, no bone loss	Arthroscopic Bankart repair	Age Number of dislocations Shoulder laxity Activity level
Isolated humeral bone loss	Arthroscopic Bankart repair and remplissage	
Glenoid bone loss maximum 10–15%	Arthroscopic Bankart repair and remplissage	
Glenoid bone loss more than 10–15%	Bone block procedures	

most important. Some investigation methods can give us information regarding bone loss. X-ray is useful for screening, but the accuracy is insufficient. The computed tomography (CT) scan is the most reliable method to assess the corresponding bone loss on the glenoid and humeral side. Nevertheless, there is no consensus on the measuring technique and no clarity as to what constitutes a clinically significant bony lesion. Besides bone loss, additional factors are important to consider that can modify our decision toward soft-tissue or bone block procedures, as proposed in the algorithm of Table 10.4. Thus, treatment selection is based on the degree of bone injury, patient expectations, patient age, shoulder laxity, expected tissue quality, and the expected postoperative activity level.

References

1. Boileau P, Villalba M, Héry JY, Balg F, Ahrens P, Neyton L. Risk factors for recurrence of shoulder instability after arthroscopic Bankart repair. J Bone Joint Surg Am. 2006;88:1755–63.
2. Burkhart SS, De Beer JF. Traumatic glenohumeral bone defects and their relationship to failure of arthroscopic Bankart repairs: significance of the inverted-pear glenoid and the humeral engaging Hill–Sachs lesion. Arthroscopy. 2000;16:677–94.
3. Lee SH, Lim KH, Kim JW. Risk factors for recurrence of anterior-inferior instability of the shoulder after arthroscopic Bankart repair in patients younger than 30 years. Arthroscopy. 2018;34:2530–6.
4. Nakagawa S, Mae T, Sato S, Okimura S, Kuroda M. Risk factors for the postoperative recurrence of instability after arthroscopic Bankart repair in athletes. Orthop J Sports Med. 2017;5:2325967117726494.
5. Porcellini G, Campi F, Pegreffi F, Castagna A, Paladini P. Predisposing factors for recurrent shoulder dislocation after arthroscopic treatment. J Bone Joint Surg Am. 2009;91:2537–42.
6. Voss JE, Livermore RW, Feeley BT, Altcheck DW, Williams RJ, Warren RF, Cordasco FA, Allen AA, HSS Sports Medicine Service. Prospective evaluation of arthroscopic Bankart repairs for anterior instability. Am J Sports Med. 2010;38:302–7.
7. Hovelius L, Augustini BG, Fredin H, Johansson O, Norlin R, Thorling J. Primary anterior dislocation of the shoulder in young patients. A ten-year prospective study. J Bone Joint Surg. 1996;78:1677–84.
8. Dumont GD, Russell RD, Robertson WJ. Anterior shoulder instability: a review of pathoanatomy, diagnosis and treatment. Curr Rev Musculoskelet Med. 2011;4:200–7.
9. Lippitt S, Matsen F. Mechanisms of glenohumeral joint stability. Clin Orthop Relat Res. 1993;291:20–8.
10. Olds M, Ellis R, Donaldson K, Parmar P, Kersten P. Risk factors which predispose first-time traumatic anterior shoulder dislocations to recurrent instability in adults: a systematic review and meta-analysis. Br J Sports Med. 2015;49:913–22.
11. Balg F, Boileau P. The instability severity index score. A simple pre-operative score to select patients for arthroscopic or open shoulder stabilization. J Bone Joint Surg Br. 2007;89:1470–7.
12. Milano G, Grasso A, Russo A, Magarelli N, Santagada DA, Deriu L, Baudi P, Bonomo L, Fabricciani C. Analysis of risk factors for glenoid bone defect in anterior shoulder instability. Am J Sports Med. 2011;39:1870–6.
13. Randelli P, Ragone V, Carminati S, Cabitza P. Risk factors for recurrence after Bankart repair: a systematic review. Knee Surg Sports Traumatol Arthrosc. 2012;20:2129–38.
14. Rouleau DM, Hébert-Davies J, Djahangiri A, Godbout V, Pelet S, Balg F. Validation of the instability shoulder index score in a multicenter reliability study in 114 consecutive cases. Am J Sports Med. 2013;41:278–82.
15. Seybold D, Schliemann B, Heyer CH, Muhr G, Gekle C. Which labral lesion can be reduced with external rotation of the shoulder after a first-time traumatic anterior shoulder dislocation? Arch Orthop Trauma Surg. 2009;129:229–304.
16. Kandziora F, Jäger A, Bischof F, Herresthal J, Starker M, Mittlmeier T. Arthroscopic labrum refixation for post-traumatic anterior shoulder instability: suture anchor versus transglenoid fixation technique. Arthroscopy. 2006;16:359–66.
17. Taylor DC, Arciero RA. Pathologic changes associated with shoulder dislocations. Arthroscopic and physical examination findings in first-time, traumatic anterior dislocations. Am J Sports Med. 1997;25:306–11.
18. Yiannakopoulos CK, Matargas E, Antonogiannakis E. A comparison of the spectrum of intra-articular lesions in acute and chronic anterior shoulder instability. Arthroscopy. 2007;23:985–90.

19. Provencher MT, Bhatia S, Ghodadra NS, Grumer RC, Bach BR Jr, Dewing CB, LeClere L, Romeo AA. Recurrent shoulder instability: current concepts for evaluation and management of glenoid bone loss. J Bone Joint Surg Am. 2010;92(Suppl 2):133–51.
20. Skendzel JG, Sekiya JK. Diagnosis and management of humeral head bone loss in shoulder instability. Am J Sports Med. 2012;40:2633–44.
21. Itoi E, Lee SB, Berglund LJ, Berge LL, An KN. The effect of a glenoid defect on anteroinferior stability of the shoulder after Bankart repair: a cadaveric study. J Bone Joint Surg Am. 2000;82:35–46.
22. Yamamoto N, Itoi E, Abe H, Kikuchi K, Seki N, Minagawa H, Tuoheti Y. Effect of an anterior glenoid defect on anterior shoulder stability: a cadaveric study. Am J Sports Med. 2009;37:949–54.
23. Piasecki DP, Verma NN, Romae AA, Levine WN, Bach BR Jr, Provencher MT. Glenoid bone deficiency in recurrent anterior shoulder instability: diagnosis and management. J Am Acad Orthop Surg. 2009;17:482–93.
24. Provencher MT, Frank RM, Leclere LE, Metzger PD, Ryu JJ, Bernhardson A, Romeo AA. The Hill–Sachs lesion: diagnosis, classification, and management. J Am Acad Orthop Surg. 2012;20:242–52.
25. Saliken DJ, Bornes TD, Bouliane MJ, Sheps DM, Beaupre LA. Imaging methods for quantifying glenoid and Hill–Sachs bone loss in traumatic instability of the shoulder: a scoping review. BMC Musculoskelet Disord. 2015;16:164.
26. Arciero RA, Parrino A, Bernhardson AS, Diaz-Doran V, Obopilwe E, Cote MP, Golijanin P, Mazzocca AD, Provencher MT. The effect of a combined glenoid and Hill–Sachs defect on glenohumeral stability: a biomechanical cadaveric study using 3-dimensional modeling of 142 patients. Am J Sports Med. 2015;43:1422–9.
27. Di Giacomo G, Itoi E, Burkhart SS. Evolving concept of bipolar bone loss and the Hill–Sachs lesion: from "engaging/non-engaging" lesion to "on-track/off-track" lesion. Arthroscopy. 2014;30:90–8.
28. Yamamoto N, Itoi E, Abe H, Minagawa H, Seki N, Shimada Y, Okada K. Contact between the glenoid and the humeral head in abduction, external rotation, and horizontal extension: a new concept of glenoid track. J Shoulder Elb Surg. 2007;16:649–56.

11 Arthroscopic Bankart Repair: How It Looks Today

Nuno Gomes, Mikel Aramberri, and Helder Fonte

11.1 Introduction

Shoulder instability is a common pathology and several treatment approaches are possible, from conservative to surgical. Still, several surgical techniques have been described to address this condition, each with different indications according to the pathological findings, patient's age, activity level and expectations [1].

Anterior instability of the shoulder results from different types of soft tissue alterations (Fig. 11.1), with or without bony defects. They may range from a classic Bankart lesion to other variants of capsulolabral lesions such as the Perthes lesion, a labral peel off to the glenoid neck also occurring with acute anterior instability, and the anterior labro-ligamentous periosteal sleeve avulsion (ALPSA) that has also been termed 'medialized Bankart lesion', which is more common in cases of recurrent than with first-time traumatic dislocations of the shoulder. The gleno labral articular disruption (GLAD) lesion is present when a superficial tear of the antero-inferior labrum is combined with a portion of articular cartilage of the contiguous quadrant of the glenoid and the humeral avulsion of glenohumeral ligaments (HAGL) lesion does not involve the labro-ligamentous complex at the glenoid, but represents an isolated tear of the IGHL at its humeral insertion following vigorous shoulder dislocation.

Besides the capsulolabral detachment from the glenoid leading to these well-described labral lesions, a plastic deformation of the capsule also occurs every time a shoulder dislocates, particularly at the first event. It is a phenomenon that is similar to what happens to a simple plastic bag that is stretched with the fingers. The deformation of the plastic after the first time it is stretched will never recover back to the previous condition.

It is this variability in the type and extent of the imaging and arthroscopic findings, along with the natural clinical history of each unstable shoulder, that makes it of utmost importance to precisely define the instability pattern in order to select the most appropriate treatment.

11.2 Background

Surgical treatment of the unstable shoulder has evolved significantly since the first descriptions of open techniques. With the increasing popularity of arthroscopy and improved techniques and implants, arthroscopic stabilization has

N. Gomes (✉)
Hospital das Forças Armadas and Hospital da Luz, Porto, Portugal

M. Aramberri
Alai Sport Medicine Clinic, Madrid, Spain

H. Fonte
Hospital das Forças Armadas and Centro Hospitalar do Porto, Porto, Portugal

R. Brzóska et al. (eds.), *360° Around Shoulder Instability*,
https://doi.org/10.1007/978-3-662-61074-9_11

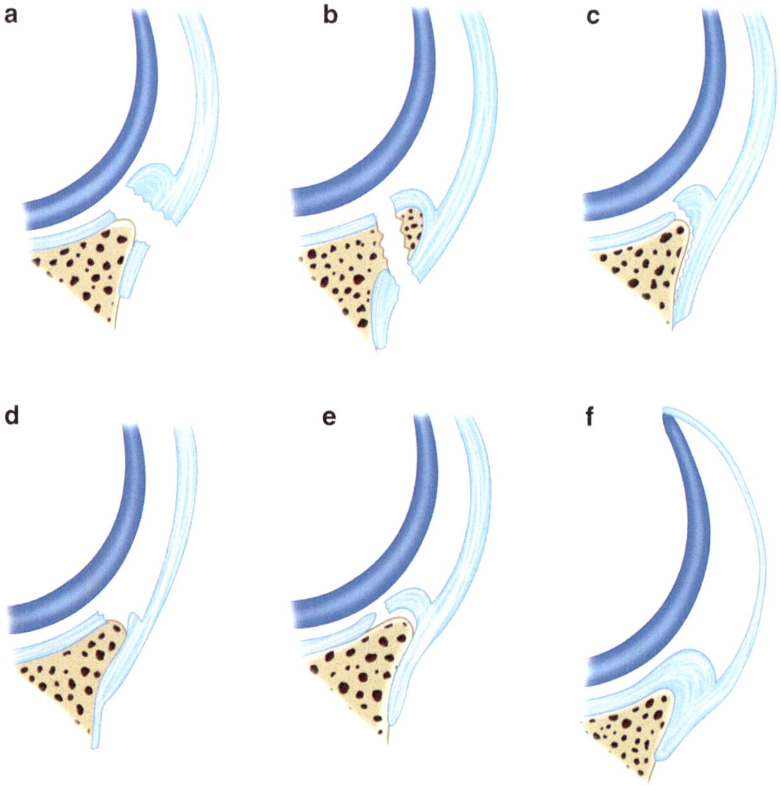

Fig. 11.1 Variants of labroligamentous lesions in the shoulder. (**a**) Bankart lesion; (**b**) Bony Bankart; (**c**) Perthes lesion; (**d**) ALPSA (Anterior Labro-ligamentous Periosteal Sleeve Avulsion); (**e**) GLAD (Gleno Labral Articular Disruption); (**f**) HAGL (Humeral Avulsion of Glenohumeral Ligaments)

very rapidly become an appealing and effective choice for the treatment of traumatic shoulder instability.

Early series on the results of arthroscopic repairs reported failure rates that were quite high, despite initial success rates [2, 3]. Later studies with longer follow-ups and updated surgical techniques comparing open and arthroscopic approaches reported variable results, from 3 to 18% after open techniques and 9 to 31% after arthroscopic techniques [4–8]. However, many others would state that there are no statistical differences between the two groups [9, 10]. One reason for such differences in results is the heterogeneity of the groups that were studied, considering that the indications for simple labral reconstruction are, for some, controversial. Furthermore, the techniques and implants used may have varied, offering today a higher potential for success.

11.3 Indications for Capsulolabral Repair

Whichever surgical technique is performed to address shoulder instability, the potential success of the arthroscopic or open procedures is similar as long as the surgeon is able to recognize and address all underlying relevant contributory pathologies. Many of the failures after isolated Bankart repair reported in the literature are probably due to improper patient selection and one must bear this fact in mind when interpreting scientific evidence.

Several pre-operative risk factors for failure after surgery have been recognized, namely, younger patient age, involvement in contact sports, important bony lesions in the glenoid and/or humeral head, hyperlaxity and concomitant rotator cuff or deltoid insufficiency. Still, even with correct recognition and consideration of these factors, it seems that underestimated capsular tears and deformation are the most common cause of failure after arthroscopic Bankart repair [1, 11–13] along with inadequate correction of an excessively large anteroinferior capsular pouch and detached capsulolabral complex with poor quality tissue, more common after multiple episodes of dislocations or subluxations.

Bony lesion assessment is of utmost importance. The presence of a bony Bankart defect is very frequent in revision patients [13] and one should clearly distinguish between loss of glenoid contour such as the 'classic inverted pear glenoid' and an avulsion fracture of the anterior glenoid. While the latter may be treated arthroscopically by an anatomical reconstruction with no major increase in the failure rate [1], the former often has an associated attenuation of the anteroinferior capsulolabral complex that contribute to further erosion of the anteroinferior glenoid. In such cases, it is generally accepted that when a bony loss of over 20% is present, surgery should ideally include a bony reconstruction procedure [14–17].

Besides glenoid bony amputations, bone defects on the humeral head side, which are present in virtually all cases of shoulder dislocations, can also contribute to recurrent instability. The volume and the location of a Hill–Sachs lesion will interfere in the likelihood of repetitive dislocations, and several attempts to quantify it in the most effective way have been described.

The concept of an 'engaging' Hill–Sachs was introduced in order to qualify the humeral head lesion as one at a higher risk of recurrence if treated with a classic arthroscopic capsulolabral repair [18], which only addresses the restoration of the anteroinferior soft tissues. Such 'engagement' would have to be checked under anaesthesia or arthroscopically as the locking of the humeral head bone defect on the anterior glenoid rim in external rotation and abduction of the shoulder. In fact, as many would say, all dislocating shoulders are 'engaging' before performing the Bankart repair, voiding this concept of its major value and potentially leading to overtreatment of 'engaging' Hill–Sachs lesions. Yamamoto [19] therefore introduced the 'glenoid track' concept, which evaluates the zone of contact between the glenoid and the humeral head that is modified according to the arm position. The need for specific calculations under imaging, such as MRI or CT scan with 3D reconstruction, has certainly compromised wide acceptance of this method for routine usage despite allowing an objective identification of those patients with bipolar lesions at a higher risk of recurrence following isolated Bankart repair.

11.4 Techniques and Hardware

Surgical repair of a Bankart lesion follows steps that have been thoroughly described. The main discussion today is over the correct indications and whether there is place or not for associated procedures. However, enhancements in the technique and evolutions on implants and instrumentation have offered the orthopaedic surgeon a broader set of options to manage this lesion.

Current evidence would argue that there is hardly room for open repair of the labrum today. Still, variations in the arthroscopic approach may be necessary to be able to offer the most safe and effective method.

Both lateral decubitus and beach chair positioning allow for excellent visualization but the former may be advantageous for intra-articular procedures—which include instability repairs—due to the permanent double traction to the arm (Fig. 11.2), which will maintain the head retracted with a spacious joint.

A standard posterior viewing portal is established, which allows for a first intra-articular observation and diagnosis, followed by one or two additional anterior portals.

An anterior–inferior portal, ideally chosen using an outside-in technique with a needle, is located right superior to the subscapularis tendon through the rotator interval and slightly lateral to the glenoid plan, in a fashion that permits drilling and placement of an anchor at around 45° angulation in respect to the glenoid surface and as low as possible on the anteroinferior glenoid rim (Fig. 11.3).

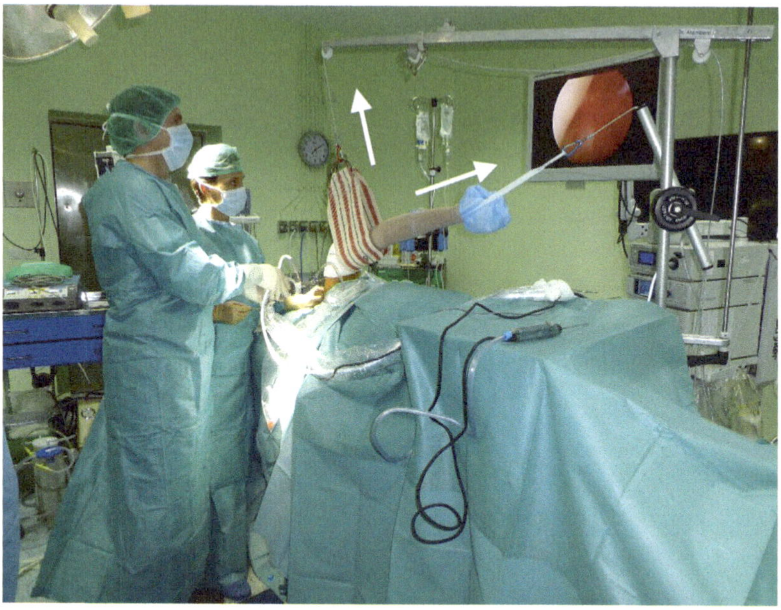

Fig. 11.2 Patient in lateral decubitus with permanent double traction to the arm, offering good joint distraction for hassle-free intra-articular arthroscopic procedures. According to the case, traction between 2 and 3 kg may be used on each vector

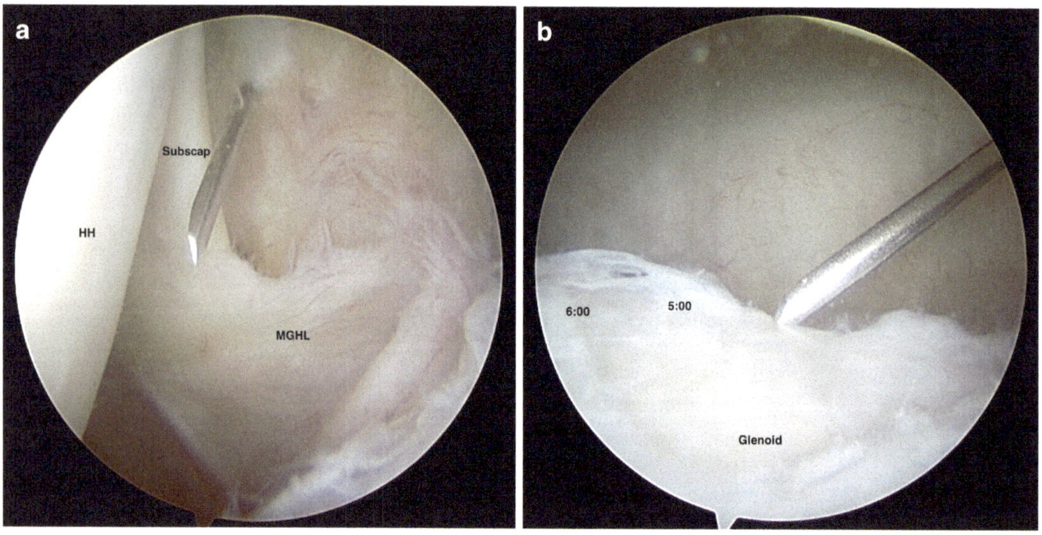

Fig. 11.3 Anterior-inferior rotator interval portal in a left shoulder; (**a**) located using an outside-in technique with a needle, right superior to the subscapularis tendon and slightly lateral to the glenoid plan, (**b**) allowing drilling and placement of the most inferior anchor at around 45° angulation in respect to the glenoid surface

A second anterior portal may be useful for both instrumentation and viewing (Fig. 11.4). It is placed at the superior border of the rotator interval, right behind the long biceps tendon, or directly through the pulley on top of the long biceps. Viewing from this portal may identify anterior labrum lesions more properly, allowing an easy mobilization and tensioning of the soft tissues, invaluable for a proper capsulolabral plication.

An alternative to this, in case a SLAP lesion repair is planned, is using a transcuff approach instead (Fig. 11.5), which can be used for both instrumentation and anchor placement in the superior labrum.

The use of a percutaneous 5:30 o'clock portal [20] through the subscapularis muscle is an option that can be very useful to place the lowest anterior anchor. It allows a safe drilling into the glenoid vault and avoids the risks of marginal drilling when using a rotator interval portal for that purpose.

It has been demonstrated that drilling for the most inferior anchor from a standard rotator interval portal will most likely perforate the far cortex on the inferior glenoid neck [21], with risks of iatrogenic lesion to the axillary nerve and of impairment of the anchor fixation. Following the placement of the anchor through this portal, subsequent handling of the sutures and soft tissue repairs are performed in a classical way using other portals.

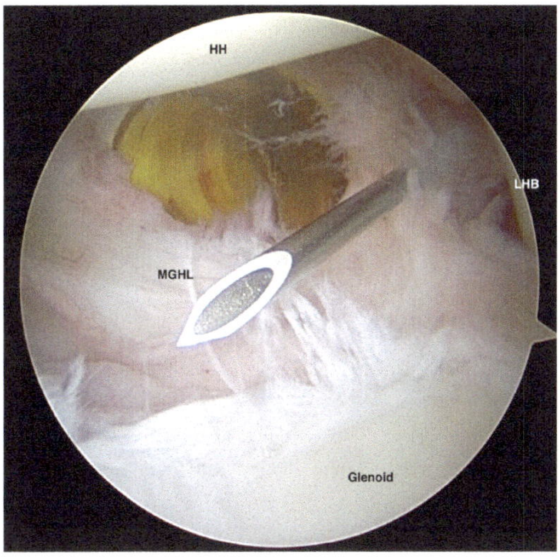

Fig. 11.4 A second anterior portal may be useful for both instrumentation and viewing at the superior border of the rotator interval, right behind the long biceps tendon, or directly through the pulley on top of the long biceps. Viewing from this portal may identify anterior labrum lesions more properly, allowing an easy mobilization and tensioning of the soft tissues, invaluable for a proper capsulolabral plication

To minimize this risk of missing the best drilling direction for the most inferior anchor, some companies offer the possibility of using a curved guide and a flexible drill, enabling an effective perforation of a tunnel inside bone, dispensing the 5:30 portal.

Fixation of the capsulolabral tissue to the glenoid rim can be effectively achieved by the usage of different types of anchors and suture configurations. Evolutions on these have been the rule since the advent of shoulder arthroscopy, with various reports contributing to a better knowledge of the biomechanical properties of the fixation today.

The recognition of the capsulolabral footprint led to the description of double-row fixations on the glenoid by Lafosse et al.—the Cassiopeia technique—and later by other surgeons [22–25], with significant improvement in functional outcomes with no major complications. However, in spite of laboratorial studies and a few low-strength studies with patients showing the time-zero strength of this technique, there is no clinical evidence that this option has advantages over the single row and the higher risks of complications and increased costs must not be underestimated.

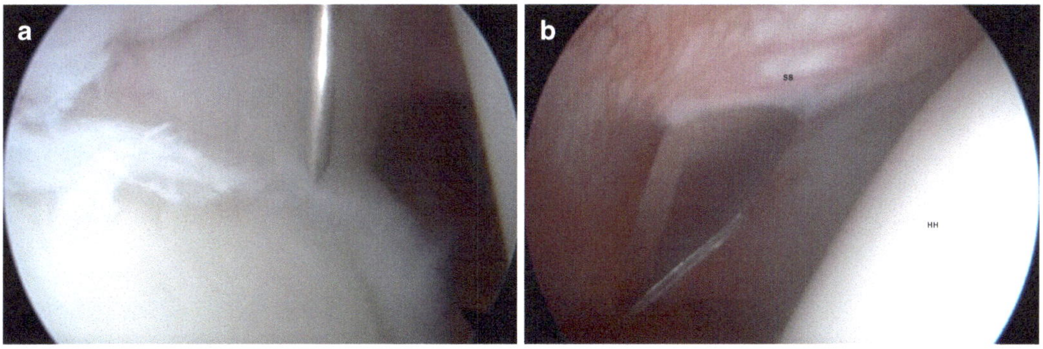

Fig. 11.5 Right shoulder. In the case of a SLAP lesion, a transcuff approach can be used for anchor placement in the superior labrum. The same portal can also be used for instrumentation for a 360° labral repair. (**a**) choosing the location; (**b**) one stab incision in line with the supraspinatus fibers

Other Bankart repair configurations are widely used and have deserved a dedicated comparison (Fig. 11.6). Classical knotted and knotless fixations, simple vertical stitch, horizontal mattress stitch, Mason–Allen (a combination of a mattress and single stitch with a double-loaded anchor) [11, 26], double-row and purse-string [27] techniques have all been presented as viable options but there is a lack of strong clinical evidence of advantages of one over another.

Double-row repair techniques have been shown to provide better coverage of the native footprint of the labrum but have not provided superior biomechanical properties in the lab compared to single-row repair techniques. There is no clear difference in footprint coverage, gapping, stiffness or biomechanical strength between the simple suture and horizontal mattress suture repair techniques [28]. Likewise, the same authors did not find any additional strength by using labral tape in double-row fixations.

Mattress type repairs are reportedly more effective in achieving a more anatomical reconstruction of the labral stump, potentially more similar to the native labral slope with a bumper effect, but they have been shown to offer identical biomechanical characteristics when compared to simple suture repairs [29]. In fact, laboratorial and post-operative studies with MRI have shown that the labral slope, height and morphology are reliably restored at 15 months after using bioabsorbable knotless anchors, similar to controls and other reports on simple knotted repairs [30]. There is also no difference in the radiological and clinical outcomes at, respectively, 6 months and at least 2 years after surgery between using a simple stitch and a modified Mason-Allen stitch in arthroscopic Bankart repairs [26].

The availability of different types of anchors in the market for this purpose today is very wide and they definitely deserve an overview, considering their role in the final clinical result. Major evolutions have taken place concerning this matter since the advent of shoulder arthroscopy in order to increase its success and limit the risk of complications.

Despite the good results of the first reports on arthroscopic Bankart repairs, the rate, pattern and extent of the complications due to the usage of metallic suture anchors in the glenoid

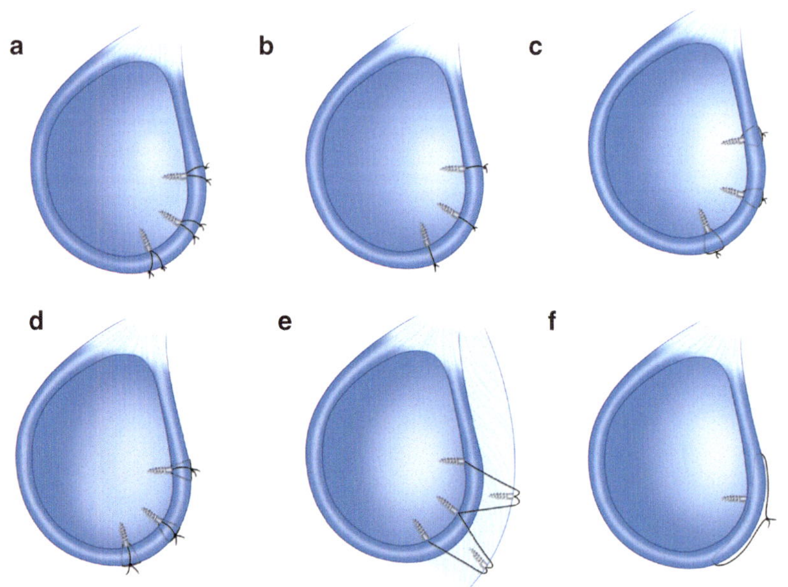

Fig. 11.6 Bankart repair configurations: (**a**) vertical stitch with double-loaded anchor, (**b**) simple vertical stitch with single-loaded anchor (knotted or knotless), (**c**) horizontal mattress stitch, (**d**) Mason–Allen, a combination of a mattress and single stitch with a double-loaded anchor [11, 26], (**e**) double-row and (**f**) purse-string [27] techniques

lead to a shift from metallic to bioabsorbable implants [31–33]. The acceptance of 'arguably' biodegradable suture anchors, such as the slowly degrading pure PLLA (poly-L-lactic acid) or more rapidly degrading biocomposite PLLA/β-tricalcium phosphate-based anchors was, for that reason, very high among orthopaedic surgeons. Nevertheless, even these are not risk-free, with reports on breakage, osteolysis, chondrolysis and synovitis after using them [34] and therefore the constant evolution in implant types and profiles, with older anchors and techniques being replaced with newer ones as technology develops. Besides biodegradable lactide-containing suture anchors, other innovations included the use of polyetheretherketone (PEEK) as the anchor material, the addition of multiple high-strength sutures made in part or entirely with ultrahigh molecular weight polyethylene (UHMWPE) and the development of 'knotless' designs.

PEEK is a radiolucent but not biodegradable plastic suitable for a variety of implants that has the advantages of being high strength, enabling good post-operative imaging and facilitating revision surgery because it is soft enough to be drilled through [35]. However, complications due to the fact that it is a rigid implant are not negligible and therefore the appeal for newer options, such as the all-suture anchors.

All-suture anchors are made using UHMWPE—the material of which virtually all the anchors' sutures currently in the market are made of—and perform very well in terms of pull-out strength in the lab, in some cases better than their rigid counterparts [35, 36]. However, some biomechanical concerns have been reported with the use of these newer anchors, namely, the first-generation ones [37], concerning load to failure and bone cyst formation [38]. A direct comparison between an all-soft and a rigid biocomposite glenoid anchor revealed a histologic and biomechanical response in dogs [38] that brought some concern about the former, by means of a large cyst-like cavity formation with a rim of dense lamellar bone in the anchor sites. This potential risk for clinical failure has motivated further studies and another group found satisfying radiological and clinical outcomes after arthroscopic instability surgery using first-generation all-suture anchors in human patients [39]. Unlike the canine models of the previous report, these patients followed a classical post-op protocol that included immobilization, and imaging at early follow-up (12–28 months) revealed good labral healing without important bony reaction or the formation of large cysts.

In spite of some differences in displacement after cyclic loading between different all-soft anchors for the glenoid [40], it has been demonstrated that this phenomenon can be minimized by slightly reducing the insertion depth for the anchor [41] which will minimize the amount of bone stock that is destroyed with a deep drilling. At the end of the day, its overall efficacy compares favourably to standard solid anchors for labral repairs.

Knotless anchors for labral repair have been an appealing option for some time now and have been subject to several comparisons in the literature. They offer the advantage of a quicker and easier repair, diminishing the potential for errors, and absence of a bulky knot stack that may lead to early osteoarthritis when present and rubbing against the chondral surface. Furthermore, the rate of glove and skin lacerations is lower, recognized as a risk for both the patient and the surgeon when tying knots. [42]

While some studies report no significant differences between the two options [43, 44], others report worse clinical results using knotless anchors when compared to classical knot-tying suture anchors [45].

But one must be judicious when interpreting these scientific conclusions. Generally speaking, there are two different kinds of knotless labral anchors available, demanding either an 'anchor first' or 'suture first' technique for their usage. All the comparisons available in the literature consider the 'suture first' technique anchors, which, as recurrently reported, do not allow the best estimation of the tension to give the sutures and respective soft tissues fixation.

However, an 'anchor first' technique, due to its different method of application and tissue fixation, does not present with the same issue and may be a valuable option without such limitation (Fig. 11.7).

Regardless of the type of anchor that is used, a satisfactory capsular shift is mandatory whenever there is a need to reduce the capsular volume, which is normally the case. Previous reports have demonstrated that a minimum of three double-loaded suture anchors had to be used for that purpose [1] but another one states that one or two anchors could be enough, as long as the capsulolabral tissue is plicated as desired [27].

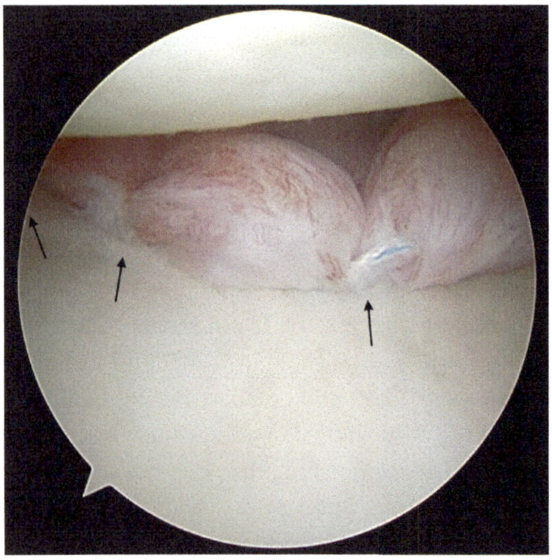

Fig. 11.7 Capsulolabral repair in a left shoulder using a knotless 'anchor first' technique, showing two out of three all-soft anchors with no proud knot stack

It seems today that all-soft anchors, being less invasive and requiring a significantly smaller bone tunnel than rigid suture anchors, may reduce the risk of hardware complications such as secondary joint damage or glenoid fracture, and at the same time allow a safer drilling for multiple anchors into a small anatomic area, in case of failure of a previous one or in the revision setting. Besides, in the event of marginal tunnel drilling or perforation of the far cortex, the fact that these anchors only require an intact cortical surface for proper seating will likely diminish the risk of their loosening (Fig. 11.8).

These facts may eventually lead to better clinical results in the long run and widen the indications for soft tissue repairs, compared to bony procedures.

Still, objective criteria are necessary in order to take a better-informed decision on the treatment of an unstable shoulder.

11.5 Discussion and Conclusion

Given the subjectivity and lack of consensus on the surgical management of shoulder instability, Balg and Boileau [46] proposed a simple ten-

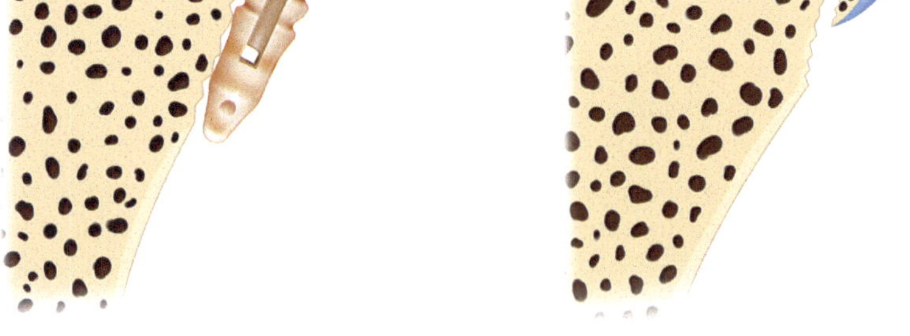

Fig. 11.8 The thin tunnel for all-soft anchors allows multiple anchors into a small anatomic area, in case of failure of a previous one or in the revision setting. In the event of marginal tunnel drilling or perforation of the far cortex, the sole requirement for an intact cortical surface for proper seating, usage of a soft anchor will likely diminish the risk of their loosening

point scale Instability Severity Index Score (ISIS) to determine the risk of recurrence following isolated arthroscopic Bankart repair. It considers several prognostic factors, which, if present, add up 1 or 2 points to the final score: age below 20, being into competitive, contact or overhead sports, hyperlaxity and important bony losses either on the humeral head (Hill–Sachs lesion) or the glenoid. A score of 3 or less was associated with a 5% recurrence rate and a score above 4 was associated with an unacceptable recurrence rate after an isolated Bankart repair and therefore a bony reconstruction should be performed. In spite of some recognized weaknesses [47, 48], the ISIS is a useful tool for the surgeon to choose the optimal surgical treatment and minimize the risk of recurrent instability.

Still, many questions remain unanswered concerning this matter, despite substantial progress made in the understanding of risk factors for recurrence following surgical treatment of anterior shoulder instability.

Arthroscopic remplissage for anterior instability has become an adjunct to Bankart repairs since it was first described in 2008 as a means to augment the labral repair in patients with subcritical glenoid bone loss.

However, the critical level of glenoid bone loss requiring bone grafting or coracoid transfer is not clearly defined, ranging from 10 to 25% according to different researchers [49]. This led to the definition of the glenoid track concept as a means for defining the need for isolated Bankart with or without remplissage versus Latarjet [50] as described in another chapter of this book. It is a valid tool to guide the surgeon but, like other tools available for the same purpose, has limitations, since it is often difficult, inaccurate and not very practical to calculate and does not account for soft tissue quality and patient factors such as age and sex.

Taking this into account as well as evidence that the soft tissues repair is of undeniable importance, even when performing a Latarjet [51], it is clear that a proper capsulolabral reconstruction has a major place in shoulder instability treatment today.

References

1. Boileau P, Villalba M, Héry JY, Balg F, Ahrens P, Neyton L. Risk factors for recurrence of shoulder instability after arthroscopic Bankart repair. J Bone Joint Surg Am. 2006;88(8):1755–63.
2. Grana WA, Buckley PD, Yates CK. Arthroscopic Bankart suture repair. Am J Sports Med. 1993;21:348–53.
3. Green MR, Christensen KP. Arthroscopic Bankart repair: two to five year follow-up with clinical correlation to severity of glenoid labral lesion. Am J Sports Med. 1995;23:276–81.
4. Bacilla P, Field LD, Savoie FH. Arthroscopic Bankart repair in a high demand patient population. Arthroscopy. 1997;13:51–60.
5. Gartsman GM, Roddey TS, Hammerman SM. Arthroscopic treatment of anterior-inferior glenohumeral instability. J Bone Joint Surg. 2000;82:991–1003.
6. Cole BJ, L'Insalata J, Irrgang J, Warner JJP. Comparison of arthroscopic and open anterior shoulder stabilization. J Bone Joint Surg. 2000;82:1108–14.
7. Sperber A, Hamberg P, Karlsson J, et al. Comparison of an arthroscopic and an open procedure for posttraumatic instability of the shoulder: a prospective randomized multicenter study. J Shoulder Elbow Surg. 2001;10:105–8.
8. Provencher MT. Editorial commentary: is it time to take a stand? When arthroscopic Bankart repair is no longer a viable option for anterior shoulder instability. Arthroscopy. 2018;34(9):2537–40.
9. Fabbriciani C, Milano G, Demontis A, Fadda S, Ziranu F, Mulas PD. Arthroscopic versus open treatment of Bankart lesion of the shoulder: a prospective randomized study. Arthroscopy. 2004;20:456–62.
10. Harris JD, Gupta AK, Mall NA, et al. Long-term outcomes after Bankart shoulder stabilization. Arthroscopy. 2013;29(5):920–33.
11. Castagna A, Conti M, Moushine E, Delle Rose G, Massazza G, Garofalo R. A new technique to improve tissue grip and contact force in arthroscopic capsulolabral repair: the MIBA stitch. Knee Surg Sports Traumatol Arthrosc. 2008;16:415–9.
12. Mologne TF, McBride MT, Lapoint JM. Assessment of failed arthroscopic anterior labral repairs: findings at open surgery. Am J Sports Med. 1997;25:813–7.
13. Tauber M, Resch H, Forstner R, Raffl M, Schauer J. Reasons for failure after surgical repair of anterior instability. J Shoulder Elbow Surg. 2004;13(3):279–85.
14. Arce G, Arcuri F, Ferro D, Pereira E. Is selective arthroscopic revision beneficial for treating recurrent anterior shoulder instability? Clin Orthop Relat Res. 2012;479(4):965–71.
15. Bartl C, Schumann K, Paul J, Vogt S, Imhoff AB. Arthroscopic capsulolabral revision repair for

recurrent anterior shoulder instability. Am J Sports Med. 2011;39:511–8.
16. Mologne TS, Provencher MT, Menzel KA, et al. Arthroscopic stabilization in patients with an inverted pear glenoid: results in patients with bone loss of the anterior glenoid. Am J Sports Med. 2007;35(8):1276–83.
17. Provencher MT, Arciero RA, Burkhart SS, Levine WN, Ritting AW, Romeo AA. Key factors in primary and revision surgery for shoulder instability. Instr Course Lect. 2010;59:227–44.
18. Burkhart SS, De Beer JF. Traumatic glenohumeral bone defects and their relationship to failure of arthroscopic Bankart repairs: significance of the inverted-pear glenoid and the humeral engaging Hill–Sachs lesion. Arthroscopy. 2000;16:677–94.
19. Yamamoto N, Itoi E, Abe H, et al. Contact between the glenoid and the humeral head in abduction, external rotation, and horizontal extension: a new concept of glenoid track. J Shoulder Elbow Surg. 2007;16(5):649–56.
20. Imhoff AB, Ansah P, Tischer T, et al. Arthroscopic repair of anterior-inferior glenohumeral instability using a portal at the 5:30 o'clock position: analysis of the effects of age, fixation method, and concomitant shoulder injury on surgical outcomes. Am J Sports Med. 2010;38(9):1795–803.
21. Lim TK, Koh KH, Lee SH, Shon MS, Bae TS, Park WH, Yoo JC. Inferior anchor cortical perforation with arthroscopic bankart repair: a cadaveric study. Arthroscopy. 2013;29(1):31–6.
22. Lafosse L, Baier GP, Jost B. Footprint fixation for arthroscopic reconstruction in anterior shoulder instability: the Cassiopeia double-row technique. Arthroscopy. 2006;22(2):231.e1–6.
23. Iwaso H, Uchiyama E, Sakakibara S, Fukui N. Modified double-row technique for arthroscopic Bankart repair: surgical technique and preliminary results. Acta Orthop Belg. 2011;77(2):252–7.
24. Wade R, Reddy PVB. Functional outcome of arthroscopic double row repair for Bankart lesion. J Orthop. 2018;15(3):792–7. https://doi.org/10.1016/j.jor.2018.03.021. eCollection 2018 Sep
25. McDonald LS, Thompson M, Altchek DW, McGarry MH, Lee TQ, Rocchi VJ, Dines JS. Doublerow capsulolabral repair increases load to failure and decreases excessive motion. Arthroscopy. 2016;32(11):2218–25. https://doi.org/10.1016/j.arthro.2016.03.025. Epub 2016 May 18
26. Park JY, Chung SW, Lee JS, Oh KS, Lee JH. Comparison of clinical and radiographic outcomes of vertical simple stitch versus modified Mason-Allen Stitch in arthroscopic Bankart repairs: a prospective randomized controlled study. Am J Sports Med. 2019;47(2):398–407.
27. Witney-Lagen C, Perera N, Rubin S, Venkateswaran B. Fewer anchors achieves successful arthroscopic shoulder stabilization surgery: 114 patients with 4 years of follow-up. J Shoulder Elbow Surg. 2014;23(3):382–7.
28. Judson CH, Voss A, Obopilwe E, Dyrna F, Arciero RA, Shea KP. An anatomic and biomechanical comparison of Bankart repair configurations. Am J Sports Med. 2017;45(13):3004–9.
29. Boddula MR, Adamson GJ, Gupta A, McGarry MH, Lee TQ. Restoration of labral anatomy and biomechanics after superior labral anterior-posterior repair - comparison of mattress versus simple technique. Am J Sports Med. 2012;40(4):875–81.
30. Stein T, Mehling AP, Reck C, Buckup J, Efe T, Hoffmann R, Jaeger A, Welsch F. MRI assessment of the structural labrum integrity after Bankart repair using knotless bio-anchors. Knee Surg Sports Traumatol Arthrosc. 2011;19:1771–9.
31. Papalia R, Franceschi F, Diaz Balzani L, D'Adamio S, Denaro V, Maffulli N. The arthroscopic treatment of shoulder instability: bioabsorbable and standard metallic anchors produce equivalent clinical results. Arthroscopy. 2014;30(9):1173–83.
32. Silver MD, Daigneault JP. Symptomatic interarticular migration of glenoid suture anchors. Arthroscopy. 2000;16(1):102–5.
33. Ozbaydar M, Elhassan B, Warner JJ. The use of anchors in shoulder surgery: a shift from metallic to bioabsorbable anchors. Arthroscopy. 2007;23(10):1124–6.
34. Cobaleda AF, Sanders EJ, Barber FA. Adverse events associated with biodegradable lactide-containing suture anchors. Arthroscopy. 2014;30(5):555–60.
35. Barber FA, Herbert MA, Hapa O, Rapley JH, Barber CA, Bynum JA, Hrnack SA. Biomechanical analysis of pullout strengths of rotator cuff and glenoid anchors: 2011 update. Arthroscopy. 2011;27(7):895–905.
36. Barber FA, Herbert MA. Cyclic loading biomechanical analysis of the pullout strengths of rotator cuff and glenoid anchors: 2013 update. Arthroscopy. 2013;29(5):832–44.
37. Erickson J, Chiarappa F, Haskel J, Rice J, Hyatt A, Monica J, Dhawan A. Biomechanical comparison of a first- and a second-generation all-soft sutureglenoid anchor. Orthop J Sports Med. 2017;5(7):2325967117717010. https://doi.org/10.1177/2325967117717010. eCollection 2017 Jul
38. Pfeiffer FM, Smith MJ, Cook JL, Kuroki K. The histologic and biomechanical response of two commercially available small glenoid anchors for use in labral repairs. J Shoulder Elbow Surg. 2014;23(8):1156–61.
39. Willemot L, Elfadalli R, Jaspars KC, Mark H, Ahw MH, Peeters J, Jansen N, Declerq G, Verborgt O. Radiological and clinical outcome of arthroscopic labral repair with all-suture anchors. Acta Orthop Belg. 2016;82:174–8.
40. Ruder JA, Dickinson EY, Peindl RD, Habet NA, Fleischli JE. Cyclic and load-to-failure properties of all-suture anchors in human cadaveric shoulder glenoid bone. Arthroscopy. 2019. pii: S0749-8063(19)30061-1.
41. Ruder JA, Dickinson EY, Habet N, Peindl RD, D'Alessandro DF, Fleischli JE. Slight reduction in the insertion depth for an all-suture anchor decreases

cyclic displacement in the shoulder glenoid. Arthroscopy. 2018;34(5):1384–90.
42. Ng DZ, Kumar VP. Arthroscopic Bankart repair using knot-tying versus knotless suture anchors: is there a difference? Arthroscopy. 2014;30(4):422–7.
43. Martinez A, Han Y, Sardar ZM, Beckman L, Steffen T, Miller BS, Martineau PA. Risk of glove perforation with arthroscopic knot tying using different surgical gloves and high-tensile strength sutures. Arthroscopy. 2013;29(9):1552–8.
44. Kocaoglu B, Guven O, Nalbantoglu U, Aydin N, Haklar U. No difference between knotless sutures and suture anchors in arthroscopic repair of Bankart lesions in collision athletes. Knee Surg Sports Traumatol Arthrosc. 2009;17(7):844–9.
45. Cho NS, Lubis AM, Ha JH, Rhee YG. Clinical results of arthroscopic Bankart repair with knot-tying and knotless suture anchors. Arthroscopy. 2006;22(12):1276–82.
46. Balg F, Boileau P. The instability severity index score. A simple pre-operative score to select patients for arthroscopic or open shoulder stabilisation. J Bone Joint Surg Br. 2007;89(11):1470–7.
47. Rouleau DM, Hebert-Davies J, Djahangiri A, Godbout V, Pelet S, Balg F. Validation of the instability shoulder index score in a multicenter reliability study in 114 consecutive cases. Am J Sports Med. 2013;41(2):278–82.
48. Ruiz Ibán MA, Asenjo Gismero CV, Moros Marco S, Ruiz Díaz R, Del Olmo Hernández T, Del Monte Bello G, García Navlet M, Ávila Lafuente JL, Díaz Heredia J. Instability severity index score values below 7 do not predict recurrence after arthroscopic Bankart repair. Knee Surg Sports Traumatol Arthrosc. 2019;27(12):3905–11. https://doi.org/10.1007/s00167-019-05471-w.
49. Lazarides AL, Duchman KR, Ledbetter L, Riboh JC, Garrigues GE. Arthroscopic remplissage for anterior shoulder instability: a systematic review of clinical and biomechanical studies. Arthroscopy. 2019;35:617–28.
50. Di Giacomo G, Itoi E, Burkhart SS. Evolving concept of bipolar bone loss and the Hill-Sachs lesion: from "engaging/ non-engaging" lesion to "on-track/ off-track" lesion. Arthroscopy. 2014;30:90–8.
51. Cuéllar A, Cuéllar R, de Heredia PB. Arthroscopic revision surgery for failure of open latarjet technique. Arthroscopy. 2017;33(5):910–7.

ASA, an Arthroscopic Technique for Recurrent Anterior Dislocations Using Partial Subscapularis Tenodesis in Association with Bankart Repair

12

Marco Maiotti, Raffaele Russo, Giuseppe Della Rotonda, and Cecilia Rao

12.1 Introduction

Over the past decades, arthroscopic treatment of recurrent anterior dislocations has become the most popular method to repair the atraumatic or post-traumatic capsulo-labral defect [1]. In fact, these techniques achieved good results in terms of restoration of joint function and a relapse rate comparable with open surgery, especially if the glenoid and humeral head bone morphology are quite normal [2–4]. In case of glenohumeral bone defects, such as anterior glenoid bone loss and engaging Hill Sachs lesions, the percentage of re-dislocation grows up to a higher percentage until 67% [5–7]. Other techniques such as Bankart repair plus Remplissage [8, 9] to the open or all-arthroscopic Bristow-Latarjet [10–13] and bone graft procedures [14–16] are used as an effective alternative to treat shoulder instability, with gleno-humeral defects.

M. Maiotti (✉)
Shoulder-Knee Unit, Mediterranea Clinic, Napoli, Italy

R. Russo · G. Della Rotonda
Orthopaedics and Traumatology Unit, Pineta Grande Hospital, Caserta, Italy

C. Rao
Orthopaedics and Traumatology Unit, San Giovanni Evangelista Hospital, Rome, Italy

No study demonstrates actually which arthroscopic technique should be used in young and sportive patients with subsidence of capsulo-labral structures or hyperlaxity without severe anterior glenoid bone loss.

In 1986, Johnson described an arthroscopic technique for recurrent shoulder dislocation in patients with 'virtually nonexistent glenohumeral ligaments' using the articular portion of the subscapularis tendon [17]. Despite the numerous advantages of the arthroscopic approach, Johnson's technique was abandoned because of potential complications related to the placement of metal staples for tendon fixation adjacent to the level of the glenoid edge.

Starting from Johnson' idea, Maiotti and Massoni in 2010 developed a new surgical technique that was a combination of a Bankart repair and an arthroscopic subscapularis augmentation (ASA) (Fig. 12.1) consisting of a tenodesis of the upper third of the tendon [18]. The number of patients treated with this technique is increasing over time, with more than 600 cases in different hospitals. The surgical skills have been implemented in a biomechanical study to attest the stability, and have been perfomed [19] using ASA in association with Bankart with relative glenoid bone loss inferior to 20%, and a series of 72 patients have been studied to attest arthropathy at mid-term follow-up.

R. Brzóska et al. (eds.), *360° Around Shoulder Instability*,
https://doi.org/10.1007/978-3-662-61074-9_12

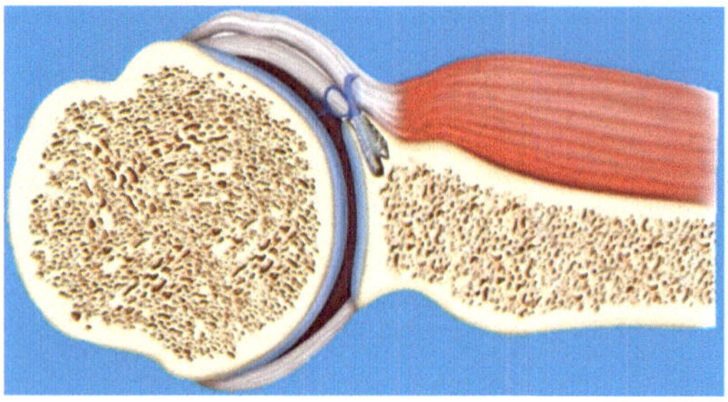

Fig. 12.1 Tenodesis of the upper third of the subscapularis

Table 12.1 Indication and contraindication for ASA technique

Indication	Contraindication
Hyperlaxity or capsular insufficiency associated with glenoid bone defect of less than 10% in patients practising contact sports	Multi-directional instability
Hyperlaxity or capsular insufficiency associated with glenoid bone defect between 10 and 20% in patients who do not practise contact sport	Gleno-humeral osteoarthritis Throwing sports Subscapular tendon lesions

12.2 Algorithm of Treatment

Given the several pathomechanical aspects of chronic anterior instabilities, we are working to rationalize the use of the upper part of subscapularis tendon among other treatment techniques. The common parameters to be considered for the most suitable use of the subscapularis tendon in association with a simple Bankart repair are: clinical observation of more than 90° of external rotation position at ER1 in the supine position; pain and positive apprehension test also in ER1 position between 80° and 90° of external rotation; intraoperative observation of inadequate soft tissues anatomy due to the chronic instability or high superior traction mobility of the subscapularis tendon.

The indications for Bankart repair associated with ASA are (Table 12.1):

- Hyperlaxity or capsular insufficiency associated with glenoid bone defect of less than 10% in patients practising contact sports
- Hyperlaxity or capsular insufficiency associated with glenoid bone defect between 10 and 20% in patients who do not practise contact sport

Contraindications to perform this type of procedure are the following: multi-directional instability, gleno-humeral osteoarthritis, throwing sports, subscapular tendon lesions.

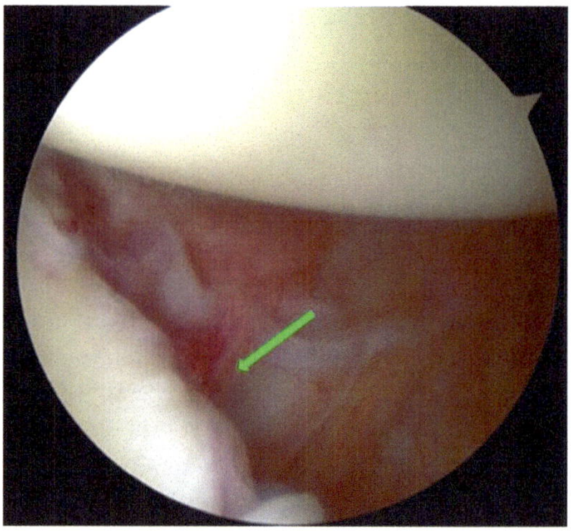

Fig. 12.2 Capsulo-labral lesion

12.3 Bankart Repair and Subscapularis Augmentation: Surgical Technique

The procedure was performed with the patient under an inter-scalene block or under a blended anaesthesia in the lateral decubitus position.

Standard anterior and posterior portals were used. The anterior and posterior gleno-humeral joint structures were inspected to assess any anteroinferior labral insufficiency (Fig. 12.2), superior labrum anterior-posterior (SLAP) lesions, anterior glenoid defects and Hill–Sachs

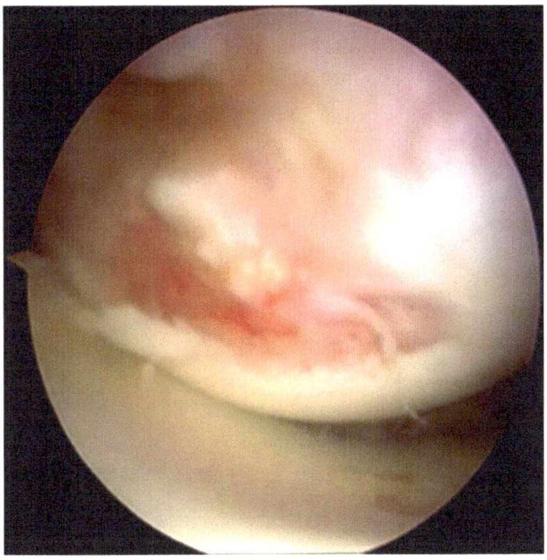

Fig. 12.3 Hill–Sachs lesion

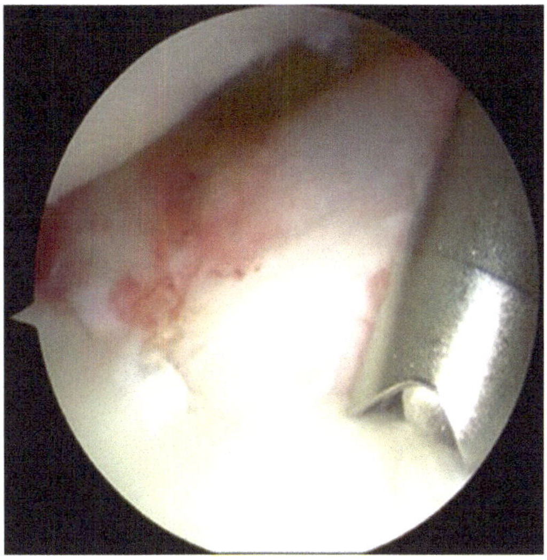

Fig. 12.4 Glenoid hole for subscapularis fixation

lesions (Fig. 12.3) and to confirm the anterior displacement of the humeral head with respect to the glenoid cavity. An additional anterior–superior portal was used.

A lower capsular repair was performed with 2.9 mm non-absorbable knotless suture anchors loaded with multi-strand sutures.

The subscapularis fixation bone hole should be done over the top of the glenoid corner (Fig. 12.4). We systematically performed the superior subscapular is traction test (SSTT) to test with a graduate gripper the elasticity of the subscapularis tubular part of tendon in order to fix and give it the proper tension between 2 and 3 o'clock in a right shoulder or 10 and 11 in the left side (Figs. 12.5 and 12.6).

After testing, the upper third of the subscapularis tendon was penetrated at least 5 mm from its superior border with a penetrator punch loaded with multi-strand tape (Labral tape, Arthrex); the tape is then retrieved from the upper cannula and then passed again in the lower cannula so that the free ends of the tape remain accessible through the same lower cannula (Fig. 12.7).

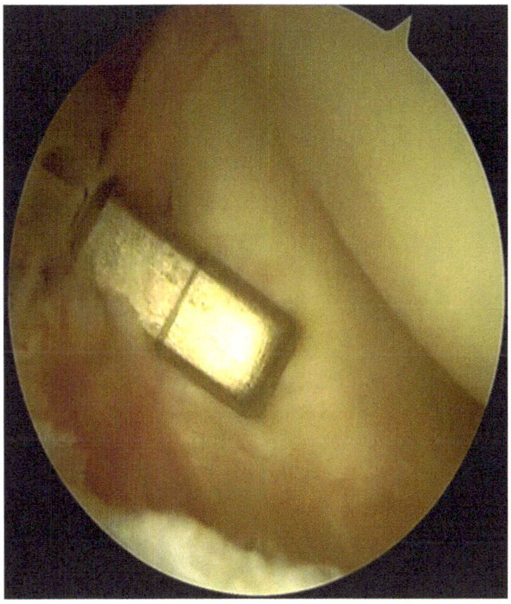

Fig. 12.5 Non-elastic tendon

A loop is created by passing the two ends of the tape through the loop in the middle of the suture (Fig. 12.8).

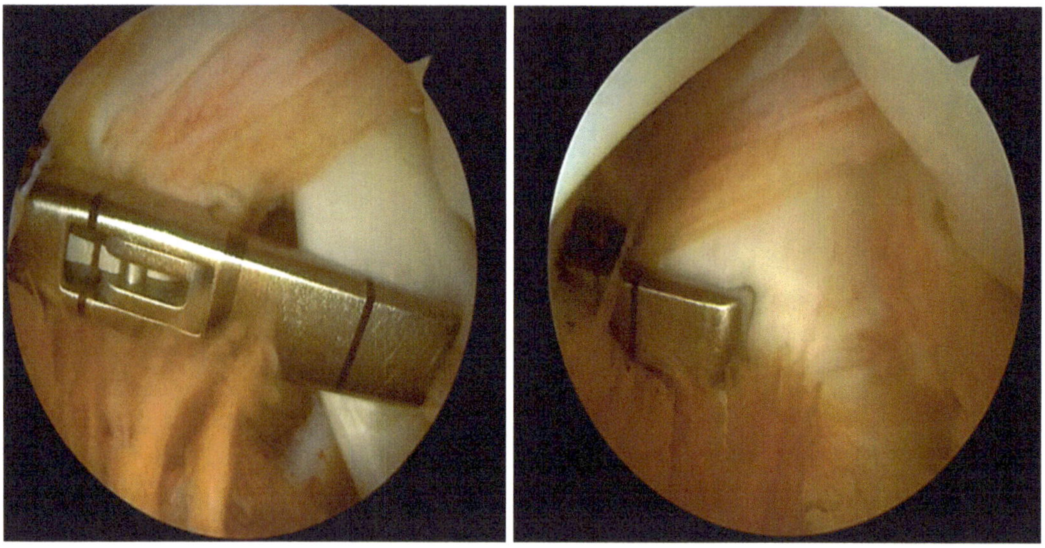

Fig. 12.6 Elastic tendon

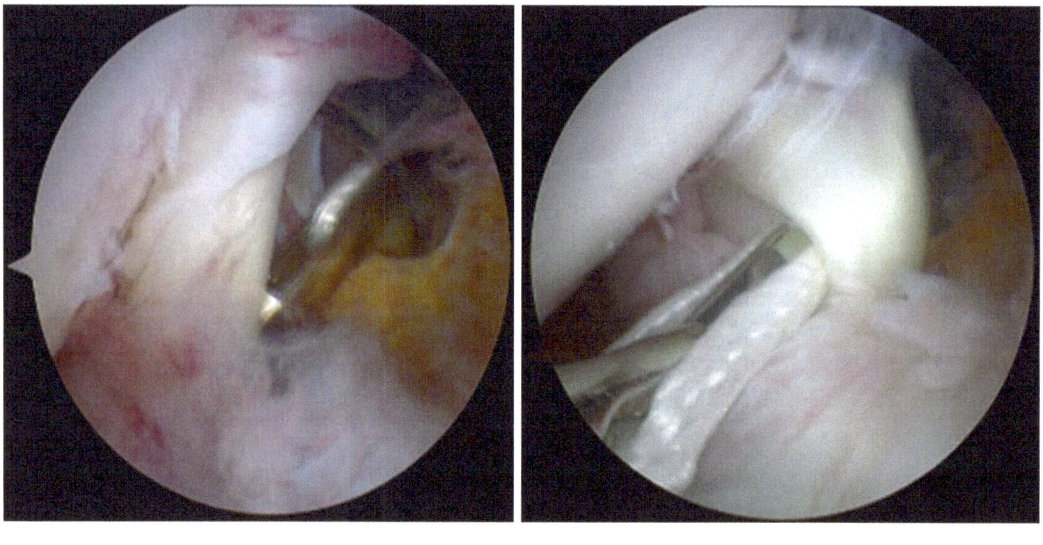

Fig. 12.7 Penetrator punch loaded with multi-strand tape through the subscapularis

At this point, both free ends of the tape are passed through the eyelet's anchor (3.5 mm knotless PEEK suture anchor [PushLock]) that is pushed along the tape towards the bone hole.

While impacting the anchor (Fig. 12.9), care is taken to keep the patient's arm in neutral rotation to avoid excessive tensioning on the tenodesis. The repair, including complete closure of the anterior pouch and centring of the humeral head in the glenoid cavity, was assessed by arthroscopic examination from the antero-superior portal (Figs. 12.10 and 12.11).

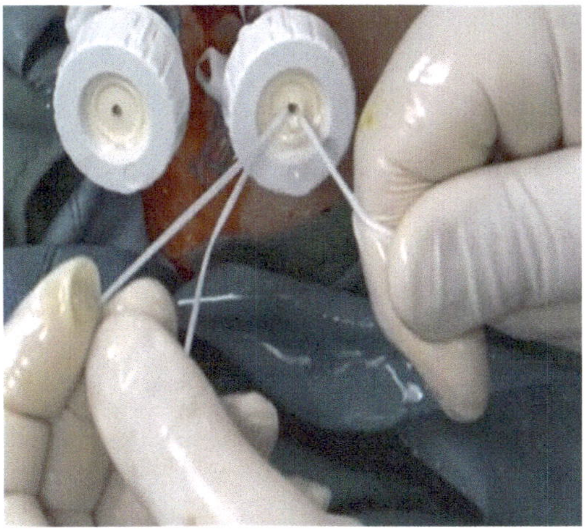

Fig. 12.8 A loop made outside to grab the subscapularis

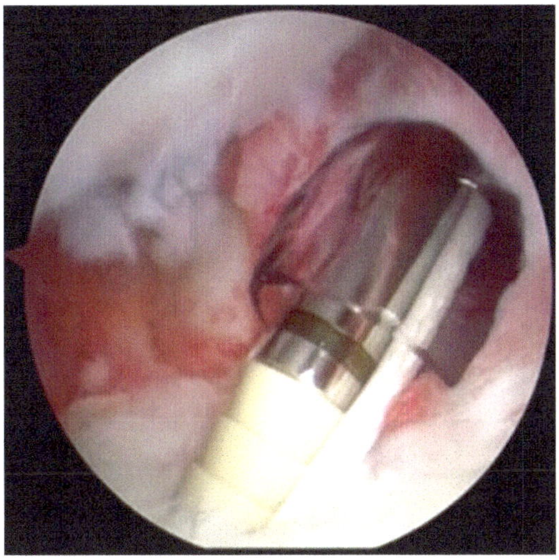

Fig. 12.9 Anchor insertion-loaded multi-strand tape

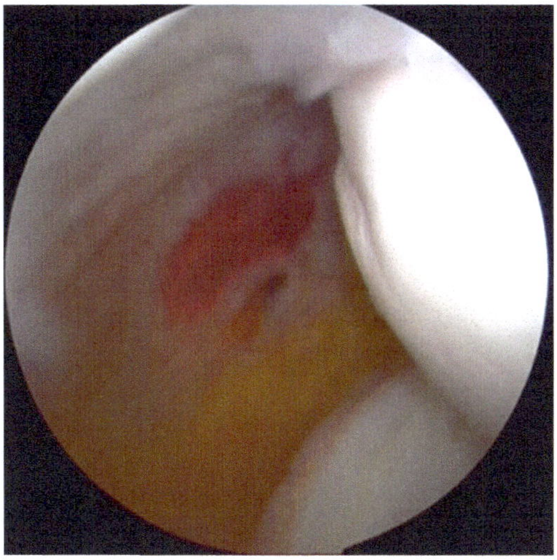

Fig. 12.10 Final view from posterior portal

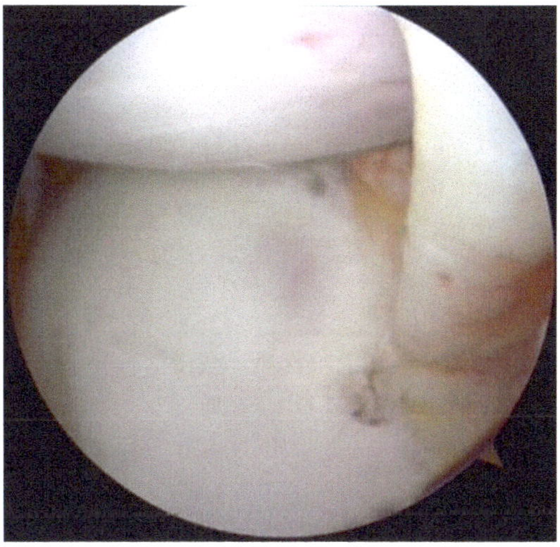

Fig. 12.11 Final view from antero-superior portal

12.4 Biomechanical Study

In order to examine the biomechanical effect of the ASA procedure on gleno-humeral joint motion and stability, a biomechanical study has been performed to investigate the stabilizing effect of the ASA procedure on translation and rotation in the gleno-humeral joint after Bankart lesion with additional bony defect [20].

Eight human cadaver shoulder specimens, without evidence of rotator cuff tear and shoulder injury in their medical history, were investigated and tested using a robot based on a shoulder simulator (Fig. 12.12).

Translational stability and range of motion was tested in each specimen in four different configurations: physiologic, Bankart lesion with bony defect, simple Bankart repair and Bankart repair plus ASA.

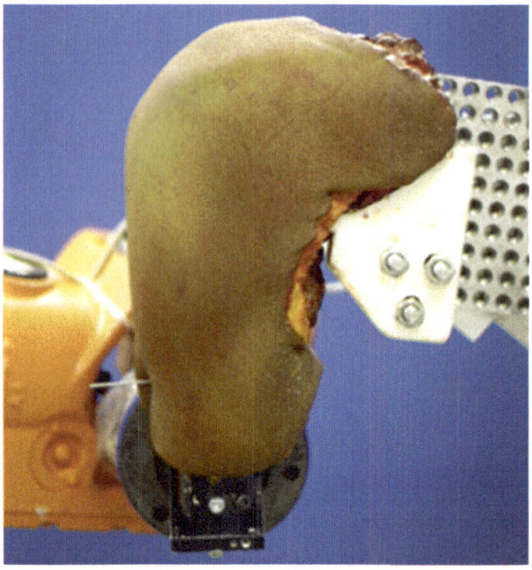

Fig. 12.12 The specimen is mounted on the robot

The results of the study showed that the Bankart plus ASA procedure has a higher stabilizing effect than a simple Bankart repair in anterior and anteroinferior translation, preventing the joint from dislocations; the limitation of external rotation decreased from 0° and 30° of abduction, to 60° abduction.

12.5 Clinical Retrospective Studies of ASA and Bankart Repair

The recently published clinical results at medium term follow-up are encouraging. A retrospective clinical study on 89 patients engaged in sports has been performed at 2–5 years' follow-up [19]. All patients underwent a computed tomography scan to assess the percentage of glenoid bone loss by the Pico method. A prior stabilization procedure had failed in 20 patients. Only 3 of 89 patients had a post-traumatic re-dislocation (3.3%). Clinical scores showed significant improvements: the VAS score decreased from a mean of 3.1 to 0.5 ($P < 0.0157$), the Rowe score increased from 58.9 to 94.1 ($P < 0.0215$) and the ASES score increased from 68.5 to 95.5 ($P < 0.0197$). No limitation in internal rotation as well as in abduction and flexion were found. In contrast, there was a difference of 6° in external rotation with the arm at the side of the trunk and 3° with the arm at 90°of abduction, to the contralateral side.

A multi-centre study has been performed on 110 patients treated for chronic anterior shoulder instability with arthroscopic Bankart repair and ASA at four different European hospitals [21]. Patients selected for this study were involved in contact sports, with a history of traumatic recurrent shoulder dislocations and a minimum of 2-year follow-up. Three patients (2.7%) had a traumatic re-dislocation. At final follow-up, the mean scores were as follows: VAS scale decreased from a mean of 3.5 to 0.5 ($P < 0.015$), Rowe score increased from 57.4 to 95.3 ($P < 0.035$) and ASES score increased from 66.5 to 96.5 ($P < 0.021$). The mean deficit of external rotation was 8° ± 2.5° with the arm at the side of the trunk and 4° ± 1.5° with the arm at 90° of abduction.

Another study has been published to compare the ASA procedure with the open Latarjet in case of glenoid bone loss [22] in two groups of 20 homogeneous but randomly selected patients. At a mean follow-up of 24 months (range, 20–39 months), no statistically significant differences were found between the two groups according to QuickDash, Constant and Rowe shoulder scores.

12.6 Discussion

In the last decades, many studies have reported a variable rate of recurrence from 0 up to 40% when a standard Bankart repair was performed in patients with anterior shoulder instability and quite normal glenoid shape. Based on this consideration, the necessity to program, in patients with a moderate glenoid damage, the 'Bankart plus' [23] procedure with a higher number of anchors in order to achieve a good stabilization and better healing of the capsulo-labral complex was underlined. The other option for decreasing the number of failures was the association of the Bankart plus the Remplissage, which consists of tenodesis of the infraspinatus tendon in the posterior humeral defect. New studies have shown the pathomechanics of the bipolar defect in the shoulder instability and underlined the necessity to use a graft in cases of on–off track Hill Sachs lesions; moreover, the role of the capsular deficiency and the constitutional hyperelasticity of the anterior soft tissue capsular complex was not considered. Our failure rate of 3%, also in case of mild glenoid defect and Hill Sachs lesions, suggests that the ASA plus Bankart could be considered as a Remplissage plus Bankart addressing the pathology from the front, instead of the back. Furthermore, the arthroscopic test for the Subscapularis elasticity could demonstrate an important role of the tendon in shoulder hyperlaxity. We think that ASA could improve the biological healing of the Bankart repair, reduce the anterior capsular elasticity, strengthen with scar tissue the coraco-humeral ligament acting in the opposite site of the Remplissage. The loss of external rotation (6° with the arm at the side of the trunk and 3° with the arm in 90° of abduction) was significantly lower compared with the ER loss resulting from Bankart repair plus Remplissage, and open or arthroscopic bone-block transfers [9, 24–26]. Another important observation is that with this technique we did not observe any early osteochondral damage, as reported with other procedures [27, 28].

12.7 Conclusions

The ASA technique associated with a Bankart repair represents a new technique for the treatment of recurrent anterior dislocations. It is a reproducible, safe and effective technique for patients with hyperlaxity or capsular insufficiency and low glenoid bone loss where the Latarjet could be considered an overtreatment, going to fill the grey area between Bankart repair and bone-block procedures.

References

1. Voos JE, Livermore RW, Feeley BT, Altchek DW, Williams RJ, Warren RF, Cordasco FA, Allen AA, HSS Sports Medicine Service. Prospective evaluation of arthroscopic bankart repairs for anterior instability. Am J Sports Med. 2010;38:302–7. https://doi.org/10.1177/0363546509348049.
2. Fabbriciani C, Milano G, Demontis A, Fadda S, Ziranu F, Mulas PD. Arthroscopic versus open treatment of Bankart lesion of the shoulder: a prospective randomized study. Arthroscopy. 2004;20:456–62. https://doi.org/10.1016/j.arthro.2004.03.001.
3. Kim SJ, Kim SH, Park BK, Chun YM. Arthroscopic stabilization for recurrent shoulder instability with moderate glenoid bone defect in patients with moderate to low functional demand. Arthroscopy. 2014;30:921–7. https://doi.org/10.1016/j.arthro.2014.03.023.
4. Lenters TR, Franta AK, Wolf FM, Leopold SS, Matsen FA. Arthroscopic compared with open repairs for recurrent anterior shoulder instability. A systematic review and meta-analysis of the literature. J Bone Joint Surg Am. 2007;89:244–54. https://doi.org/10.2106/JBJS.E.01139.
5. Burkhart SS, De Beer JF. Traumatic glenohumeral bone defects and their relationship to failure of arthroscopic Bankart repairs: significance of the inverted-pear glenoid and the humeral engaging Hill-Sachs lesion. Arthroscopy. 2000;16:677–94. https://doi.org/10.1053/jars.2000.17715.
6. Boileau P, Villalba M, Héry JY, Balg F, Ahrens P, Neyton L. Risk factors for recurrence of shoulder instability after arthroscopic Bankart repair. J Bone Joint Surg Am. 2006;88:1755–63. https://doi.org/10.2106/JBJS.E.00817.
7. Russo R, Cautiero F, Della Rotonda G. Risk factors for recurrent shoulder dislocation arthroscopically managed with absorbable knotless anchors. Adv Orthop Surg. 2014;2014:964358. https://doi.org/10.1155/2014/964358.
8. Boileau P, O'Shea K, Vargas P, et al. Anatomical and functional results after arthroscopic Hill-Sachs remplissage. J Bone Joint Surg Am. 2012;94:618–26.
9. Wolf EM, Arianjam A. Hill-Sachs remplissage, an arthroscopic solution for the engaging Hill-Sachs lesion: 2-to 10 year follow-up and incidence of recurrence. J Shoulder Elbow Surg. 2014;23:814–20.
10. Walch G, Boileau P. Latarjet-Bristow procedure for recurrent anterior instability. Tech Shoulder Elbow Surg. 2000;1:256–61.
11. Lafosse L, Lejeune E, Bouchard A, et al. The arthroscopic Latarjet procedure for the treatment of anterior shoulder instability. Arthroscopy. 2007;23:1242–5.
12. Lafosse L, Boyle S. Arthroscopic Latarjet procedure. J Shoulder Elbow Surg. 2010;19:2–12.
13. Russo R, Togo F, Jannelli E. The surgical treatment of recurrent anterior dislocation of the shoulder. Ital J Orthop Traumatol. 1990;16(2):183–9.
14. Taverna E, Golano P, Pascale V, et al. An arthroscopic bone graft procedure for treating anterior–inferior glenohumeral instability. Knee Surg Sports Traumatol Arthrosc. 2008;16:872–5.
15. Mizuno N, Denard PJ, Raiss P, et al. Long term results of the Latarjet procedure for anterior instability of the shoulder. J Shoulder Elbow Surg. 2014;23(11):1691–9.

16. Provencher MT, Ghodadra N, LeClere L, et al. Anatomic osteochondral glenoid reconstruction for recurrent glenohumeral instability with glenoid deficiency using a distal tibia allograft. Arthroscopy. 2009;25(4):446–52.
17. Johnson LL. Arthroscopic surgery: principle and practice, Chap 15. St. Louis: Mosby; 1986. p. 1420–4.
18. Maiotti M, Massoni C. Arthroscopic augmentation with subscapularis tendon in anterior shoulder instability with capsulolabral deficiency. Arthrosc Tech. 2013;2(3):e303–10.
19. Maiotti M, Russo R, Zanini A, et al. Arthroscopic Bankart repair and subscapularis augmentation: an alternative technique treating anterior shoulder instability with bone loss. J Shoulder Elbow Surg. 2016;25(6):898–906.
20. Schröter S, Krämer M, Welke B, et al. The effect of the arthroscopic augmentation of the subscapularis tendon on shoulder instability and range of motion: A biomechanical study. Clin Biomech. 2016;38:75–83.
21. Maiotti M, Massoni C, Russo R, et al. Arthroscopic subscapularis augmentation of Bankart repair in chronic anterior shoulder instability with bone loss less than 25% and capsular deficiency: clinical multicenter study. Arthroscopy. 2016;S0749–8063(16):30710–1.
22. Russo R, Della Rotonda G, Cautiero F, et al. Arthroscopic Bankart repair associated with subscapularis augmentation (ASA) versus open Latarjet to treat recurrent anterior shoulder instability with moderate glenoid bone loss: clinical comparison of two series. Musculoskelet Surg. 2017;101(1):75–83. https://doi.org/10.1007/s12306-016-0446-8.
23. Gordey EE, Wong IH. Using Bankart "plus" techniques to tackle anterior shoulder instability with bone loss: can newer arthroscopic adjuncts provide long-term stability? Arthroscopy. 2018;34(8):2294–7.
24. Longo UG, Loppini M, Rizzello G, Ciuffreda M, Berton A, Maffulli N, et al. Remplissage, humeral osteochondral grafts, Weber osteotomy, and shoulder arthroplasty for the management of humeral bone defects in shoulder instability: systematic review and quantitative synthesis of the literature. Arthroscopy. 2014;30:1650–66.
25. Meulen PD, Weening AA, Derek FP, Van Deurzen DF, Van den Bekerom MP. The relevance of the Latarjet procedure for the management of humeral bone defects in anterior shoulder instability. Arthroscopy. 2015;3:393–4.
26. Taverna E, Golano P, Pascale V, Battistella F. Anarthroscopicbone graft procedure for treating anterior–inferior glenohumeral instability. Knee Surg Sports Traumatol Arthrosc. 2008;16:872–5.
27. Griesser MJ, Harris JD, McCoy BW, Hussain WM, Jones MH, Bishop JY, et al. Complications and reoperations after Bristow- Latarjet shoulder stabilization: a systematic review. J Shoulder Elbow Surg. 2013;22:286–92.
28. Shah AA, Butler RB, Romanowski J, Karadagli D, Warner JJ. Short-term complications of the Latarjet procedure. J Bone Joint Surg Am. 2012;94:495–501.

13 Anterior Shoulder Instability Treatment with BLS Method

Roman Brzóska and Hubert Laprus

13.1 Introduction

Treatment of anterior shoulder instability is currently a subject of debate. Several different operative techniques, with various effectiveness, have been proposed and there is yet no consensus of which technique provides the best outcome. For many years, open or arthroscopic Bankart repair procedure was the proposed treatment for every case [1, 2]. Unfortunately, studies showed that approximately one-third of patients had instability recurrence after arthroscopic Bankart repair and among patients younger than 21 years, the risk of failure was shown to be even higher, with a reported failure rate of more than 50% [2–5]. In the pursuit for a surgical technique that could prevent recurrent anterior shoulder instability, the authors of this article developed a new arthroscopic technique, which could be seen as a modification of the classic Bankart procedure [6, 7]. This non-anatomic technique relies on augmentation of the damaged anterior wall soft tissues by a part of the subscapularis muscle and was named 'between glenohumeral ligaments and subscapularis muscle stabilization' (BLS). This technique enables restoration of the original capsulolabral footprint while protecting the articular surface by extracapsular knots placement, thus reducing the risk of future articular damage by abrasion.

13.2 Surgical Technique

For performance of the BLS procedure, the patient is placed in the beach chair position under general anaesthesia following interscalene block. The standard posterior portal is performed. Two additional portals, anterolateral and anterior, are created. During the initial arthroscopic examination a Hill–Sachs lesion should be identified. In case of arthroscopically confirmed engaging Hill–Sachs lesion [8], remplissage standard technique was performed [9]. Viewing through the posterior portal, the glenoid labrum pouch (GLP) and ligament subscapularis pouch (LSP) are marked with electrothermal cautery inserted through the anterolateral portal (Fig. 13.1). The GLP is prepared first in the standard fashion, using a rasp to approximate the 6-o'clock position. The LSP is then marked through the direct anterior portal, viewing through the anterolateral portal (Fig. 13.1). To create this space, the capsule must be separated from the overlying subscapularis, and this delicate dissection is carried out medially and inferiorly until subscapularis muscle fibres are visualized. Care must be taken to orient the electrothermal cautery towards subscapularis and away from the anterior capsule, which might

R. Brzóska · H. Laprus (✉)
St Luke's Hospital, Bielsko-Biała, Poland

R. Brzóska et al. (eds.), *360° Around Shoulder Instability*,
https://doi.org/10.1007/978-3-662-61074-9_13

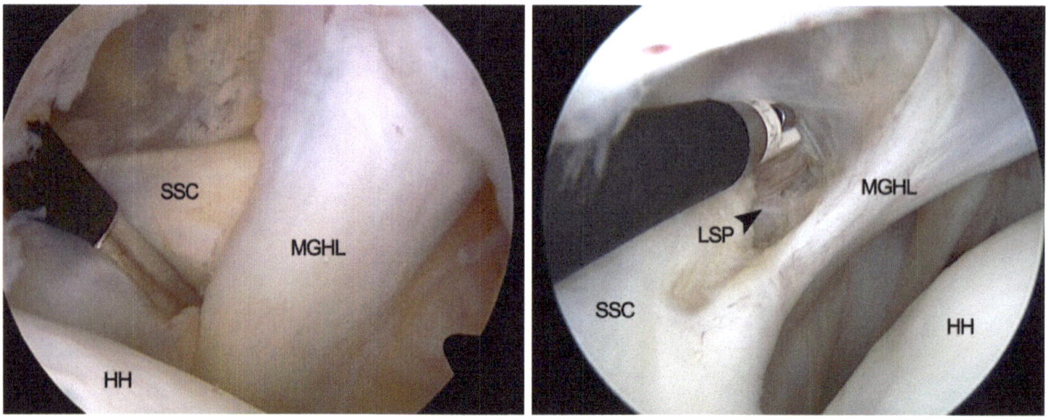

Fig. 13.1 Arthroscopic view of marked glenoid labrum pouch (GLP) and ligament subscapularis pouch (LSP) and arthroscopic view of LSP through the anterolateral portal

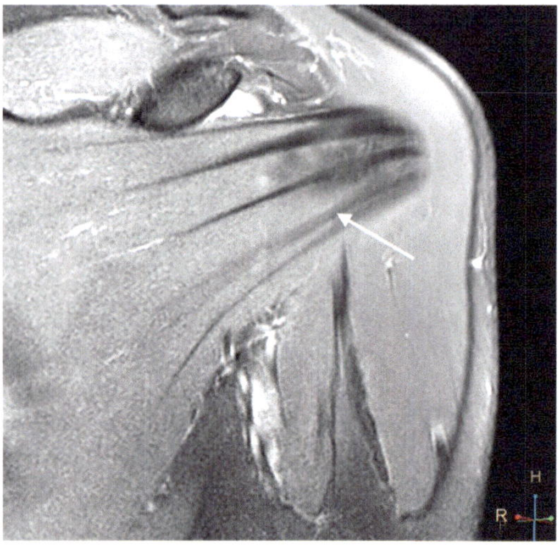

Fig. 13.2 Subscapularis muscle tendinous cords in MRI imaging. White arrow indicates proper cord used for anterior wall augmentation

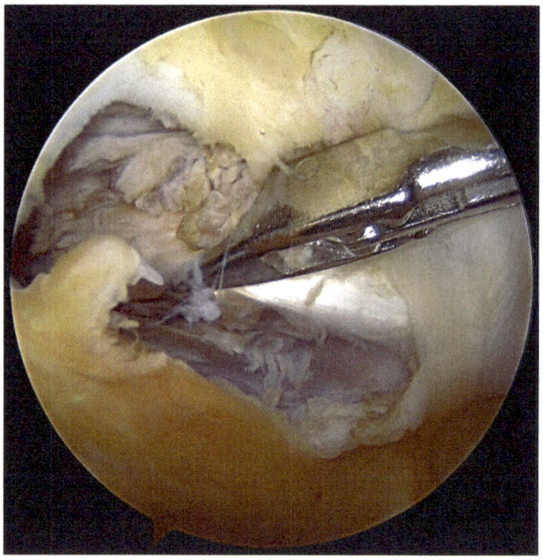

Fig. 13.3 Lower cord of subscapularis muscle used in anterior wall augmentation

otherwise become injured. Because the anterior capsular tissues are usually deficient, a lower third or fourth tendinous cord of subscapularis muscle is separated with a grasper in order to augment the repair without affecting motion (Figs. 13.2 and 13.3). Double-loaded suture anchor is inserted into the glenoid rim at the 5:30. The threads from anchor must pass through the centre of the labrum, anterior capsule and glenohumeral ligaments and finally attach a silver cord of subscapularis tendon to augment the repaired anterior stabilizers. Using the grasper through the posterior portal to pull up the anterior wall complex and hold it in position, a second double-loaded suture anchor is placed at 4-o'clock, and two additional mattress sutures are placed. Previously dissected third or fourth tendinous cord of subscapularis muscle has to surrounded and stitched by thread from the lowest anchor (Figs. 13.4 and 13.5). It should be underlined that thread passing through the tendon and knots tying should be performed with the shoulder in external rotation, which is crucial, so that after the suturing this part of the subscapularis muscle, there is no restriction in the external rotation. If necessary, another anchor is placed as in the standard arthro-Bankart procedure (Fig. 13.6).

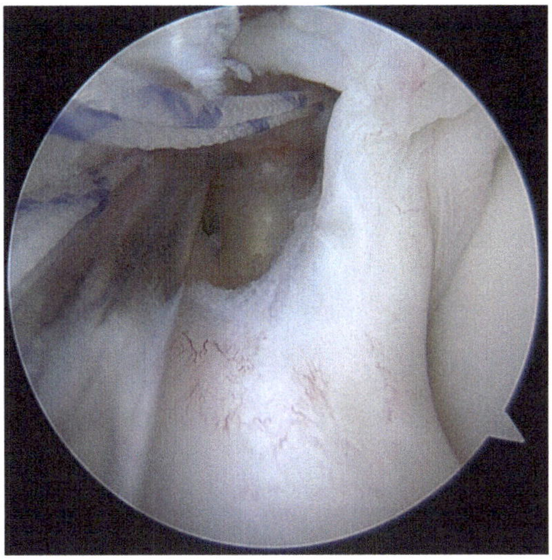

Fig. 13.4 Cord of subscapularis muscle used for anterior wall augmentation

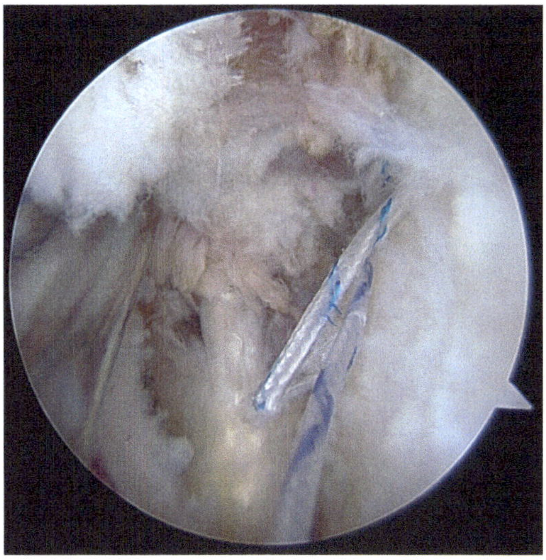

Fig. 13.6 BLS technique before knot tying

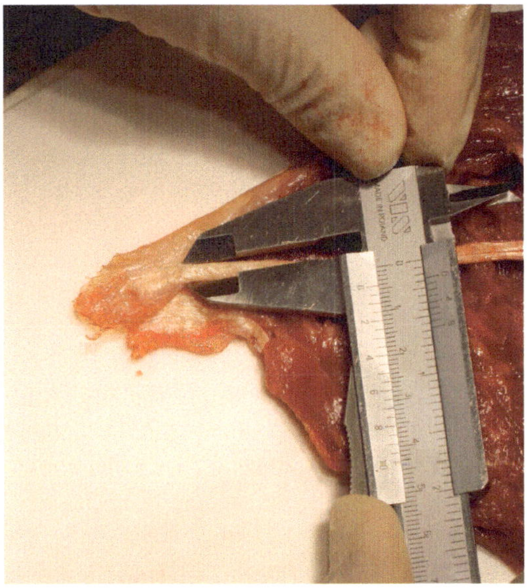

Fig. 13.5 Cadaveric view of subscapularis muscle tendinous cord

After suture tying, tendinous cord dissected previously from subscapularis muscle is parallel to the lower glenohumeral ligament, thus strengthening the anterior capsulo-ligamentous complex. The use of mattress sutures helps to position the suture material away from the articular surface, and the knots used to control the LSP are truly extracapsular, lying between the capsule and subscapularis (Fig. 13.7).

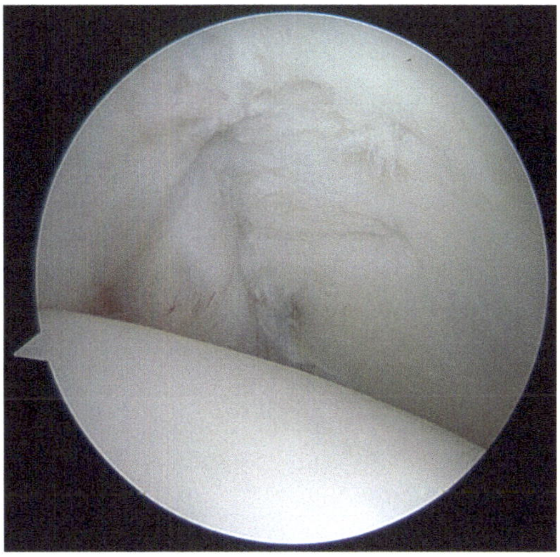

Fig. 13.7 Final intraarticular view after BLS technique

13.3 Results After BLS

A total of 150 patients underwent arthroscopic BLS surgery. During the study period, 50 patients were lost to follow-up, leaving 100 patients for final analysis in the present study. There were no statistically significant differences between lost-in-follow-up group and analysed group of patients in measured parameters [ns]. The study cohort consisted of 74 men and 26 women with a

Table 13.1 Variables of GBL groups

Baseline variables of patients' GBL	
Variable	Number of patients
Glenoid bone loss group	
Group 1 (0–5%)	34
Group 2 (6–10%)	32
Group 3 (11–15 %)	24
Group 4 (>15%)	10

mean age of 27.5 years [SD 10.3] at the time of surgery. The dominant shoulder was affected in 62 cases. The mean follow-up was 82.9 [SD 29.4] months.

The Constant Score increased statistically significantly from mean 82.89 [SD 9.1], pre-operatively, to mean 88.2 [SD 10.3] ($p < 0.001$) at the final follow-up. The corresponding numbers for the Walch–Duplay Score were mean 52.0 [SD 11.1], pre-operatively, and mean 81.1 [SD 19.0] ($p < 0.001$) at the final follow-up. At the final follow-up, there was no statistically significant difference in shoulder ER [ns] or IR [ns] compared with the pre-operative range of motion. Analysis of outcome between the different GBL groups (Table 13.1) did not show any statistically significant differences in the Constant score [ns], Walch–Duplay score [ns], shoulder ER [ns] or shoulder IR [ns]. Patients whose affected shoulder was the non-dominant arm improved more in the Walch–Duplay score compared with patients whose dominant arm was affected, mean 34.8 points [SD 14.9] and 25.4 points [SD 19.2] ($p = 0.01$), respectively.

At the final assessment, 86 patients (86%) were categorized as having a positive outcome, with full restoration of joint stability. These patients did not experience any dislocation or subluxation episodes during the follow-up period and had a negative apprehension test at the final clinical examination or did not report apprehension in questionnaire.

Failure of the treatment was observed in 14 patients (14%). In six cases, the reason of recurrence of anterior dislocation was a major trauma during sport activity. Patients with recurrent dislocation were younger compared to patients without recurrent dislocation, mean age 23.9 years [SD 6.7] compared with mean age 28.1 years [SD 10.7]; however, this age differences was not statistically significant (ns). The frequency of failure was higher in patients with a more severe GBL [$p = 0.001$]. In GBL group 1, only one case of recurrence was observed, and the reason for re-dislocation was major trauma. In GBL group 2, there were three cases of failure including two after trauma. In GBL group 3, five cases of failure were observed, including one post-traumatic case. In GBL group 4, there were five instability recurrences, including two cases of post-traumatic patients. Failure distribution according to size of GBL was presented in Fig. 13.8. Patients who failed had also greater baseline range of ER compared with patients with a positive outcome [mean 87.1° vs. 76.8°, $p = 0.02$].

No severe complications, like post-operative infection or persistent pain were observed.

13.4 Discussion

The most important finding for study on BLS technique was that this technique was shown to provide good clinical outcome with high shoulder stability and functional improvement, without decreasing shoulder range of motion. After a mean follow-up of 82.9 months, 86% of the patients who underwent surgery with the BLS technique regained a satisfactory stability of the shoulder. Furthermore, among the 14 failures observed in present study, six were the consequence of high energy trauma during sport activity. Thus, the BLS technique presented high effectiveness as an arthroscopic anterior instability treatment technique. Another important finding was that no patient developed post-operative mobility limitation or infection, which indicates a high safety of this technique.

Complications after traditional arthroscopic Bankart repair has been reported to occur in 21–68% of cases and typically involve significant labral damage and cartilage destruction, partially due to suture knot placement too close to the articular surface [3, 6, 9–12]. The BLS method described in the present study, relies on placing the sutures and the knots that are harmful for car-

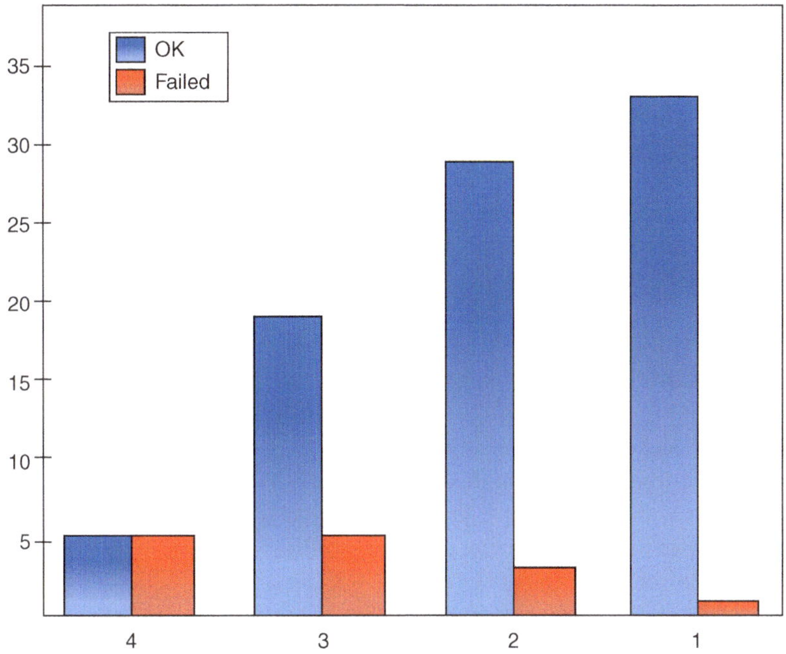

Fig. 13.8 Failure distribution according to size of GBL

tilage outside the joint and, instead, place them in the space between the medial glenohumeral ligament (MGHL) and subscapularis muscle. Thus, similarly to the open Bankart technique, all suture materials are placed outside the joint and the risk of cartilage and labrum abrasion is reduced. The improvement in constant score showed that satisfactory patient-reported outcome could be expected 2–9 years post-operatively. Future study comparing pre-operative and post-operative radiographs in long-time follow-up is necessary to prove that extracapsular suture placing reduces the risk of osteoarthritis after Bankart repair.

Several modified Bankart techniques have been described previously. For instance, Maiotti et al. [13] reported satisfactory results after an arthroscopic Bankart repair augmented by subscapularis muscle tenodesis even in case of chronic anterior shoulder instability, with GBL less than 25% and capsular joint deficiency [13]. However, Maiotti et al. also reported a significant reduction in shoulder joint ER, which is an inevitable complication of whole subscapularis muscle tenodesis. The BLS technique is advantageous since it results in a significant increase in the anterior joint stabilization, while not limiting the ER, as shown in the present study.

Another important part of this study was the assessment of GBL and its effect on outcome. According to Owens recommendations [14] concerning GBL measurement, the authors of this study divided GBL into four groups based on MRI examination to abandon the harmful CT radiation in pre-operative diagnosis, especially after considering the young age of patients (Table 13.1). Patients with GBL > 15% or with an intraoperatively observed 'flat-line' shaped front wall of the glenoid were considered to have the largest defect. The 'flat-line' term refers to the bony loss of the antero-medial glenoid, resulting in the lack of the anterior curvature, thereby creating a straight vertical cut-off line. It is possible that this type of glenoid damage predisposes to recurrent dislocations to a similar extent as the 'inverted pear' described by Burkhart [15] and can be a severe risk factor for treatment failure. In this study, a statistically significant correlation between the GBL level and higher frequency of treatment failure was noticed as well. Taking into consideration the size of the GBL in particular groups, patients with recurrent instability had a median GBL group of 3 (11–15%), while patients with a positive outcome had a median GBL group of 2 (6–10%). Burkhart et al. and other studies investigating the effect of the GBL size reported that a GBL size of 21–25% predisposes recurrence of anterior shoulder instability [15–17]. However, a later study by Shaha et al. suggested a GBL of 13.5% to be sufficient to predispose recurrent instability [18]. The finding in the present study with a higher recurrence rate of shoulder instability among patients with a GBL of 11% or more is in line with the study by Shaha et al. [18].

13.5 Conclusions

The BLS technique has been shown to be an effective method to anterior shoulder instability in patients without significant glenoid bone loss. It was shown that this technique provides significant improvement in shoulder function without reducing shoulder range of motion.

References

1. Bankart AS. Recurrent or habitual dislocation of the shoulder. BMJ. 1923;2:1132–3.
2. Fabbriciani C, Milano G, Demontis A, Fadda S, Ziranu F, Mulas PD. Arthroscopic versus open treatment of Bankart lesion of the shoulder: a prospective randomized study. Arthroscopy. 2004;20:456–62.
3. Flinkkilä T, Knape R, Sirniö K, Ohtonen P, Leppilahti J. Long-term results of arthroscopic Bankart repair: Minimum 10 years of follow-up. Knee Surg Sports Traumatol Arthrosc. 2018:26:94–9.
4. Privitera DM, Bisson LJ, Marzo JM. Minimum 10-year follow-up of arthroscopic intra-articular Bankart repair using bioabsorbable tacks. Am J Sports Med. 2012;40:100–7.
5. Owens BD, DeBernandino TM, Nelson BJ, Thurman J, Cameron KL, Taylor DC, et al. Long-term follow-up of acute arthroscopic repair for initial anterior shoulder dislocations in young athletes. Am J Sports Med. 2009;37:669–73.
6. Brzoska R, Blasiak A, Hldaki W, Streit JJ, Toussaint B, Solecki W. Arthroscopic Bankart repair using extracapsular suture between the glenohumeral ligaments and subscapularis tendon (BLS technique): a technical note. Tech Shoulder Surg. 2012;13:86–9.
7. Brzóska R, Laprus H, Michniowski P, et al. Novel and effective arthroscopic extracapsular stabilization technique for anterior shoulder instability-BLS. Knee Surg Sports Traumatol Arthrosc. 2019;27(12):3897–904. https://doi.org/10.1007/s00167-019-05496-1.
8. Yamamoto N, Itoi E, Abe H, Minagawa H, Seki N, Shimada Y, Okada K. Contact between the glenoid and the humeral head in abduction, external rotation, and horizontal extension: a new concept of glenoid track. J Shoulder Elbow Surg. 2007;16:649–56.
9. Purchase RJ, Wolf EM, Hobgood ER, Pollock ME, Smalley CC. Hill-Sachs "remplissage": an arthroscopic solution for the engaging Hill-Sachs lesion. Arthroscopy. 2008;24:723–6.
10. Franceschi F, Papalia R, Del Buono A, Vasta S, Maffulli N, Denaro V. Glenohumeral osteoarthritis after arthroscopic Bankart repair for anterior instability. Am J Sports Med. 2011;39:1653–9.
11. Kavaja L, Pajarinen J, Sinisaari I, Savolainen V, Björkenheim J-M, Haapamäki V, et al. Arthrosis of glenohumeral joint after arthroscopic Bankart repair: a long-term follow-up of 13 years. J Shoulder Elbow Surg. 2012;21:350–5.
12. Kowalsky MS, et al. Evaluation of suture abrasion against rotator cuff tendon and proximal humerus bone. Arthroscopy. 2008;24(3):329–34.
13. Maiotti M, Massoni C, Russo R, Schroter S, Zanini A, Bianchedi D. Arthroscopic subscapularis augmentation of Bankart repair in chronic anterior shoulder instability with bone loss less than 25% and capsular deficiency: clinical multicenter study. Arthroscopy. 2017;33:902–9.
14. Owens BD, Burns TC, Campbell SE, et al. Simple method of glenoid bone loss calculation using ipsilateral magnetic resonance imaging. Am J Sports Med. 2013;41:622–4.
15. Burkhart SS, De Beer JF. Traumatic glenohumeral bone defects and their relationship to failure of arthroscopic Bankart repairs: Significance of the inverted-pear glenoid and the humeral engaging Hill-Sachs lesion. Arthroscopy. 2000;16:677–94.
16. Griffith JF, Antonio GE, Tong CW, Ming CK. Anterior shoulder dislocation: quantification of glenoid bone loss with CT. Am J Roentgenol. 2003;180:1423–30.
17. Griffith JF, Antonio GE, Yung PS, et al. Prevalence, pattern, and spectrum of glenoid bone loss in anterior shoulder dislocation: CT analysis of 218 patients. Am J Roentgenol. 2008;190:1247–54.
18. Shaha JS, Cook JB, Song DJ, Rowles DJ, Bottoni CR, Shaha SH, Tokish JM. Redefining "critical" bone loss in shoulder instability: functional outcomes worsen with "subcritical" bone loss. Am J Sports Med. 2015;43:1719–25.

14 Trans-subscapular Tenodesis and Labroplasty by the Long Head of the Biceps Graft

Oleg Milenin and Ruslan Sergienko

14.1 Introduction

Traumatic chronic anterior instability is a common pathology of the shoulder joint. The frequency of recurrent dislocation in patients 20–30 years old reaches 75%. In the case of a bone defect in the glenoid, the Latarjet procedure [1] or bone block is the method of choice [2, 3]. The arthroscopic Bankart procedure and its modifications are still the preferred method in the absence of significant bone lesions in glenoid and humeral head [4]. Nevertheless, the number of revisions of Bankart procedure performed according to optimal indications and without technology errors can reach 20% after 5 years of observation [5, 6]. One of the main reasons for recurrence in this case is the poor quality and weakness of the glenohumeral ligaments and labrum [7, 8].

For the prophylaxis of recurrence, a number of methods have been proposed such as using allografts and augmentation by a part of the tendon of the subscapular muscle [9–11]. Some authors suggested using the tendon of the short head of the biceps muscle without the bone block [12]. Nevertheless, the recurrence rate of this procedure is quite high. Therefore, some authors recommend Latarjet procedure in this case [6].

Several authors proposed the use of dynamic stabilization by transposition of the long biceps head tendon for additional stabilization in the repair of Bankart injury and fixation in the bone channel with the suture button or biotenodesis anchor [13, 14].

We proposed an alternative technique for performing shoulder stabilization by biceps transposition, which has the same triple stabilization mechanism as the Latarjet procedure. It consists of using the tendon of the long head of the biceps as static and dynamic stabilizer by transposition of the biceps through the subscapularis split with simultaneous labroplasty of the anterior segment of the labrum and subsequent fixation of the glenohumeral ligaments to the same anchors.

14.2 Materials and Methods

The procedure is performed with the patient in the beach chair position and the injured arm (right arm herein) in a traction of 1.5 kg. We use three standard portals [15], the posterior portal, anterosuperior, and anteromedial portal, and an additional suprapectoral portal, which is located 3–4 cm inferior from the standard anterosuperior portal in the projection of the cross-section of the biceps groove at the insertion site of the superior edge of the pectoralis major tendon.

After diagnostic arthroscopy and mobilization of the capsule and labrum, the arthroscope is

O. Milenin (✉)
Pirogov's National Medical Surgical Center, Moscow, Russia

R. Sergienko
Medical Center of Modern Orthopedics, Kyiv, Ukraine

R. Brzóska et al. (eds.), *360° Around Shoulder Instability*, https://doi.org/10.1007/978-3-662-61074-9_14

transferred to the anterior-superior portal, and then on the front edge of the glenoid, two anchors are placed with a double thread at 3 and 5 o'clock positions (Fig. 14.1).

The threads of anchors are captured in the standard posterior portal. After tenotomy of the long head of the biceps, the arthroscope is transferred into the subdeltoid space. The tendon of the long head is mobilized, captured (Fig. 14.2), and passed through an additional lateral portal. The end of the tendon of the long head of the biceps is stitched with the nonabsorbable thread (Fig. 14.3).

After the dissection of the space between conjoint tendon and the subscapular muscle, we inspect the axillary nerve. The subscapular muscle is perforated opposite the lower anchor under the labrum using a suture manipulator inserted through the posterior portal (Fig. 14.4), which captures the threads attached to the tip of the long head of the biceps through the subscapular muscle split and passed into the joint (Fig. 14.5).

Then, the tendon of the biceps is attached to the lower anchor (Fig. 14.6). The upper part of

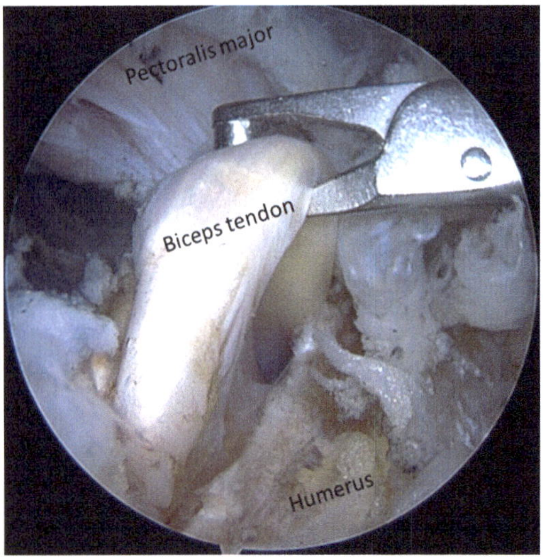

Fig. 14.1 View of the subdeltoid space of the right shoulder from the anterosuperior portal. The long head of the biceps tendon is grasped from the additional suprapectoral portal

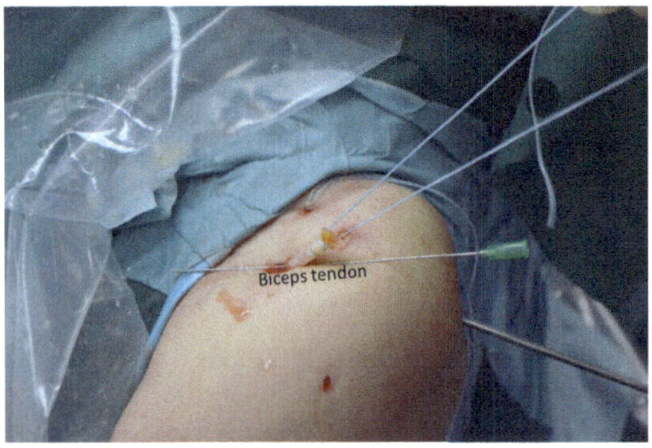

Fig. 14.2 Extraarticular view of the right shoulder. The end of the tendon of the long head of the biceps is sewn with nonabsorbable thread

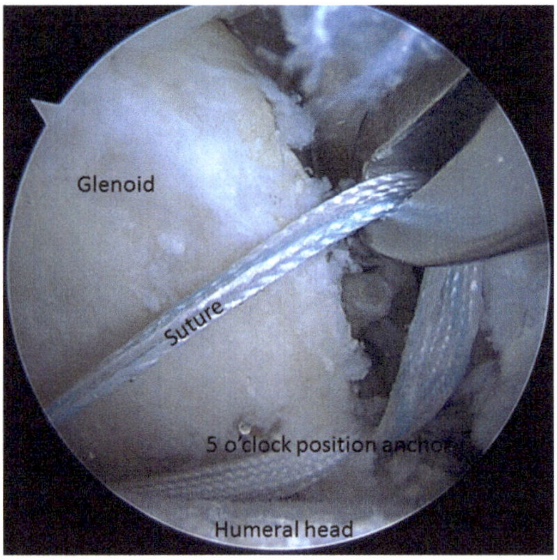

Fig. 14.3 Intraarticular view of the right shoulder. The 5 o'clock position anchor is placed

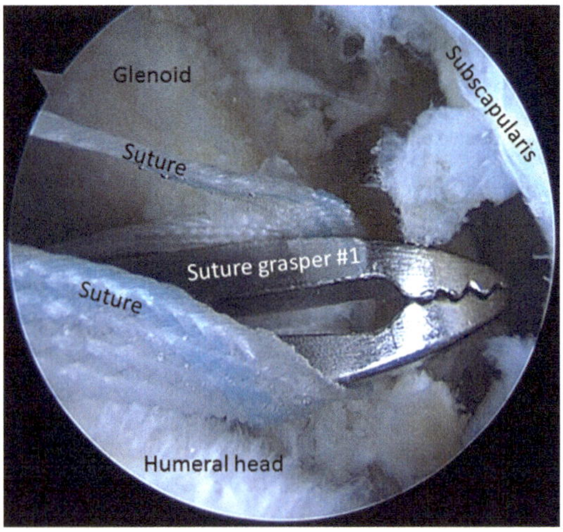

Fig. 14.4 The suture grasper #1 starts to perforate subscapularis muscle from the posterior portal between two sutures

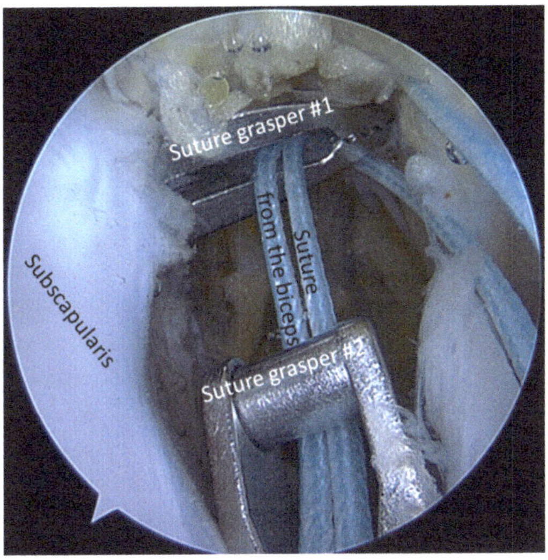

Fig. 14.5 View of the subdeltoid space of the right shoulder from the anterosuperior portal. The suture grasper #1 is inserted from the posterior portal, perforates the subscapular muscle at 5 o'clock position of the glenoid, and captures the sutures attached to the tip of long head of the biceps tendon with the suture grasper #2

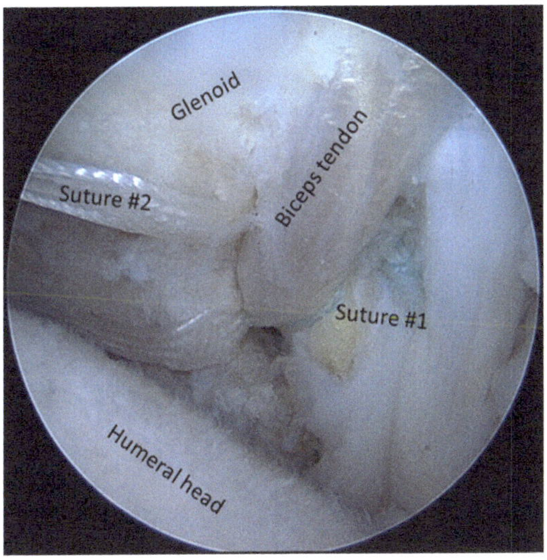

Fig. 14.6 Intraarticular view of the right shoulder. Biceps tendon is fixed at 5 o'clock position with suture #1. Suture #2 corresponds to posterior portal for additional capsule fixation at the end of the procedure

the biceps tendon is attached to the upper segment of the glenoid at 1 o'clock position with a knotless anchor (Fig. 14.7) and finally at 3 o'clock position (Fig. 14.8). The next step is

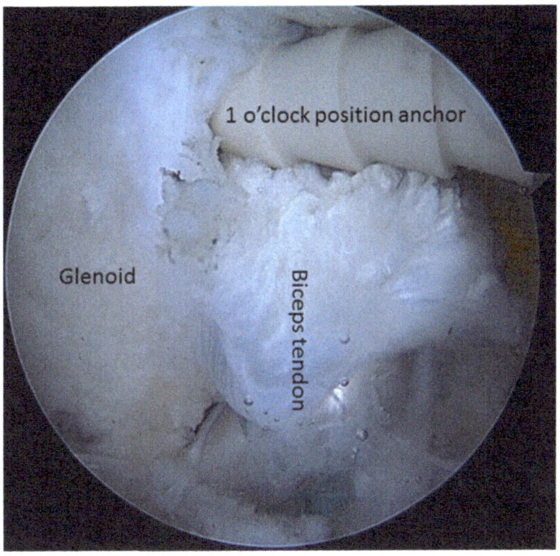

Fig. 14.7 Intraarticular view of the right shoulder. The tip of the long head of the biceps tendon is fixed at 1 o'clock position with 3.5 knotless anchor

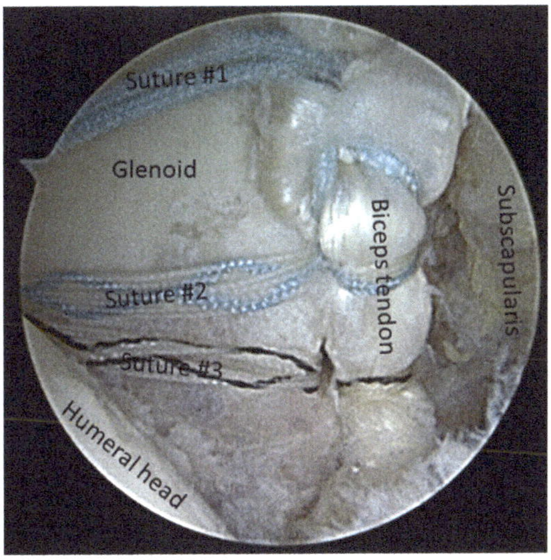

Fig. 14.8 Intraarticular view of the right shoulder. Sutures #1, #2, and #3 are placed around the graft and grasped through the anteromedial portal. The biceps tendon is fixed with another pair of sutures

fixation of the glenohumeral ligaments and the labrum to the glenoid in anatomical position to the second pair of anchor threads over the soft tissue graft (Fig. 14.9).

All steps of the procedure are presented in Table 14.1.

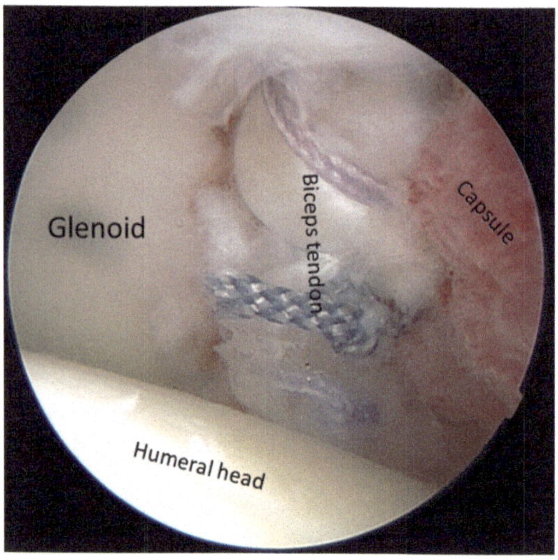

Fig. 14.9 Final view from the anterosuperior portal of the anterior labroplasty before closure of the capsular ligaments in the right shoulder

Table 14.1 Surgical technique

Number of the step	Step description
Step 1	Diagnostic arthroscopy and mobilization of capsule and labrum
Step 2	Tenotomy of the long head of the biceps
Step 3	The arthroscope is transferred to the subdeltoid space, the long head of the biceps tendon is mobilized and grasped from the additional suprapectoral portal
Step 4	The end of the long head of the biceps tendon stitched with a nonabsorbable suture
Step 5	Placement of two double-load anchors at 3 and 5 o'clock positions
Step 6	Perforation of subscapularis muscle from the posterior portal with the suture grasper #1
Step 7	Biceps tendon is fixed at 5 o'clock position
Step 8	The tip of the long head of the biceps tendon is fixed at 1 o'clock position with a 3.5 knotless anchor and then the graft fixed at 3 o'clock positon
Step 9	Fixation of the glenohumeral ligaments and labrum to glenoid in the anatomical position with the second pair of anchor sutures across the biceps soft tissue graft

14.3 Results

We performed 21 procedures with 12- to 24-month follow-up. We inspected pain in biceps groove, range of motions, apprehension test, incidences of dislocations, level of sport activity, and 3 T MRI studies after 6 months.

All the patients achieved full range of motion as well as the absence of pain in biceps groove after 3 months; 2 patients had slight restriction of external rotation (from 10° to 15°) compared to the healthy hand. Repeated dislocations and subluxations were not observed in follow-up. Slight apprehension was observed in two cases; 3 patients successfully came back to professional sport. MRI revealed a complete reintegration of glenohumeral ligament to the edge of the glenoid and good sling effect (Figs. 14.10 and 14.11); 2 patients were missed from the study.

Early follow-up has shown us very optimistic results; thus, the proposed method can be effec-

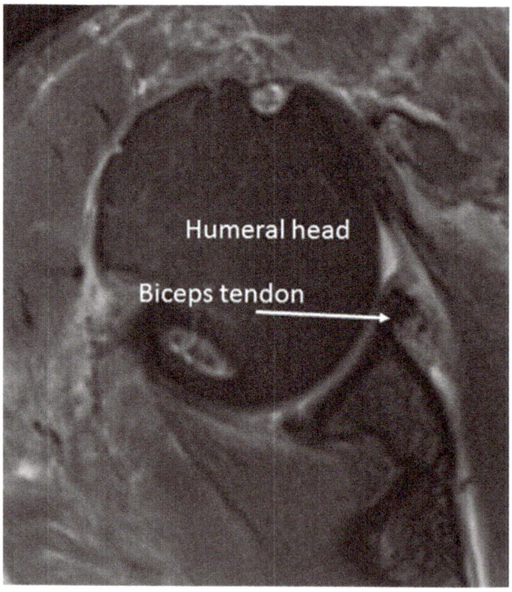

Fig. 14.10 Coronal view of the right shoulder MRI 6 months after the surgery shows good healing of biceps tendon and transformation to neolabrum

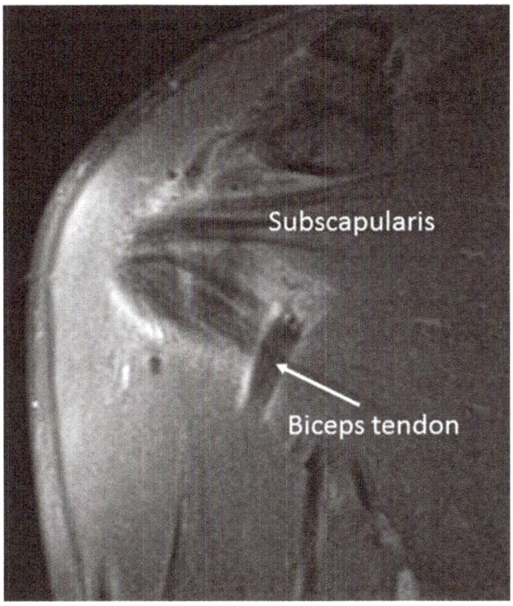

Fig. 14.11 Frontal view of MRI 6 months after the surgery shows significant sling effect after the procedure

tive for labral repair augmentation for patients with sick capsule and poor quality of glenohumeral ligament.

14.4 Case Report

A 25-year-old professional skater with chronic shoulder instability (more than 10 cases of dislocation) was examined in 3 months after the last episode of dislocation. The forward elevation abduction and adduction, and internal and external rotations were significantly decreased. On MRI and CT, there was no significant bone loss (less than 10% in glenoid and humerus). Significant apprehension test was observed on 90° forward elevation and external rotation (Fig. 14.12).

We performed an anterior labroplasty and transposition of the long head of the biceps graft. After the surgery, we inspected the patient on MRI (Fig. 14.13).

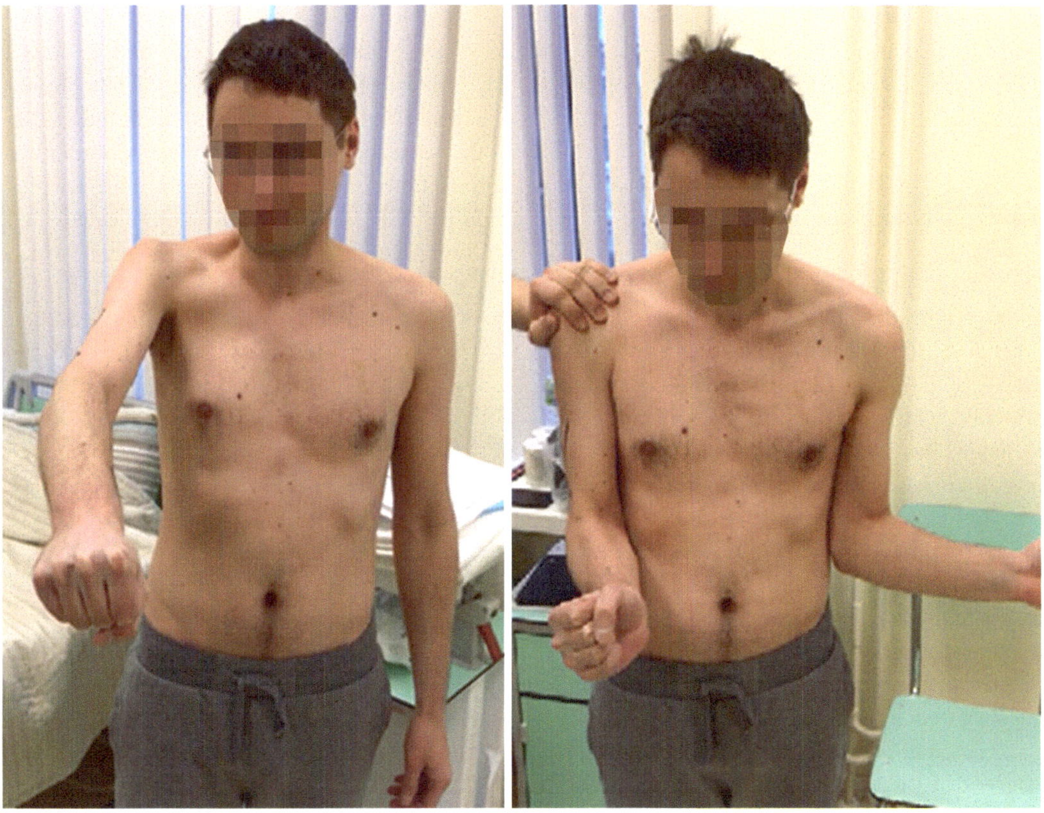

Fig. 14.12 Maximal active forward elevation and external rotation before the surgery

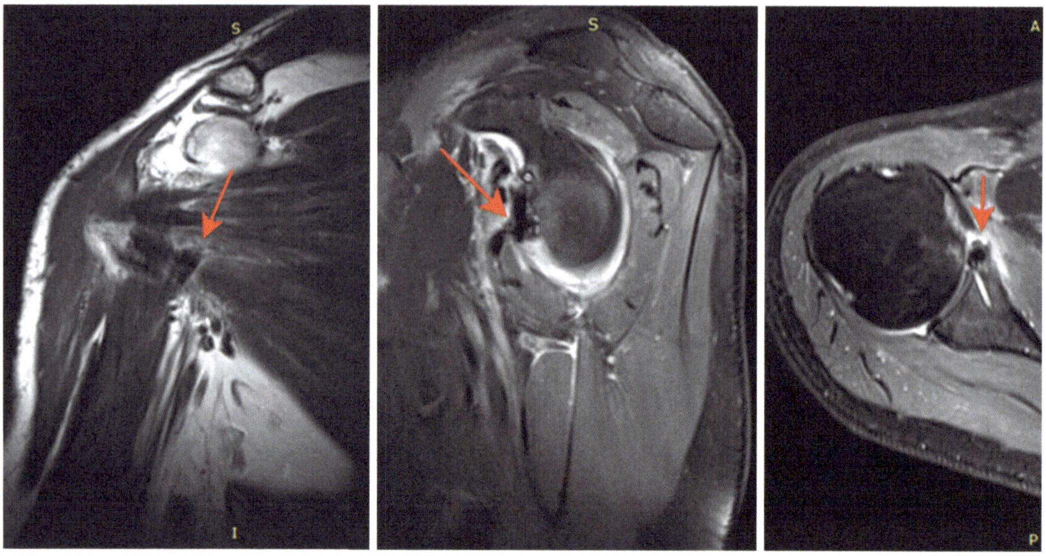

Fig. 14.13 View of MRI 6 months after the surgery. The arrow shows long head of biceps graft

In 6 months after the procedure, allograft is completely healed. In a year, the range of motion and muscle strength were completely restored (Fig. 14.14), there was no apprehension and biceps pain, and the patient came back to professional skating.

14.5 Discussion

One of the preferred methods of treatment of anterior inferior shoulder instability is Bankart procedure [16]. Therefore, the treatment option is plasty of the joint labrum with autograft and allograft, which is effective [17]. However, this technique has several disadvantages. Firstly, this procedure is complicated, technically demanding, and requires allograft or autograft harvesting. In addition, it requires a large number of anchor fixators and sutures that can damage the cartilage. Besides, the presence of strong glenohumeral ligaments and absence of their plastic deformation make this procedure ineffective for capsular deficit.

The "Belt-and-suspenders" technique [12] consists of transposition of the conjoint tendon through splitting the scapular muscle and fixing the tendon in the bone tunnel with an interferential screw. This technique does not use the advantages of bone block like Latarjet procedure [7]. The Maiotti technique [11] that involves tenodesis of the tendon of the scapular muscle solves the problem of capsular deficiency while biomechanically "killing" the upper third of the tendon of the subscapularis, which is most important for normal function. The arthroscopic Latarjet procedure [18] is technically complicated and requires release of the pectoralis minor, which can cause scapulothoracic dyskinesis [19] and there is a potential risk of injuring neurovascular structures [20]. Incorrect positioning of the screws and lysis of the coracoid graft are possible complications after arthroscopic Latarjet procedure too [21].

Our procedure is different from the techniques by Collin's et al. [13] and Tang and Zhao's [14] techniques in the direction of the biceps tendon fixation. In these techniques, the graft is placed and fixed perpendicular to the glenoid rim to create a mostly dynamic stabilization effect as in the Bristow procedure. In our technique, we fix the graft parallel to the glenoid rim and create a neolabrum and anterior static bumper effect as a soft tissue block that is analogous to the bone block in the Latarjet procedure. The grasping and passing of the long head of the biceps tendon are

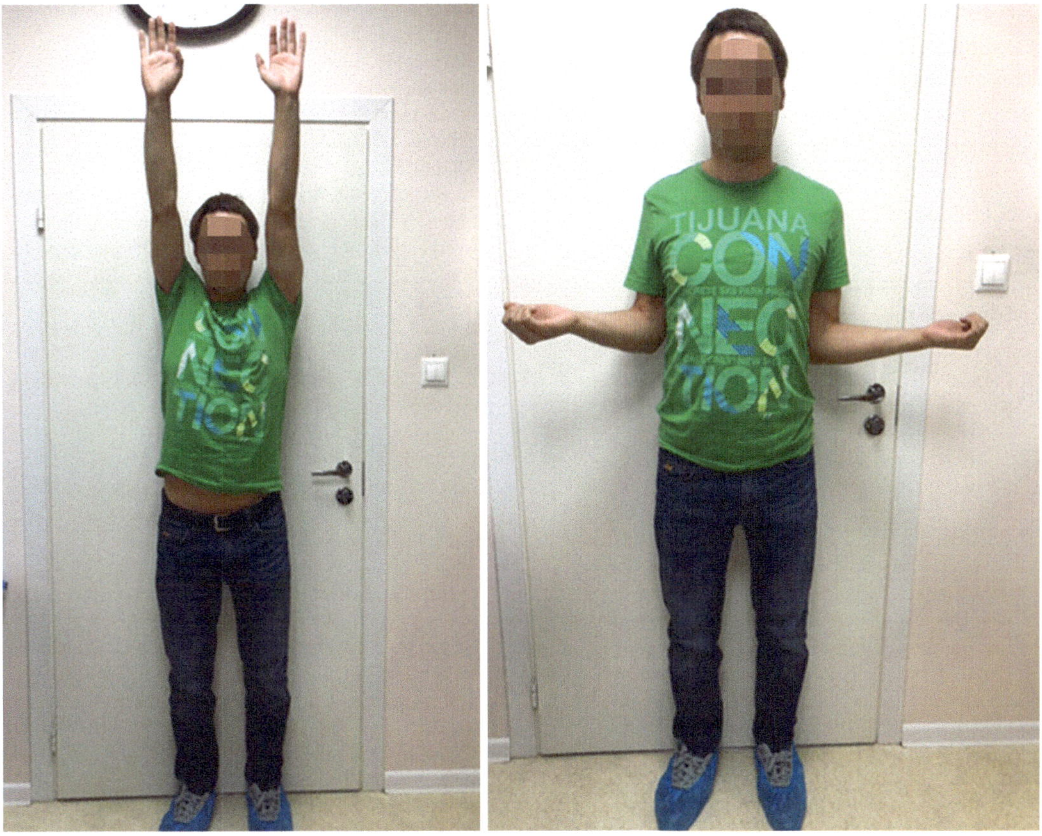

Fig. 14.14 Maximal active forward elevation and external rotation 12 month after the surgery

performed from the inside-outward direction by perforation with a suture grasper, causing less damage to the subscapularis than standard arthroscopic subscapular splitting with a radiofrequency.

In case of absence of significant bone loss, this procedure has a number of advantages over arthro-Latarjet. With triple mechanism of stability like Latarjet, it can significantly reinforce the Bankart procedure in case of sick glenohumeral ligaments. It is less traumatic, easier, and faster, and can easily revise using standard Latarjet procedure. In addition, the procedure can be used together with the bone block in revision cases after Latarjet or for MDI treatment. In case of superior labral lesion from anterior to posterior tears, our procedure simultaneously treats this pathology. Our procedure can be performed in lateral decubitus or "beach chair" position (depending on the surgeon's preference). And last but not least, it can be performed in cases of subcritical glenoid bone loss if there are any doubts in choosing soft tissue or bone reconstruction procedure.

There are some disadvantages of this procedure as well. We do not recommend our procedure in case of significant glenoid or humeral head bone loss and total absence of the capsule because the long head of the biceps does not generate so much power like conjoint tendon. Besides, the procedure is not recommended in cases of poor quality of the biceps tendon or previous procedures with biceps tenodesis or tenotomy. There is a theoretical possibility of biceps pain after the procedure. There is a risk of axillary nerve injury during the perforation of subscapularis muscle perforation from inside-outward direction. And finally, our procedure requires significant surgical skills.

To conclude, the main stabilizing effect of our procedure is created by the synergy of the anterior labroplasty due to the soft-tissue bumper, sling effect of dynamic tenodesis, and refixation of the glenohumeral ligaments. Future research is necessary to study incidents of recurrence, and range of motion restrictions, and the possibility of using this technique for professional athletes.

References

1. Latarjet M. Treatment of recurrent dislocation of the shoulder. Lyon Chir. 1954;49:994–7.
2. Boileau P, Mercier N, Roussanne Y, Thelù CE, Old J. Arthroscopic Bankart-Bristow-Latarjet procedure: the development and early results of a safe and reproducible technique. Arthroscopy. 2010;26:1434–50.
3. Burkhart SS, De Beer JF. Traumatic glenohumeral bone defects and their relationship to failure of arthroscopic Bankart repairs: significance of the inverted-pear glenoid and the humeral engaging Hill-Sachs lesion. Arthroscopy. 2000;16:677–94.
4. Frank RM, Romeo AA. Arthroscopic soft tissue reconstruction in anterior shoulder instability. Orthopade. 2018;47:121–8.
5. Bliven KCH, Parr GP. Outcomes of the Latarjet procedure compared with Bankart repair for recurrent traumatic anterior shoulder instability. J Athl Train. 2018;53:181–3.
6. Lafosse L, Lejeune E, Bouchard A, Kakuda C, Gobezie R, Kochhar T. The arthroscopic Latarjet procedure for the treatment of anterior shoulder instability. Arthroscopy. 2007;23:1242.e1–5.
7. Giles JW, Boons HW, Elkinson I, et al. Does the dynamic sling effect of the Latarjet procedure improve shoulder stability? A biomechanical evaluation. J Shoulder Elbow Surg. 2013;22:821–7.
8. Phadnis J, Arnold C, Elmorsy A, Flannery M. Utility of the instability severity index score in predicting failure after arthroscopic anterior stabilization of the shoulder. Am J Sports Med. 2015;43(8):1983–8.
9. Denard PJ, Narbona P, Lädermann A, Burkhart SS. Bankart augmentation for capsulolabral deficiency using a split subscapularis tendon flap. Arthroscopy. 2011;27:1135–41.
10. Iannotti JP, Antoniou J, Williams GR, Ramsey ML. Iliotibial band reconstruction for treatment of glenohumeral instability associated with irreparable capsular deficiency. J Shoulder Elbow Surg. 2002;11:618–23.
11. Maiotti M, Massoni C, Russo R, Schroter S, Zanini A, Bianchedi D. Arthroscopic subscapularis augmentation of Bankart repair in chronic anterior shoulder instability with bone loss less than 25% and capsular deficiency: clinical multicenter study. Arthroscopy. 2017;33:902–9.
12. Boileau P, Bicknell RT, El Fegoun AB, Chuinard C. Arthroscopic Bristow procedure for anterior instability in shoulder with a stretched or deficient capsule: the "belt-and suspenders" operative technique and preliminary results. Arthroscopy. 2007;23:593–601.
13. Collin P, Lädermann A. Dynamic anterior stabilization using the long head of the biceps for anteroinferior glenohumeral instability. Arthrosc Tech. 2018;7:e39–44.
14. Tang J, Zhao J. Arthroscopic transfer of the long head of the biceps brachii for anterior shoulder instability. Arthrosc Tech. 2017;6:e1911–7.
15. Snyder SJ. Shoulder arthroscopy, vol. 1. Philadelphia: Lippincott Williams & Wilkins; 2003.
16. Thomazeau H, Courage O, Barth J, et al. Can we improve the indication for Bankart arthroscopic repair? A preliminary clinical study using the ISIS score. Orthop Traumatol Surg Res. 2010;96:S77–83.
17. Gervasi E, Sebastiani E, Spicuzza A. Multidirectional shoulder instability: arthroscopic labral augmentation. Arthrosc Tech. 2017;6:e219–25.
18. Lafosse L, Boyle S. Arthroscopic Latarjet procedure. J Shoulder Elbow Surg. 2010;19:2–12.
19. Carbone S, Moroder P, Runer A, Resch H, Gumina S, Hertel R. Scapular dyskinesis after Latarjet procedure. J Shoulder Elbow Surg. 2016;25:422–7.
20. Lädermann A, Denard PJ, Burkhart SS. Injury of the suprascapular nerve during Latarjet procedure: an anatomic study. Arthroscopy. 2012;28:316–21.
21. Di Giacomo G, Costantini A, De Gasperis N, et al. Coracoid graft osteolysis after the Latarjet procedure for anteroinferior shoulder instability: a computed tomography scan study of twenty-six patients. J Shoulder Elbow Surg. 2011;20:989–95.

15 Revision After Soft Tissue Procedure in Anterior Shoulder Instability

Przemysław Lubiatowski

15.1 Introduction

Soft tissue procedures have a long record in the treatment of anterior shoulder instability, including classic open Bankart repair followed later by arthroscopic equivalent of capsulolabral repair using suture anchors. Arthroscopic approach has been reported to have a variable rate of success to keep the shoulder stable long term and regain function. The rate of recurrence of instability has been reported from 10 to 22% [1, 2]. Complication risk is still low with need to reoperation reaching 5% [1]. Most common complications included infections, implant-related problems (malposition, impingement), secondary osteoarthritis, and nerve lesions. However, the most common reason for revision surgery has been the failure to provide stable shoulder, including the recurrence of instability. The current chapter focuses on this particular issue.

Various authors have identified the most common reasons for failure after soft tissue repair in anterior shoulder instability. They mostly include young age of patient (<20–22 years), male sex, number of previous dislocations, participation in contact (mostly collision) sports, inherent capsular laxity of glenohumeral joint, and capsular stretching over time [3, 4]. Well-known risk factors include bone loss on both glenoid and humeral side. More recently, special attention has been brought to not only the presence of osseous deficiency but also its location and bipolar interplay of defects (engaging or off-track) [5, 6]. In Tauber's study, 59% of failed stabilizations had traumatic event to cause the recurrence, including 40% injuries occurring while doing sports. In the case of soft tissue sport-related trauma, possible soft tissue technique was not adequate for the athlete [7]. However, 41% had no significant trauma and the episode occurred during "clumsy" movement. Authors identified 42% of cases in bony Bankart lesion, 5% had glenoid erosion, and 12% would have an enlarged capsule. A worrying observation was that 51% of patients had already osteoarthritic changes based on the radiological appearance. When analyzing the reasons of failure, either initial diagnosis was not appropriate (did not include the risk factors of recurrence), the lesions were not addressed (bone, soft tissues), or there was a technical error (number and location of anchors) (Fig. 15.1), suture and tissue management, inadequate release and reposition of the labrum, inadequate re-tensioning of glenohumeral ligaments. Eighty percent of failures have been related to bone deficiency. Others included also soft tissue-related problems including a myriad of labral tear types (SLAP, ALPSA), humeral avulsion of ligaments and cuff tears. Other problems might have come from capsular laxity, capsular stretching, failure to heal or retear of Bankart (Fig. 15.3) and tear at the margin of bone.

P. Lubiatowski (✉)
Sport Trauma and Biomechanics Unit, Rehasport Clinic, University of Medical Sciences in Poznan, Poznan, Poland
e-mail: p.lubiatowski@rehasport.pl

R. Brzóska et al. (eds.), *360° Around Shoulder Instability*,
https://doi.org/10.1007/978-3-662-61074-9_15

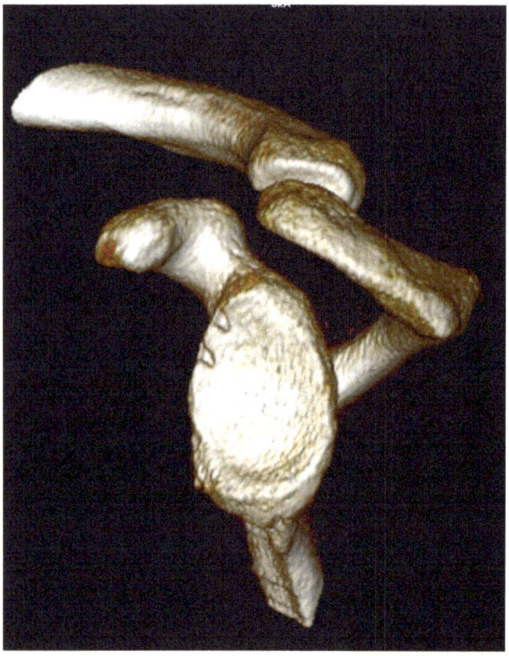

Fig. 15.1 3D computed tomography of glenoid with anterior bone deficiency and failed arthroscopic Bankart repair. Clear malposition of the anchors in the anterosuperior margin of glenoid

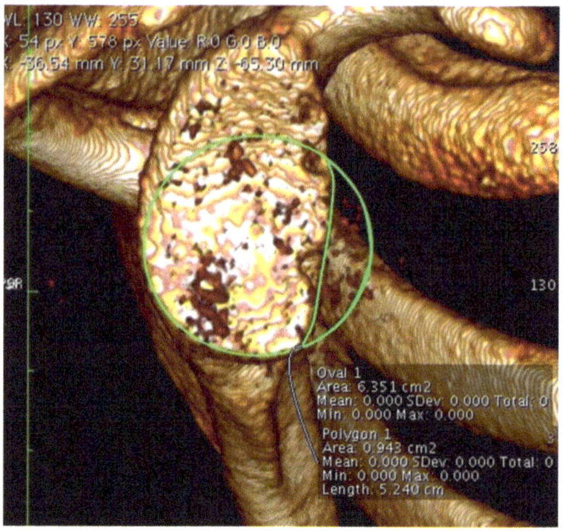

Fig. 15.2 Anterior glenoid deficit as shown with circle area measurement acc. to Sugaya (10% deficit)

15.2 Evaluation of the Patient with Failed Surgery

Appropriate and thorough evaluation is the key to plan the treatment. Attempt should be made to explain the reason for failure. History will reveal whether the recurrence was due to traumatic event (collision, fall) or due to daily activities (reaching for the object, at night). Traumatic event my just indicate fresh injury of a previously healed repair, whereas an atraumatic or low energy incident could mean that the shoulder was unstable before the event (not healed, not repaired properly, bone deficiency ignored, and repair biomechanically incompetent) (Fig. 15.1). Risk factors for recurrence need to be identified. The most important ones include young age, male sex, collision sport, existing bone deficiency (both amount and interplay) laxity, and the number of previous dislocations or subluxations. Clinical evaluation might already indicate suspected bone deficiency. Positive "bony" apprehension (at low angle of abduction or external rotation) has a high level of sensitivity and specificity to detect significant (>25%) anterior glenoid deficiency or engaging Hill–Sachs lesions [8]. Imaging will help to evaluate the current status of tissues. X-ray is the first to identify bone deficiency to some extent and will allow for the identification of osteoarthritic changes [3, 9, 10]. In order to quantify bone lesions, computed tomography (CT) scan has been a golden standard [11, 12] (Fig. 15.2). In acute scenario, MR may rely on natural arthrography form the hematoma and will allow to identify fresh lesions (edema, fracture, labral tear). Magnetic resonance arthrography may also allow for bone deficiency measurements and in case of chronic case may help evaluate soft tissue status (Fig. 15.3).

In general, MR has some limitations. It is less accurate for bone evaluation, unless specific protocol with high resolution will be used [13]. I am routinely using "circle" techniques to measure glenoid deficiency and on-track-off-track concept for Hill–Sachs defect (both size and relation to glenoid) [5, 14, 15].

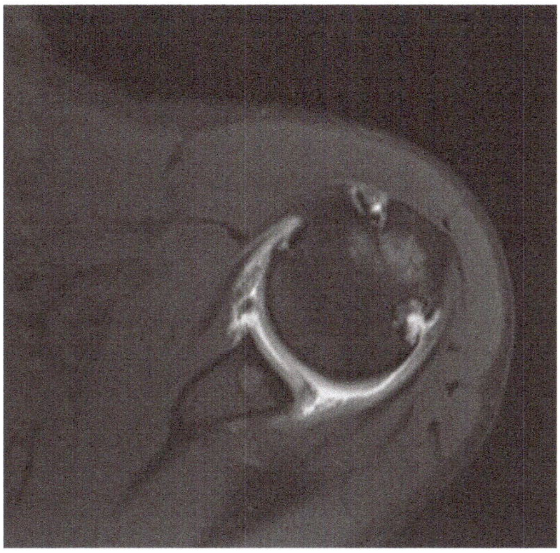

Fig. 15.3 Magnetic resonance arthrography depicting anterior labrum retear following prior stabilization with suture anchors

15.3 Management

The treatment options for patient with recurrent instability include both nonoperative and operative treatment. Nonoperative treatment can be an option for some patients. In case of acute event and high risk of redislocation (age, sports), I tend to do early MR. If patient has partial labral tear and the tear that is not displaced, a short period of sling rest and early rehabilitation might be effective [16]. If the patient within 3-month evaluation continues to be apprehensive or has another incident surgical management should be considered.

In general, revision surgery may indicate the choice of either repeated soft-tissue procedure or the choice of bone reconstruction. Unfortunately, both approaches have the risk of being less successful as a revision surgery when compared with primary procedure. Arthroscopy can initially be used as a diagnostic tool to identify tissue lesions and the assessment of reparability (quality of soft tissues). Previous anchors and sutures can be removed (Fig. 15.4).

Soft tissue may be addressed, including laxity (with capsular shift) and array of labral tears (SLAP, GLAD, labral tear extending beyond anterior part) (Fig. 15.4c). Major limitations and contraindications for arthroscopic soft tissue revision procedures include voluntary dislocators, subscapularis deficiency, bone deficiency, severe osteoarthritis, and low quality of anterior capsulolabral complex (degenerative labrum, ALPSA). Adjunct to labral repair may be infraspinatus tenodesis to address the Hill–Sachs lesions (remplissage). This has been shown to reduce the risk of recurrence [17]. Another technical option is labroplasty with transfer of long head of the biceps [18]. Results have been mixed. DeGorgi showed low value for arthroscopic soft tissue revision repair with 21% recurrence rate and 36% if persistent apprehension was included [19]. However, a systematic review performed by Friedman at al. showed that in properly selected cases (no bone deficiency), the success rate was the same as for coracoid transfer in revision cases (14.7% vs. 14.3% recurrence rate) [20].

There is no doubt that significant bone deficiency and interplay of both glenoid deficit and engaging Hill–Sachs cannot be addressed with the soft tissue repair. Golden standard in such case seems to be coracoid transfer [Latarjet, Bristow] (Fig. 15.5). It has proved its value for revision on the failed Bankart repair (Fig. 15.4). *Schmidt* et al. presented 88% good and excellent results, with 4% recurrent subluxations and 10% of patient having persistent positive apprehension [21]. They have reported 12% complication rate, but of minor clinical importance. None of the patients needed revision. Recently, arthroscopic Latarjet brings more options [22, 23], mostly using the advantages of thorough evaluation and intraoperative decision-making. It has also an advantage of performing some pre-reconstructive procedures (debridement, removal of suture/implants). Then appropriate coracoid transfer may be performed. With recent modification and techniques, capsulolabral complex can be addressed as well (Fig. 15.6). That may potentially improve proprioception ability and decrease the chance of persistent apprehension [24, 25].

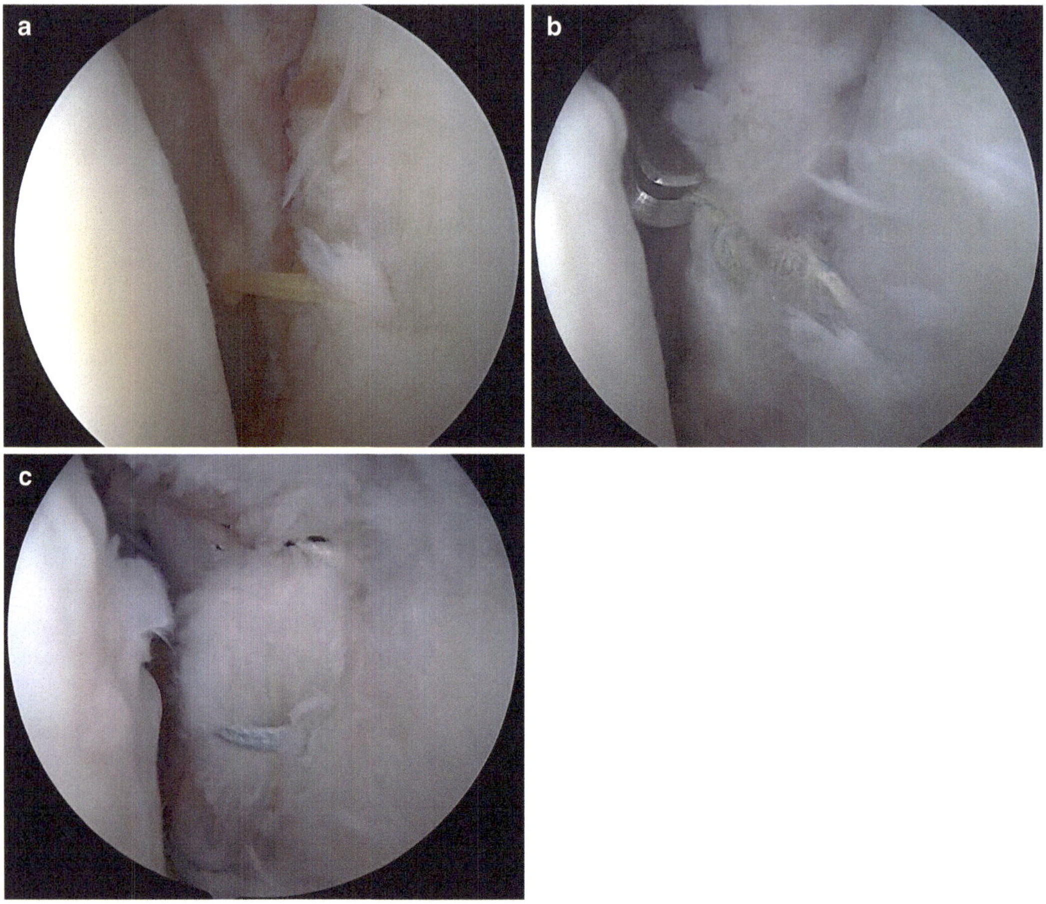

Fig. 15.4 Shoulder arthroscopy in failed Bankart repair: evaluation (**a**), suture removal (**b**) and suture anchor fixation with three double-loaded anchors (**c**)

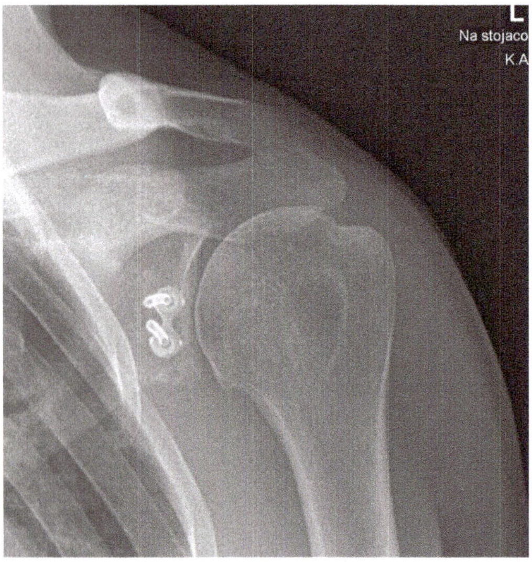

Fig. 15.5 Ragiographic picture of coracoid transfer fixed with 2 canulated screws

Surgeons may sometimes face more severe cases (several failed surgeries, significant bipolar bone deficiency, existent osteoarthritis, and congenital generalized laxity). Armamentarium should include procedures like grafting of humeral head, partial or resurfacing arthroplasty. Finally, arthrodesis could be valuable solution in rare severe cases. Diaz et al. showed a series of 8 patients with an average of 7 failed previous repair attempts with pain, dysfunction and disability that have been treated with shoulder fusion. They have reported 100% satisfaction rate and 73% subjective improvement. The range of movement allowed to reach above the head and wash lower back [26].

In order to summarize the chapter, a shoulder surgeon needs to be prepared to be confronted with patients with a failed stabilization proce-

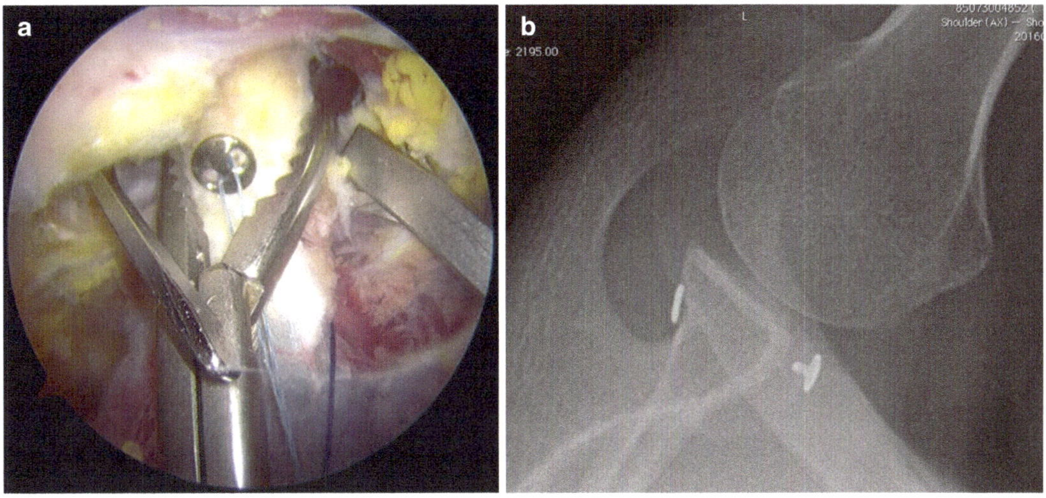

Fig. 15.6 Arthroscopic Coracoid transfer (Latarjet-Bankart) with endobutton fixation and labral repair ((**a**) arthroscopic picture, (**b**) postoperative X-ray)

dure. A thorough preoperative evaluation is the key for successful management and proper choice of treatment methods. Risk factors of possible failure need to be addressed, as well as patients' expectations. Conservative treatment may be considered in some cases. Arthroscopic repeated repair with adjunct procedures may be an option. However, in majority of cases due to frequently coexisting osseous deficiencies and poor soft-tissue quality, bone reconstructive procedures should be considered (coracoid transfer). Arthroscopically assisted coracoid transfer approach has many advantages, but its ultimate value and safety are still to be proved.

References

1. An VV, Sivakumar BS, Phan K, Trantalis J. A systematic review and meta-analysis of clinical and patient-reported outcomes following two procedures for recurrent traumatic anterior instability of the shoulder: Latarjet procedure vs. Bankart repair. J Shoulder Elbow Surg. 2016;25(5):853–63. https://doi.org/10.1016/j.jse.2015.11.001.
2. Blonna D, Bellato E, Caranzano F, Assom M, Rossi R, Castoldi F. Arthroscopic Bankart repair versus open Bristow-Latarjet for shoulder instability: a matched-pair multicenter study focused on return to sport. Am J Sports Med. 2016;44(12):3198–205. PMID: 27501835
3. Balg F, Boileau P. The instability severity index score. A simple pre-operative score to select patients for arthroscopic or open shoulder stabilisation. J Bone Joint Surg Br. 2007;89(11):1470–7.
4. Boileau P, Villalba M, Héry JY, Balg F, Ahrens P, Neyton L. Risk factors for recurrence of shoulder instability after arthroscopic Bankart repair. J Bone Joint Surg Am. 2006;88(8):1755–63. PMID: 16882898
5. Di Giacomo G, Itoi E, Burkhart SS. Evolving concept of bipolar bone loss and the Hill-Sachs lesion: from "engaging/non-engaging" lesion to "on-track/off-track" lesion. Arthroscopy. 2014;30(1):90–8. https://doi.org/10.1016/j.arthro.2013.10.004.
6. Yamamoto N, Itoi E, Abe H, et al. Contact between the glenoid and the humeral head in abduction, external rotation, and horizontal extension: a new concept of glenoid track. J Shoulder Elbow Surg. 2007;16:649–56.
7. Tauber M, Resch H, Forstner R, Raffl M, Schauer J. Reasons for failure after surgical repair of anterior shoulder instability. J Shoulder Elbow Surg. 2004;13(3):279–85.
8. Bushnell BD, Creighton RA, Herring MM. The bony apprehension test for instability of the shoulder: a prospective pilot analysis. Arthroscopy. 2008;24(9):974–82. https://doi.org/10.1016/j.arthro.2008.07.019.
9. Bouliane MJ, Chan H, Kemp K, Glasgow R, Lambert R, Beaupre LA, Sheps DM. The intra- and inter-rater reliability of plain radiographs for Hill–Sachs and bony glenoid lesions: evaluation of the radiographic portion of the instability severity index score. Shoulder Elbow. 2013;5:33–8. https://doi.org/10.1111/j.1758-5740.2012.00208.x.
10. Rouleau DM, Hébert-Davies J, Djahangiri A, Godbout V, Pelet S, Balg F. Validation of the instability shoulder index score in a multicenter reliability study in 114

consecutive cases. Am J Sports Med. 2013;41(2):278–82. https://doi.org/10.1177/0363546512470815.
11. Bishop JY, Jones GL, Rerko MA, Donaldson C, MOON Shoulder Group. 3-D CT is the most reliable imaging modality when quantifying glenoid bone loss. Clin Orthop Relat Res. 2013;471(4):1251–6. https://doi.org/10.1007/s11999-012-2607-x.
12. Kubicka AM, Stefaniak J, Lubiatowski P, Długosz J, Dzianach M, Redman M, Piontek J, Romanowski L. Reliability of measurements performed on two dimensional and three dimensional computed tomography in glenoid assessment for instability. Int Orthop. 2016;40(12):2581–8. Epub 2016 Aug 5
13. Friedman LG, Ulloa SA, Braun DT, Saad HA, Jones MH, Miniaci AA. Glenoid bone loss measurement in recurrent shoulder dislocation: assessment of measurement agreement between CT and MRI. Orthop J Sports Med. 2014;2(9):2325967114549541. https://doi.org/10.1177/2325967114549541.
14. Baudi P, Righi P, Bolognesi D, Rivetta S, Rossi Urtoler E, Guicciardi N, Carrara M. How to identify and calculate glenoid bone deficit. Chir Organi Mov. 2005;90(2):145–52.
15. Sugaya H, Moriishi J, Dohi M, Kon Y, Tsuchiya A. Glenoid rim morphology in recurrent anterior glenohumeral instability. J Bone Joint Surg Am. 2003;85(5):878–84.
16. Marquardt B, Garmann S, Schulte T, Witt KA, Steinbeck J, Pötzl W. Outcome after failed traumatic anterior shoulder instability repair with and without surgical revision. J Shoulder Elbow Surg. 2007;16(6):742–7.
17. Wolf EM, Arianjam A. Hill-Sachs remplissage, an arthroscopic solution for the engaging Hill-Sachs lesion: 2- to 10-year follow-up and incidence of recurrence. J Shoulder Elbow Surg. 2014;23(6):814–20. https://doi.org/10.1016/j.jse.2013.09.009.
18. Milenin O, Toussaint B. Labral repair augmentation by labroplasty and simultaneous trans-subscapular transposition of the long head of the biceps. Arthrosc Tech. 2019;8(5):e507–12. https://doi.org/10.1016/j.eats.2019.01.010.
19. de Giorgi S, Garofalo R, Tafuri S, Cesari E, Rose GD, Castagna A. Can arthroscopic revision surgery for shoulder instability be a fair option? Muscles Ligaments Tendons J. 2014;4(2):226–31.
20. Friedman LG, Griesser MJ, Miniaci AA, Jones MH. Recurrent instability after revision anterior shoulder stabilization surgery. Arthroscopy. 2014;30(3):372–81. https://doi.org/10.1016/j.arthro.2013.11.019.
21. Schmid SL, Farshad M, Catanzaro S, Gerber C. The Latarjet procedure for the treatment of recurrence of anterior instability of the shoulder after operative repair: a retrospective case series of forty-nine consecutive patients. J Bone Joint Surg Am. 2012;94(11):e75.
22. Boileau P, Saliken D, Gendre P, Seeto BL, d'Ollonne T, Gonzalez JF, Bronsard N. Arthroscopic latarjet: suture-button fixation is a safe and reliable alternative to screw fixation. Arthroscopy. 2019;35(4):1050–61. https://doi.org/10.1016/j.arthro.2018.11.012.
23. Lafosse L, Boyle S, Gutierrez-Aramberri M, Shah A, Meller R. Arthroscopic latarjet procedure. Orthop Clin North Am. 2010;41(3):393–405. https://doi.org/10.1016/j.ocl.2010.02.004.
24. Kordasiewicz B, Kicinski M, Małachowski K, Wieczorek J, Chaberek S, Pomianowski S. Comparative study of open and arthroscopic coracoid transfer for shoulder anterior instability (Latarjet)-computed tomography evaluation at a short term follow-up. Part II. Int Orthop. 2018;42(5):1119–28. https://doi.org/10.1007/s00264-017-3739-0.
25. Lädermann A, Tirefort J, Zanchi D, Haller S, Charbonnier C, Hoffmeyer P, Cunningham G. Shoulder apprehension: a multifactorial approach. EFORT Open Rev. 2018;3(10):550–7. https://doi.org/10.1302/2058-5241.3.180007.
26. Diaz JA, Cohen SB, Warren RF, Craig EV, Allen AA. Arthrodesis as a salvage procedure for recurrent instability of the shoulder. J Shoulder Elbow Surg. 2003;12(3):237–41.

16 Algorithm in Acute Glenoid Fractures: From Imaging to Decision Making

Boris Poberaj

16.1 Introduction

Glenoid has specific anatomical structure with thick subchondral bone plate conveying load onto a relatively small amount of cancellous bone. It has a stronger posterior vault compared with a thinner and steeper anterior vault. The mean articular cartilage thickness is 3.8 mm [1].

Glenoid fractures represent up to 20% of all scapular fractures. The usual mechanism of a glenoid fracture is the direct impact of humeral head onto glenoid fossa or humeral head dislocation with anterior rim fracture. The prevalence of rim fractures at first-time dislocation ranges from 16 to 22%, whereas in recurrent dislocations from 38 to 73%.

Most of the bone fragments are tightly connected to the labrum and maintain their blood supply [2], which makes absorption unlikely. On the opposite side, Nakagawa [3] reported that most of the bone fragments show severe absorption within 1 year after the primary traumatic episode and bone fragment absorption and glenoid defects are more frequent in patients with recurrent anterior shoulder instability. The possible mismatch between the glenoid defect size and the bone fragment size would be due to the glenoid defect enlarging by recurrent erosions from dislocations.

Nakagawa et al. [4] reported that the postoperative bone union rate was lower when the residual bone fragment was small or medium sized.

16.2 Exploration

Plain X-rays in different planes are routinely carried out, but they are not enough to evaluate the real extent of fracture. It is reported that plain radiographs alone miss 60% of anterior glenoid rim fractures found during surgery. Computed tomography (CT) scanning, both two-dimensional (2D) and three-dimensional (3D), gives the most accurate assessment of the size of the fracture fragment(s) [5] and the relationship between the humeral head and the main fragment of the glenoid. Magnetic resonance imaging (MRI) reliability and consistency with higher magnetic field machines are improving in comparison to CT and 3D-CT.

16.3 Treatment Guidelines

The goal of surgical treatment is anatomical and concentric joint restoration. The main question pertains as to what are the size of the fragment and the size of displacement when there is an absolute indication for surgery.

B. Poberaj (✉)
Aspetar Orthopaedic and Sports Medicine Hospital, Doha, Qatar

R. Brzóska et al. (eds.), *360° Around Shoulder Instability*,
https://doi.org/10.1007/978-3-662-61074-9_16

The fact is that even large, displaced glenoid rim fractures can be successfully treated nonoperatively, if the glenohumeral joint is concentrically reduced [6]. Salomonsson et al. [7] found that bony Bankart lesions were associated with good functional outcomes in cases of first-time dislocations and conservative therapy. On the other hand, when the humeral head is mainly in contact with the displaced fractured fragment or the joint congruency is completely lost, then surgical intervention is mandatory.

Definition for surgical indication based on millimeters of fragment displacement is not clearly put forth or validated. The proposed relative indication is ≥5 mm of intra-articular fragment displacement with subchondral bone exposure or step-off fracture displacement for ≥5 mm, which depends on the size and location of the fragments. In these cases, the risk of nonunion, malunion, and posttraumatic osteoarthritis was increased.

16.4 Algorithm

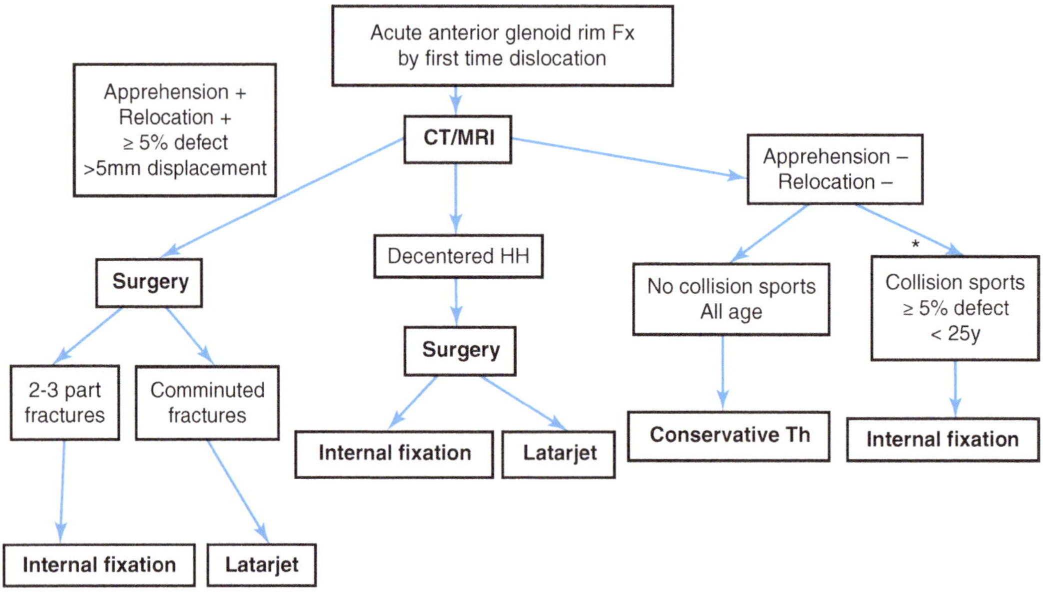

*The indication is further dependent on the age of the player, the size of the anterior bony defect >5% of glenoid width, and the presence of bipolar lesion with important Hill–Sachs lesion.

16.5 Surgery Techniques

The technique selection for anterior glenoid rim fractures can be open or arthroscopic, or combined. Different implants are available like Titanium and bio-compression screws and variety of suture anchors. Usually, a combination of screws and anchors is necessary to completely restore the glenoid and soft tissue anatomy. Advanced arthroscopic techniques are used to reconstruct multifragmented or large (>21% of glenoid length) solitary fractures with good and excellent results [8]. The technique using suture anchors as the single point or suture bridge has shown equivalent failure strengths and load transfers [9]. Care should be taken not to compromise the glenoid osseous integrity by greater number of anchors in the same line. The advantages of primary repair versus bone grafting are better viability of fracture fragments due to their attachment to labrum and more physiological position of the reconstructed labrum. One of the disadvantages is that the bone fragment is usually shifted cranially, due to vertical shift of the labrum. Bone fragment enlargement and remodeling are seen up to 2 years after reconstruction [10].

16.6 Summary

There is no consensus on the operative treatment of anterior glenoid rim fractures.

The absolute indication for surgery is the loss of joint congruence with humeral head in contact with a displaced fractured fragment.

Values showing ≥5 mm intra-articular fragment displacement or ≥5 mm step-off displacement relatively to the fragment size are indications for surgery.

Special attention must be given to anterior glenoid fractures with mechanism of humeral head dislocation, as the recurrence can be particularly high in the young age group with concomitant bipolar lesions. In this group of patients with bone fragments, which represent >5% of glenoid defect and patients are clinically unstable, the surgical stabilization is indicated with incorporation of bone fragment to restore the glenoid anatomy.

References

1. Frich LH, Larsen MS. How to deal with glenoid fracture. EFORT Open Rev. 2017;2:151–7.
2. Fuji Y, Yoneda M, Wakitani S, Hayashida K. Histologic analysis of bony Bankart lesions in recurrent anterior instability of the shoulder. J Shoulder Elbow Surg. 2006;15:218–23.
3. Nakagawa S, Mizuno N, Hiramatsu K, Tachibana Y, Mae T. Absorption of the bone fragment in shoulders with bony Bankart lesions caused by recurrent anterior dislocations or subluxations. Am J Sports Med. 2013;41(6):1380–6.
4. Nakagawa S, Mae T, Yoneda K, Kinugasa K, Nakamura H. Influence of glenoid defect size and bone fragment size on the clinical outcome after arthroscopic Bankart repair in male collision/contact athletes. Am J Sports Med. 2017;45(9):1967–74.
5. Milano G, Saccomanno MF, Magarelli N, Bonomo L. Analysis of agreement between computed tomography measurements of glenoid bone defects in anterior shoulder instability with and without comparison with the contralateral shoulder. Am J Sports Med. 2015;43(12):2918–26.
6. Maquieira GJ, Gerber C, Eid K. Non-operative treatment of large anterior glenoid rim fractures after traumatic anterior dislocation of the shoulder. J Bone Joint Surg Br. 2007;89:1347–51.
7. Salomonsson B, Von Heine A, Dahlborn M, Abbaszadegan H, Ahlstrom S, Dalen N, Lillkrona U. Bony Bankart is a positive predictive factor after primary shoulder dislocation. Knee Surg Sports Traumatol Arthrosc. 2010;18:1425–31.
8. Scheibel M, Hug K, Gerhardt C, Krueger D. Arthroscopic reduction and fixation of large solitary and multifragmented anterior glenoid rim fractures. J Shoulder Elbow Surg. 2016;25(5):781–90.
9. Giles JW, Puskas GJ, Welsh MF, Johnson JA, Athwal GS. Suture anchor fixation of bony Bankart fractures. Am J Sports Med. 2013;41(11):2624–31.
10. Nakagawa S, Ozaki R, Take Y. Bone fragment union and remodeling after arthroscopic bony Bankart repair for traumatic anterior shoulder instability with glenoid defect: influence on postoperative recurrence. Am J Sports Med. 2015;43:1438–49.

17 Glenoid Fractures

Adrian Błasiak, Hubert Laprus, Roman Brzóska, and Pascal Gleyze

17.1 Introduction

The topic of this chapter is the management of glenoid fracture accompanying the shoulder instability. These mostly referred to the anterior glenoid rim.

Bone defects of the anteroinferior glenoid can be the main cause of recurrences in glenohumeral instability. Glenoid bone loss is a result of acute fracture during shoulder dislocation or erosion of anterior glenoid rim in cases of chronic anterior instability.

The prevalence of anterior glenoid rim fractures has been reported from 22% after first-time anterior shoulder dislocation and up to 73% in recurrent instability with an increased prevalence in male patients [1–7].

Arciero et al. observed the recurrence of dislocation in 80% of patients with classic or bony Bankart lesion treated with nonsurgical methods [8].

Although the incidence of glenoid bony lesions is high and their treatment is widespread, there is still lack of clear distinction between the bony Bankart lesion and the fracture of anterior glenoid rim. Usually, most of the authors tend to define a small bony fragment as bony Bankart lesion and larger one as fracture.

Therefore, fractures of the anterior–inferior glenoid rim associated with instability or bony Bankart lesions are quite common but lead to failures after arthroscopic Bankart repairs [9–11].

Osseous glenoid injury is particularly common in patients who have undergone high-energy trauma and patients with recurrent instability, up to 90% of whom have some degree of glenoid bony injury.

Also, cadaveric studies showed us the consequences of glenoid bone loss. Itoi et al. recognized that a bony defect of at least 21% of the glenoid length will significantly decrease stability [12].

In the same manner, Yamamoto et al. created a model with an osseous defect at 3 o'clock and stated that the defect equal to or greater than 20% of the glenoid length significantly decreases anterior stability [13].

17.2 Evaluation and Classification

The radiological assessment comprises conventional X-ray examination and includes standard anteroposterior (AP) and transscapular (Y projection) views. Sometimes double contour of anterior glenoid rim can be visible (Fig. 17.1). However, these fractures can be easily missed on plain radiographs, so computed tomography (CT) scans are crucial for correct diagnosis [14, 15] (Fig. 17.2).

A CT examination should be performed in all patients for further evaluation and treatment.

A. Błasiak · H. Laprus · R. Brzóska
Shoulder and Upper Limb Department,
St. Luke's Hospital, Bielsko-Biala, Poland
e-mail: blasiak@lukasza.pl

P. Gleyze (✉)
Sport Trauma Center - Saint Louis Hospital,
Saint Louis, France

R. Brzóska et al. (eds.), *360° Around Shoulder Instability*,
https://doi.org/10.1007/978-3-662-61074-9_17

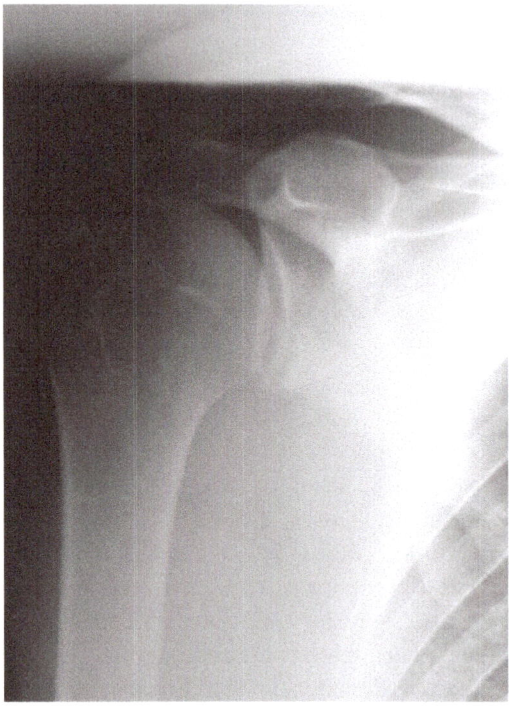

Fig. 17.1 Small fracture of the anterior glenoid—double contour visible on AP X-ray

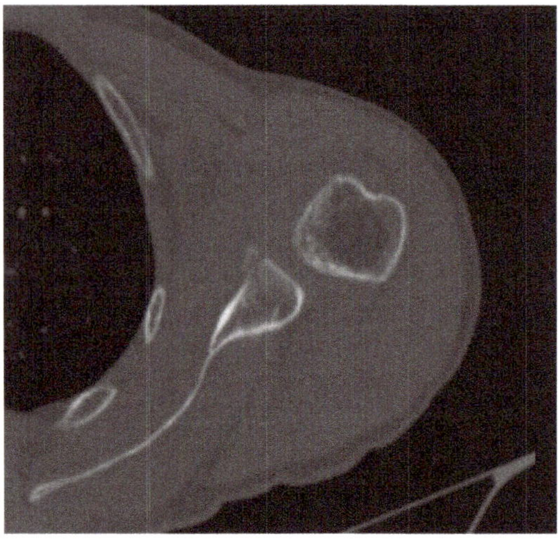

Fig. 17.2 CT transverse scan

The fracture size is quantified by CT using three-dimensional (3D) reconstruction and an estimation of fracture configuration (solid or comminuted), orientation, and alignment is performed (Figs. 17.3, 17.4, and 17.5).

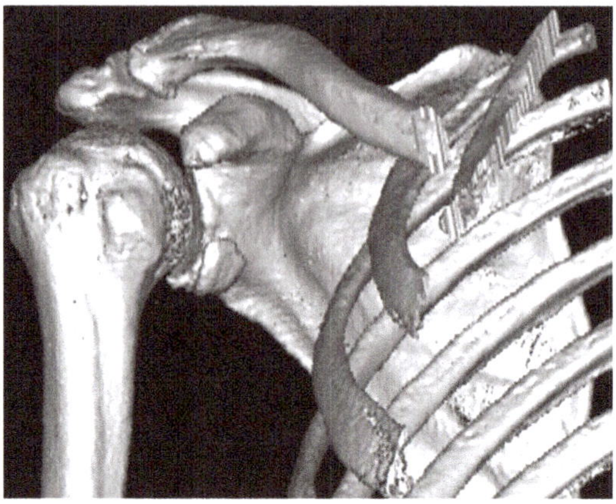

Fig. 17.3 3D-CT reconstruction 1

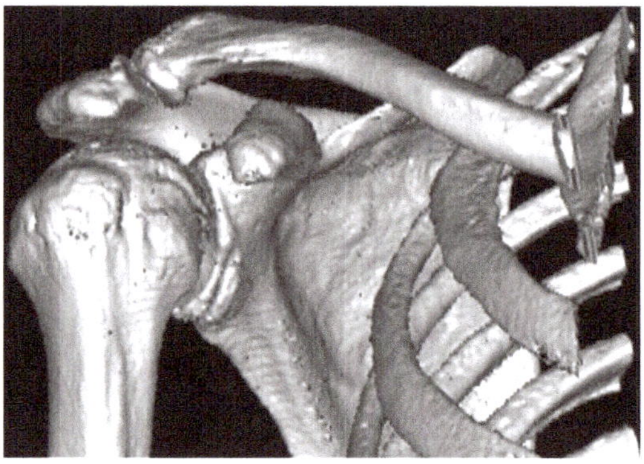

Fig. 17.4 3D-CT reconstruction 2

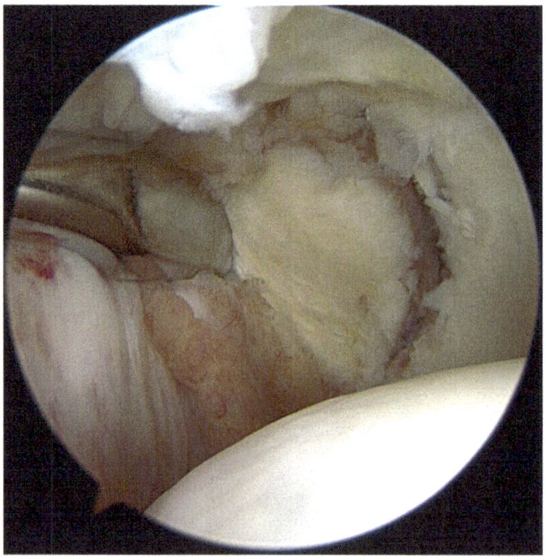

Fig. 17.5 Mobilization of the bony fragment

Magnetic resonance imaging (MRI) is also used as a diagnostic tool and this examination is rationalized by the detection of existing intra-articular co-injuries.

Several classification systems for glenoid fractures have been described, but none of these have been proven to be superior. The Ideberg classification is the most widely used and cited one [16].

Fractures of anterior glenoid correspond to type IA in the Ideberg classification.

These types of injuries have also been classified by Bigliani et al. into three types according to the fracture morphology. Type I represents an avulsion fracture with attached capsulolabral complex, type II a medially displaced fragment and united with the glenoid neck, and type III an erosion of the inferior glenoid with less (IIIA) or more (IIIB) than 25% bone loss [17].

One of the latest classification systems was proposed by Sugaya et al. He divided glenoid rim lesions in patients with recurrent anterior shoulder instability in small (<5%), medium (5–20%), and large lesions (>20%) by assessment of the bone loss percentage with 3D-CT reconstruction. He recommended reduction and internal fixation of small- or medium-sized lesions and grafting procedures in large defects [18].

17.3 Treatment

There exist, as always, either conservative or surgical treatment options.

Some authors report good and excellent results of the conservative treatment of anterior–inferior glenoid followed by a high rate of osseous healing of the bony Bankart lesion [19–22].

On the other hand, De Palma recommended that anterior glenoid fractures displaced by at least 10 mm and involving 25% of the glenoid surface should be treated surgically, with open reduction and internal fixation [23].

Sugaya et al. go further and suggest reduction and internal fixation of small- or medium-sized lesions (<20% bone loss), as well as grafting procedures in large defects (>20%) [18].

More recently, Spiegl et al. recommend a conservative treatment strategy in active patients with small osseous Bankart lesions (<5%), whereas patients with medium-sized or large Bankart fractures were suggested a surgical treatment strategy [24].

According to Mologne et al. when a bony Bankart lesion is present, in either the acute or chronic case, the best treatment is to reattach that fragment into anterior glenoid rim. Such repair can heal reliably and reduce the risk of redislocation [25].

The time of surgery seems to be of great importance, because the quality of capsulolabral complex of the anterior joint wall deteriorates with time and number of dislocations [26].

Furthermore, shoulders treated after multiple dislocations have a longer trauma-to-surgery interval and the clinical outcomes are less satisfactory [27–30].

The good results achieved while operating acute dislocations and the worse outcomes of chronic lesions repairs are reflected in the literature. The latter outcomes are related to histopathologic bone, capsule, and ligament changes due to repeatable dislocations [30–32].

There is some evidence in the literature for superior results of osseous Bankart repair in acute cases compared to chronic ones [7].

Furthermore, Nakagawa et al. proved the high chance of partial absorption of the bony fragment during the first year after fracture that reduces the chance of healing of the postponed refixation of the fracture [33].

17.3.1 Surgical Treatment

Treatment includes open or arthroscopic repair with use of either suture anchors or metal cannulated and bioabsorbable screws [34–36].

Indications for use of suture anchors are situations, when the osseous fragment is relatively small (<25% of the glenoid width) and can be reliably incorporated into anterior glenoid together with the capsulolabral complex [7, 37].

Internal fixation with screws is recommended for larger bony fragments (>25% of the anteroposterior diameter of glenoid) [38, 39].

Although both open and arthroscopic approaches are recommended for that purpose, arthroscopy theoretically has some advantages. These are intra-articular visualization of the reduction, preservation of the bony fragment blood supply, decreased soft-tissue dissection, lower blood loss, cosmetic issues, and the possibility of prompt rehabilitation. Another extremely important advantage is the possibility of recognition and treatment of other concomitant intra-articular injuries.

Scheibel et al. report the incidence of such lesions in 78.3% (18 of 23) of the cases [36].

The most common concomitant findings are Hill–Sachs lesion, partial or full-thickness supraspinatus tendon tear, traumatic or degenerative lesion of the long head of the biceps tendon, superior and posteroinferior labral tear, acromion or coracoid fracture, and osteochondral lesions. Other additional injuries, like avulsion fracture of the greater tuberosity or proximal humerus fracture, have also been described [40, 41].

17.3.2 Surgical Technique

The position of the patient could be lateral decubitus or beach chair and is operator dependent.

The arthroscope is introduced via a standard posterior portal. Next, an accessory anterolateral (suprabicipital) portal using an outside-in technique is established. The probe is inserted through this portal and the diagnostic arthroscopy is performed. Meticulous visualization of the anterior glenoid rim and assessment of concomitant lesions are the next steps of the procedure. With the use of the shaver, introduced through the anterolateral portal, hematoma, fibrin clot, and small loose fragments of fractured gleonid are evacuated. Then, an anterior portal (above the superior margin of the subscapularis tendon) is established and the bony fragment along with the capsuloligamentous complex is mobilized with a rasp or elevator, and initially reduced (Fig. 17.5). At this moment, other concomitant lesions diagnosed during the arthroscopy can be addressed. The most common procedures include labrum repair, long head of biceps tenodesis, stabilization of other fractures, and rotator cuff reconstruction. All the above-mentioned procedures inevitably prolong the duration of surgery.

Accessory procedures are performed, if needed.

After accessory procedures are finished, stabilization of the fracture is performed. Depending on the size of the bony fragment or fragments and their integrity with the labral complex, a screw osteosynthesis or an anchor fixation technique has to be performed.

The goal of that stage is anatomical fracture reduction without step formation of the articular cartilage with preservation of the capsulolabral complex (Fig. 17.6). For that purpose, an additional anteroinferior portal through the inferior part of the subscapularis tendon should be used [42].

First, the scope should be switched into anterolateral portal and the space between anterior surface of the subscapularis tendon and deltoid fascia is created with the use of shaver. Under the direct visualization, an anteroinferior portal is established using a spinal needle. Only a skin incision is created to avoid bleeding and a potential injury to the cephalic vein. The entrance point of this portal is placed about 5 cm distally and 1 cm laterally to the coracoid tip. This portal is mandatory to allow a proper screw insertion, almost perpendicular to the fracture line. It should be performed only under direct visualization. The potential structure under risk is the conjoined tendon musculocutaneous and axillary nerve,

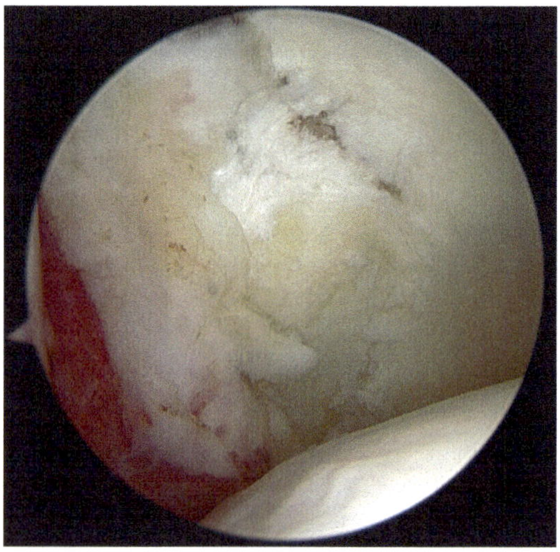

Fig. 17.6 View of fixed fragment

anterior circumflex humeral vessels. The tissue grasper is inserted through the posterior portal to hold the bony soft-tissue complex. Then with the vapor inserted through the same portal, the subscapularis tendon and muscle is cut partially along the muscle fibers and afterwards a capsule is detached from the anterior surface of the fragment to fully visualize it. A drill sleeve is then introduced through the anteroinferior portal and placed on the fragment. Now, reduction is performed using a tissue grasper inserted through posterior portal pulling the capsulolabral complex superiorly and laterally. Accessory anterior portal (above the superior border of the subscapularis tendon) can be established to facilitate the reduction of the fracture. A switching-stick or rasp may be inserted through that portal. This stage of the operation is a four-hand surgery, so the help of an experienced assistant is valuable. Then, the K wire is placed through the drill sleeve and driven into a bony fragment. The K wire can be used as a joystick in order to pinpoint the reposition (Figs. 17.7, 17.8, 17.9 and 17.10). The tip of the wire is placed medially to the labrum just a few millimeters away from the cartilage surface and drilled into glenoid. The entrance point of the wire is dependent on the fragment size. When the fragment is relatively small and we plan to put only one screw, the wire should be placed above or below the planned entrance point for the screw. In the case of a large bony fragment, the first wire is placed in its upper part and the second parallel and below with a distance of 5–7 mm from each other. The first K wire serves as a temporary fixation. The reduction of the fracture is again checked with a probe. The K wire followed by the drill bit is driven in as far as the posterior cortex of the scapular neck. Then, the central wire in the small fragment or the lower wire in larger ones is drilled through the protective drill sleeve. After removing the cannulated drill bit, the screw is inserted over the remaining guide wire into the fragment. Usually, the length of screws ranges between 24 and 32 mm. The first person who described this technique was Cameron in 1998 [43].

After fracture fixation, complementary labrum fixation using suture anchor is performed, if needed.

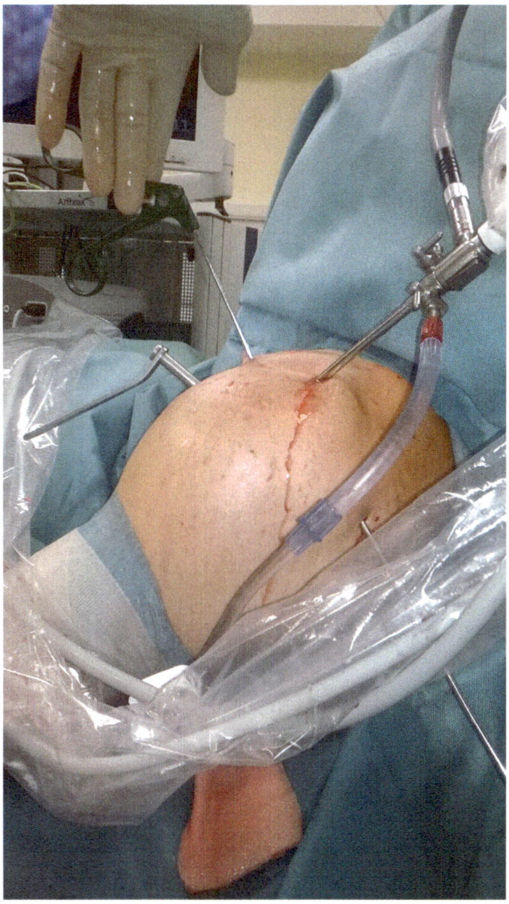

Fig. 17.7 Anterior–inferior portal

In cases of small bony fragments, when the risk of breakage of fragment with a screw exists, reconstruction with suture anchors is an alternative [34, 35].

Anchors are placed superiorly and inferiorly to the fragment into the glenoid. The capsulolabral complex is sutured with simple stitches inferiorly and superiorly or the fragment is penetrated using an awl. The mattress stitches are performed and knots are tied as far from the glenoid surface as possible to avoid contact with the cartilage of either glenoid or humeral head. Embracing of the fragment with the treads from anchors is undesirable for the same reason.

Managing multifragmented fractures is challenging. The fragments should be fully mobilized and all small free fragments

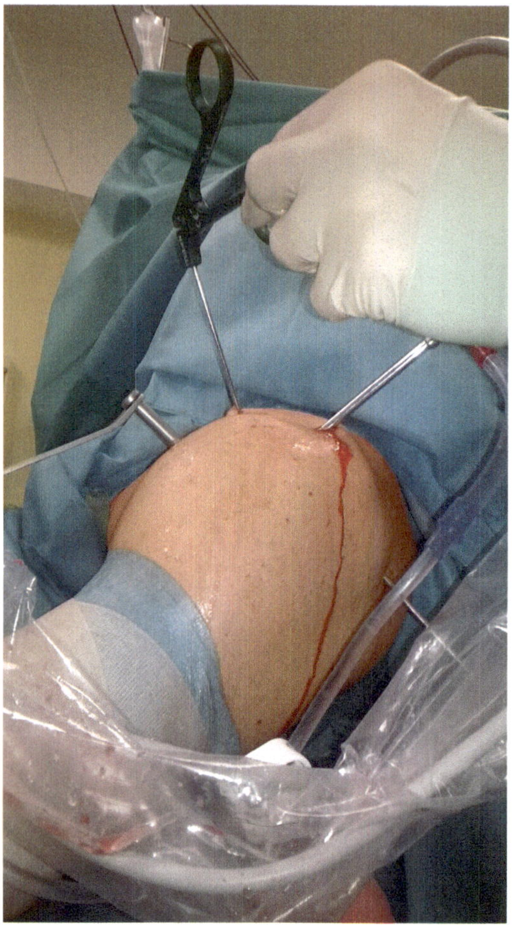

Fig. 17.8 Anterior–inferior portal

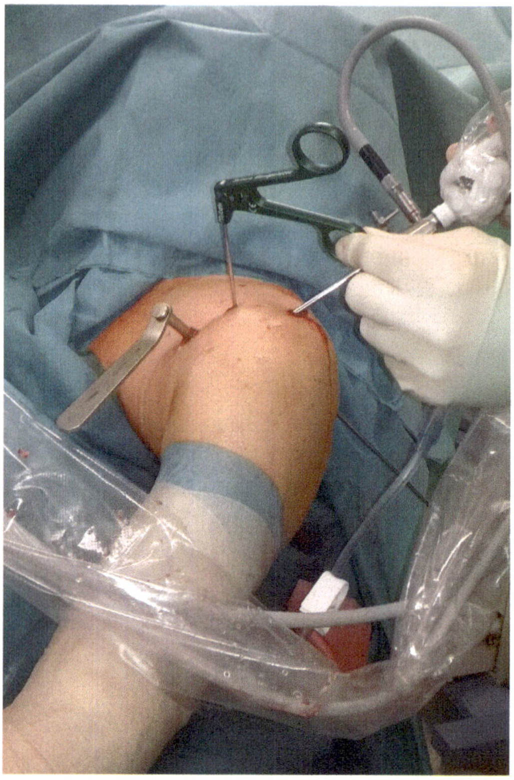

Fig. 17.9 Anterior–inferior portal

removed. Every bony fragment attached to the labrum should be reduced and fixed with suture anchors in a manner as described above. Temporary traction sutures, switching-stick and rasp, may be helpful in reducing main fragments.

Additional procedures, like rotator cuff repair, reduction of other fractures, and long head of biceps tenodesis, are applied afterwards.

Recently, alternative stabilization system was described by Taverna et al. [44]. Depending on the size of the bony fragment, authors suggest to place one or two pairs of round endobuttons. By the use of a dedicated tensioner, a good fixation that is achieved with strong compression of the fracture is described.

17.4 Postop Treatment

After performing postop X-rays confirming the proper bony fragment fixation, rehabilitation protocol is implemented (Figs. 17.11 and 17.12). According to most of the authors, the patients are advised to wear a shoulder sling for 3–4 weeks. During this period, beginning from the second postoperative day on, passive exercises were introduced. Forward flexion, abduction, internal rotation up to 60°, and 10° of external rotation are allowed. From week 4, the sling is removed and active assisted range-of-motion exercises in all planes begin within pain limit. From week 6 to 7, free range of motion is allowed. Practicing noncontact sports is allowed after 3 months, and full return to manual work and contact or throwing sports after 6 months. When associated rotator cuff or labral repairs are performed, the time of immobilization is extended to 6 weeks [7, 36, 40].

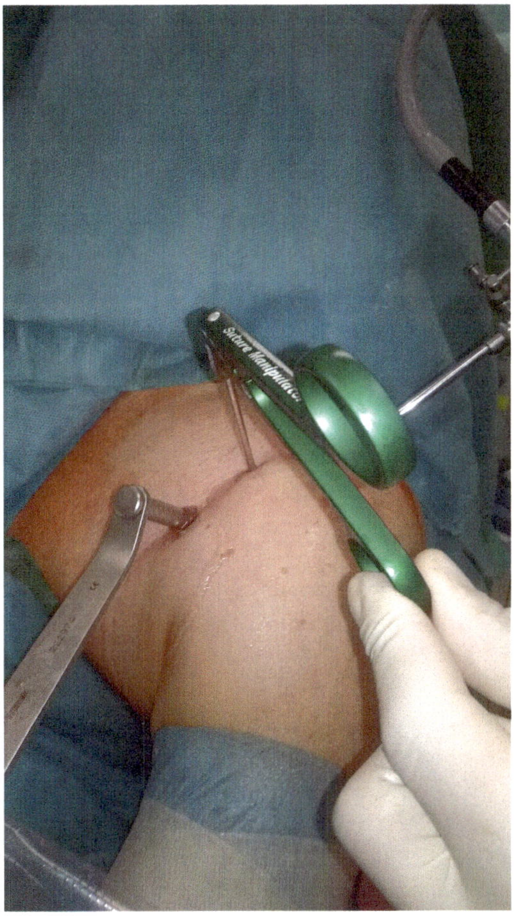

Fig. 17.10 Anterior–inferior portal

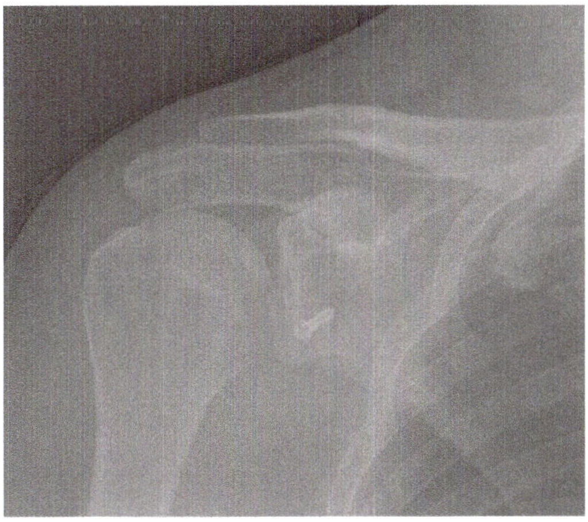

Fig. 17.11 Postoperative X-ray—AP view

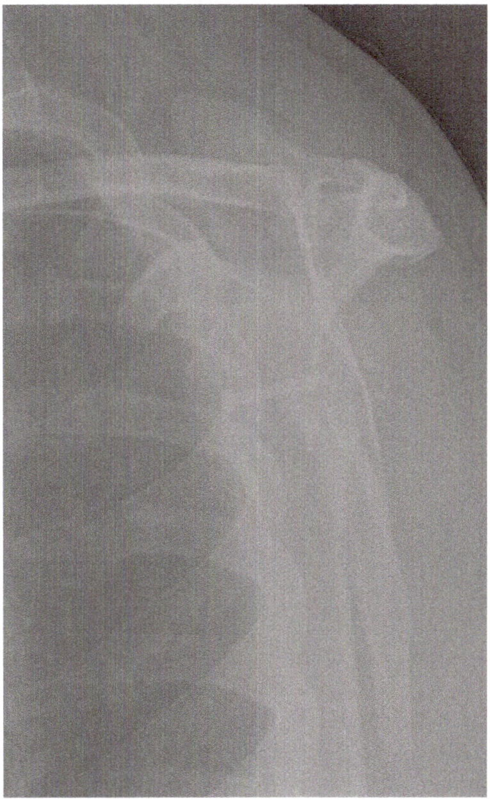

Fig. 17.12 Postoperative X-ray—Y view

17.5 Results

Overall, the results of arthroscopic treatment of anterior glenoid fractures are satisfying.

A redislocation rate occurs from 0 to 6.6% in either acute or chronic lesions [7, 36, 45].

A nonunion rate of the bony fragment ranges in the literature from 8.0 to 16% [7, 34, 45–47].

However, in a study of Plath et al., clinical outcome and stability were not affected by glenoid bone deficiency or nonunion. Furthermore, nonanatomic glenoid fossa reconstruction did not influence any of the evaluated osteoarthritis features [45].

In one of the largest case series, Porcellini et al. found that osseous integration of the refixed bony fragment was significantly dependent on the injury to surgery time. Furthermore, they observed significantly worse clinical results in chronic cases than in acute cases, with redislocation rates of 2.4% and 4.2%, respectively, but still there was one patient in each group [7].

On the contrary, Plath et al. did not detect differences regarding shoulder scores and external rotation between cases of acute instability and cases of chronic instability. They stated that chronic lesions may have an inferior healing potential; therefore, early surgical stabilization of acute Bankart fragments is suggested to avoid possible nonunion [45].

The same authors, in their research, took into account the sporting activity of patients. They stated that although 95% of patients returned to some level of sporting activity, a significant reduction in sporting activities concerning the number of sports disciplines, hours per week, sports level, and participation in risky activities was observed [45].

Scheibel et al. evaluated radiological signs of osteoarthritis and found in seven cases, which was preexisting in 1 patient. Also in seven cases, a postoperative step-off of the glenoid was noticed and it ranged from 1 to 3 mm, but there was no correlation between the step-off and the presence of osteoarthritis [36].

A similar remaining step-off was detected by Plath. In the same series, anatomic reduction was achieved in 72%, and the remaining glenoid defect size averaged 6.8 ± 7.3%. The final conclusion was that the reconstruction of the articular surface did not influence the clinical outcome [45].

17.6 Complications

Few reports were published on complications during arthroscopic reconstruction of anterior glenoid fractures. Among them must be listed damage to the cartilage in the anterior region of the humeral head due to mechanical impingement with the screw head, implant loosening, postop stiff shoulder, etc. Nonunion does not influence the final result according to most of the papers, therefore it is not considered as a complication. Overall, the surgical treatment is a safe procedure characterized by a low number of complications [40].

17.7 Posterior Bony Bankart Lesion

In contrast to anterior instability, posterior instability is uncommon. Authors estimate it at 2 and 12% of all the patients with glenohumeral instability [48, 49].

Goss et al. reported an arthroscopically assisted reduction and internal fixation of a displaced posterior glenoid fracture (Ideberg type Ib) along with an associated comminuted scapular body fracture. Authors fixed the glenoid fracture with a cannulated screw [50].

Full arthroscopic repair of posterior bony Bankart with the use of suture anchors and accomplished with a reverse remplissage procedure was described by Luedke et al. [51].

A similar technique with the use of knotless anchors was recently published by Baxter et al. [52].

17.8 Conclusions

Appropriate management of bony pathology in terms of acute anterior glenohumeral dislocation and chronic instability is critical to prevent recurrent dislocation. Arthroscopic techniques, like suture anchor repair, cannulated screws, or combination of these two methods, may enable an anatomic reduction of bony Bankart lesions or acute fractures with no or with only minimal articular steps and provide successful outcomes and patient satisfaction. The return to activity is possible in most of the cases.

References

1. Hovelius L, Eriksson K, Fredin H, Hagberg G, Hussenius A, Lind B, Thorling J, Weckstrom J. Recurrences after initial dislocation of the shoulder. Results of a prospective study of treatment. J Bone Joint Surg. 1983;65:343–9.
2. Itoi E, Lee SB, Berglund LJ, Berge LL, An KN. The effect of a glenoid defect on anteroinferior stability of the shoulder after Bankart repair: a cadaveric study. J Bone Joint Surg. 2000;82:35–46.
3. Rowe CR, Patel D, Southmayd WW. The Bankart procedure: a long-term end-result study. J Bone Joint Surg. 1978;60:1–16.

4. Bigliani LU, Newton PM, Steinmann SP, Connor PM, McLlveen SJ. Glenoid rim lesions associated with recurrent anterior dislocation of the shoulder. Am J Sports Med. 1998;26:41–5.
5. Hovelius L, Augustini BG, Fredin H, Johansson O, Norlin R, Thorling J. Primary anterior dislocation of the shoulder in young patients. A ten-year prospective study. J Bone Joint Surg. 1996;78:1677–84.
6. Griffith JF, Antonio GE, Yung PS, Wong EM, Yu AB, Ahuja AT, et al. Prevalence, pattern, and spectrum of glenoid bone loss in anterior shoulder dislocation: CT analysis of 218 patients. AJR Am J Roentgenol. 2008;190:1247–54.
7. Porcellini G, Paladini P, Campi F, Paganelli M. Long-term outcome of acute versus chronic bony Bankart lesions managed arthroscopically. Am J Sports Med. 2007;35:2067–72.
8. Arciero RA, Wheeler JH, Ryan JB, McBride JT. Arthroscopic Bankart repair versus nonoperative treatment for acute, initial anterior shoulder dislocations. Am J Sports Med. 1994;22:589–94.
9. Burkhart SS, De Beer JF. Traumatic glenohumeral bone defects and their relationship to failure of arthroscopic Bankart repairs: significance of the inverted-pear glenoid and the humeral engaging Hill-Sachs lesion. Arthroscopy. 2000;16:677–94.
10. Tauber M, Resch H, Forstner R, Raffl M, Schauer J. Reasons for failure after surgical repair of anterior shoulder instability. J Shoulder Elbow Surg. 2004;13:279–85.
11. Meehan RE, Petersen SA. Results and factors affecting outcome of revision surgery for shoulder instability. J Shoulder Elbow Surg. 2005;14:31–7.
12. Itoi E, Lee SB, Berglund LJ, Berge LL, An KN. The effect of a glenoid defect on anteroinferior stability of the shoulder after Bankart repair: a cadaveric study. J Bone Joint Surg Am. 2000;82(1):35–46.
13. Yamamoto N, Itoi E, Abe H, et al. Effect of an anterior glenoid defect on anterior shoulder stability: a cadaveric study. Am J Sports Med. 2009;37(5): 949–54.
14. Chuang TY, Adams CR, Burkhart SS. Use of preoperative three-dimensional computed tomography to quantify glenoid bone loss in shoulder instability. Arthroscopy. 2008;24:376–82.
15. Griffith JF, Antonio GE, Tong CW, Ming CK. Anterior shoulder dislocation: Quantification of glenoid bone loss with CT. AJR Am J Roentgenol. 2003;180:1423–30.
16. Ideberg R, Grevsten S, Larsson S. Epidemiology of scapular fractures: incidence and classification of 338 fractures. Acta Orthop Scand. 1995;66:395–7.
17. Bigliani LU, Newton PM, Steinmann SP, Connor PM, McIlveen SJ. Glenoid rim lesions associated with recurrent anterior dislocation of the shoulder. Am J Sports Med. 1998;26(1):41–5.
18. Sugaya H, Moriishi J, Dohi M, Kon Y, Tsuchiya A. Glenoid rim morphology in recurrent anterior glenohumeral instability. J Bone Joint Surg. 2003;85-A:878–84.
19. Ideberg R. Fractures of the scapula involving the glenoid fossa. In: Bateman JE, Welsh RP, editors. Surgery of the shoulder. Philadelphia: Decker; 1984. p. 63–6.
20. Kraus N, Gerhardt C, Haas N, Scheibel M. Conservative therapy of antero-inferior glenoid fractures. Unfallchirurg. 2010;113:469–75.
21. Maquieira GJ, Espinosa N, Gerber C, Eid K. Non-operative treatment of large anterior glenoid rim fractures after traumatic anterior dislocation of the shoulder. J Bone Joint Surg Br. 2007;89:1347–51.
22. Salomonsson B, Von Heine A, Dahlborn M, Abbaszadegan H, Ahlstrom S, Dalen N, Lillkrona U. Bony Bankart is a positive predictive factor after primary shoulder dislocation. Knee Surg Sports Traumatol Arthrosc. 2010;18:1425–31.
23. DePalma AF. Fracture and fracture-dislocation of the shoulder girdle. In: Jacob RP, Kristainsen T, Mayo K, et al., editors. Surgery of the shoulder. 3rd ed. Philadelphia: JB Lippincott; 1983. p. 366–7.
24. Spiegl U, Ryf C, Hepp P, Paavo R. Evaluation of a treatment algorithm for acute traumatic osseous Bankart lesions resulting from first time dislocation of the shoulder with a two year follow-up. BMC Musculoskelet Disord. 2013;14:305.
25. Mologne TS, Provencher MT, Menzel KA, Vachon TA, Dewing CB. Arthroscopic stabilization in patients with an inverted pear glenoid: results in patients with bone loss of the anterior glenoid. Am J Sports Med. 2007;35:1276–83.
26. McMahon PJ, Dettling JR, Sandusky MD, Lee TQ. Deformation and strain characteristics along the length of the anterior band of the inferior glenohumeral ligament. J Shoulder Elbow Surg. 2001;10:482–8.
27. Buscayret F, Edwards TB, Szabo I, Adeleine P, Coudane H, Walch G. Glenohumeral arthrosis in anterior instability before and after surgical treatment: Incidence and contributing factors. Am J Sports Med. 2004;32:1165–72.
28. Larrain MV, Botto GJ, Montenegro HJ, Mauas DM. Arthroscopic repair of acute traumatic anterior shoulder dislocation in young athletes. Arthroscopy. 2001;17:373–7.
29. Pollock RG, Wang VM, Bucchieri JS, et al. Effects of repetitive sub-failure strains on the mechanical behavior of the inferior glenohumeral ligament. J Shoulder Elbow Surg. 2000;9:427–35.
30. Urayama M, Itoi E, Sashi R, Minagawa H, Sato K. Capsular elongation in shoulders with chronic anterior dislocation: quantitative assessment with magnetic resonance arthrography. Am J Sports Med. 2003;31:64–7.
31. Fujii Y, Yoneda M, Wakitani S, Hayashida K. Histologic analysis of bony Bankart lesions in recurrent anterior instability of the shoulder. J Shoulder Elbow Surg. 2006;15:218–23.
32. Larrain MV, Botto GJ, Montenegro HJ, Mauas DM. Arthroscopic repair of acute traumatic anterior shoulder dislocation in young athletes. Arthroscopy. 2001;17:373–7.

33. Nakagawa S, Mizuno N, Hiramatsu K, Tachibana Y, Mae T. Absorption of the bone fragment in shoulders with bony Bankart lesions caused by recurrent anterior dislocations or subluxations: when does it occur? Am J Sports Med. 2013;41:1380–6.
34. Porcellini G, Campi F, Paladini P. Arthroscopic approach to acute bony Bankart lesion. Arthroscopy. 2002;18:764–9.
35. Sugaya H, Kon Y, Tsuchiya A. Arthroscopic repair of glenoid fractures using suture anchors. Arthroscopy. 2005;21:635.
36. Scheibel M, Hug K, Gerhardt C, Krueger D. Arthroscopic reduction and fixation of large solitary and multifragmented anterior glenoid rim fractures. J Shoulder Elbow Surg. 2016;25:781–90.
37. Yamamoto N, Muraki T, Sperling JW, et al. Stabilizing mechanism in bone-grafting of a large glenoid defect. J Bone Joint Surg Am. 2010;92:2059–66.
38. Bushnell BD, Creighton RA, Herring MM. Bony instability of the shoulder. Arthroscopy. 2008;24:1061–73.
39. Lynch JR, Clinton JM, Dewing CB, Warme WJ, Matsen FA III. Treatment of osseous defects associated with anterior shoulder instability. J Shoulder Elbow Surg. 2009;18:317–28.
40. Tauber M, Moursy M, Eppel M, Koller H, Resch H. Arthroscopic screw fixation of large anterior glenoid fractures. Knee Surg Sports Traumatol Arthrosc. 2008;16:326–32.
41. van Dijkman BA, Schep NWL, Luitse JSK, Ponsen KJ, Kloen P, Goslings JC. Patient related functional outcome of glenoid rim fractures treated with open reduction and internal fixation. Acta Orthop Belg. 2010;76:730–4.
42. Resch H, Wykypiel HF, Maurer H, Wambacher M. The antero-inferior (transmuscular) approach for arthroscopic repair of the Bankart lesion: an anatomic and clinical study. Arthroscopy. 1996;12:309–19.
43. Cameron SE. Arthroscopic reduction and internal fixation of an anterior glenoid fracture: case report. Arthroscopy. 1998;14:743–6.
44. Taverna E, Guarrella V, Freehill MT, Garavaglia G. Arthroscopic reduction with endobutton fixation for glenoid fracture. Joints. 2017;05(02):127–30.
45. Plath JE, Feucht MJ, Bangoj R. Arthroscopic suture anchor fixation of bony Bankart lesions: clinical outcome, magnetic resonance imaging results, and return to sports. Arthroscopy. 2015;31:1472–81.
46. Jiang CY, Zhu YM, Liu X, Li FL, Lu Y, Wu G. Do reduction and healing of the bony fragment really matter in arthroscopic bony Bankart reconstruction?: A prospective study with clinical and computed tomography evaluations. Am J Sports Med. 2013;41:2617–23.
47. Park JY, Lee SJ, Lhee SH, Lee SH. Follow-up computed tomography arthrographic evaluation of bony Bankart lesions after arthroscopic repair. Arthroscopy. 2012;28:465–73.
48. Maffulli N, Longo UG, Gougoulias N, Caine D, Denaro V. Sport injuries: a review of outcomes. Br Med Bull. 2011;97:47–80.
49. Maffulli N, Longo UG, Spiezia F, Denaro V. Aetiology and prevention of injuries in elite young athletes. Med Sport Sci. 2011;56:187–200.
50. Goss DA Jr, Trplet JJ, Taylor BC, Long N. Arthroscopically assisted reduction and internal fixation of a displaced posterior glenoid fracture: a case report. JBJS Case Connect. 2017;7(4):e84.
51. Luedke C, Tolan SJ, Tokish JM. Arthroscopic repair of posterior bony Bankart lesion and subscapularis remplissage. Arthrosc Tech. 2017;6:e689–94.
52. Baxter JA, Tyler J, Bhamber N, Arnander M, Pearse E, Tennent D. Arthroscopic posterior glenoid fracture fixation using knotless suture anchors. Arthrosc Tech. 2017;6(5):e1933–6.

18 Arthroscopic Distal Tibial Allograft Reconstruction Using Double-Button Suture Fixation for Anterior Shoulder Instability with Glenoid Bone Loss

Alexis Lo, Michael James, and Ian K. Y. Lo

18.1 Introduction

The shoulder is the most frequently dislocated joint in the body, with anteroinferior instability accounting for over 90% of dislocations [1]. While many factors can contribute to anterior shoulder instability, glenoid bone loss is a well-known and well-researched risk factor for both recurrent instability [2] and failure of arthroscopic soft tissue (e.g., Bankart) repairs [3, 4].

Glenoid bone loss is common and has been reported in 5–56% of traumatic anterior instability cases and is found in nearly all cases of recurrent anterior glenohumeral instability [5, 6]. In a consecutive series of 100 patients with anterior shoulder instability, 90% demonstrated varying degrees of glenoid bone loss on preoperative three-dimensional computed tomography (3D CT) [7]. The degree of bone loss does appear to be related to the number of instability episodes. In a study by Nakagawa et al. (Am J Sports Medicine 2019), 144 patients undergoing arthroscopic Bankart repair were evaluated with preoperative CT [8]. Glenoid defects were detected in 68% of patients, with an increasing degree of glenoid bone loss with repeated instability episodes and an increasing degree of bipolar (i.e., concomitant Hill–Sachs) bone loss [8].

While most authors agree that glenoid bone loss is a risk factor for failure of an arthroscopic Bankart repair [3, 4], it is unclear what the "critical" glenoid bone loss must be when considering alternative surgical treatments. Traditionally, many authors have recommended bone grafting procedures when the glenoid bone loss defect reaches 20–25% [6, 9]. However, recently a number of authors have suggested that the threshold for "critical bone loss" may be even lower [9–11]. In a study by Shaha et al. (2015), researchers noted that patients with "subcritical" bone loss (bone loss of 13.5% with stability of the shoulder maintained (i.e., no redislocation at follow-up)) had significantly lower Western Ontario Stability Index (WOSI) when compared to patients with less bone loss [12].

While the exact percentage of "critical" bone loss may be debated, it is clear that glenoid bone loss is not the only factor. Other factors, such as humeral bone loss [8], patient age [13], activity level (e.g., competitive versus noncompetitive), sport (contact versus noncontact), and hyperlaxity, should be considered when determining the appropriate surgical procedure for a particular patient [3].

A. Lo
Lewis Katz School of Medicine at Temple University, Philadelphia, PA, USA

M. James · I. K. Y. Lo (✉)
Section of Orthopaedic Surgery, Department of Surgery, University of Calgary, Calgary, AB, Canada
e-mail: michael.james@albertahealthservices.ca; ikylo@ucalgary.ca

R. Brzóska et al. (eds.), *360° Around Shoulder Instability*,
https://doi.org/10.1007/978-3-662-61074-9_18

18.2 Treatment Options

When augmentation of the glenoid bone is indicated, a number of treatment options may be considered. The Latarjet procedure has long been considered the standard of care when glenoid bone augmentation is required or alternatively there is a risk of failure of an arthroscopic Bankart repair [14]. The Latarjet procedure has had a long history of documented clinical success, with a recent meta-analysis of long-term outcomes demonstrating a recurrent dislocation rate of only 3.2% and a recurrent instability rate of 8.5% [15]. Similarly, approximately 86.1% of patients reported "good/excellent" outcomes, and with about the same percentage (84.9%) able to return to sport [15]. These long-term outcomes represent the gold standard of instability treatment for which other treatment options must be compared.

Although an excellent option for repair, some authors have been concerned of the disadvantages and complications associated with coracoid transfer and the Latarjet procedure. Indeed in a meta-analysis, coracoid transfer was associated with a high complication rate of ~30% [16]. While many complications are relatively minor (e.g., hematoma, hardware complications), other complications including intraoperative- or postoperative fracture, infection, nonunion, coracoid lysis, osteoarthritis, subscapularis rupture, and neurovascular injury [16] have limited wide acceptance of the Latarjet procedure in North America. In addition, revision of failed Latarjet procedure or for arthritis following Latarjet procedure can be extremely complex due to the altered anatomy associated with coracoid transfer [14, 17].

To limit the disruption in local anatomy, other autograft or allograft options can be considered. While iliac crest autograft (e.g., Eden-Hybinette procedure) has the disadvantage of donor site morbidity, this procedure has demonstrated excellent clinical outcomes, with a high rate of patient satisfaction, a low redislocation rate, and low incidence of secondary arthrosis [18–20]. However, the use of allograft and in particular distal tibial allograft (DTA) has recently gained wide attention.

Distal tibal allograft offers the advantages of no donor site morbidity, and relatively abundant graft availability, with early results comparable to other bone restoration options. In addition, the articular surface curvature and concavity of the lateral distal tibia closely mimic the natural curvature of the glenoid, making this graft relatively congruent to the humeral articular surface when compared to other graft options [21, 22]. In a study by Bhatia et al. (2013), distal tibial allograft reconstruction demonstrated improved glenohumeral contact areas and significantly lower glenohumeral peak forces, when compared to other procedures such as the Latarjet reconstruction [23]. In addition, the dense corticocancellous bone of the weight-bearing distal tibia is advantageous when placing fixation through the graft.

While screw fixation remains the most common method of fixation for glenoid grafts (i.e., iliac crest, distal tibia, Latarjet procedure), screws have been specifically associated with a number of complications. These include nonunion, bone resorption, graft fracture, screw breakage, screw bending, and screw impingement [16, 24]. Due to these potential complications, alternative methods of fixation have been investigated. In 2016, Gendre et al. reported on 35 patients following double suture button fixation during Latarjet reconstruction [25]. This method utilizes no screws but instead two buttons spanned by sutures similar to the suspensory fixation utilized for coracoclavicular ligament reconstruction. Despite nonrigid fixation, the authors reported excellent graft positioning and a 91% healing rate on CT. For these reasons, it is the authors' preferred method of fixation for arthroscopic distal tibial allograft reconstruction using two, double-button suture fixation (Smith & Nephew, Andover, MA). In addition, due to the soft fixation there is no necessity to establish a medial pectoralis (e.g., Halifax) portal [26].

In our clinical practice, arthroscopic distal tibial allograft reconstruction is indicated in patients with risk of failure of an arthroscopic Bankart repair. We consider distal tibial allograft reconstruction in patients with >15% glenoid bone loss, contact and competitive athletes, revision procedures, and those with bony Bankart lesions. Other reconstructive procedures (e.g., Latarjet reconstruction) are only considered in revision surgery or in specialized circumstances (e.g., rugby players).

18.3 Surgical Technique

Arthroscopic distal tibial allograft reconstruction with double-button fixation may be performed in a beach chair or lateral decubitus position as per surgeon's preference. In our experience, we prefer lateral decubitus position for all arthroscopic instability procedures, which allows superior visualization of the anterior, inferior, and posterior aspects of the glenohumeral joint. Thus, we prefer to perform arthroscopic distal tibial allograft reconstruction in the lateral decubitus position.

The patient is placed in the lateral decubitus position with the body tilted ~20° posteriorly which places the glenoid face parallel to the floor. The patient's body is secured with a beanbag and the arm in placed in a spider arm positioning device with lateral attachment (Smith & Nephew, Andover, MA). The arm is positioned in approximately 20° of forward flexion and 20° of abduction.

The patient is prepared and draped in the usual fashion and a posterior and anteroinferior and anterosuperolateral portals are established. The posterior portal is usually created approximately 1 cm distal and 1 cm medial to the posterolateral corner of the acromion. This portal is more lateral and superior than commonly established but usually provides a more direct angle of approach for the drilling of glenoid tunnels later in the procedure. The anterosuperolateral portal is utilized primarily as a visualization portal while the anteroinferior and posterior portals are utilized for instrumentation and suture management.

A diagnostic arthroscopy is performed and the extent of labral pathology and bone pathology is determined. In our experience, bone pathology and in particular glenoid bone pathology is best viewed through the anterosuperolateral portal, which provides an en face view of the glenoid. The size of the glenoid defect may be measured arthroscopically, although in our experience it is not reproducible as preoperative CT measurements. Importantly, the arm is removed from the traction device and brought into the position of 90° of abduction and 90° of external rotation to determine the interaction between the glenoid bone defect and the Hill–Sachs lesion.

When the indication for distal tibial allograft reconstruction is confirmed, the glenoid neck is then prepared. The Bankart lesion is mobilized and the anterior labrum is detached from the anterior glenoid neck from ~2 o'clock position to the 7 o'clock position. A large detachment and mobilization is required to ensure an adequate "pocket" is created to accommodate the size of the graft (Fig. 18.1). The labrum is mobilized, so that the underlying subscapularis muscle belly is revealed and the labrum naturally floats to the level of the glenoid articular surface. A traction suture is placed in the labrum at approximately the 4:30 position and retrieved through a separate anterior percutaneous portal. This facilitates retraction of the labrum during graft passage.

Unlike standard Bankart repair, the bony glenoid must now be prepared to a flat surface. While viewing through the anterosuperolateral portal, a combination of instruments (e.g., arthroscopic burr, rasp) is introduced through

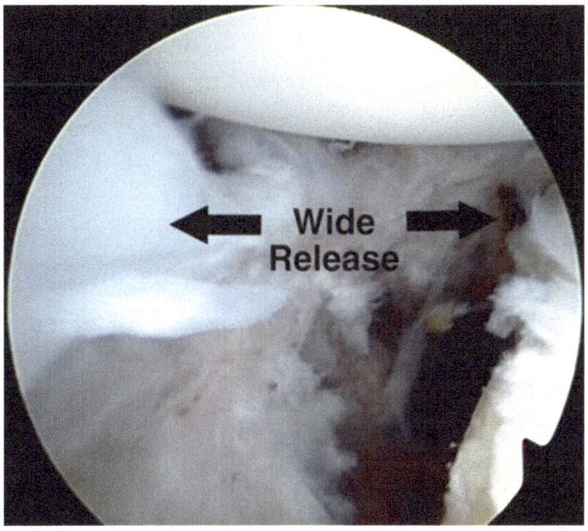

Fig. 18.1 Arthroscopic view through the anterosuperolateral portal of a right shoulder demonstrating the wide Bankart release required creating a "pocket" to accommodate the distal tibial graft

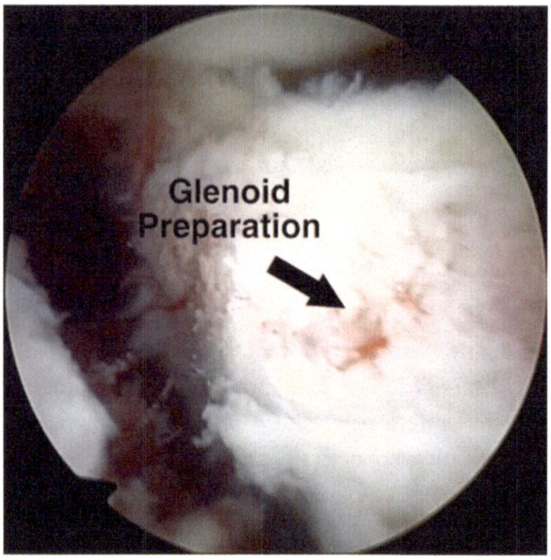

Fig. 18.2 Arthroscopic view through the anterosuperolateral portal of a right shoulder demonstrating bony preparation of the anterior glenoid neck to a flat bleeding bone surface

the anteroinferior portal and the anterior glenoid neck is prepared. Care is taken to remove any residual anchor material or sutures and to create a bleeding bone surface (Fig. 18.2).

Once the bone preparation is complete, the glenoid drill guide is inserted through the posterior portal. While viewing through the anterosuperolateral portal, the angle of approach for the glenoid drill guide is evaluated. If the previously established posterior portal is inadequate for tangential placement of the drill guide, a second posterior portal may be established. The goal is to place the drill guide tangential to the face of the glenoid with the hook below the 3 o'clock position and the arm of the hook contacting both the anterior and posterior rims of the glenoid articular surface just inferior to the bare area (Fig. 18.3). This usually places the hook and therefore the distal tibial allograft at the center of the defect.

While holding the glenoid drill guide, the double-barrel glenoid drill sleeves or "bullets" are aligned by an assistant. Two small skin incisions are made to allow the bullets to percutaneously pass through the soft tissues and contact the posterior aspect of the glenoid neck. A 2.8 mm drill is the used to drill parallel tunnels through the glenoid. The two bullets and glenoid drill guide are designed so that the two tunnels exit

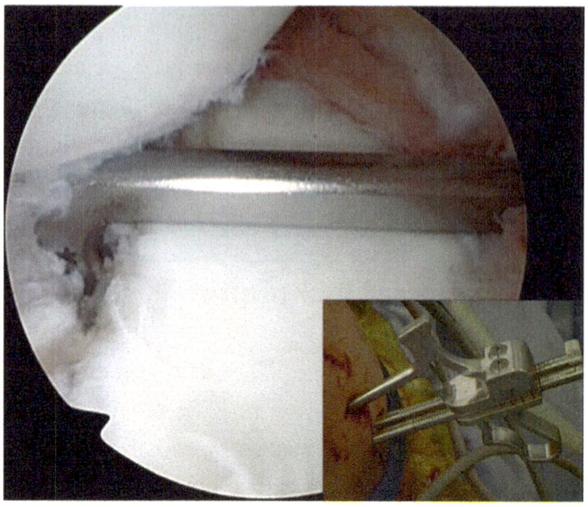

Fig. 18.3 Arthroscopic view through the anterosuperolateral portal and outside views of a right shoulder (inset) demonstrating position of the double barrel guide tangential to the glenoid face

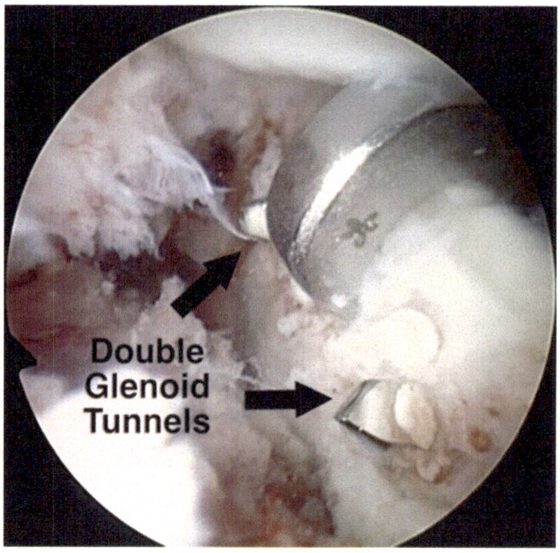

Fig. 18.4 Arthroscopic view through the anterosuperolateral portal demonstrating parallel double tunnel placement on the anterior glenoid neck approximately 10 mm apart and 5 mm medial to the glenoid surface

the anterior glenoid neck approximately 10 mm apart and 5 mm medial to the glenoid articular surface (Fig. 18.4). The guide is removed leaving the outer drill sleeves in the glenoid neck.

Two or three suture anchors (1.8 mm Q-Fix Anchors (Smith & Nephew, Andover, MA)) are then placed along the native glenoid rim for later Bankart repair over the distal tibial allograft. Sutures are retrieved through the posterior portal for suture management. It is important to drill and insert the suture anchors after the glenoid tunnels have been drilled and with the outer drill sleeves still within the glenoid vault. This prevents inadvertent entanglement of the anchor drill with the double-button suture fixation if anchors are inserted after the distal tibial allograft has been secured.

With the tunnels drilled, the distal tibial allograft is then prepared. To save time, a second team of surgeons or an assistant may prepare the tibial allograft on a separate table. To ensure adequate bone quality, we use fresh frozen nonirradiated distal tibial allografts from donors <60 years of age. The lateral third of the distal tibia is utilized, which usually provides the best matching contour to the humeral articular surface. The size of the graft is estimated by preoperative CT measurements.

In general, a graft is utilized to restore the anterior to posterior width of the glenoid ~2–3 mm larger than the native size compared to normative data or the opposite side as measured by CT. Grafts are typically 2 cm in superior-to-inferior direction, 10 mm in an anterior-to-posterior direction, and 10–15 mm in a medial-to-lateral direction. In order to recreate the normal version of the glenoid, it is important to angle the posterior cut of the graft (e.g., the surface that mates with the anterior glenoid neck) approximately 15–20° away from perpendicular. This will allow a smooth extension of the articular arc of the glenoid. A 0.5 mm sagittal saw is used to make the cuts as the assistant holds the allograft using bone-holding forceps. Any final contouring of the graft is performed and the graft is clamped with the graft preparation tool. Two 2.8 mm drill holes are then drilled 10 mm apart and ~5 mm from each edge and the suture button constructs are fed through each drill hole to rest flat on the anterior portion of the graft. To aid in orientation of the graft intraarticularly, the superior surface of the graft is marked.

With the graft prepared, the rotator interval is then resected to accommodate a larger 10 mm metal cannula. Alternatively, a 20 cc syringe or half pipe cannulas may be utilized for passing the graft through the anteroinferior portal. Looped passing wires are then fed through the outer glenoid drill sleeves from posterior to anterior and grasped through the anteroinferior cannula. Care is taken to ensure there is no entanglement of the sutures. The outer drill sleeves are then removed.

Using the looped passing wires, the endobutton sutures are then shuttled via the anteroinferior cannula through the glenoid (from an anterior to posterior direction) and out through the posterior skin incisions (Fig. 18.5). By placing traction on the endobutton sutures, the graft is shuttled intraar-

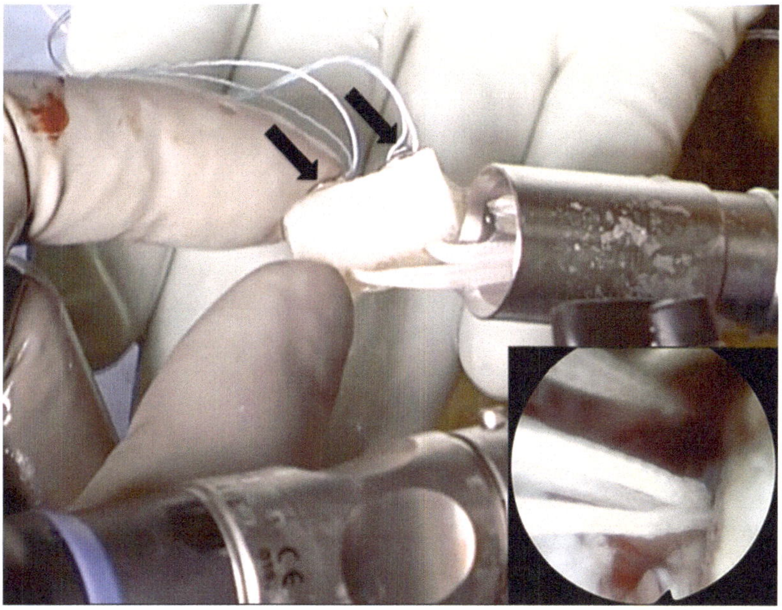

Fig. 18.5 Outside view and arthroscopic view through the anterosuperolateral portal (inset) of a right shoulder demonstrating the distal tibial allograft with suture buttons (arrows) and sutures shuttled through the double glenoid tunnels

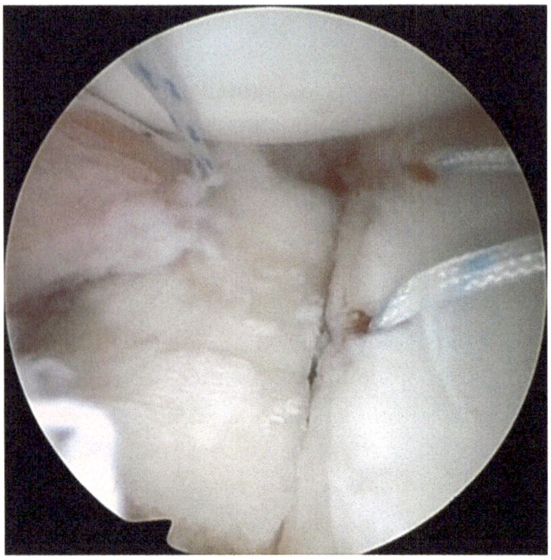

Fig. 18.6 Arthroscopic view through the anterosuperolateral portal of a right shoulder demonstrating reduction of the distal tibial allograft to the anterior glenoid neck

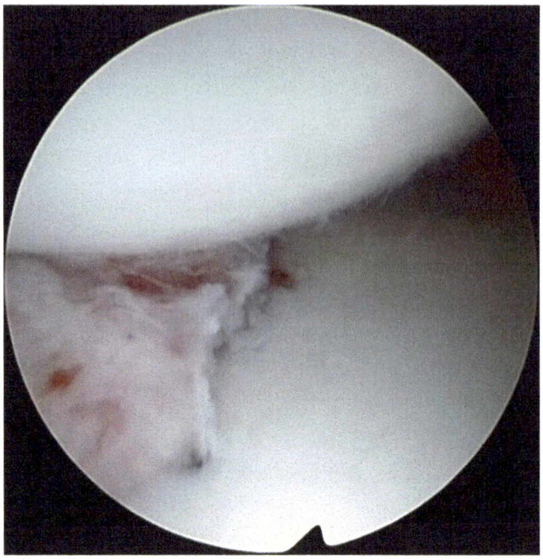

Fig. 18.7 Arthroscopic view through the anterosuperolateral portal of a right shoulder demonstrating final repair with the Bankart repair completed creating an extra-articular graft

ticularly, and against the anterior glenoid neck. A grasper introduced through the anteroinferior portal may also be utilized to assist in graft passage. We prefer to advance the inferior portion of the graft first by placing traction on the inferior sutures. In addition, it is important to place traction on the labrum suture to widen the "pocket" and to ensure the labrum is not interposed between the graft and the anterior glenoid neck. If still difficult, a radial "episiotomy" incision may be made through the labrum at the ~2 o'clock position which greatly widens the pocket and facilitates graft passage.

With the bone block provisionally reduced (Fig. 18.6), the endobutton suture loops are cut making two free ends. The two free ends are passed through the eyelets of the posterior suture button and a sliding Nice knot is tied reducing the posterior button against the posterior glenoid neck. The process is repeated for the other suture. The final position of the graft is confirmed when the knots are tightened using a tensiometer. A switching stick through the posterior portal can be used to ensure the graft is not prominent or lateralized. The tensiometer is used to alternatively tighten the superior and inferior sutures to 50N and 100N. The double endobutton sutures are then finally secured with three reversing half-hitches on alternating posts.

The labrum is then reattached to the native glenoid rim in a standard fashion using simple or mattress sutures (Fig. 18.7). This restores the tension of the capsuloligamentous structures and results in an extra-articular graft.

Postoperatively, patients are rehabilitated in a similar fashion to a standard Bankart repair. Patients are immobilized for 4 weeks allowing hand, wrist, and elbow range of motion. External rotation is limited to 0° for the first 4 weeks. After 4 weeks, the sling is discontinued and progressive active range of motion is achieved in forward elevation and external rotation. Rotator cuff strengthening exercises are permitted 8 weeks following surgery with progressive strengthening after 12 weeks. Full return to sports is allowed approximately 6–8 months following surgery once healing of the graft is confirmed on postoperative CT.

18.4 Results

Due to the relative novelty of the procedure, the results of distal tibial allograft reconstruction of anterior glenoid defects are relatively sparse when compared to other methods (e.g., Latarjet reconstruction). However, the limited research on distal tibial allograft reconstruction has been reported by a number of authors with excellent clinical outcomes.

In 2017, Provencher et al. reported on 27 patients for an average of 45 months following open distal tibial allografting and demonstrated excellent outcomes in joint stability and functional improvement. Patients reported significant improvements in American Shoulder and Elbow Surgeons (ASES) scores from 63 preoperatively to 91 postoperatively ($p = 0.02$) significant improvement in Western Ontario Stability Index (WOSI) score from 46% preoperatively to 11% postoperatively ($p = 0.02$), and significant improvement in the Single Assessment Numeric Evaluation (SANE) score from 50 preoperatively to 90.5 postoperatively ($p = 0.0001$). In addition, CT scanning demonstrated at mean of 1.4 years postoperatively an 89% allograft healing rate (range: 80–100%) with the mean allograft lysis of 3% (0–25%) [27].

In addition, open distal tibial allografting is a relatively safe procedure. In a study by Frank et al., an overall 90-day complication rate of 7.9% was reported [28]. Complications included hardware failure, subscapularis repair, debridement for a foreign body, postoperative pain requiring a subacromial injection, and a stitch abscess. Importantly, the 90-day short-term complication rate is significantly less than that of the Latarjet procedure (25%) for recurrent anterior glenohumeral instability. However, although the short-term complication rate at 90 days is significantly different between open distal tibial allografting and Latarjet procedures, with a longer term follow-up, similar overall complication rates (10%) and reoperation rates (6%) have been reported [29].

The outcomes of arthroscopic distal tibial allograft reconstruction using screw fixation have also been reported. In one study of 55 patients, Wong et al. (2016) reported excellent outcomes at 12 months postoperatively with no recurrent dislocations, no nonunions, one malunion due to screw fracture, and only two patients demonstrated bone resorption (without overt instability) [30]. Similarly in a later study by the same group, Amar et al. (2018) studied the safety profile and radiologic outcomes in patients undergoing arthroscopic DTA reconstruction with screws in a case series of 42 patients [31]. The authors noted the safe nature of the operation, reporting no intraoperative complications, adverse events, or neurovascular injuries with the procedure. In addition, CT scans at a mean of 6.31 ± 1.20 months postoperatively demonstrated no cases of nonunion or partial union. Graft resorption <50% was seen in 13 patients (42%), graft resorption >50% was seen in 5 patients (16%), and there was no graft resorption in 13 patients (42%) [31].

Due to the relative novelty of the described technique, there are currently no peer-reviewed studies specifically reporting on the outcomes of distal tibial allografts with double suture button fixation. In the authors' experience, double-button fixation results in a similar healing rate to rigid screw fixation without the disadvantages of screw fixation. In addition, the learning curve required for double-button suture fixation is shorter than that required for screw fixation [32].

18.5 Conclusion

In conclusion, there are many different surgical options, which may be considered when reconstructing the anterior aspect of the glenoid. Arthroscopic distal tibial allograft with double endobutton suture fixation is a promising technique that eliminates many of the disadvantages of screw fixation while extending the articular arc in an anatomic fashion. Further studies are required to determine the long-term clinical outcomes and healing of this procedure.

References

1. Levy DM, Cole BJ, Bach BR Jr. History of surgical intervention of anterior shoulder instability. J Shoulder Elbow Surg. 2016;25(6):e139–50.
2. Sasek CA. Recurrent anterior glenohumeral instability with glenoid bone loss: evaluation and management. JBJS J Orthop Physician Assistants. 2018;6(1):e5.
3. Balg F, Boileau P. The instability severity index score (ISIS score): a rational approach for patient selection

in arthroscopic Bankart repair. Paper presented at the Orthopaedic Proceedings; 2009.
4. Burkhart SS, De Beer JF. Traumatic glenohumeral bone defects and their relationship to failure of arthroscopic Bankart repairs: significance of the inverted-pear glenoid and the humeral engaging Hill-Sachs lesion. Arthroscopy. 2000;16(7):677–94.
5. Frank RM, Romeo AA, Provencher MT. Glenoid reconstruction with distal tibia allograft for recurrent anterior shoulder instability. Orthopedics. 2017;40(1):e199–205.
6. Lynch JR, Clinton JM, Dewing CB, Warme WJ, Matsen Iii FA. Treatment of osseous defects associated with anterior shoulder instability. J Shoulder Elbow Surg. 2009;18(2):317–28.
7. Sugaya H, Moriishi J, Dohi M, Kon Y, Tsuchiya A. Glenoid rim morphology in recurrent anterior glenohumeral instability. J Bone Joint Surg. 2003;85(5):878–84.
8. Nakagawa S, Iuchi R, Mae T, Mizuno N, Take Y. Clinical outcome of arthroscopic Bankart repair combined with simultaneous capsular repair. Am J Sports Med. 2017;45(6):1289–96.
9. Provencher MT, Bhatia S, Ghodadra NS, Grumet RC, Bach BR Jr, Dewing LCB, LeClere L, Romeo AA. Recurrent shoulder instability: current concepts for evaluation and management of glenoid bone loss. J Bone Joint Surg Am. 2010;92(Suppl 2):133–51.
10. Rabinowitz J, Friedman R, Eichinger JK. Management of glenoid bone loss with anterior shoulder instability: indications and outcomes. Curr Rev Musculoskelet Med. 2017;10(4):452–62.
11. Tokish JM, Fitzpatrick K, Cook JB, Mallon WJ. Arthroscopic distal clavicular autograft for treating shoulder instability with glenoid bone loss. Arthrosc Tech. 2014;3(4):e475–81.
12. Shaha JS, Cook JB, Song DJ, Rowles DJ, Bottoni CR, Shaha SH, Tokish JM. Redefining "critical" bone loss in shoulder instability: functional outcomes worsen with "subcritical" bone loss. Am J Sports Med. 2015;43(7):1719–25.
13. Mohtadi NGH, Chan DS, Hollinshead RM, Boorman RS, Hiemstra LA, Lo IKY, Hannaford HN, Fredine J, Sasyniuk TM, Paolucci EO. A randomized clinical trial comparing open and arthroscopic stabilization for recurrent traumatic anterior shoulder instability: two-year follow-up with disease-specific quality-of-life outcomes. J Bone Joint Surg. 2014;96(5):353–60.
14. Fortun CM, Wong I, Burns JP. Arthroscopic iliac crest bone grafting to the anterior glenoid. Arthrosc Tech. 2016;5(4):e907–12.
15. Hurley ET, Jamal MS, Ali ZS, Montgomery C, Pauzenberger L, Mullett H. Long-term outcomes of the Latarjet procedure for anterior shoulder instability: a systematic review of studies at 10-year follow-up. J Shoulder Elbow Surg. 2018;28(2):e33–9.
16. Griesser MJ, Harris JD, McCoy BW, Hussain WM, Jones MH, Bishop JY, Miniaci A. Complications and re-operations after Bristow-Latarjet shoulder stabilization: a systematic review. J Shoulder Elbow Surg. 2013;22(2):286–92.
17. Willemot LB, Elhassan BT, Sperling JW, Cofield RH, Sánchez-Sotelo J. Arthroplasty for glenohumeral arthritis in shoulders with a previous Bristow or Latarjet procedure. J Shoulder Elbow Surg. 2018;27(9):1607–13.
18. Haaker RGA, Eickhoff U, Klammer H-L. Intraarticular autogenous bone grafting in recurrent shoulder dislocations. Mil Med. 1993;158(3):164–9.
19. Piasecki DP, Verma NN, Romeo AA, Levine WN, Bach BR Jr, Provencher MT. Glenoid bone deficiency in recurrent anterior shoulder instability: diagnosis and management. J Am Acad Orthop Surg. 2009;17(8):482–93.
20. Steffen V, Hertel R. Rim reconstruction with autogenous iliac crest for anterior glenoid deficiency: forty-three instability cases followed for 5-19 years. J Shoulder Elbow Surg. 2013;22(4):550–9.
21. Provencher MT, Ghodadra N, LeClere L, Solomon DJ, Romeo AA. Anatomic osteochondral glenoid reconstruction for recurrent glenohumeral instability with glenoid deficiency using a distal tibia allograft. Arthroscopy. 2009;25(4):446–52.
22. Willemot LB, Shandiz MA, Zhao KD, Sanchez-Sotelo J, Verborgt O. Distal tibia and glenoid allografts are best for restoration of overall glenoid congruency in scapulae with an anterior glenoid rim defect. J Shoulder Elbow Surg. 2017;26(5):e165–6.
23. Bhatia S, Van Thiel GS, Gupta D, Ghodadra N, Cole BJ, Bach BR Jr, Shewman E, Wang VM, Romeo AA, Verma NN. Comparison of glenohumeral contact pressures and contact areas after glenoid reconstruction with Latarjet or distal tibial osteochondral allografts. Am J Sports Med. 2013;41(8):1900–8.
24. Butt U, Charalambous CP. Complications associated with open coracoid transfer procedures for shoulder instability. J Shoulder Elbow Surg. 2012;21(8):1110–9.
25. Gendre P, Thélu CE, d'Ollonne T, Trojani C, Gonzalez JF, Boileau P. Coracoid bone block fixation with cortical buttons: an alternative to screw fixation? Orthop Traumatol Surg Res. 2016;102(8):983–7.
26. Wong IH, Urquhart N. Arthroscopic anatomic glenoid reconstruction without subscapularis split. Arthrosc Tech. 2015;4(5):e449–56.
27. Provencher MT, Frank RM, Golijanin P, Gross D, Cole BJ, Verma NN, Romeo AA. Distal tibia allograft glenoid reconstruction in recurrent anterior shoulder instability: clinical and radiographic outcomes. Arthroscopy. 2017;33(5):891–7.
28. Frank RM, Richardson C, Gregory B, Sumner S, O'Brien MC, Bernardoni E, Verma NN, Cole BJ, Nicholson GP, Provencher MT. 90-Day complications following the distal tibia allograft procedure. Orthop J Sports Med. 2018;6(7_suppl 4):2325967118S2325900090.
29. Frank RM, Romeo AA, Richardson C, Sumner S, Verma NN, Cole BJ, et al. Outcomes of latarjet versus distal tibia allograft for anterior shoulder instability

repair: a matched cohort analysis. Am J Sports Med. 2018;46(5):1030–8.
30. Wong I, Amar E, Coady CM, Dilman DB, Smith B. Arthroscopic treatment for shoulder instability with glenoid bone loss using distal tibia allograft augmentation-short term results. Orthop J Sports Med. 2016;4(7_suppl 4):2325967116S2325900098.
31. Amar E, Konstantinidis G, Coady C, Wong IH. Arthroscopic treatment of shoulder instability with glenoid bone loss using distal tibial allograft augmentation: safety profile and short-term radiological outcomes. Orthop J Sports Med. 2018;6(5):2325967118774507.
32. Moga I, Konstantinidis G, Coady C, Ghosh S, Wong IH-B. Arthroscopic anatomic glenoid reconstruction: analysis of the learning curve. Orthop J Sports Med. 2018;6(11):2325967118807906.

Open Latarjet Procedure

19

E. Gervasi, R. Castricini, and O. Galasso

19.1 History and Rationale

Current free bone grafting techniques for treatment of recurrent anterior shoulder instability are based on the initial descriptions by Eden in 1918 [1] and Hybinette in 1932 [2]. Noeske conducted the first coracoid transfer in 1921 [3]; in this procedure, coracoid process is harvested near its base proximal to the pectoralis minor insertion but maintaining a bony periostal connection of the inferior aspect allowing it to be bent inferiorly into the subcoracoid fossa. The coracoids process was secured in this position merely by sutures to the soft tissue of the subcoracoid fossa and joint capsule and by the coracobrachialis and pectoralis minor muscles. Because of an observed excessive graft resorption, in 1944 Lange [4] and in 1951, Alvik [5] began fixing the bone graft to the scapular neck by impaction. In 1954, Michel Latarjet introduced a new procedure [6]. In the original description proposed by Latarjet, the coracoid was drilled for the single screw used for fixation prior to osteotomy. The horizontal limb of the coracoid process was then sectioned between the insertions of coracobrachialis and pectoralis minor using a chisel. Latarjet's preference was to perform a subscapularis tenotomy allowing shortening of the tendon during closure and stated that a longitudinal approach parallel to the muscle fibers could also be performed. The scapula neck was cleared, and the coracoid laid flat with its posterior surface against the glenoid neck, fixed in place outside the joint using a single screw. Subscapularis and the capsule were repaired by suture over the bone graft. In 1958, Helfet [7] published his results using a similar procedure that he attributed to his mentor, Rowley Bristow; this technique became known as the Bristow operation in the English language. In the original Bristow procedure, the coracoid process is sutured to the anterior part of the scapular neck through a transversely sectioned subscapularis muscle. The rationale for the Latarjet procedure was described by Patte as the "triple blocking" effect [8]. First, the "bone block" introduced by positioning of the coracoids at the anterior inferior glenoid rim serves as a static restraint for translation before dislocation (*bony effect*). Although the Latarjet, like the Bristow, is traditionally thought of as a "bone block" procedure, in reality, most of the stability gained from this procedure is more likely attributable to the conjoined tendon sling. When the arm is placed in

E. Gervasi (✉)
Shoulder Surgery Unit, Casa di cura Giovanni XXIII, Monastier di Treviso, Italy

R. Castricini
Orthopaedic and Trauma Surgery Unit, Villa Maria Cecilia Hospital, Cotignola, Italy

O. Galasso
Department of Medical and Surgical Sciences, "Mater Domini" University Hospital, "Magna Græcia" University, V.le Europa, Catanzaro, Italy
e-mail: galasso@unicz.it

R. Brzóska et al. (eds.), *360° Around Shoulder Instability*,
https://doi.org/10.1007/978-3-662-61074-9_19

the abducted and externally rotated position, the conjoined tendon, in its new position, acts to reinforce the inferior subscapularis and anterior inferior capsule (*belt or sling effect*). Finally, repair of the capsule and inferior glenohumeral ligament to the stump of the coracoacromial ligament provides a third mechanism of stability to the glenohumeral joint. This portion of the procedure emulates a capsulolabral reconstruction such as a Bankart procedure (*bumper effect*) [9].

19.2 Indications

Bone blocks are not the procedure of choice for routine cases of recurrent anterior glenohumeral instability. Soft-tissue repairs and reconstructions are safer and more effective for dealing with the usual case of recurrent traumatic instability. However, when a major anterior glenoid deficiency reduces the anterior or anteroinferior balance stability angle, reconstruction of the anterior glenoid lip may be necessary [10]. For these reasons, Latarjet procedure is proposed in cases of traumatic recurrent anterior shoulder instability associated with shoulder pain and bone defects that confirm instability.

Contraindications include patients with a subscapularis tear and patients with fractures of the anterior glenoid involving more than one third of the articular surface. In the case of a large glenoid fracture, the coracoid does not provide enough bone for glenoid reconstruction. In these cases, the fracture should be fixed, if possible, or reconstruction should be undertaken.

Plain radiographs should include AP views in neutral, internal, and external rotation, as well as bilateral glenoid profile views for comparison, as described by Bernageau et al. [11]. Radiographs should be performed under fluoroscopic control, if possible. With this method, a glenoid rim lesion will be apparent in 85% of patients with anterior instability and a Hill–Sachs lesion will be visualized in 75% [9, 12]. A computed tomography arthrogram or magnetic resonance imaging is recommended if exists the possibility of a concomitant rotator cuff tear and may assist if the diagnosis is in doubt or in cases of subtle instability [13].

19.3 Surgical Technique

19.3.1 Patient Positioning and Surgical-Site Preparation

After an interscalene block and general anesthesia, the patient is placed in a modified beach-chair position with the head of the bed elevated 60°. A thick folded sheet can be placed under the scapula on the affected side in order to flatten and stabilize the scapula, making the coracoid process readily palpable. A specialized arm holder should be used to prevent the arm from dangling. The arm should be draped free to allow for intraoperative manipulation of the upper extremity, particularly abduction and external rotation.

19.3.2 Skin Incision and Surgical Exposure

A limited deltopectoral approach is used. The skin incision is vertical from the tip of the coracoid extending 4–5 cm down the deltopectoral groove to the superior portion of the axillary fold. The cephalic vein, when identified, should be protected and gently retracted laterally. Any branches of the cephalic vein (typically, there is a large medial branch) that appear in the operative field may be carefully ligated with absorbable suture to prevent postoperative hematoma. A self-retaining retractor is then placed between the pectoralis major and the deltoid, completing the operative exposure. The arm is placed in abduction and external rotation, and a Hohmann retractor is placed over the top of the coracoid process (Fig. 19.1).

19.3.3 Harvesting Coracoid Process

The coracoacromial ligament is identified and completely transected 1 cm lateral to its coracoid insertion with electrocautery. Some authors [13] suggested that it is advantageous to harvest a small cuff of this ligament attached to the coracoid because it can later be incorporated into the capsular repair. The arm is now placed in adduction and internal rotation to improve exposure on

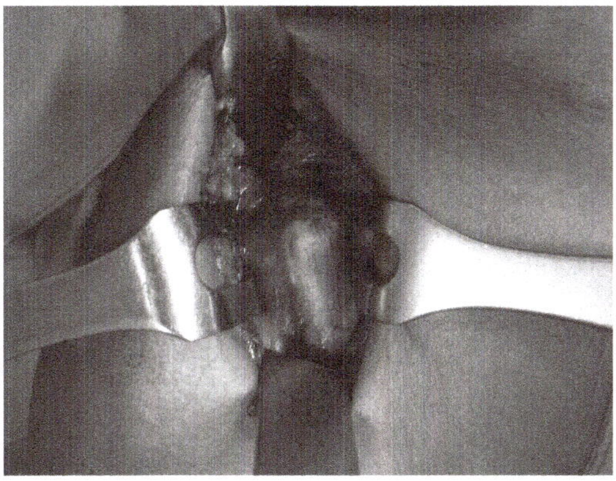

Fig. 19.1 Coracoid exposure. A Hohmann retractor is placed over the top of the coracoid process to facilitate the surgical exposure

the medial side of the coracoid. The pectoralis minor is released directly from the coracoid with electrocautery, taking care not to continue the release past the tip of the coracoid and thereby risking the blood supply to the coracoid graft. A periosteal elevator is used to remove any soft tissue from the undersurface of the coracoid. To harvest the coracoid bone graft, a 90° oscillating saw blade is used to perform osteotomy of the coracoid from a medial-to-lateral direction at a line just anterior to the coracoclavicular ligament insertion at the coracoid base [14] (Fig. 19.2). This typically allows for the harvesting of a 2.5- to 3-cm coracoid graft (Fig. 19.3). It is important to perform the osteotomy perpendicular to the coracoid process, so that it is not accidentally extended to the glenoid articular surface; an angled saw is preferred over an osteotome because the saw is less likely to cause iatrogenic glenoid fracture. To protect vital neurovascular structures including the musculocutaneous nerve, axillary nerve and artery, and brachial plexus, Chandler elevators should be positioned inferior and medial to the coracoid. During osteotomy, care should be taken not to disturb the blood supply to the graft, which enters the coracoid at the medial aspect of the insertion of the conjoined tendon. Grasping forceps are used to hold the coracoid process, and the arm is returned to the abducted and externally rotated position. The coracohumeral ligament is released from the coracoid, liberating the coracoid process.

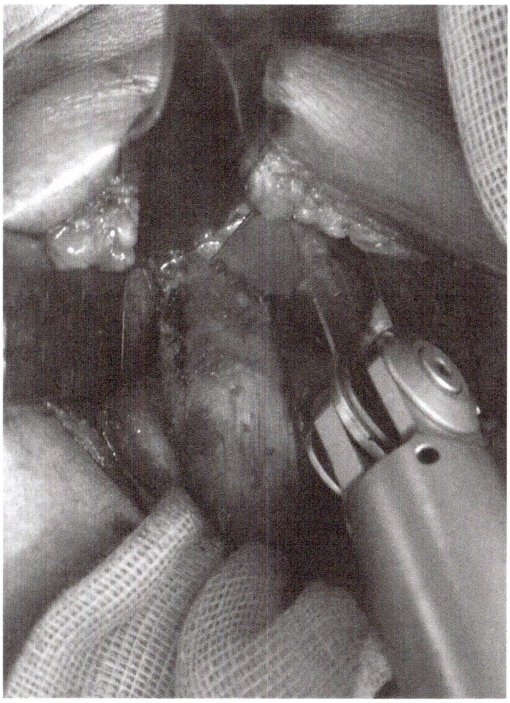

Fig. 19.2 A 90° oscillating saw blade is used to perform coracoid osteotomy from a medial-to-lateral direction

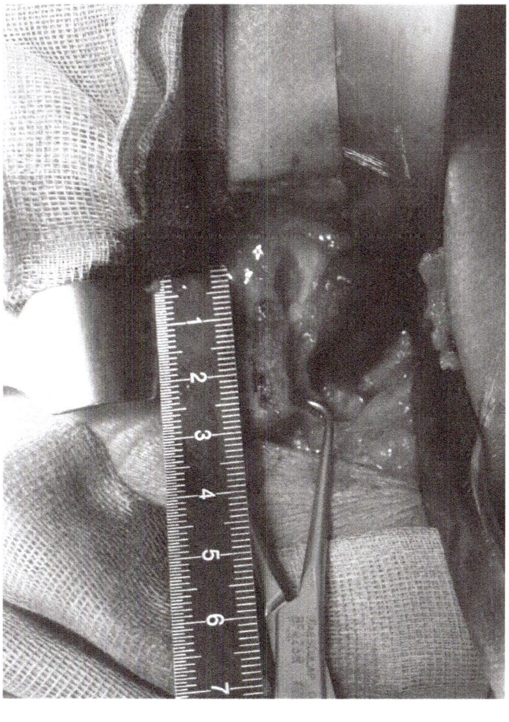

Fig. 19.3 A 2.5-cm coracoid graft is harvested

19.3.4 Coracoid Preparation

With the grasping forceps gripping the medial and lateral aspects of the coracoid, any remaining soft tissue is removed from the deep surface of the coracoid process, taking care not to disrupt the stump of the coracoacromial ligament. Decortication of the coracoid's deep surface may be performed with a sagittal saw. Ideally, to allow for optimal fit, the inferior surface should be a flat cancellous surface to optimize graft healing. An osteotome is placed beneath the coracoid to protect the skin and a 3.2-mm drill is used to place two bicortical drill holes perpendicular to longitudinal axis of the coracoid graft about 1 cm apart and centered with respect to its width (Fig. 19.4). Electrocautery is used to clear any soft tissue from the holes, and drilling can be repeated in the opposite direction to complete the tunnels. The arm is then externally rotated, at which time the lateral border of the conjoined tendon can be further released to additionally mobilize the coracoid process if necessary. The arm is returned to the neutral position, and the coracoids process is placed beneath the arm of the self-retaining retractor holding the pectoralis major.

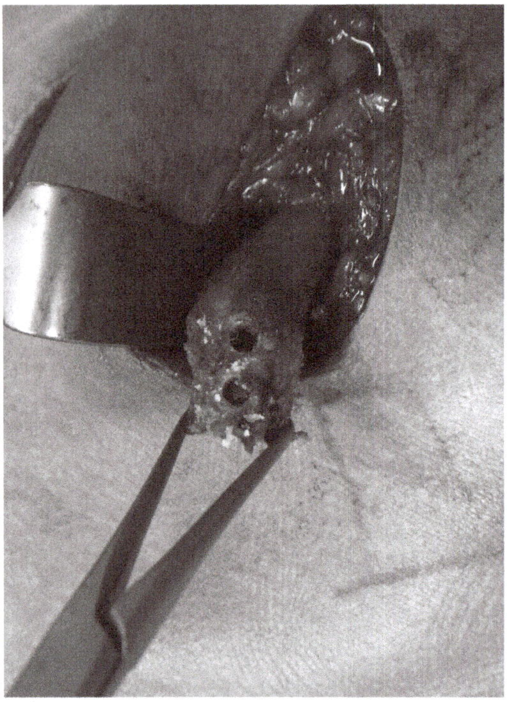

Fig. 19.4 Two bicortical drill holes perpendicular to longitudinal axis of the coracoid graft are performed about 1 cm apart

19.3.5 Glenoid Exposure

With the arm by the side and externally rotated, the subscapularis is exposed. The superior and inferior borders of the muscle should be identified. The subscapularis muscle is divided in line with its fibers using Mayo scissors. The location of the subscapularis split is at the junction of the superior two-thirds and the inferior one-third avoiding detaching it distally at the insertion. However, in the case of the hyperlax patient, the junction of the superior and inferior half is selected to maximize the effect of the conjoined tendon sling [15].

The scissors are opened vertically, exposing the underlying anterior capsule, and a swab is pushed in a superior and medial direction into the subscapular fossa. A Hohmann retractor is then placed over the swab in the subscapularis fossa as far medial as possible. A Bennett retractor is used on the inferior part of the subscapularis, and the lateral aspect of the split is extended to the lesser tuberosity with a scalpel in order to expose underlying capsule and glenohumeral joint line. A 1- to 2-cm vertical incision in the capsule is made at the level of the joint line; a needle can be used to identify the joint line. Capsulotomy should be performed 1 cm medial to the glenoid rim to preserve length and facilitate placement of a humeral head retractor such as Trillat or Fukuda retractors. Superior exposure is improved by placing a 4-mm Steinman pin into the superior scapular neck. The Hohmann retractor is now placed inferiorly between the capsule on the inferior neck and the inferior part of the subscapularis.

19.3.6 Glenoid Preparation

Electrocautery excises the anteroinferior labrum and periosteum off the glenoid neck in the region where the coracoid graft will sit commencing at the 5-o'clock position in a right shoulder (or the 7-o'clock position in a left shoulder) and con-

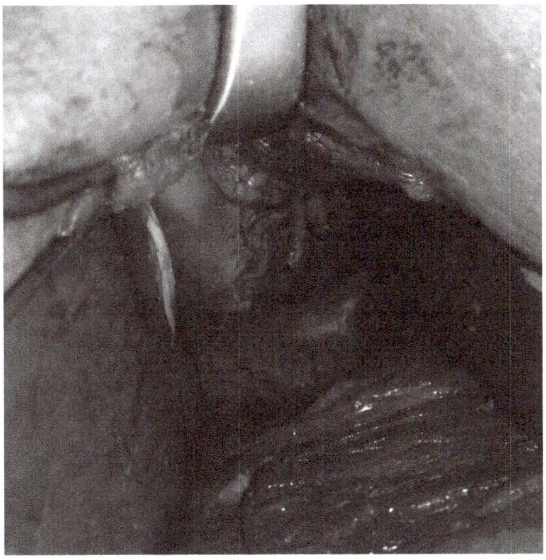

Fig. 19.5 Glenoid exposure. The anterior glenoid neck has been decorticated to create a flat bleeding surface to receive the graft

tinuing medially on to the glenoid for about 2 cm, then directing the incision superiorly for a distance of 2–3 cm, and lastly turning laterally to complete the incision by dividing the labrum again, this time at the 2-o'clock position (10 o'clock in a left shoulder) (Fig. 19.5). Scissors can be used to retract the incised labrum medially, exposing glenoid neck and an eventually Bankart lesion. Once subperiosteal dissection is complete, the anterior glenoid neck should be lightly decorticated by use of a high-speed burr to create a flat, bleeding surface to receive the graft. Care should be taken to remove only minimal amounts of bone because osseous tissue in the glenoid may already be deficient.

19.3.7 Coracoid Fixation

Positioning of the coracoid graft is often regarded as the most critical aspect of the Latarjet procedure. As noted by Allain et al. [16], excessive lateral placement of the coracoids may lead to a higher-than-expected rate of postoperative degenerative changes. However, an excessively medialized graft will fail to correct recurrent instability. The graft should be positioned flush with the glenoid margin; however, a slightly medial position (1–2 mm) is acceptable. A Fukuda retractor is inserted inside the glenohumeral joint to retract the humeral head and control the articular surface of the glenoid during drilling. The 3.2-mm drill is used to create an anterior to posterior hole in the scapula between the 4- and 5-o'clock position (7 o'clock in a left shoulder) and 7 mm medial to the articular border of the glenoid but can vary depending on the coracoid size. The drill is directed parallel to the glenoid articular surface, and drilling is continued until the hole passes through the posterior glenoid cortex. The depth of the hole can be measured with a depth gauge, and the measurement is usually between 30 and 45 mm. A partially threaded 4.5-mm malleolar screw is inserted into the inferior hole in the coracoid graft close to the tip of the coracoid. The screw is then placed into the already drilled hole in the glenoid and tightened into position, ensuring that the coracoid does not overhang the articular margin of the glenoid. Forceps can be used to check for the orientation of the coracoid. Thereafter, the drill is used to go through the superior coracoid hole parallel to the glenoid surface. The appropriately size malleolar screw is selected and placed in the superior hole. The screws should be snug, using the "2-finger" technique according to Walch and Boileau [17]. Overtightened should be avoided because of the risk of coracoid fracture. Final position of the coracoid must be evaluated (Fig. 19.6), and any lateral overhang of the coracoid should be removed with high-speed burr. Alternatively, the graft can be rotated after removing one screw and loosening the other, and then the glenoid is drilled in a slightly different direction.

19.3.8 Capsular Repair

The capsular repair is an additional possible stabilizing procedure. It is unclear whether the repair of the capsule to the transferred portion of the coracoacromial ligament after coracoid fixation has any harmful effects, such as restriction of range of motion [18]. Repairing the capsule to the anterior glenoid rim decreases external rotation but makes the coracoid block extra-articular,

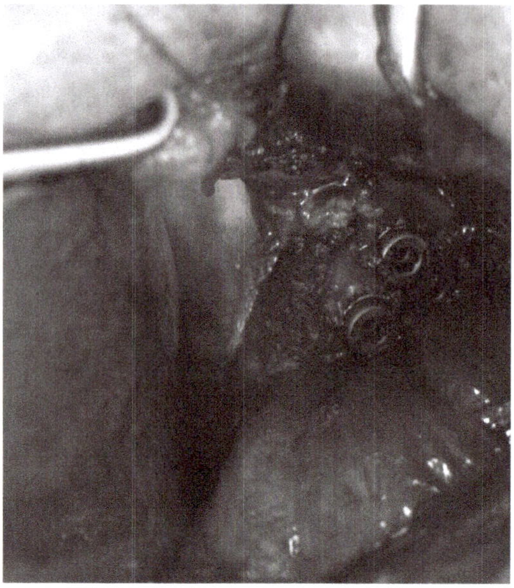

Fig. 19.6 Final position of the coracoid graft

and this has been shown to lower the rate of osteoarthritis after 13 years of follow-up [19].

The stump of the coracoacromial ligament is repaired to the capsule using absorbable sutures. The first suture is placed inferiorly in the coracoacromial ligament before the retractor is removed. Then, the humeral head retractor is removed, and the arm is placed in adduction and full external rotation with the elbow by the side to allow immediate postoperative range of motion exercises in external rotation, without risking failure of the repair. The suture is then passed through the capsule and inferior glenohumeral ligament and tied. A second suture is placed superior to the first, completing the repair of the coracoacromial ligament to the inferior glenohumeral ligament and capsule. Bhatia et al. [13] described that three suture anchors should be placed at the 3-, 4-, and 5-o'clock positions (in right shoulders) in the native glenoid to assist with capsular repair after Latarjet coracoids transfer. The sponge previously placed in the subscapularis fossa, the Steinmann pin, and remaining retractors are removed. It is not necessary to suture the horizontal split in the subscapularis even if some surgeons [13] suggested the subscapularis reparation over the coracoids transfer. Drain is typically not used, unless excessive bleeding is noted.

19.4 Postoperative Management

After surgery, a sling is maintained for 3 weeks. Active motion of the fingers, hand, and elbow is encouraged. No resisted elbow flexion is allowed for at least 4–5 weeks to reduce the risk of nonunion. All activities of daily living are allowed by 6 weeks postoperative. Patients are encouraged to swim starting at postoperative week 3 and continuing through the third postoperative month. Progressive return to sporting activities, including contact sports, is allowed at 3 months after clinical and radiographic evaluation confirms healing of the coracoid graft.

19.5 Results and Complications

A systematic review [20] of studies at 10-year follow-up found high patient-reported functional outcome scores after the Latarjet procedure, with 86% of patients achieving good to excellent outcomes and more than 90% satisfied with the procedure at an average of 16 years postoperatively. The high level of satisfaction might be attributable to the high rate of return to play, because Warth et al. [21] found that the greatest concern in patients undergoing surgery for anterior shoulder instability was the ability to return to sporting activity. In addition, the rate of return to play at the previous level was high in more than 75% of patients. Several studies have compared the results of return to play between the Latarjet procedure and Bankart repairs, with similar results reported between the two techniques [22–24].

Intraoperatively, coracoid fracture can occur if the screws are overtightened or too large such as a 4.5-mm cortical screw that requires a 4.5-mm hole for compression. Use of the partially threaded malleolar screw permits interosseous compression and only requires a 3.2-mm hole. Complication rate has been reported as high as 30% and includes residual pain and/or instability, partial recovery of previous sport activity, glenohumeral osteoarthritis. Overall, 5% of patients undergo a revision procedure and the most common reason for revision is recurrent instability, although this occurs in less than 2% of patients.

In the absence of complications such as fracture of the coracoid process, the recurrences are often related to voluntary instability or in patients with poorly controlled epilepsy. Recurrence after a Latarjet procedure can be successfully treated with a modified Eden–Hybbinette procedure [25]. Loss of external rotation and postoperative stiffness are rare after the Latarjet procedure if the coracoacromial ligament is sutured to the capsule with the arm in maximal external rotation. Risk factors for progressive arthropathy are older age, high-demand sports, and lateral positioning of the transferred coracoid in relation to the glenoid rim [26].

19.6 Open Latarjet, Open Latarjet Arthroscopically Assisted, All-Arthroscopic Latarjet: 2019 State of the Art

The open Latarjet bone block procedure is widely considered mainstay for surgical treatment of recurrent anterior shoulder instability. The low rate of recurrence after Latarjet technique made this technique the benchmark against which were measured all the other surgical procedures to treat recurrent anterior instability of the shoulder [27]. The overall 90-day complication rate following the Latarjet procedure for anterior shoulder stabilization was 7.5% [28], and with increased surgeon experience, fewer associated complications, decreased operative time, and higher functional outcomes have been reported. However, open questions remain unanswered as for the use of arthroscopy to address the procedure.

19.6.1 Drawbacks of Open Latarjet Through the Anterior Approach

Missed treatment of concomitant soft of bone tissue injuries can occur after open Latarjet [29]. A Hill–Sachs lesion can be missed. Notably, glenoid bony defects do not occur in isolation, but in association with humeral bone defects that are also present in 80–90% of the cases [30]. The presence of humeral bone loss can still lead to an "off-track" situation with persistent shoulder instability from engagement of the Hill–Sachs on the anterior glenoid. In these cases, the combination of a Hill–Sachs remplissage and the Latarjet procedure can be effective in preventing persistent instability. The arthroscopic remplissage procedure has gained popularity in recent years as an excellent and safe procedure to perform in patients with large engaging Hill–Sachs lesions. Thereby, the Hill–Sachs becomes an extra-articular defect, eliminating the potential engagement of the anterior glenoid and contribution to recurrent instability. The disadvantage of this additional procedure can be the decreased shoulder motion.

A further limitation of the open technique is that the use of a Fukuda retractor to expose the anterior glenoid rim conceals concomitant injuries to the posterior labrum and bicipital anchor.

19.6.2 The Advantages of Arthroscopically Assisted Latarjet Procedure

The arthroscopy allows the diagnosis of possible concomitant injuries and allows treatment of posterosuperior labrum lesions. Moreover, the Latarjet procedure can be combined to an arthroscopic Hill–Sachs remplissage, if required. If this is the case, the sutures of the anchor placed into the bony defect are tightened once the coracoid graft has been fixed.

19.6.3 All-Arthroscopic Latarjet

Lafosse et al. proposed that the arthroscopic approach offers advantages such as more accurate bone graft placement, quicker functional recovery, decreased stiffness, and cosmetic benefits [31]. In detail, the variability of scapular inclination in relation to the thorax may be an important factor that distorts the final perioperative evaluation of glenoid retroversion and may affect the placement of the screws to fix the coracoid graft and thus the surgical outcomes. Graft nonunion resulting in recurrent instability was the main indication for open revision surgery after Latarjet procedure, followed by resorption, malpositioning, and graft fracture [32]. Coracoid bone graft osteolysis is more pronounced in cases without glenoid bone loss, which may be due to a diminished mechanotransduction effect of the humeral head on the graft influencing its remodeling and the bone healing process. The larger is the glenoid bone loss, the smaller is the conical shape of the scapular neck, and thus, the greater is the contact surface between the graft and the scapular neck [33]. The direction of the screws to fix the graft also influences the graft resorption. The choice of an arthroscopic procedure allows to guide through the posterior view the screw positioning, thus improving the direction of screws. Although as of today there is no proven advantage of the arthroscopic procedure over an open one [34], a clear benefit for the use of a guide with an arthroscopically assisted technique in terms of graft and hardware placement has been reported [35]. Theorized disadvantages of the arthroscopic Latarjet include increased cost, longer surgery time, and learning curve [36].

19.6.4 The Authors' Choice

The treatment of recurrent anterior shoulder instability is a challenge we need to take up in the next years. Several variables such as the age, gender, number of preoperative dislocations, time of surgery after the first episode, sport activity, and glenoid or humeral bone loss drawing an on-track or off-track lesion influence the choice of treatment and the surgical outcomes [37].

The open or arthroscopic Latarjet procedure represents our preferred surgical techniques to treat recurrences, patients with an ISIS score over 6 points or >15% glenoid bone loss [38, 39].

References

1. Eden R. Zur Operation der habituellen Schulterluxation unter Mitteilung eines neuen Verfahrens bei Abriß am inneren Pfannenrande. Dtsch Z Chir. 1918;144:269.
2. Hybinette S. De la transplantation d'un fragment osseux pour remidier aux luxations recidivantes de l'epaule. Constatations et resultants operatoires. Acta Chir Scand. 1932;71:411–45.
3. Noesske. Zur habituellen Schulterluxation. Zbl Chir. 1924;51:2402–4.
4. Lange M. Orthopädisch-chirurgische Operationslehre. München: Bergmann; 1944. p. 162–6.
5. Alvik I. Hybinette's operation in three cases of habitual dislocation of the shoulder. Nord Med. 1951;45:96–7.
6. Latarjet M. Treatment of recurrent dislocation of the shoulder. Lyon Chir. 1954;49:994–7.
7. Helfet AJ. Coracoid transplantation for recurring dislocation of the shoulder. J Bone Joint Surg Br. 1958;40:198–202.
8. Patte D, Bernageau J, Bancel P. The anteroinferior vulnerable point of the glenoid rim. In: Bateman JE, Welsch RP, editors. Surgery of the shoulder. New York, NY: Marcel Dekker; 1985. p. 94–9.
9. Edwards TB, Walch G. Latarjet procedure for recurrent anterior shoulder instability: rationale and technique. Oper Tech Sports Med. 2012;20:57–64.
10. Rockwood CA, Wirth MA, Matsen FA, Lippitt SB. The shoulder, vol. 1. 4th ed. Amsterdam: Elsevier; 2009.
11. Bernageau J, Patte D, Bebeyre J. Interet du profile glenoidien dans le luxations recidivantes de l'epaule. Rev Chir Orthop. 1976;62:142–7.
12. Edwards TB, Boulahia A, Walch G. Radiographic analysis of bone defects in chronic anterior shoulder instability. Arthroscopy. 2003;19:732–9.
13. Bhatia S, Frank RM, Ghodadra NS, Hsu AR, Romeo AA, Bach BR Jr, Boileau P, Provencher MT. The outcomes and surgical techniques of the Latarjet procedure. Arthroscopy. 2014;30:227–35.
14. Young AA, Walch G. Open bony augmentation of glenoid bone loss–the Latarjet and variants. In: Provencher MT, Romeo AA, editors. Shoulder instability: a comprehensive approach. Philadelphia: Elsevier; 2011. p. 197–208.
15. Young AA, Maia R, Berhouet J, Walch G. Open Latarjet procedure for management of bone loss in anterior instability of the glenohumeral joint. J Shoulder Elbow Surg. 2011;20:S61–9.9.
16. Allain J, Goutallier D, Glorion C. Long-term results of the Latarjet procedure for the treatment of anterior instability of the shoulder. J Bone Joint Surg Am. 1998;80:841–52.
17. Walch G, Boileau P. Latarjet-Bristow procedure for recurrent anterior instability. Tech Shoulder Elbow Surg. 2000;1:256–61.
18. Itoigawa Y, Hooke AW, Sperling JW, Steinmann SP, Zhao KD, Yamamoto N, Itoi E, An KN. Repairing the capsule to the transferred coracoid preserves external rotation in the modified latarjet procedure. J Bone Joint Surg Am. 2016;98(17):e75.
19. Bouju Y, Gadéa F, Stanovici J, Moubarak H, Favard L. Shoulder stabilization by modified Latarjet-Patte procedure: results at a minimum 10 years' follow-up,

and role in the prevention of osteoarthritis. Orthop Traumatol Surg Res. 2014;100:S213–8.
20. Hurley ET, Jamal MS, Ali ZS, Montgomery C, Pauzenberger L, Mullett H. Long-term outcomes of the Latarjet procedure for anterior shoulder instability: a systematic review of studies at 10-year follow-up. J Shoulder Elbow Surg. 2019;28(2):e33–9.
21. Warth RJ, Briggs KK, Dornan GJ, Horan MP, Millett PJ. Patient expectations before arthroscopic shoulder surgery: correlation with patients' reasons for seeking treatment. J Shoulder Elbow Surg. 2013;22:1676–81.
22. Bessière C, Trojani C, Carles M, Mehta SS, Boileau P. The open Latarjet procedure is more reliable in terms of shoulder stability than arthroscopic Bankart repair. Clin Orthop Relat Res. 2014;472:2345–51.
23. Blonna D, Bellato E, Caranzano F, Assom M, Rossi R, Castoldi F. Arthroscopic Bankart repair versus open Bristow-Latarjet for shoulder instability: a matched-pair multicenter study focused on return to sport. Am J Sports Med. 2016;44:3198–205.
24. Cho NS, Yoo JH, Rhee YG. Management of an engaging Hill-Sachs lesion: arthroscopic remplissage with Bankart repair versus Latarjet procedure. Knee Surg Sports Traumatol Arthrosc. 2016;24:3793–800.
25. Lunn JV, Castellano-Rosa J, Walch G. Recurrent anterior dislocation after the Latarjet procedure: outcome after revision using a modified Eden-Hybinette operation. J Shoulder Elbow Surg. 2008;17:744–50.
26. Gordins V, Hovelius L, Sandstrom B, Rahme H, Bergstrom U. Risk of arthropathy after the Bristow-Latarjet repair: a radiologic and clinical thirty-three to thirty-five years of follow-up of thirty-one shoulders. J Shoulder Elbow Surg. 2014;24:691–9.
27. Smolen D, Went P, Tomala D, Sternberg C, Lafosse L, Leuzinger J. Identification of a remodeled neo-tendon after arthroscopic Latarjet procedure. Arthroscopy. 2017;33:534–42.
28. Frank RM, Gregory B, O'Brien M, Bernardoni E, Verma NN, Cole BJ, Nicholson GP, Romeo AA. Ninety-day complications following the Latarjet procedure. J Shoulder Elbow Surg. 2019;28:88–94.
29. Arrigoni P, Huberty D, Brady PC, Weber IC, Burkhart SS. The value of arthroscopy before an open modified Latarjet reconstruction. Arthroscopy. 2008;24:514–9.
30. Boileau P, Saliken D. Editorial Commentary: The Wake of the Dragon: will the orthopaedic community adopt the shoulder arthroscopic Latarjet procedure as we adopted the arthroscopic rotator cuff repair? Arthroscopy. 2017;33:2139–43.
31. Lafosse L, Boyle S. Arthroscopic Latarjet procedure. J Shoulder Elbow Surg. 2010;19:2–12.
32. Willemot L, De Boey S, Van Tongel A, Declercq G, De Wilde L, Verborgt O. Analysis of failures after the Bristow-Latarjet procedure for recurrent shoulder instability. Int Orthop. 2019;43(8):1899–907.
33. Di Giacomo G, de Gasperis N, Costantini A, De Vita A, Beccaglia MA, Pouliart N. Does the presence of glenoid bone loss influence coracoid bone graft osteolysis after the Latarjet procedure? A computed tomography scan study in 2 groups of patients with and without glenoid bone loss. J Shoulder Elbow Surg. 2014;23:514–8.
34. Lädermann A. Editorial commentary: arthroscopic Latarjet shoulder stabilization: where are we? where are we going? Arthroscopy. 2017;33:2136–8.
35. Taverna E, Guarrella V, Cartolari R, Ufenast H, Broffoni L, Barea C, Garavaglia G. Arthroscopically-assisted Latarjet: an easy and reproducible technique for improving the accuracy of graft and screw placement. Shoulder Elbow. 2018;10:99–106.
36. Castricini R, De Benedetto M, Orlando N, Rocchi M, Zini R, Pirani P. Arthroscopic Latarjet procedure: analysis of the learning curve. Muscoloskelet Surg. 2013;97(S1):93–8.
37. Gasparini G, De Benedetto M, Cundari A, De Gori M, Orlando N, McFarland EG, Galasso O, Castricini R. Predictors of functional outcomes and recurrent shoulder instability after arthroscopic anterior stabilization. Knee Surg Sports Traumatol Arthrosc. 2016;24:406–13.
38. Shaha JS, Cook JB, Song DJ, Rowles DJ, Bottoni CR, Shaha SH, Tokish JM. Redefining "Critical" bone loss in shoulder instability: functional outcomes worsen with "Subcritical" bone loss. Am J Sports Med. 2015;43:1719–25.
39. Shin SJ, Kim RG, Jeon YS, Kwon TH. Critical value glenoid bone loss that leads to recurrent glenohumeral instability after arthroscopic Bankart repair. Am J Sports Med. 2017;45:1975–81.

20 "New" Graft Procedures

A. Kwapisz, A. Sibilska, and J. M. Tokish

Bone loss is considered as a critical issue in the treatment of glenohumeral instability [1]. Many authors have already correlated unsatisfactory clinical outcomes, failure risk, and increased cost with arthroscopic surgical stabilization in the setting of significant bone loss. Bone loss can be monopolar or bipolar, which refers both to glenoid and humeral bone loss [1–3].

Glenoid bone loss is present in up to 22% in initial anterior traumatic dislocation and up to 72% in recurrent dislocations cases [4, 5].

Consequently, failure to identify glenoid bony pathology may lead to loss of glenohumeral congruence and, therefore, to failure of management of shoulder dislocation. There is still much discussion about the critical amount of bone loss that is clinically important and contributes to poorer results [2].

Glenoid diameter is on average 24–26 mm. Lo and Burkhart proposed an "inverted pear" concept which corresponds to a bone defect of around 6–8 mm. Generally, loss greater than 20% has been shown to negatively affect biomechanical stability and clinical results [6]. More currently, the term "subcritical" bone loss proposed by Shaha et al. appeared in the literature. They reported that bone loss above 13.5% lead to clinically significant decrease in WOSI scores consistent with an unacceptable outcome, even in patients who did not sustain a recurrence of their instability [7].

Glenoid bone loss may also interplay with Hill–Sachs (HS) lesions of the humerus, which is called a bipolar bone deficiency. The Hill–Sachs lesion is a posttraumatic impaction injury along the posterolateral aspect of the humeral head. It has been shown that the Hill–Sachs lesion is fairly common and is demonstrated in 67–93% of anterior dislocations and may reach an incidence rate of 100% in patients with recurrent anterior shoulder instability [8].

Burkhart and De Beer reported that anatomic relation of the humeral head and the glenoid bone loss is one of the risk factors for arthroscopic stabilization failure. They were also first to use the term "engaging Hill–Sachs" to describe a lesion that may "engage" glenoid defects of all sizes in functional positions and have been proven to negatively affect arthroscopic capsuloligamentous repairs [1].

More recently, both glenoid and humeral bone defects have been combined into an "on-track" and "off-track" concept. Itoi et al. identified bipolar bone losses and their interaction in abduction-external rotation, and they clarified the contact area of the humeral head and glenoid. They called this contact the glenoid track. This model assumes that the individual lesions can influence each

A. Kwapisz (✉) · A. Sibilska
Medical University of Lodz, Lodz, Poland

J. M. Tokish
Department of Orthopedics, Mayo Clinic Arizona, Phoenix, AZ, USA

R. Brzóska et al. (eds.), *360° Around Shoulder Instability*,
https://doi.org/10.1007/978-3-662-61074-9_20

other and as a consequence reduce shoulder joint stability [9, 10].

The "on-track" and "off-track" concept has been clinically confirmed, and it has been shown that applying this model is highly predictive of outcome and more predictive than glenoid bone loss alone [11].

Considering all the above, correct recognition and selection of treatment are critical to ensure the successful management of anterior shoulder instability. Several bone-grafting options have been described so far to solve this deficiency including coracoid bone transfer, iliac crest bone autograft (ICBG), distal tibia autograft, and distal clavicle osteochondral autograft (DCA). Each of these techniques has its advantages and disadvantages. A brief comparison of the discussed techniques is presented in Table 20.1. The following should be taken into consideration in decision-making for graft selection: graft size, whether it has an inherent cartilage source, immunocompatibility, availability, and eventually cost. The ideal graft should be able to restore the bone and cartilage loss seen in erosive glenoid bone loss, be readily available, free, and without donor-site morbidity.

20.1 Coracoid Bone Autograft

Coracoid bone autograft was first proposed in 1954 by Latarjet [12]. He described his technique of coracoid bone transfer to the anterior glenoid for the treatment of shoulder anterior dislocations. A few years later, an alternative coracoid tip transfer, the Bristow technique, was proposed by Helfet in 1958 [13]. Although more than a half century passed, the open coracoid transfer is still considered as a gold standard technique for the treatment of glenoid bone loss.

Besides restoring glenoid articular bone, this technique provides further stabilization via capsuloligamentous reconstruction and inferior subscapularis myodesis from tightening of the conjoined tendon in the provocative position (the so-called sling effect), and collectively, the coracoid transfer performs stability through a mechanism referred to as the "triple blocking effect."

Biomechanical studies showed that this surgical procedure is efficient in terms of restoring shoulder stability. Moreover, clinical outcome studies published so far demonstrated that the recurrence rate is relatively low with excellent patient-reported outcomes [14–17].

Nevertheless, there are also many disadvantages of this technique. First, coracoid transfer is a nonanatomic approach. This may make future revision surgery more challenging with an overall complication rate of up to 30% reported by Griesser et al. [18].

Moreover, the amount of glenoid surface that can be restored is limited. Paladini et al. stated that this technique may be insufficient to restore defects exceeding 31% [19]. Modification of the traditional Latarjet procedure, the congruent arc technique, may be used to reconstruct bone loss of an approximate size of 54% according to Giles et al. [20]. However, this modification was shown to result in greater graft displacement and lower clinical failure load. Some authors demonstrated that up to 60% of the graft may undergo osteolysis [21].

Another significant drawback to coracoid transfer is the lack of articular cartilage on the transferred graft. This is said to be potential reason for high incidence of osteoarthritis development after Latarjet procedure. In literature, it is reported in up to 62% of cases [22].

Probably, the most worrying aspect of this technique is its potential for complications. Unplanned reoperations have been reported at a higher rate

Table 20.1 Comparison of available techniques for bone loss in shoulder

Graft choice characteristic	Availability	Cartilage source	Cost	Donor-site morbidity	Rejection/ infection	Sling effect
Distal clavicle autograft	+	+	+	+	+	–
Latarjet	+	–	+	+	+	+
Distal tibial allograft	–	+	–	+	–	–
Iliac crest bone graft	+	–	+	–	+	–

than that of the traditional Bankart, and the overall complication rate has been reported up to 25% [18, 23]. Delaney et al. have reported nerve alert in 77% patients using neuromonitoring during Latarjet, and postoperatively 21% of them had clinically detectable nerve deficit [24].

Moreover, cost-effectiveness analysis of the arthroscopic Bankart and the open Latarjet in the treatment of primary shoulder instability performed by Min et al. showed that Bankart is more cost-effective than the Latarjet, primarily because of a lower health utility state after a failed Latarjet [25]. According to authors, the clinical scenario may favor Latarjet (i.e., critical glenoid bone loss) in certain circumstances and that is why decisions should be made on a case-by-case basis.

20.2 Iliac Crest Bone Autograft (ICBG)

The first reports of using bone block to restore glenoid bone loss were made by Eden in 1918 and later by Hybinette in 1932 [26, 27]. Many years later in 2006, Warner et al. reported autogenous tricortical iliac crest bone to be effective in the treatment of recurrent instability in the setting of glenoid bone loss [28].

It is said that this graft could restore defects up to 35 mm in length, which is significantly more surface than in the case of coracoid graft. Warner et al. also reported excellent short-term result with only a few complications in 4% of patients. Summarizing this technique, being readily available, essentially free and having an autograft source of bone are said to be the main advantages [28].

However, there are several potential drawbacks. First, due to the fact that the iliac crest is nonarticular, it cannot restore the osteoarticular loss seen in the glenoid. This may lead to secondary osteoarthritis, which has been already reported after this procedure [29, 30].

Another disadvantage is potential for donor-site morbidity. Persistent pain lasting more than 1 year after procedure is described in up to 100% of cases. Other, less frequent complications such as local infection (14%) and anterior superior spine fracture (3%) have been also reported [28, 31, 32]. Finally, the ICBG graft does not, in itself, address the soft-tissue pathology that is frequently present in instability cases where it is applied [33].

20.3 Distal Tibia Allograft (DTA)

Distal tibial allografts have been introduced as an osteochondral source for glenoid bone loss treatment. Studies proved that they can provide at least equivalent biomechanical properties to the iliac crest bone graft. What is more, it has been shown that this technique produces a better articular pressure than the Latarjet. Frank et al. and Provencher et al. reported in their reports that articular conformity of glenoid arc can be reproduced with this source of graft [34, 35]. Naturally, this method has some limitations. The original article of this procedure stated that the distal tibia is well matched to the humerus, but more recent studies reported conflicting results.

Decker et al. reported that the chance of a random pairing of a distal tibial allograft matching the radius of curvature of recipient glenoid was low [36]. How precise a match is necessary to achieve optimal results remains to be studied. The possibility of graft resorption as well as immunologic response after this procedure has not been investigated yet, but these concerns have plagued allograft usage in other transplant settings [37–40].

Comparing outcomes of DTA versus Latarjet for anterior shoulder instability repair, Frank et al. reported no significant differences in postoperative patients who reported outcomes measurement scores between those groups [41]. They concluded that fresh DTA reconstruction results in a clinically stable joint with similar clinical outcomes as the Latarjet procedure, but more long-term studies are needed.

20.4 Distal Clavicle Osteochondral Autograft (DCA)

The most recent method is one described by Tokish et al. [42]. They have proposed usage of the distal clavicle as a fresh, osteochondral autograft in glenoid bone loss treatment. DCA is the first reported method that provides an autograft source of bone and cartilage to replace similar loss tissue on the glenoid. The advantages of such option are ready availability with minimal cost. In addition, it can be placed arthroscopically as well as employed in both anterior and posterior cases of bone loss. Donor-site morbidity has not been reported yet; however, graft harvest is comparable to the Mumford technique which is reported to give excellent or good outcome in up to 85% treated patients with dissatisfaction correlated with clavicle over or under resection. Excising 5–10 mm of a distal clavicle is suggested to be a safe method in both mentioned procedures [43].

When comparing to traditional coracoid transfer, DCA reproduces up to 44% of the glenoid radius and coracoid transfer up to 31% [44]. Moreover, the distal clavicle graft is capped with articular cartilage which is within 1 mm of native glenoid cartilage thickness. According to Kwapisz et al., it is a fresh, unprocessed tissue source that is immediately transplant, so concerns about chondrocyte viability, immunorejection, or infection are minimized. Although encouraging anatomic result has been reported, there is still a lack of clinical outcome studies. Thus, while this procedure has been an effective option in the senior author's hands, no clinical series has been published in the peer-reviewed literature. However, supporting biomechanical data have been published by Petersen et al. They demonstrated that contact pressure differences between clavicular grafting and congruent arc coracoid transfer are favorable to the DCA. It is the preference of the senior author to use to the DCA in young patients who have glenoid bone loss as the primary reason for their instability, with defects from 15% to 30%, and relatively preserved soft-tissue structures [45]. A summarized summary of the benefits of this method is given in Table 20.2.

This technique has also several limitations. First, it is does not augment or address anterior capsular structures that are often a part of complex instability cases. Thus, in cases of collagenopathies, such as Ehlers–Danlos syndrome, previous thermal capsulorrhaphy or multiply operated patients, other techniques addressing these issues are preferred.

Table 20.2 Benefits of distal clavicle in glenoid bone loss usage

Characteristic	Benefit
Source	Autograft: no risk of disease transmission or host issues
Osteochondral	Cartilage source quickly accessible, similar to the thickness of native glenoid
Cost	Free
Availability	Quickly available source, no waiting time for serologic testing, etc
Versatility	Can be used for both posterior and anterior bone loss in glenoid

20.5 DCA Surgical Technique

20.5.1 Preoperative Preparation

Patients with glenohumeral instability should undergo a standard history and physical examination, as well as preoperative advanced imaging such as CT or MRI. Glenoid bone loss is calculated in every patient, and this calculation aids in determining the operative approach to the patient according to the "on-track off-track" concept. As relative indications for bony augmentation of either anterior or posterior instability, bone loss of greater than 15% of the glenoid diameter or the existence of significant retroversion in the presence of posterior instability is considered. Other factors such as age, athletic status, capsular laxity, and patient preferences are weighed when deciding between different treatment options.

20.5.2 Arthroscopic Portal Positioning

After the induction of general anesthesia, examination under anesthesia to confirm the preoperative diagnosis is performed. The patient is positioned in the lateral decubitus position on a beanbag with a padded axillary roll, with the use of a padded arm sleeve (STAR sleeve; Arthrex, Naples, FL), with balanced suspension.

A standard posterior portal is established approximately 1 cm medial and 2 cm distal to the posterolateral acromial border. The arthroscope is introduced, and additional portals are established using an outside–in technique under direct visualization with the use of a switching stick. The anterosuperior portal is established first, approximately 1 cm inferior to the clavicle and lateral to the coracoid. The mid-glenoid portal is created just superior to the superior border of the subscapularis. In cases of posterior augmentation, a 7-o'clock portal is created approximately 4 cm off of the posterolateral corner of the acromion, bisecting the angle created by the posterior and lateral borders of the acromion, respectively, under direct visualization. To allow efficient switching of the camera and instruments throughout the case, 8.25-mm cannulas are liberally used.

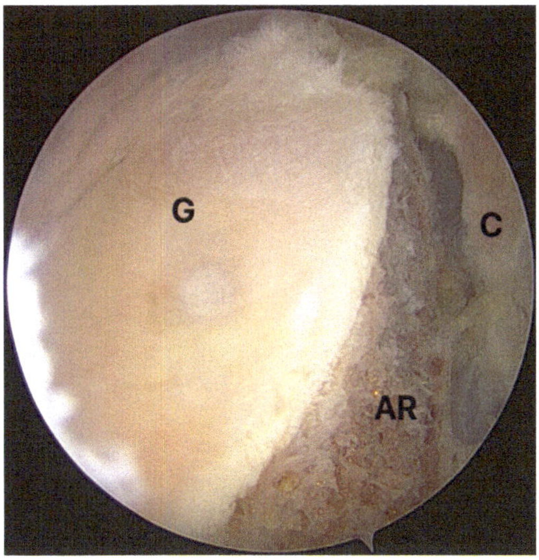

Fig. 20.1 Anterior rim of the glenoid after the bone stock preparation. *G* glenoid, *AR* anterior rim, *C* capsule

20.5.3 Diagnostic Arthroscopy and Biologic Preparation

After the diagnostic arthroscopy is performed with particular attention to the pathology, the arthroscope is switched to the anterosuperior portal and a 3-mm graduated probe is placed to confirm our preoperative measurements of glenoid bone loss. Biologic preparation includes a wide release of the glenoid labrum to ensure its mobility for accurate reduction, especially once the bone block reconstitutes the glenoid shape. This is performed with arthroscopic liberators and ablators. The glenoid is also biologically prepared with either an arthroscopic rasp or high-speed cylindrical burr, with the goal to create a healthy bed of bleeding cancellous bone, as well as to create a flat surface perpendicular to the glenoid surface to ensure a flush fit with graft placement (Fig. 20.1).

20.5.4 Graft Harvest

A single 3-cm horizontal incision is made over the subcutaneous border of the acromioclavicular joint, along the midline of the clavicular axis. The skin and subcutaneous tissues are divided, and thick periosteal flap is raised to expose the joint and approximately 1 cm of the distal clavicle. A 1-cm-wide saw blade is used to remove the distal 1 cm of clavicle, and soft tissue is cleaned from around the bone. The graft is placed on the back table, and the periosteal flap is closed with nonabsorbable No. 2 interrupted stitches. The remainder of the soft tissue is closed in two layers, and the wound is dressed at the completion of the case.

20.5.5 Graft Preparation

The distal clavicle is a versatile graft, with a variable amount of version and an articular surface that is generally 19 mm long and 13 mm wide. The graft is evaluated based on its best fit and cut perpendicular to its articular surface to a width that matches the measurement of bone loss that was determined preoperatively and confirmed arthroscopically. In most cases, 7–8 mm of augmentation is normally sufficient to reconstruct up to 30% bone loss, and the graft is fashioned to anatomically fit and replace the loss. At this point, the method of fixation for the graft is chosen. If we decide on screw fixation, the graft is

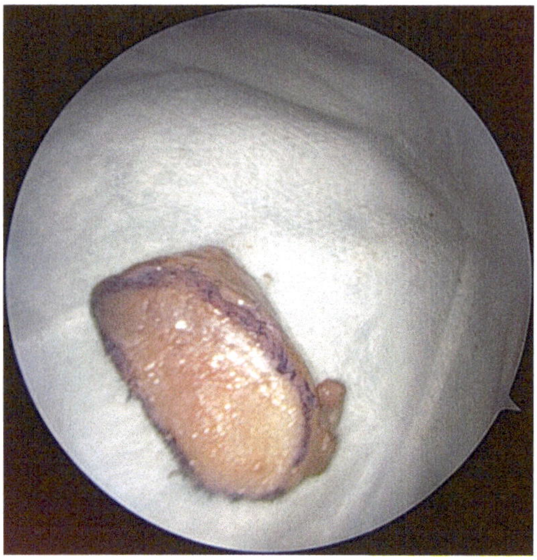

Fig. 20.2 Harvested distal clavicle osteochondral autograft (DCA)

predrilled in a lag construct with pilot holes allowing compression of the autograft with the screw. Alternatively, we often use suture anchors to secure the graft; in these cases, three 1-mm holes are drilled in a triangular formation, with two drill holes, 1 mm in diameter, 3–4 mm off of the articular surface, at the superior and inferior borders of the graft. The third hole is drilled medial with respect to the graft's final position on the glenoid (Fig. 20.2).

20.5.6 Delivery and Fixation of Graft

Screw Fixation. If the graft is to be fixed with screw fixation, it can be passed either freely into the joint or along a K-wire guide predrilled in the glenoid. The advantage of a free pass is that the graft may fit down a standard mid-glenoid cannula and, once inserted, can be flipped 90 and advanced through the rotator interval inferiorly to match its resting position at the anterior–inferior glenoid, where it can be held in place with a liberator introduced from the posterior portal for anterior bone augmentation. Trying to pass the graft down, a K-wire will require a wider exposure through the subscapularis to obtain a proper position. Another option is to pass a graft through a "Halifax portal" as described by Wong et al. [46]. At that moment, this is our technique of choice. Likewise, the graft can be introduced through a posterior cannula and held in place with a liberator from the mid-glenoid portal. Once in place, a K-wire is placed through the pilot holes of the clavicle graft and advanced into the native glenoid. This is usually not difficult for posterior grafts, but with anterior screw placement, the standard mid-glenoid portal may not be sufficient to achieve the appropriate angle. In such situations, an additional 5-o'clock portal is established through the subscapularis to ensure the correct trajectory.

We perform a medial "Halifax" portal with by means of the inside-out technique, the subscapularis tendon is then retracted distally and conjoined tendon medial as to protect the nerve structures including the axillary nerve. This is performed by using a large channeler that follows the slotted cannula. Once the portal is established, a cannulated drill is advanced into the glenoid to allow lag fixation of the graft, with a cannulated, titanium 3.75-mm screw (Arthrex, Naples, FL). If the graft is too large to easily be delivered, the cannula can be removed, the portal expanded, and the graft delivered directly. The proper trajectory should be easy to achieve with wire provisional fixation; however, if it is difficult, one can still consider using a suture anchor as an alternative or conversion to an open approach.

Suture Anchor Fixation. If suture anchor fixation is selected, the previously drilled holes in the graft are noted by their measurements from the articular surface and from each other. From these measurements, two 3.0-mm BioComposite SutureTaks (Arthrex) are placed at the superior and inferior borders of the bone defect at the corresponding distances from the articular surface and each other, respectively. All limbs are delivered out of the working portal. One limb from each suture anchor is passed through the medial "conjoined" drill hole. The other two sutures are passed, one each, through the superior and inferior articular drill holes. These latter sutures are tied in a square-knot fashion over the intervening bone bridge with three stacked half-hitches. The

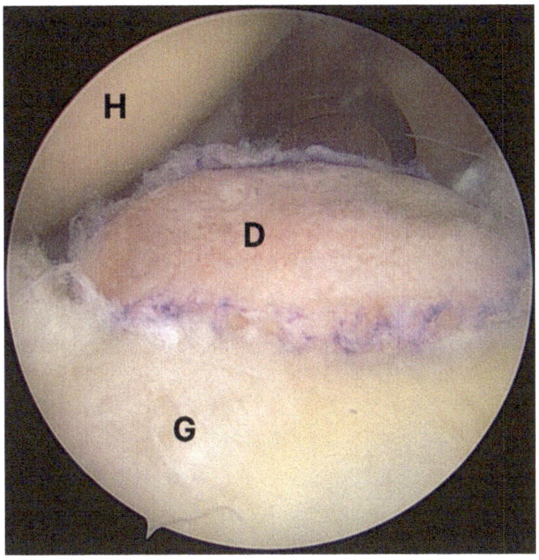

Fig. 20.3 The DCA after its fixing to the anterior rim of the native glenoid. *D* DCA, *G* glenoid, *H* humerus

excess suture is not cut. Graft delivery is then accomplished through the cannula by a "double-pulley" technique whereby the free limbs are pulled, which brings the graft to the suture anchor eyelets because of the knotted ends of the opposite limbs of suture. Either the graft can be assisted with a switching stick through a cannula or, if the graft is too large, the portal can be enlarged slightly, and the graft can be introduced with the assistance of a curved hemostat. Once the slack is pulled out of the anchor system, an arthroscopic knot with three additional half-hitches is tied and the graft is secured to the native glenoid across two bone bridges in a "double-row" fashion (Fig. 20.3).

20.5.7 Incorporation of Native Labrum to Graft

The remaining tails are passed through the native labrum to bring it up to the neo-articular surface with the aid of retrograde suture lassos and tied down with secondary similar knots.

If screw fixation has been used, supplemental suture anchors can be placed either through grafts of larger size or at the superior and inferior borders of the graft if there is concern about there being enough accommodating graft. All arthroscopic instrumentation is removed, and the skin is closed and dressed sterilely.

20.5.8 Postoperative Rehabilitation

The patient is placed in a neutral rotation sling for 6 weeks. Pendulums are allowed immediately, and passive motion is started at 3 weeks, with a goal to obtain full range of motion by 8 weeks. At 8 weeks of follow-up, imaging is obtained, and if the graft looks incorporated, active motion is begun. Strengthening is added at 4 months postoperatively, and return to full activity is assessed at 6 months. Final radiographs are obtained at this point to ensure graft incorporation.

20.6 Conclusion

Glenoid bone loss can be addressed by a variety of different techniques. Each has unique advantages and limitations. In this chapter, we detail the use of the distal clavicle osteochondral graft. This autograft provides a readily available and almost noncost method for anatomical reconstruction of glenoid bone loss. The graft restores both the radius of the native glenoid and comparable amount of its native cartilage thickness. It also compares favorably to the coracoid in terms of arc of restoration, providing a corticocancellous buttress for glenoid restoration. While this graft provides promising theoretical, anatomic, and biomechanical promises, longer term clinical studies are necessary to validate its use in the clinical setting.

References

1. Burkhart SS, Joe F, Beer D. Traumatic glenohumeral bone defects and their relationship to failure of arthroscopic Bankart repairs: significance of the inverted-pear glenoid and the humeral engaging Hill-Sachs lesion. Arthroscopy. 2000;16(7):677–94.
2. Provencher CDR, Matthew T, et al. Recurrent shoulder instability: current concepts for evaluation and management of glenoid bone loss. J Bone Joint Surg Am. 2010;92(Supplement 2):133–51.

3. Balg F, Boileau P. The instability severity index score. Bone Joint J. 2007;89(11):1470–7.
4. Taylor DC, Arciero RA. Pathologic changes associated with shoulder dislocations. Arthroscopic and physical examination findings in first-time, traumatic anterior dislocations. Am J Sports Med. 1997;25(3):306–11.
5. Hovelius LK, Sandstrom BC, Rosmark DL, Saebo M, Sundgren KH, Malmqvist BG. Long-term results with the Bankart and Bristow-Latarjet procedures: recurrent shoulder instability and arthropathy. J Shoulder Elbow Surg. 2001;10(5):445–52.
6. Lo IKY, Parten PM, Burkhart SS. The inverted pear glenoid: an indicator of significant glenoid bone loss. Arthroscopy. 2004;20(2):169–74.
7. Shaha JS, et al. Redefining "Critical" bone loss in shoulder instability functional outcomes worsen with "Subcritical" bone loss. Am J Sports Med. 2015;43(7):1719–25.
8. Fox JA, Sanchez A, Zajac TJ, Provencher MT. Understanding the Hill-Sachs lesion in its role in patients with recurrent anterior shoulder instability. Curr Rev Musculoskelet Med. 2017;10(4): 469–79.
9. Itoi E, et al. The effect of a glenoid defect on anteroinferior stability of the shoulder after Bankart repair: a cadaveric study. J Bone Joint Surg Am. 2000;82(1):35–46.
10. Di Giacomo G, Eiji I, Burkhart SS. Evolving concept of bipolar bone loss and the Hill-Sachs lesion: from "engaging/non-engaging" lesion to "on-track/off-track" lesion. Arthroscopy. 2014;30(1):90–8.
11. Shaha JS, Cook JB, Song DJ, Rowles DJ, Bottoni CR, Shaha SH, Tokish JM. Clinical validation of the "On-Track" vs. "Off-Track" concept in anterior glenohumeral instability. J Bone Joint Surg Am. 2016;98(22):1918–23.
12. Latarjet M. A propos du traitement des luxations récidivantes de l'épaule. Lyon Chir. 1954;49(994–997):27.
13. Helfet AJ. Coracoid transplantation for recurring dislocation of the shoulder. Bone Joint J. 1958;40(2):198–202.
14. Giles JW, et al. Does the dynamic sling effect of the Latarjet procedure improve shoulder stability? A biomechanical evaluation. J Shoulder Elbow Surg. 2013;22(6):821–7.
15. Yamamoto N, et al. The stabilizing mechanism of the Latarjet procedure. J Bone Joint Surg Am. 2013;95(15):1390–7.
16. Neyton L, et al. Surgical treatment of anterior instability in rugby union players: clinical and radiographic results of the Latarjet-Patte procedure with minimum 5-year follow-up. J Shoulder Elbow Surg. 2012;21(12):1721–7.
17. Burkhart SS, et al. Results of modified Latarjet reconstruction in patients with anteroinferior instability and significant bone loss. Arthroscopy. 2007;23(10):1033–41.
18. Griesser MJ, et al. Complications and re-operations after Bristow-Latarjet shoulder stabilization: a systematic review. J Shoulder Elbow Surg. 2013; 22(2):286–92.
19. Paladini P, et al. Latarjet procedure: is the coracoid enough to restore the glenoid surface? Int Orthop. 2016;40:1675–81.
20. Giles JW, et al. Do the traditional and modified Latarjet techniques produce equivalent reconstruction stability and strength? Am J Sports Med. 2012;40(12):2801–7.
21. Di Giacomo G, et al. Coracoid graft osteolysis after the Latarjet procedure for anteroinferior shoulder instability: a computed tomography scan study of twenty-six patients. J Shoulder Elbow Surg. 2011;20(6):989–95.
22. Allain J, Goutallier D, Glorion C. Long-term results of the Latarjet procedure for the treatment of anterior instability of the shoulder. J Bone Joint Surg Am. 1998;80(6):841–52.
23. Shah AA, et al. Short-term complications of the Latarjet procedure. J Bone Joint Surg Am. 2012;94(6):495–501.
24. Delaney RA, et al. Neer Award paper: neuromonitoring the Latarjet procedure. J Shoulder Elbow Surg. 2014;23(10):1473–80.
25. Min K, Fedorka C, Solberg MJ, Shaha SH, Higgins LD. The cost-effectiveness of the arthroscopic Bankart versus open Latarjet in the treatment of primary shoulder instability. J Shoulder Elbow Surg. 2018;27(6S):S2–9.
26. Eden R. Zur Operation der habituellen Schulterluxation unter Mitteilung eines neuen Verfahrens bei Abriss am inneren Pfannenrande. Langenbecks Arch Surg. 1918;144(3):269–80.
27. Hybbinette SR. De la transplantation d'un fragment osseux pour remédier aux luxations récidivantes de l'épaule: Constatations et résultats opératoires. Acta Chir Scand. 1932;71(411–445):26.
28. Warner JJP, et al. Anatomical glenoid reconstruction for recurrent anterior glenohumeral instability with glenoid deficiency using an autogenous tricortical iliac crest bone graft. Am J Sports Med. 2006;34(2):205–12.
29. Bouju Y, et al. Shoulder stabilization by modified Latarjet-Patte procedure: results at a minimum 10 years' follow-up, and role in the prevention of osteoarthritis. Orthop Traumatol Surg Res. 2014;100(4):S213–8.
30. Hovelius L, Sandström B, Saebö M. One hundred eighteen Bristow-Latarjet repairs for recurrent anterior dislocation of the shoulder prospectively followed for fifteen years: study II—the evolution of dislocation arthropathy. J Shoulder Elbow Surg. 2006;15(3):279–89.
31. Almaiman M, Al-Bargi HH, Manson P. Complication of anterior iliac bone graft harvesting in 372 adult patients from May 2006 to May 2011 and a literature review. Craniomaxillofac Trauma Reconstr. 2013;6(04):257–66.
32. Calori GM, et al. Incidence of donor site morbidity following harvesting from iliac crest or RIA graft. Injury. 2014;45:S116–20.
33. Kleiner MT, et al. Biomechanical comparison of the Latarjet procedure with and without capsular repair. Clin Orthop Surg. 2016;8(1):84–91.

34. Frank RM, et al. Comparison of glenohumeral contact pressures and contact areas after posterior glenoid reconstruction with an iliac crest bone graft or distal tibial osteochondral allograft. Am J Sports Med. 2014;42(11):2574–82.
35. Provencher MT, et al. Anatomic osteochondral glenoid reconstruction for recurrent glenohumeral instability with glenoid deficiency using a distal tibia allograft. Arthroscopy. 2009;25(4): 446–52.
36. Decker MM, et al. Distal tibia allograft for glenohumeral instability: does radius of curvature match? J Shoulder Elbow Surg. 2016;25(9):1542–8.
37. Aponte-Tinao LA, et al. What are the risk factors and management options for infection after reconstruction with massive bone allografts? Clin Orthop Relat Res. 2016;474(3):669–73.
38. Lozano-Calderón SA, et al. Predictors of soft-tissue complications and deep infection in allograft reconstruction of the proximal tibia. J Surg Oncol. 2016;113(7):811–7.
39. Chapovsky F, Kelly JD. Osteochondral allograft transplantation for treatment of glenohumeral instability. Arthroscopy. 2005;21(8):1007–e1.
40. Stevenson SDVM, Li XQ, Martin B. The fate of cancellous and cortical bone after transplantation of fresh and frozen tissue-antigen-matched and mismatched osteochondral allografts in dogs. J Bone Joint Surg Am. 1991;73(8):1143–56.
41. Frank RM, Romeo AA, Richardson C, Sumner S, Verma NN, Cole BJ, Nicholson GP, Provencher MT. Outcomes of Latarjet versus distal tibia allograft for anterior shoulder instability repair: a matched cohort analysis. Am J Sports Med. 2018;46(5):1030–8.
42. Tokish JM, Fitzpatrick K, Cook JB, Mallon WJ. Arthroscopic distal clavicular autograft for treating shoulder instability with glenoid bone loss. Arthrosc Tech. 2014;3(4):e475–81.
43. Strauss EJ, et al. The evaluation and management of failed distal clavicle excision. Sports Med Arthrosc Rev. 2010;18(3):213–9.
44. Kwapisz A, Fitzpatrick K, Cook JB, Athwal GS, Tokish JM. Distal clavicular osteochondral autograft augmentation for glenoid bone loss: a comparison of radius of restoration versus Latarjet graft. Am J Sports Med. 2018;46(5):1046–52.
45. Petersen SA, et al. Autologous distal clavicle versus autologous coracoid bone grafts for restoration of anterior-inferior glenoid bone loss: a biomechanical comparison. J Shoulder Elbow Surg. 2016;25(6):960–6.
46. Wong IH, Urquhart N. Arthroscopic anatomic glenoid reconstruction without subscapularis split. Arthrosc Tech. 2015;4(5):e449–56.

Anteroinferior Shoulder Instability Treatment with Arthroscopic Latarjet

21

Leonard Achenbach, Christian Moody, and Laurent Lafosse

21.1 Introduction

Shoulder anterior instability may present with different symptoms: shoulder dislocation, subluxation, or simple pain. As soon as the shoulder dislocates, the inferior glenohumeral ligament (IGHL) can be damaged along with labral detachment and a potential bony lesion. These problems when combined commonly lead to recurrent instability. In cases of isolated labrum detachment, arthroscopic reattachment provides excellent result, but in our experience, as soon as the IGHL is involved during a dislocation, long-term result of soft-tissue reattachment is poor. Management of shoulder instability in young collision athletes with soft-tissue stability alone remains problematic with high revision and recurrent dislocation rates [1, 2]. A variety of open and arthroscopic treatment methods exist and are described in this textbook. Our preferred technique for not only athletes but also for patients with recurrent anterior instability, instability secondary to any bony Bankart lesions, off-track lesions including bipolar lesions, and humeral avulsions of the glenohumeral ligament (HAGL) is an arthroscopic Latarjet. The arthroscopic Latarjet has several advantages over the traditional open Latarjet that described in 1954 [3]. These advantages include better visualization of the entire joint, which allows for optimum graft placement as well as management of concomitant lesions of the posterior and superior labrum. In addition, direct visualization of the axillary nerve and surrounding hypervascular tissue allows for reducing the change of a neurovascular injury [4, 5].

The Latarjet procedure is successful in stabilizing the shoulder through several key mechanisms. First, the coracoid transfer provides static stability by increasing the glenoid surface area, which results in a greater articular arc, thus preventing a Hill–Sachs lesion from engaging the anterior rim. Second, the conjoint tendon serves as a dynamic reinforcement of the inferior capsule providing a "hammock" effect, particularly when the shoulder is in its most vulnerable position of abduction, external rotation. Lastly, the intersection between the split subscapularis tendon and the conjoint tendon provides further dynamic tension to the inferior portion of the subscapularis tendon, again with the most tension during the position of highest vulnerability [4, 5]. Further details describing all pathology and mechanisms of stabilization will be described in the following text.

L. Achenbach (✉)
ALPS Surgery Institute, Annecy, France

Department of Trauma, Hand, Plastic and Reconstructive Surgery, University Hospital Wuerzburg, Wuerzburg, Germany
e-mail: leonard@dr-achenbach.eu

C. Moody
ALPS Surgery Institute, Annecy, France

Prisma Health System, Greenville, SC, USA

L. Lafosse
ALPS Surgery Institute, Annecy, France

R. Brzóska et al. (eds.), *360° Around Shoulder Instability*,
https://doi.org/10.1007/978-3-662-61074-9_21

Our technique has evolved since we first published on the arthroscopic Latarjet in 2007 [4]. It is important to note that this procedure should be reserved for surgeons with extensive arthroscopy expertise. We recommend becoming familiar with the anterior shoulder compartment, including the subcoracoid space when possible during routine arthroscopic procedures. Then, in a laboratory setting, use a cadaver to perform the full procedure for the first time, and multiple times if possible. Finally, asking a local mentor to assist in the live setting can provide tips and troubleshooting assistance that is second to none.

21.2 The Anterior Shoulder Instability Lesion

"Anterior instability of the shoulder" is commonly used to include all symptoms of pathological anteroinferior displacement of the glenohumeral joint. However, with our expanded knowledge of the shoulder, it is critical to be more precise.

One must describe the direct correlation between the severity of the symptoms and the location of the lesion.

According the severity of the symptoms, three major groups of patients have been defined:

- *Group I* (56%): Dislocation (at least one full dislocation which needs a reduction by a person other than the patient)
- *Group II* (26%): Subluxation (shoulder never fully dislocates, but the patient has a sensation of shoulder instability confirmed by physical examination)
- *Group III* (18%): Unstable painful shoulder (the patient complains of shoulder pain and the surgeon determines the origin is an issue of instability such as labral detachment)
- [French Society]

21.2.1 Further Subdifferentiation

- **Soft-tissue lesions** range from a simple Bankart lesion to more complicated capsulolabral lesions like the anterior labroligamentous periostal sleeve avulsion (ALPSA), complicated ruptures of the labrum (Detrisac II and IV), or humeral avulsion of glenohumeral ligaments. In the most frequent cases of instability with dislocation (group I) concerning only soft tissues, the humeral displacement is anterior, medial, and *inferior*. The IGHL is always involved, and most of the time, the soft tissue is badly damaged (ligament stretch or tear; humeral detachment: HAGL lesion). In addition to ligament damage, the labral ring is frequently torn, thus causing a loss of concentric forces of the intact ring that are critical to the healing process.
- Associated **bone lesions** are created on both humeral and glenoid side at the moment of the dislocation. These lesions are the Hill–Sachs lesion, at the level of the posterior humerus, and the Bankart/glenoid rim fractures with permanent loss of glenoid bone, which can further impair the remaining stability. Four of five patients who have anterior shoulder instability have a "bipolar lesion," which is defined as having both a Hill–Sachs and glenoid bone lesion. Itoi described the contact zone between the glenoid and humeral head as the "glenoid track" [6]. Based on the location of the Hill–Sachs lesion, it will either engage the glenoid and dislocate (off-track lesion) or avoid engagement and remain reduced (on-track lesion) [6].

21.3 Why a Coracoid Transfer?

Operative Bankart repair, both open and arthroscopic, has demonstrated excellent results when used for isolated soft-tissue Bankart lesions. However, in cases of unrecognized soft-tissue injury, for example, humeral avulsion of glenohumeral ligament (HAGL) lesions, complex labral disruptions, irreparable soft-tissue damage, and in cases of bony deficiency, this technique may not be sufficient to stabilize the shoulder. For young patients (<20), overhead athletes, and those involved in contact sports, soft-tissue repair alone should be avoided.

In 2006, Boileau highlighted several reasons for failure of the Bankart procedure for anterior instability [1]. The most important risk factors identified were bone loss on the glenoid or humeral sides and inferior ligament hyperlaxity. This is often a result of stretching from the initial dislocation. A combination of these abnormalities can result in up to a 75% recurrence of instability after soft-tissue repair [1, 7].

It seems clear that a simple Bankart repair, which reduces the labrum back on to the glenoid, cannot be expected to return soft-tissue stability to the shoulder when the glenohumeral ligaments are torn or attenuated. Further to this point, where there is glenoid bone loss or an engaging Hill–Sachs lesion, a soft-tissue repair does not lengthen the glenoid articular arc, which is necessary to prevent future engagement and recurrent symptoms. In these situations, another approach must be adopted.

The initial description of Bristow procedure was a simple translation into the subscapularis muscle of the conjoint tendon by sawing the bony chip of the distal part of the coracoid. The modified Bristow by Helfet uses a larger fragment of the coracoid tip which is fixed to the anterior glenoid neck with a single screw [8].

The Latarjet procedure is fixing half of the coracoid in a flat position using the advantage of congruence between the curvature of the anterior glenoid and the coracoid fragment. A larger size bone block allows for double-screw fixation with rotational stability and better compression as well as restoration of the area of glenoid bone loss. The ligamentoplasty effect is created by crossing the conjoint tendon over the inferior part of the subscapularis tendon, which is slightly reoriented in an inferior and posterior direction [4]. This creates a dynamic tension applied to the inferior capsule and subscapularis, especially in external rotation, and, therefore, reinforces the anterior restraint. By augmenting the glenoid bony contour, engagement of a Hill–Sachs lesion is prevented. At present, the subscapularis muscle is split horizontally between the upper two-thirds and lower one-third and not superiorly detached with an L-like incision as described initially.

Alternative techniques such as *autologous bone or iliac crest grafting* have been routinely performed using open techniques with success and are indicated as a salvage surgery in cases of hardware failure, recurrent dislocation, or nonunion.

The *isolated transfer of the conjoint tendon* to the glenoid neck over the subscapularis tendon has been described to replace the sling of the torn glenohumeral ligaments, but this does not address the inferior ligament weakness and/or glenoid bone loss.

The Latarjet and modified Bristow procedure are successful because they combine a bony procedure with a ligamentoplasty by the conjoint tendon transfer through the subscapularis muscle. Biomechanical studies from Itoi proved that bony reconstruction restores 100% of a native glenoid, and that association of bony reconstruction and conjoint tendon fixation provides 130% stability of a native shoulder. Capsule reconstruction on top of Latarjet does not affect the result [9].

21.4 Why an Arthroscopic Latarjet?

1. Advantages over open Latarjet include the following:
   - Placement of the bone graft is more accurate under arthroscopic control. Several views can be afforded by the arthroscopic technique that not only improve graft placement but also will reduce the chances of overhang and impingement.
   - Unlike open surgery, arthroscopic surgery allows for the treatment of concomitant pathologies such as SLAP tears and posterior labral lesions.
   - Double instabilities can be treated during the same surgical procedure using both anterior and posterior bone blocks when employing arthroscopic methods. This is not possible through a single open approach.
   - Even though the strength of the bone block fixation allows early mobilization, the risk of adhesions and shoulder stiffness is

higher with an open technique over arthroscopy.
   - If during an intended Bankart repair, the tissue is determined to not be repairable, then an arthroscopic Latarjet offers an alternative solution to traditional open surgery and potentially having to reposition the patient.
   - As in other joints, arthroscopy offers the advantages of less postoperative pain, earlier mobility, quicker rehabilitation, and faster return to sport.
   - Improved cosmetic result for the patients with an arthroscopic technique.
2. Drawbacks of arthroscopic Latarjet include the following:
   - High level of difficulty during many steps of the procedure.
   - Risks link to swelling.
   - Potential malpositioning of the graft and of the screws due to the difficulties of scapula positioning.
   - Neurologic and vascular risks.
   - Arthroscopic Latarjet is not possible if operating conditions are not optimum, which is highly dependent on a perfect fit with an anesthesiology team.
3. It is important to keep in mind that conversion from arthroscopic to open Latarjet is possible at any stage.

21.5 Indications for Arthroscopic Latarjet

Once a detailed history, clinical examination, and radiological investigations are performed, an intraoperative assessment of the ligamentous stability can determine the appropriate operation. The following scenarios will provide examples of different surgical indications.

21.5.1 Glenoid Bone Loss

Many authors have reported failure of soft-tissue repair due to the glenoid bone loss [10]. The mechanical consequences of the anteroinferior glenoid erosion have been proven by biomechanics studies and assessed by different X-ray, CT scan techniques, and arthroscopic visualization (inverted pear) [11]. In some cases, the bony fragment can be replaced and arthroscopically repaired by anchors and sutures. However, this is always a smaller than the original glenoid and is not as strong and supportive as a bony block.

This is a common cause for recurrent instability and can manifest as a bony Bankart lesion or a true fracture of the anterior or inferior glenoid rim. Standard AP x-rays may show a fracture or a more subtle loss of contour of the anteroinferior glenoid rim. A decrease in the apparent density of the inferior glenoid line often signifies an erosion of the glenoid rim between 3 and 6 o'clock. An axillary view or better, a Bernageau view, may show flattening of this area of the glenoid when bone loss has occurred [12]. Computerized tomography (CT) provides a more detailed imaging modality that is essential to quantify the bone loss preoperatively. CT reconstructions provide a more robust static measurement than those afforded by the arthroscopic view. Arthroscopically, the distance from the glenoid rim as measured from the bare spot can assist the surgeon in identifying an inverted pear glenoid, confirming substantial bone loss and the likely failure of an isolated soft-tissue repair. Even when the bony fragment is present, replacing it is not always sufficient to restore the bony glenoid articular arc due to the difficulties in the healing of this necrotic bone. In these cases, a bone reconstruction as performed by the Latarjet procedure should be considered.

21.5.2 Humeral Bone Loss

The location and the depth of the Hill–Sachs lesion are variable with each case: sometimes small and superficial; and sometimes deep, extended, and exceptionally double. Its location and depth are responsible for persistent instability, even in cases of well-done Bankart repair. Its precise assessment is difficult but can be approached by simple X-ray in internal rotation and 2D or 3D CT scan. The "remplissage" of the infraspinatus tendon has been described with satisfactory results, but external rotation is limited and long-term results have not been reported.

The location and size of the Hill–Sachs lesion determine whether the articular arc is reduced and whether this will engage on the glenoid. A dynamic arthroscopy with the shoulder in abduction and external rotation will demonstrate whether the lesion is engaging even within an athletic overhead range of movement. A bone block procedure here will increase the arc of the anterior glenoid, thereby increasing the degree of external rotation that can be achieved before the Hill–Sachs lesion approaches the glenoid rim. We believe that by enlarging the glenoid articular arc with a bone graft, there is no increased joint contact pressure during external rotation. A remplissage, however, can lead to a decrease in external rotation and may give rise to increased contact forces on the articular cartilage during external rotation.

21.5.3 Combination of Both Glenoid and Humeral Bone Loss

As stated previously, the "bipolar lesion" is responsible for many cases of recurrent instability. This combination of two lesions usually occurs with varying degrees of severity for each individual lesion. These can be assessed before the procedure by examination, plain radiographs, and CT scan. It is critical to look for both lesions during the arthroscopy exploration under dynamic visualization.

21.5.4 The Irreparable Soft-Tissue Damage/Complex Soft-Tissue Injury

The HAGL lesion is sometime possible to diagnose by an MRI or CT arthrography, but in most cases, it is discovered during the arthroscopy. Different techniques of humeral reattachment by suture and anchor are possible depending on the location of the detachment, but our results with this technique have been disappointing due to the stiffness after repair.

Furthermore, in patients with multiple dislocations, the intrinsic structure of the glenohumeral ligaments is usually deranged although this may not be evident macroscopically. Simply repairing this damaged tissue to the glenoid does not restore stability to the shoulder. This has been likened rehanging a baggy or incompetent hammock. A final situation is that of the labral tear, often in association with a glenohumeral ligament lesion. In this situation, the ring of the labrum is disrupted and the strength of a repair will be unable to match that of an intact labral ring. In these situations, there is a need for a ligamentoplasty and accompanying bone block. A complete dislocation, according to our experience, as it is correlated to an inferior ligament detachment, is a bad prognostic factor for ligament injury. Multiple complete dislocations cause even further damage to the soft-tissue structures.

21.5.5 Revision of Bankart Repair

After an open or arthroscopic Bankart repair, success is often measured by the absence of recurrent dislocations. In some cases, the joint is not sufficiently stabilized, but it does allow function for a more sedentary lifestyle without overt symptoms of instability. This can, in part, explain the excellent results seen in series with a short follow-up. After 5–7 years, we find this particular group of patients can go on to develop instability and/or arthritis. In these cases, the initial operation was considered successful although the pathological lesion was never truly corrected and the glenoid subsequently becomes increasingly eroded. Again, these patients can be successfully managed with a bone block ligamentoplasty.

21.5.6 Specific Patients

There are some patients who play high-risk sports (climbing, football, rugby) or work (carpentry) or have a high risk of recurrence due to the intensity and action or their activity (throwers). The Latarjet procedure provides a strong stabilization mechanism and fast recovery time for these individuals.

21.6 Technique for the Arthroscopic Latarjet

The arthroscopic Latarjet technique can be divided into five steps. These include joint evaluation and exposure, harvesting of the coracoid process, subscapularis split, coracoid transfer, and finally fixation of the coracoid process. Patient positioning is beach chair. The use of an arm holder helps to manage the arm and with scapula positioning.

The following seven portals are used in our practice (Fig. 21.1):

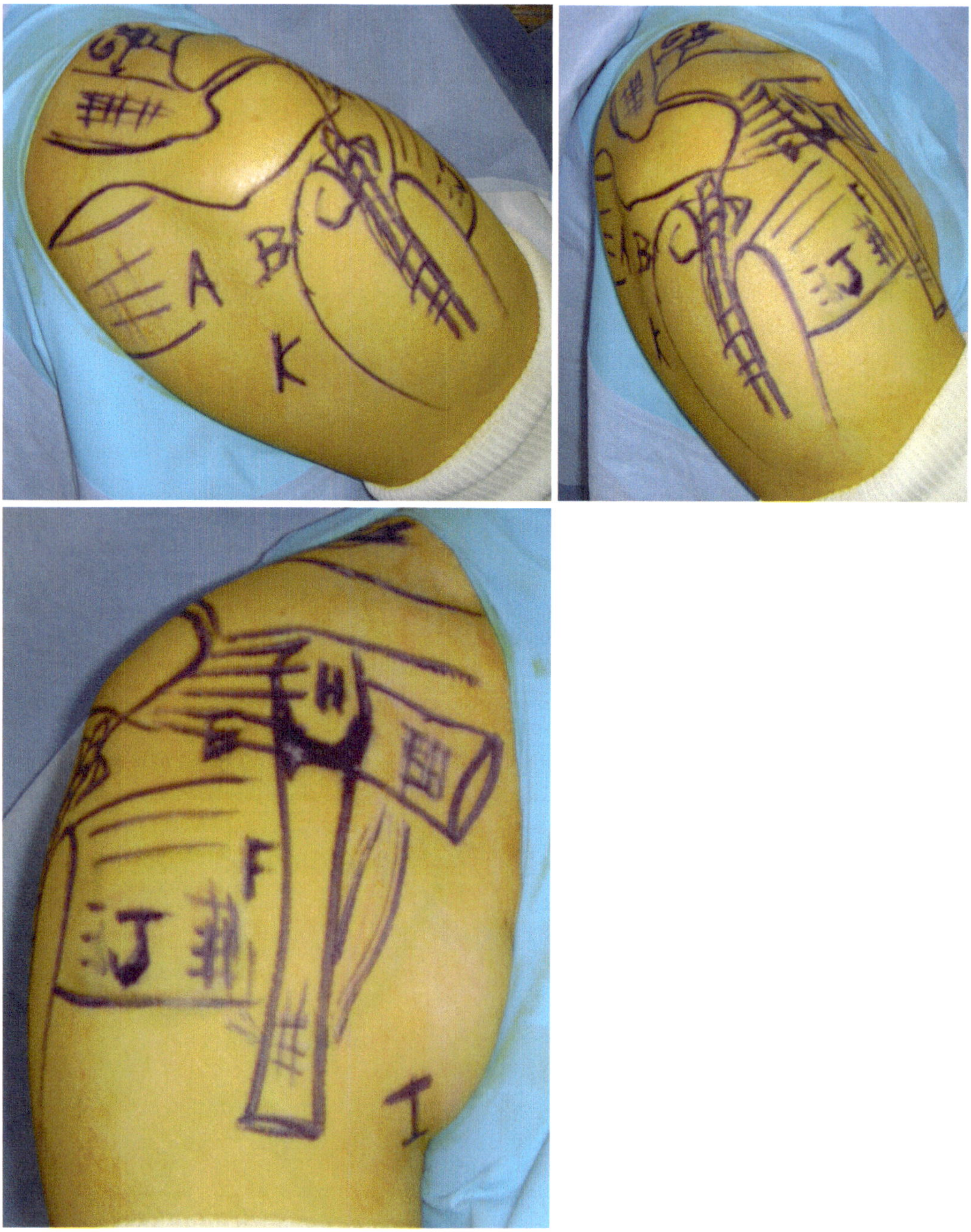

Fig. 21.1 Arthroscopic portals used for the arthroscopic Latarjet

- Portal A: standard posterior
- E: anterolateral to access the rotator interval
- D: anterolateral at the level of the anterolateral corner of the acromion
- I: aligned with the coracoid process above the axillary fold
- J: between I and D portal, parallel to the subscapularis fibers
- M: the most medial and anterior portal through the pectoralis major aligned with the glenoid surface
- H: anterosuperior portal above the coracoid

21.6.1 Step 1: Joint Evaluation and Exposure

The intraarticular approach commences through the standard A posterior portal. By means of the anterolateral E portal—which is established using an outside–in technique—a probe is introduced through the rotator interval (RI). With the probe, a diagnostic arthroscopic examination including a dynamic stability assessment is performed, specifically looking for bony glenoid lesions, humeral defects, and soft-tissue lesions, such as a HAGL.

Opening of the rotator interval (RI), exposure of both sides of subscapularis, and preparation of the glenoid neck. The glenohumeral joint is opened at the upper border of subscapularis, and the anteroinferior labrum and medial glenohumeral ligament (MGHL) are detached between 2 and 5 o'clock to expose the glenoid neck. This can be done using electrocautery. The intended graft site is exposed, and the capsule between glenoid neck and subscapularis is split. Remove the pathological anterior capsule and bony Bankart, if necessary. To provide a healthy base for graft healing, the glenoid neck is abraded with the burr. Both sides of the subscapularis tendon are then exposed, with particular attention to the articular side of subscapularis. These releases are necessary to facilitate the transfer of the coracoid graft. If case of any further intraarticular pathology, it should be addressed at this stage, for example, a posterior labral repair. The intraarticular preparation is now completed.

Coracoid Soft-Tissue Preparation. A long spinal needle is inserted parallel to the upper part of the subscapularis tendon to ensure best positioning of the D portal. The instruments are then used in this D portal. Remove the end of the bursa under the coracoid and expose the conjoint tendons down to the level of the pectoralis major.

Behind the conjoint tendon exists a medial tissue barrier, which separates the brachial plexus from the subcoracoid bursa. This is gently dissected to reveal the single nerves, such as the axillary nerve. It is important to visualize this nerve and appreciate its location when it comes to splitting the subscapularis muscle and placing the graft. Any further soft-tissue attachments to the coracoid in the bursa are released to free the coracoid for its later transfer.

The coracoacromial (CA) ligament should be located at its coracoid insertion site and subsequently detached. Attention must be paid to coagulate the terminal branch of the acromiothoracic artery. The anterior aspect of the conjoint tendon is liberated from the deltoid fascia. The inferior limit of this release should be the pectoralis major tendon. Splitting the deltoid fascia anterior of the coracoid process facilitates visualization.

The scope is now moved from the posterior A portal to the lateral D portal. Split the adhesions between the conjoint tendons and the pectoralis minor. The pectoralis minor tendon on the medial border of the coracoid is now released taking care to keep the electrocautery on bone during this step. Finalize the preparation of the coracoid process by completely debriding its superior part from any soft tissue. With this dissection completed and having an awareness of the position of the nerves, we can proceed with the knowledge that everything lateral to the conjoint tendon is safe.

21.6.2 Step 2: Harvesting the Coracoid

Preparation of the Anterior Portals. Establish the I, J, and M portals (Fig. 21.2).

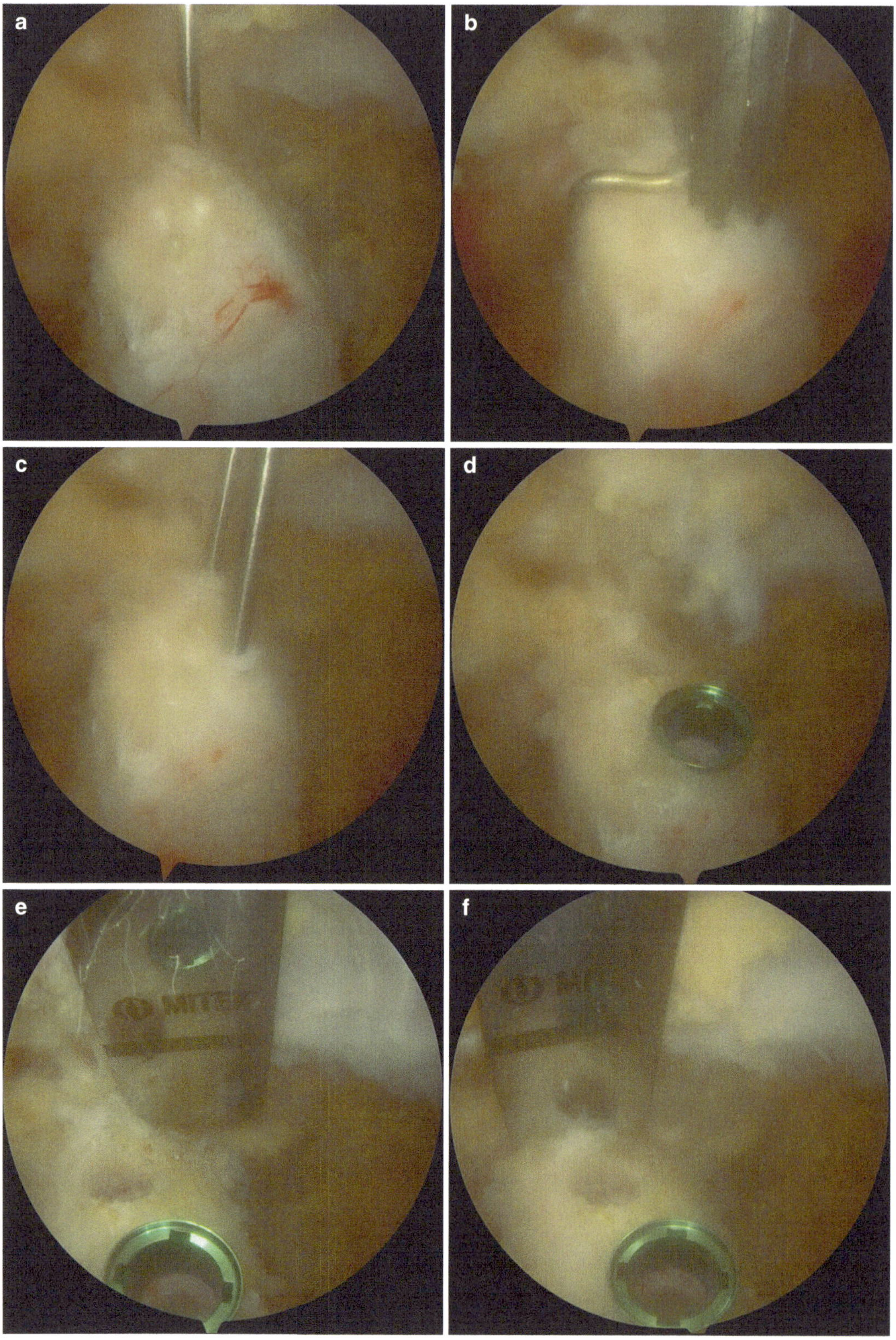

Fig. 21.2 Steps for the coracoid harvesting with (**a**) defining and establishing the H portal with a long spine needle, (**b**) placement of coracoid drill guide, (**c**) insertion of both K-wires, (**d**) insertion of top hat washer, and (**e**, **f**) osteotomy starting from exterior to interior

Using an outside–in technique, the I portal is placed above the axillary fold, aligned with the coracoid process. Manipulation of the needle used to perform this portal should anticipate visualizing the four sides of the coracoid when the scope is introduced through this I portal. The J portal is placed midway on an arc between the I and the D portals. It gives a more head on view of the coracoid, whereas the D portal gives a better lateral view. Two perpendicular views are necessary to ensure optimum coracoid preparation.

The M portal is the most medial. It should be aligned with the glenoid surface and should provide for management of the coracoid fixation parallel to the glenoid. Despite its very medial location, this portal is not dangerous as long as the pectoralis minor is not penetrated. Once this muscle is detached, the plexus is in line with the M portal and close attention should be paid with the use of this portal.

Pectoralis Minor Detachment. Once the scope is introduced in the I portal, the electrocautery is introduced into the M portal and the upper and lower parts of pectoralis minor (PM) are located. It is difficult but crucial to separate PM from the conjoint tendon. The electrocautery should remain superficial, and the split should be managed with high care until the musculocutaneous nerve is located. PM is then totally detached from the coracoid process. The plexus can be visualized at that stage, but it is not necessary to dissect the plexus.

Define the H Portal. At this point, the scope is in the J portal and the electrocautery is in the I portal. Place an arthroscopic switching stick in the D portal and elevate the space above the coracoid (like using a retractor in open surgery). I like to place the other end through the plastic fluid collection bag on the drapes to keep this "retractor" in the same position as long as I need it there. Locate the coracoid's midpoint again with a long spine needle perpendicular to the axis. This will serve to guide the position of the coracoid drill guide. Once satisfied, make a superior incision for the H portal.

Drilling the Coracoid and Inserting the Anterior Top Hat. Place the 15° coracoid drill guide flush on top of the CP. It is important to regularly change the viewing angle of the scope by rotation to ensure mediolateral alignment of the now inserted coracoid drill guide. Place the guide over junction of lateral two-thirds and medial one-third of coracoid. Use the 7-mm distance device—included in the new drill guides (DePuy-Synthes)—to ensure proper alignment to the lateral aspect of the coracoid process.

Drill the Alpha-hole (inferior and distal) with a K-wire. It is important while doing this to visualize under the coracoid to verify that the direction of the K-wires is perpendicular to the superior surface of the coracoid and to avoid penetrating too deep into the brachial plexus. Locate the final position of the Beta-hole relative to the axis. Rotationally, align the coracoid drill guide and then drill the Beta (proximal) K-wire.

Remove the drill guide, leave the K-wires, and check the wire positions. Overdrill both holes with the coracoid step drill. To ensure drilling is bicortical, place a clamp at the end of the K-wire while drilling. When the clamp (and thus the wire) begins rotating, the second cortex has been passed.

Remove the clamp and the drill but keep the K-wires.

The drill holes are now tapped to prepare for the top hat and glenoid screws. The posterior Beta K-wire is removed. The anterior top hat is now inserted in the anterior Alpha drill hole, and the K-wire is removed.

Coracoid Osteotomy. Once the coracoid is prepared, we are now ready to make the osteotomy through the H portal. First, the osteotome is placed on the medial most proximal aspect just anterior to the coracoclavicular (CC) ligaments. Here, osteotomy of the medial quarter of the coracoid is performed. The same is done on the lateral aspect. Then, in a third step, a controlled complete osteotomy is performed by placing the osteotome in the line connecting the two previous osteotomies.

At this stage, there is often facia that maintains the coracoid superiorly. It is necessary to release this facia paying attention to preserve the axillary nerve just behind.

21.6.3 Step 3: Subscapularis Split

Determine the Level of the Subscapularis Split. Remove any remaining bursa at the anterior face of the tendon and muscle by introducing the shaver in the J portal. Hemostasis by the electrocautery introduced in the M portal is managed at the same time. Locate the three sisters (one artery and two veins) and the axillary nerve running along the muscle to avoid neurovascular injury. Determine the upper two thirds and lower one third of the subscapularis muscle-tendon unit.

Subscapularis Split. The arm is placed in external rotation without causing anterior translation of the humeral head. Create the split by using electrocautery. The split is completed down to the glenoid neck in the line of fibers of subscapularis, extending from the lateral insertion of subscapularis on the lesser tuberosity, passing medially close to the axillary nerve. *Expert Tip: start medial by the axillary nerve and moving lateral in line with the fibers of the muscle, use a switching stick to elevate the upper edge of the split muscle to provide counter tension while moving to the deeper layers of muscle. A probe is introduced through the A portal and can be used to keep the subscapularis window open.*

21.6.4 Step 4: Preparation of Glenoid Bed and Graft Trimming

The shoulder is manipulated with the arm holder in slight internal rotation with scapula retropulsion in order to decrease the subscapularis tension and to facilitate the screw orientation. Use this chance to view the anterior glenoid neck and assure that the surface is flat and ready to accept the CP graft. Additional bony abrasion with a burr can be performed by introducing the burr in the M portal for this task.

Graft Trimming. Move the scope to the J portal. Insert the 15° Coracoid Process Guide (CPG) through the M portal and thread the free CP onto the CPG. Secure it to the CPG by manually screwing the coracoid positioning cannula into the top hat. The freshly harvested graft is mobilized, and all remaining adhesions of the pectoralis minor and the medial fascia are removed. Particular attention must be paid to avoid the musculocutaneous nerve while this is done. The mobile CP usually has a medial spike arising from its base that must be trimmed to permit good bony contact with the glenoid. In order to stabilize the coracoid while the burr is introduced through the D portal, a K-wire is introduced into the Alpha coracoid screw hole, through the subscapularis split and then drilled monocortically into the glenoid bone. This K-wire will insure that the coracoid does not move during its preparation and protect the plexus which is in close proximity. The guide should be placed at 5 o'clock and approximately 7 mm medial to the glenoid. To facilitate trimming, the scope is held by an assistant, and—using a two-handed technique—the graft can be controlled on the cannula with one hand and trimmed with the burr (D-portal) with the other hand. The graft is now ready for transfer and fixation to the glenoid.

21.6.5 Step 5: Coracoid Transfer and Coracoid Fixation

Manipulate the CP on the coracoid positioning cannula to the glenoid neck along the K-wire. This is made easier by elevating the subscapularis split with the switching stick. Pass the graft horizontally through the subscapularis, then turn 90° around the K-wire for its desired position on the glenoid. This position should not be prominent compared to the glenoid surface but flush with the subchondral bone.

To achieve the best position of the graft, a two-step approach will be used. First, the upper part of the graft is positioned flush at the optimal and desired position. Then, a K-wire is passed through the Beta-hole and drilled bicortically to lock the position. The wire will emerge through the skin of the posterior shoulder, at which stage, a clamp is placed on it. A minimum angulation between the K-wires and the glenoid surface should be obtained. *Expert Tip*: Good orientation of the K-wire represents approximately 2–3 cm more medial to the A portal.

In the second step, the first K-wire in the Alpha-hole is unlocked. Now, the lower part of the graft can be manipulated and turned around the upper K-wire into the desired position. The K-wire in the Alpha-hole is then also drilled bicortically and through the posterior skin. The second K-wire should emerge at close proximity to the first K-wire. This wire will also be clamped.

Overdrill the glenoid K-wire with the cannulated glenoid 3.2 drill bicortically from anterior. Remove the drill. If needed, insert the cannulated measurement device from posterior until resistance of the cortex is felt to determine screw lengths. Then, remove cannulated measurement device.

Now fixation with screws is undertaken. As a last step, both screws are passed into each predrilled hole, one screw at a time. The length of the screws was previously determined by the measurement device. The screws are inserted and alternately tightened to reduce the graft using compression onto the glenoid neck. The K-wires can then be removed posteriorly.

Final Checks. The graft and screw position are checked graft through the D and J portals, and any final trimming can be done at this stage with the burr. Any prominence of the graft, thereafter, can be burred flush to the glenoid.

After skin closure, patient is placed in a slight resting abduction pillow.

Postoperative X-rays should control that the graft is properly fixed. Only 3D CT can assess accurately the graft positioning. We usually control patient at 6 weeks and 3 months postoperatively.

21.6.6 Management of Complications

Perioperative complications are essentially coracoid breakage and neurovascular injury. When encountering excessive arthroscopic difficulties (uncontrolled bleeding, excessive swelling, and difficulties for screw positioning), these conditions should lead to an open conversion to perform the best possible Latarjet.

Early postoperative complications are extremely rare, but it is important to control and monitor swelling. Hematomas, though rare, need to be closely watched to detect any sign of possible vascular injury.

Graft nonunion occurs rarely, and this complication has decreased with the use of the top hat washer. The top hat allows greater compression to be applied to the graft.

When compression is accomplished, successful union usually occurs within 6 weeks. Long-term graft resorption, however, has been a more common problem, leading to uncovering of the screw heads anteriorly. This has resulted in pain and tendon impingement in some patients that later resolved with arthroscopic removal of the screws.

Recurrent instability is uncommon but is a difficult problem to manage; however, arthroscopic revision bone grafting with an iliac crest graft (Eden-Hybinette) has resulted in good outcomes with restored stability [13]. During this revision operation, care should be taken due its proximity to the neurovascular structures of the upper limb.

21.7 Rehabilitation and Return-to-Play Considerations

The initial strength of the bone fixation with two screws allows for early rehabilitation. Postoperative immobilization will depend on postoperative pain tolerance. Patients remain in a sling until they feel pain free. The sling can be removed at a maximum of 2 weeks, and free passive and active assisted mobilization is initiated. This management scheme has to be adapted to the profile of the patient and possible additional intraoperative procedures, such as SLAP or posterior Bankart repair.

Rehabilitation should gradually progress from closed to open chain exercises. Open chain exercises should progress from basic rotator cuff training to full throwing capacity, focusing on internal and external rotational strength and explosive capacity. Scapular rehabilitation and kinetic chain exercises are obligatory.

For high-risk (throwing) and collision sports, we recommend that they do not resume these activities before 3 months. For throwers, special attention should be given to the eccentric strength of the external rotators, being the most important decelerator mechanism for the glenohumeral joint during throwing. The Latarjet technique is, thus, beneficial for throwers as early external strength training can be initiated.

21.7.1 Results

During a symposium at the French Arthroscopic Society meeting in December 2015, we analyzed a multicentric study of open and arthroscopic Latarjet performed by the 10 members of the symposium.

We prospectively analyzed and compared complications, clinical and radiological results, positioning, and evolution of the graft by post-operative CT scans on a series of 390 patients. No significant difference was found between open and arthroscopic Latarjet. Both techniques provide excellent and good result with low complication rates. We also evaluated perioperative arthroscopic difficulties and found that the highest difficulties involved visualization, subscapularis split, and screw positioning.

Complication rates in open and arthroscopic Latarjet range from 5% [14] to 30% [15]. In the largest arthroscopic Latarjet series, 1555 patients were evaluated retrospectively and found to have a 4.2% overall complication rate and 0.2% neurologic complication rate [16].

21.7.2 Summary

Anterior shoulder instability is a common problem facing by practicing shoulder surgeons for which the operative treatment options have expanded considerably in the past 20 years. Arthroscopy has led to the improved diagnosis of previously unrecognized soft-tissue lesions underlying many cases of instability. In combination with radiological investigations, arthroscopy has also improved the awareness of bony lesions of both the glenoid and humeral head and their contribution to shoulder instability.

The arthroscopic Latarjet technique is our preferred treatment option, especially for lesions with significant bone loss and for athletes involved in contact sports or throwing. The ability of a surgeon to visualize the shoulder from different angles via various portals is crucial to the outcome of the surgery. We strongly recommend to start by the open technique, and once it becomes reliable, proceed arthroscopically and convert to the open technique if necessary. This allows progressively improving the skills of arthroscopic steps and facing difficulties with reliable solutions.

References

1. Boileau P, Villalba M, Héry JY, Balg F, Ahrens P, Neyton L. Risk factors for recurrence of shoulder instability after arthroscopic bankart repair. J Bone Joint Surg. 2006;88-A(8):1755–63.
2. Walch G, Boileau P, Levigne C, Mandrino A, Neyret P, Donell S. Arthroscopic stabilization for recurrent anterior shoulder dislocation: results of 59 cases. Arthroscopy. 1995;11:173–9.
3. Latarjet M. Treatment of recurrent dislocation of the shoulder. Lyon Chir. 1954;49:994–7.
4. Lafosse L, Lejeune E, et al. The arthroscopic latarjet procedure for the treatment of anterior shoulder instability. Arthroscopy. 2007;23:1242.e1–5.
5. Ravenscroft M, Odak S. Arthroscopic Latarjet: tips for success. Oper Tech Sports Med. 2019;27: 69–76.
6. Itoi E. 'On-track' and 'off track' shoulder lesions. EFORT Open Rev. 2017;2:343–51.
7. Gill T, Micheli L, Gebhard F, et al. Bankart repair for anterior instability of the shoulder. Long-term outcome. J Bone Joint Surg Am. 1997;79(6):850–7.
8. Helfet A. Coracoid transplantation for recurring dislocation of the shoulder. J Bone Joint Surg. 1958;40-B:198–202.
9. Itoi E, Yamamoto N, et al. Stabilizing mechanism in bone grafting of a large glenoid defect. J Bone Joint Surg. 2010;92(1):2059–66.
10. Burkhart S, De Beer J, Tehrany A. Quantifying glenoid bone loss arthroscopically in shoulder instability. Arthroscopy. 2002;18(5):488–91.
11. Burkhart S, De Beer J. Traumatic glenohumeral bone defects and their relationship to failure of arthroscopic Bankart repairs: significance of the inverted-pear glenoid and the humeral engaging Hill-Sachs lesion. Arthroscopy. 2000;88(8):677–94.
12. Bernageau J, Patte D, Debeyre J, et al. Value of the glenoid profile in recurrent luxations of the shoulder. Rev Chir Orthop Reparatrice Appar Mot. 1976;62: 142–7.

13. Lafosse L, Giannakos A, et al. All-Arthroscopic revision Eden-Hybinette procedure for failed instability surgery: technique and preliminary results. Arthroscopy. 2017;33:39–48.
14. Gartsman G, Edwards B, et al. Immediate and early complications of the open Latarjet procedure: a retrospective review of a large consecutive case series. J Shoulder Elbow Surg. 2017;26:68–72.
15. Griesser M, Bishop J, et al. Complications and re-operations after Bristow-Latarjet shoulder stabilization: a systematic review. J Shoulder Elbow Surg. 2013;22(2):286–92.
16. Walch G, Leuzinger J, Nourissat G, Lafosse L, et al. Complications of arthroscopic Latarjet: a multicenter study of 1555 cases. J Shoulder Elbow Surg. 2017;26:e148.

Bony Defects: Glenoid and Humeral Side—On-Track/Off-Track Concept

22

Giuseppe Milano, Giuseppe Frizziero, and Giacomo Marchi

22.1 Introduction

Bone loss is one of the most relevant factors affecting shoulder stability. Effective assessment of the bone loss pattern might be the key to understand the behavior of a large number of shoulder instabilities, to plan the most effective treatment, and to establish the prognosis. A great effort was made to characterize this type of lesions and their influence on the biomechanical behavior of the shoulder.

22.2 The "Glenoid Track" Concept

The "glenoid track" concept was introduced by Yamamoto et al. through a cadaveric study [1]. They began from the intuition, already expressed in other studies [2], that bony lesions of both glenoid and humeral head should be taken into account to asses shoulder instability. The physiological interaction between them at the posterior limit of the range of movement was investigated. The authors simulated the reciprocal movements and determined the track of the glenoid in respect of the articular surface of the humeral head and called it "glenoid track." This is a band on the posterior portion of the humeral head which goes from anteromedial to superolateral. It is drawn by the glenoid during abduction, external rotation, and horizontally flection at the end range of movement [1, 3] (Fig. 22.1).

Omori et al. confirmed the concept of glenoid track through an in vivo study by 3D imaging [4]. The width of the glenoid track is defined as the distance from the medial margin of the glenoid track to the medial margin of the footprint of the rotator cuff. It is expressed as a percentage of the width of the undamaged glenoid [1, 3]. The measure of the width of the track was 83% ± 12% of the glenoid width at 90° of abduction [4]. It increases with lower grade of abduction of the arm and decreases with a higher extent of abduction [4]. It is narrower if a glenoid bone defect is present [5] (Fig. 22.2).

22.3 Glenoid Bone Defects

Glenoid defects can affect shoulder instability in two ways. One concerns its behavior related to humeral head lesions. The other is directly related to the lack of support to the humeral movements

G. Milano (✉)
Department of Medical and Surgical Specialties, Radiological Sciences, and Public Health, University of Brescia, Brescia, Italy

Department of Bone and Joint Surgery, Spedali Civili, Brescia, Italy

G. Frizziero
Department of Medical and Surgical Specialties, Radiological Sciences, and Public Health, University of Brescia, Brescia, Italy

G. Marchi
Department of Bone and Joint Surgery, Spedali Civili, Brescia, Italy

R. Brzóska et al. (eds.), *360° Around Shoulder Instability*,
https://doi.org/10.1007/978-3-662-61074-9_22

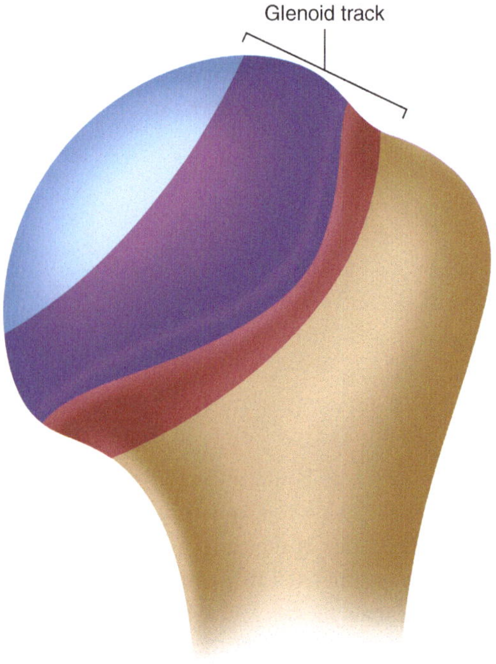

Fig. 22.1 The "glenoid track" is a band on the posterior portion of the humeral head, which goes from anteromedial to superolateral. It is drawn by the glenoid during abduction, external rotation, and horizontally flection at the end range of movement [1]

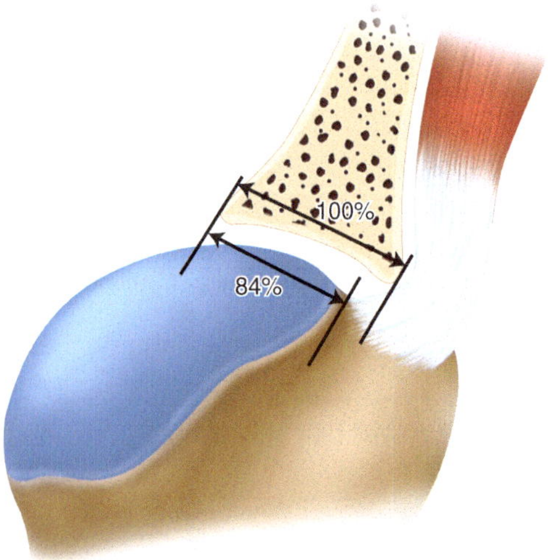

Fig. 22.2 The width of the glenoid track is about 83% of the healthy glenoid width at 90° of abduction [4]

and overload on the glenoid remnants and soft tissues.

The prevalence of glenoid bony defect ranges between 66 and 90% in anterior shoulder instability [2, 6–13], and it has been identified as a relevant risk factor for failure of soft-tissue repair procedures [14–16].

It has been studied that a lesion of 30% of the width of inferior glenoid causes a slight loss of contact area and increases the contact pressure by two times on the entire glenoid surface and by three to four times on the anteroinferior quadrant. When a Bankart repair is performed in the presence of a critical glenoid bone loss, the pressure expresses its action on soft tissues, leading to failure of the procedure [17].

Analyzing another mechanical condition, when the arm is in the mid-range of movement, the capsuloligamentous structures are lax and have no role in stabilizing the shoulder. The negative intraarticular pressure and the concavity effect created by muscle action on the glenoid are mainly active factors. In this situation, the lack of a significative portion of the glenoid and the space left by lax ligaments lead to the loss of concavity effect, thus producing mid-range instability [3].

A reduction of the glenoid width is expressed in a narrower glenoid track. In this condition, a Hill–Sachs lesion is more likely to engage the glenoid rim leading to instability [5]. The influence of a reduction of the glenoid width on the glenoid track and its relationship with the humeral head's lesions will be analyzed in detail in the main section of the chapter.

22.3.1 Pathomechanics of Glenoid Bone Defects

We can distinguish glenoid lesions in two types: fragmented type and erosion type. Fragmented type is more frequent [6, 13], but the fragment tends to be reabsorbed partially or totally in the first year after the traumatic event [13] (Fig. 22.3).

Where a traumatic event brings to an anteroinferior dislocation of the humeral head in respect of the trunk, the location of the lesion is found to

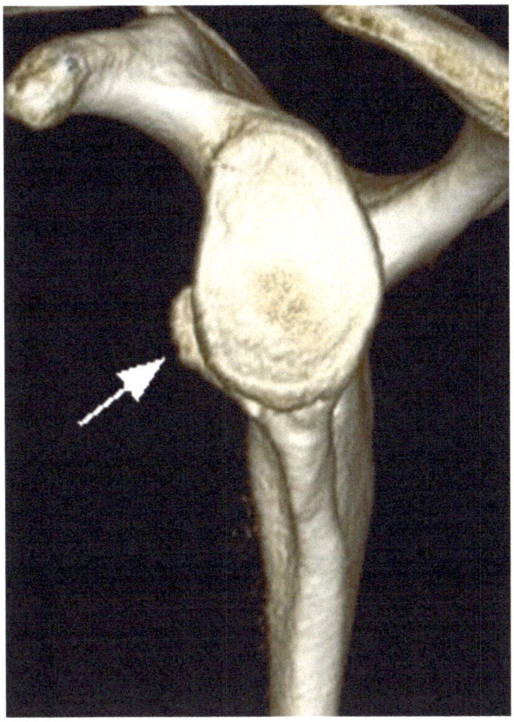

Fig. 22.3 Fragmented-type glenoid defect (arrow). The fragment tends to be partially or totally reabsorbed in the first year after the traumatic event

be anterior in respect of inferior glenoid (mean 3:01 on the "clock face" of a right shoulder) [18].

Yamamoto et al., in two biomechanical quantitative studies, evaluated the size of a glenoid bony lesion which causes measurable instability of the shoulder. They created four bony defects on cadaver shoulders on the anterior side of the glenoid with different width (2, 4, 6, and 8 mm). They found a critical value of 6 mm of the width of the lesion, which corresponds to 25% of the glenoid width [19, 20] and 20% of the best-fit circle area utilizing the ratio method of measurement [21]. These studies left a thin gray zone between 6-mm and 4-mm lesion size (25% and 17.5% of glenoid width) in which the lesion may or may not be critical [3]. Later, Shaha et al. found different values in an in vivo study [11]. They found a high recurrence of dislocation after Bankart repair if the bone loss was more than 20% in an active population. They found that with values between 13.5% and 20%, patients did not sustain recurrent instability but demonstrated decreasing in WOSI score. This range was named "subcritical" bone loss [11], and 13.5% was confirmed as a cutoff value for the successfulness of Bankart procedure in an active population by Dickens et al. [22].

22.3.2 Measurement Methods of Glenoid Bone Defects

It is highly relevant to assess the exact amount and features of glenoid bone loss. X-ray imaging has been reported to be adequate to detect bone loss, but insufficient to measure it [23, 24], consequently, many methods have been developed using computed tomography (CT) and magnetic resonance (MR).

To characterize glenoid bone loss by CT scans, it is necessary to obtain an "en face" view of the damaged glenoid and compare it to an estimate of the native bone. The "en face" view is orthogonal to the glenoid articular surface. The estimation of the native glenoid can be made by two methods: best-fit circle method and comparison with contralateral shoulder.

The lower part of the glenoid resembles a circle. This circle can be drawn along the posterior–inferior margin of the glenoid, thus estimating the anterior margin which is lacking [6].

The two glenoids have been reported to be highly similar in the same subject. The difference in width, length, and area of contralateral glenoid has been reported to be less than 1% [25]. This gives an adequate term of comparison. This method cannot be used if there is a bilateral instability or other alterations of the contralateral glenoid (Fig. 22.4).

According to data obtained with these two methods, a linear or an area method to measure bone loss can be used.

Linear measurements include the following:

- Width-to-length (*W*/*L*) ratio calculated on 2D CT-scan reconstruction: The width is defined as the distance between the anterior and posterior margin of the glenoid at its wider portion. The length is defined as the

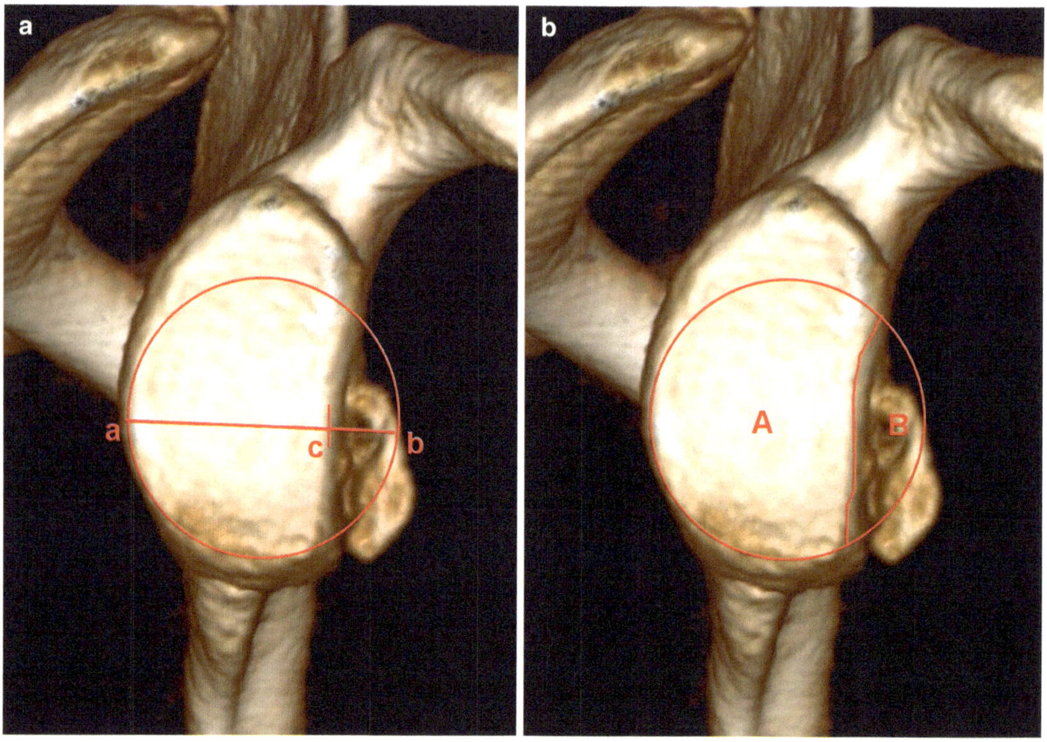

Fig. 22.4 Glenoid defect can be measured as width (**a**) or area (**b**) as difference or percentage of the healthy glenoid. The estimation of the native glenoid can be made by two methods: best-fit circle method and comparison with contralateral shoulder (**A**: area of the residual glenoid; **B**: area of the glenoid defect; **ab**: width of the residual glenoid; **bc**: width of the glenoid defect; **ac**: width of the native glenoid)

distance between the tip and the bottom of it. The referential value has been reported to be 0.7 [26].

- Glenoid index: This is the ratio of the width of the injured glenoid to the width of the uninjured one at their wider part calculated on 3D CT-scan reconstruction [27].
- Ratio method (diameter): This is the ratio of the width of the bone defect to the diameter of the best-fit circle [6, 21, 28].
- AP distance from bare area method using 3D CT scan: This calculates the percentage of bone loss. The width of the bone defect is divided by the diameter of the best-fit circle multiplied by 100 [29]. It is very similar to the former method. This method is derived from the "arthroscopic bare spot method," which is based on the founding that the bare spot area should correspond to the center of the best-fit circle, allowing the use of this formula arthroscopically [30]. Later was reported that bare spot area is not always reliable as an arthroscopic landmark [31–33] and arthroscopic measurements overestimate bone loss compared with CT [34, 35].

Area measurements include the following:

- Circle or ratio method (area): The ratio of the area of the estimated fragment to the area of the best-fit circle is calculated on 3D CT-scan reconstructions [6]. This was calculated also by the use of 2D TC-scan reconstructions [21].
- Ratio method (area) by mathematical calculation: Barchilon et al. proposed a method to estimate the area of defects by mathematical calculation. They used the ratio of the depth of injured glenoid to the radius of the best-fit circle calculated on 3D CT-scan reconstructions. The depth is defined as the line between

the center of the circle and the injured margin of the glenoid. Given these data, an estimate of the defect area can be obtained and compared to the area of the best-fit circle, by mathematical calculation [21].

- Pico method: This is based on 2D CT-scan reconstructions and gives a percentage measurement of the bone loss using the following formula: surface D/surface A × 100, where "surface D" is defined as the area of the defect directly measured as the missing bony substance in the best-fit circle and "surface A" is defined as the area of the circle in the uninjured glenoid [36]. The reliability of this method has been reported to be very high [37].

It is important to distinguish between methods that use the 3D volume-rendered technique (VRT) or the 2D multiplanar reformation (MPR). In the former, the measurements are expressed in pixels, and this allows us to calculate bone loss only as a percentage of the uninjured glenoid, so it necessary to use sophisticated software or mathematical calculations to obtain real measurements. On the contrary, MPR allows measuring directly the real size of the defect [24]. The agreement between measurements by use of the two different methods was found to be very high [38].

Similar methods can be adopted using MR instrumentation. 2D MR Pico method [39], 3D MR circle method [40–42], 3D MR anteroposterior distance from bare area method [41, 43], and 3D MR-arthrography (MRA) (fat-suppressing sequences) AP distance from bare area method [44] were tested and found to be promising alternatives to CT scan. Indeed, the use of MR has the advantage to avoid radiation exposure to the patient and to evaluate soft-tissue damage, but its use in place of CT is controversial. Many studies compared inter- and intraobserver reliability of the two methods. Some authors reported high correlation between them [39–44], albeit others found CT to be more accurate and reliable [45–47].

Recently, some controversies have been reported in glenoid bone loss measurement. Lacheta et al. reported inconsistency of 3D-CT ratio method to assess glenoid bone loss, due to poor reproducibility of estimation of the best-fit circle, which is the basis of many measurement methods. Differences have been found in the estimation of the size of the circumference of the circle and the rotational alignment of the diameter measured, thus causing a significant variation in measurements [28]. Moroder et al. reported that the impreciseness of scapula positioning for the creation of an "en face" view significantly alters glenoid defect size measurement [48].

22.4 Humeral Head Bone Defects

The humeral bone defect in anterior shoulder instability is mainly represented by the Hill–Sachs (HS) lesion, defined as a groove onto the articular surface of the humeral head caused by the impaction of the anterior ridge of glenoid on the posterosuperior humeral head during anterior glenohumeral dislocation [49]. This lesion has been reported to have a high prevalence in anterior shoulder instability [50–53], even higher if recurrent instability is considered [2, 53, 54].

22.4.1 Pathomechanics and Assessment of Humeral Head Bone Defects

Burkhart and De Beer defined a significant humeral head bone defect as an "engaging" Hill–Sachs lesion. This was a bone defect that one could arthroscopically observe to engage the glenoid rim [2]. The need to define eligibility criteria for arthroscopic surgery has brought to the search of a "critical size" of the Hill–Sachs lesion. Many clinical [55–57] and biomechanical [58, 59] studies reported different results by different methods of quantification. Nowadays, there are neither an agreement on definition of critical size nor an universally accepted method to quantify the lesion [60]. Most clinical studies focused on clinical outcome of surgical procedures for anterior shoulder instability in the presence of a Hill–Sachs lesion did not report the lesion size [60].

Cho et al. proposed a method by use of linear measurements (length, width, and depth)

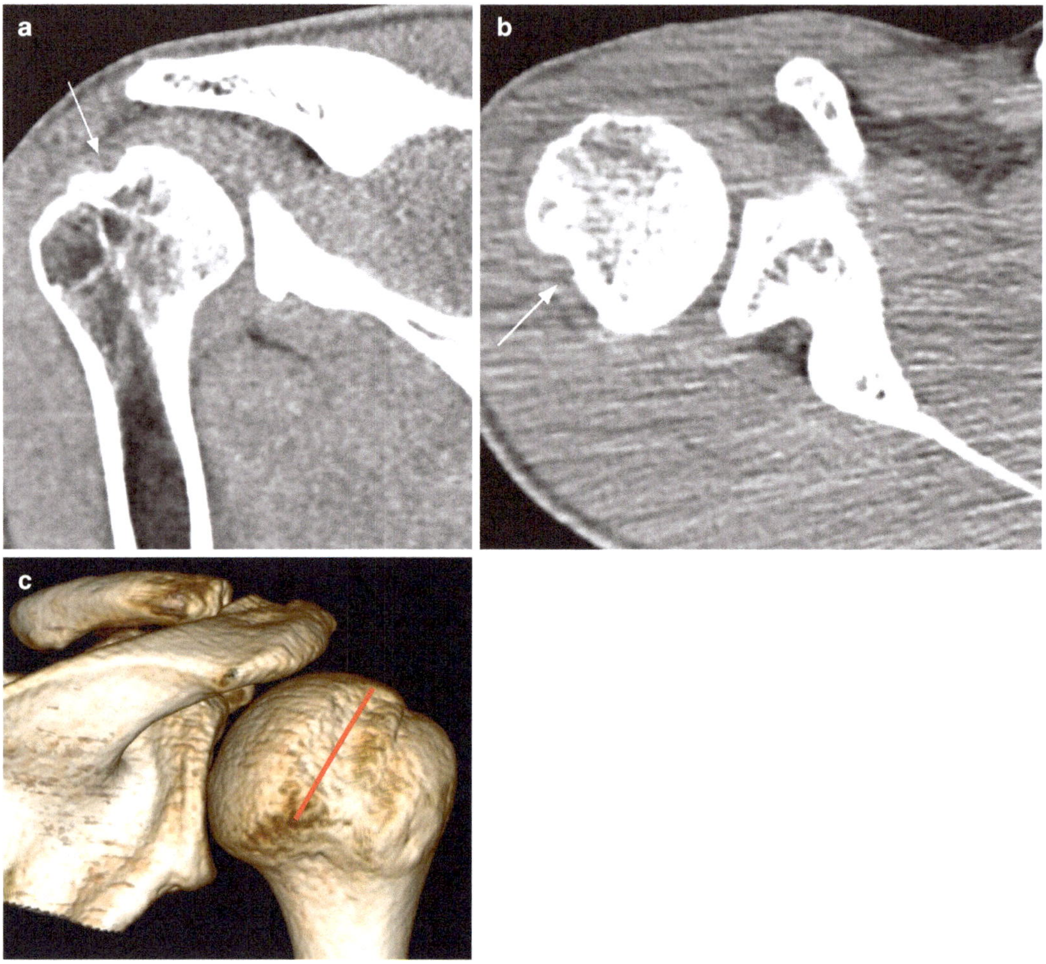

Fig. 22.5 CT scans of a right shoulder with a Hill–Sachs lesion (arrow). Linear measurements (length, width, and depth) are measured on standard 2D CT scans (**a**, **b**). Measurement of lesion orientation can be achieved on 3D CT scans (red line) (**c**)

in standard 2D CT scans (coronal, sagittal, and transverse) and measurement of lesion orientation on 3D CT scans (posterior view) [61] (Fig. 22.5).

Schneider et al. analyzed the accuracy of 3D CT reconstructions as a method to determine the size of a Hill–Sachs lesion and its position with respect to the glenoid track. They used a method based on orthogonal 3D CT reconstructions (posterior, superior, and lateral) of humeral head. They found a high variability in the measurement of the Hill–Sachs lesion. It was mostly due to the insufficient resolution of the image and the interference of soft tissues at the rotator cuff footprint [62].

Ozaki et al. proposed a method to measure the size of Hill–Sachs lesion by 3D and 2D CT scans. They measured the length and width of the lesion on an "en face" view of the 3D CT scan and its depth on 2D axial images perpendicular to the long axis of the humeral shaft [63]. This method is relatively simple and clinically useful [63]. Area or volume could be more accurate and comparable measures, but the need for sophisticated not easily available software to calculate them limits their usefulness [63]. This method has shown to have good interrater reliability [64] and has been recommended to be used in combination with the on-/off-track method for reporting measurements [60].

It was noted that the orientation of the Hill–Sachs lesion could interfere with its capability to engage the glenoid rim. Cho et al. measured it by the "Hill–Sachs angle" on 3D CT posterior scans, which was the angle between the long axis of the lesion and the axis of the humerus. They found that lesions with higher values of angle tend to be engaging [61]. Di Giacomo et al. compared the Hill–Sachs angle to the position of the arm at the time of the first dislocation. They found that shoulder that dislocated in abduction had higher angle values than shoulder that dislocated in adduction. They speculated that a lesion more parallel to the glenoid rim in an abducted and external rotation position has more chance to be engaging in that position [65].

In conclusion, it is difficult to determine a critical size of Hill–Sachs lesion: its tendency to contribute to shoulder instability has to be related to other factors, in particular to the glenoid bone loss [23, 66, 67].

22.5 Bipolar Bone Defects

The prevalence of bipolar lesions (a glenoid defect combined with a Hill–Sachs lesion) was reported to be 33.3% in shoulders with primary anterior instability and 61.8% in shoulders with recurrent anterior instability [68].

In shoulders with traumatic anterior instability, bipolar lesions were found in approximately 60% of shoulders, while monopolar lesions (an isolated glenoid defect or isolated Hill–Sachs lesion) accounted for almost 30% and were not uncommon lesions [53, 68]. Recently, a glenoid defect was found in 34%, and Hill–Sachs lesion was found in 66% of the studied shoulder at primary anterior shoulder dislocation. An isolated glenoid defect was rare and was associated with a humeral head defect in most cases. Hill–Sachs lesions were also present alone. Most recurrent cases in the same series presented bipolar bone loss, as the frequency of glenoid defect increased. It was so demonstrated that Hill–Sachs lesion occurred first followed by a glenoid defect, resulting in a bipolar bone loss [53].

It was noted that, as the glenoid defect became larger, the Hill–Sachs lesion increased in size, but there was no significant correlation between the size of the two lesions [68]. More recently, it was reported that Hill–Sachs lesions were more frequent and larger as the frequency of recurrence increased [53]. Risk factors for presence of bipolar lesions are recurrent instability [68], repetitive dislocation/subluxation [68, 69], collision/contact sports [68], and adolescence [69]. A high rate of postoperative recurrence of instability after arthroscopic Bankart repair has been reported in shoulders with bipolar lesions [2, 68]. The rate was high even with small lesions [68]. The findings support the use of bipolar assessment of shoulder dislocations [69].

Biomechanical studies have demonstrated that combined glenoid and humeral head defects have an additive and negative effect on glenohumeral stability. Arciero et al. reported that as little as a 2-mm glenoid defect with a medium-sized Hill–Sachs lesion demonstrated a compromise in soft-tissue Bankart repair, while a small-sized Hill–Sachs lesion showed compromise of soft-tissue repair with 4 mm or more glenoid bone loss. Which means that arthroscopic stabilization may be not effective and may require additional surgical strategies [70]. Gottshalk et al. reported that Bankart procedure may be not effective and bony reconstruction is indicated for humeral head defects as small as 19% of the humeral head diameter and glenoid defects as small as 10% of the glenoid width [71]. For combined defects with a humeral head bone loss greater than 31% of the diameter and 20% of glenoid width defect, coracoid transfer was found to give insufficient gain in the translation distance [72].

On identifying bipolar bone defect as a combination of lesions interacting with each other, Burkhart and De Beer introduced the concept of "significant bone loss." They defined a significant glenoid bone defect as the one that makes glenoid appear as an "inverted pear" in arthroscopy when viewed from a superior-to-inferior perspective. On the humeral side, they defined a significant bone defect to be an "engaging"

Hill–Sachs lesion, oriented in such a way that it engaged the anterior glenoid in a position of athletic function (90° of abduction combined with external rotation of approximately 90°). They found that the instabilities associated with "engaging-type" Hill–Sachs lesions were at high risk of recurrence if treated with the classic arthroscopic capsuloligamentous repair [2]. They proposed a direct visualization of the engaging mechanism by dynamic arthroscopic assessment. Arthroscopy, however, has some disadvantages. If shoulder is tested before soft-tissue repair, the test would be overestimated [5, 12]. It has been observed that a large number of lesions become "nonengaging" after Bankart repair [12]. Kurokawa et al. defined the "true engaging Hill–Sachs lesion" as either a lesion that engages after Bankart repair or a lesion that extends over the glenoid track and reported only 7.4% of true engaging lesions following this definition [12]. On the other assessing shoulder stability after Bankart repair could compromise the repair itself [5].

22.6 The "On-Track/Off-Track" Concept

Di Giacomo et al. developed a method that uses the concept of the glenoid track to determine whether a Hill–Sachs lesion will engage the anterior glenoid rim, including the influence of associated glenoid bone loss and the role of the location of the Hill–Sachs lesion with respect to the glenoid track itself [5].

The width of the glenoid track decreases if there is a glenoid bone defect. To calculate the width of the glenoid track in a patient with glenoid bone loss, the width of the defect should be subtracted from 83% of the glenoid width, which is the width of the glenoid track when there is not a glenoid defect. If the medial margin of a Hill–Sachs lesion is within the glenoid track, there is bone support adjacent to the Hill–Sachs lesion and the Hill–Sachs lesion is "on-track"; if the medial margin of the Hill–Sachs lesion is more medial than the glenoid track, there is no bone support and the Hill–Sachs lesion is "off-track" [5].

22.6.1 Assessment of On-/Off-Track Hill–Sachs Lesions

Di Giacomo et al. proposed a CT-based method to asses an on-/off-track Hill–Sachs lesion. They used the 83% value as the mean glenoid track width. With a single CT examination, data of both shoulders are recorded. The bilateral "en face" view of the glenoid is obtained. The first step is to assess the size of the glenoid bony defect. The greatest horizontal distance of the glenoid width on both shoulders is measured. Using the intact glenoid width (D) as a reference, calculate the defect size (d) as follows: d = intact glenoid width − injured glenoid width. Next, using the posterior view of the humeral head, the medial margin of the footprint of the rotator cuff and the Hill–Sachs lesion are identified. Then, a line located at a distance equivalent to 83% of the glenoid width from the medial margin of the rotator cuff footprint is drawn. If there is no bony defect of the glenoid, this line represents the medial margin of the glenoid track. If there is a bony defect of the glenoid (d), the distance d is subtracted from the 83% line to obtain the medial margin of the true glenoid track [5].

Following this method, the position of the Hill–Sachs lesion can be assessed graphically. If it is located within the glenoid track, it is called an "on-track" Hill–Sachs lesion. If it extends more medially over the medial margin of the glenoid track, it is called an "off-track" Hill–Sachs lesion [5].

On-/off-track location can be also calculated comparing two linear values which are the true width of the glenoid track (GT) and the Hill–Sachs interval (HSI). An intact bone bridge (BB) is typically observed between the rotator cuff attachments and the lateral margin of the Hill–Sachs lesion. This bone bridge width plus the width of the Hill–Sachs lesion equals what Di Giacomo et al. call the Hill–Sachs interval (HSI). If it is longer than GT, the lesion is off-track [5] (Table 22.1) (Fig. 22.6).

22.6.2 Accuracy of the Method

Validating the on-/off-track concept, Locher et al. reported that the recurrence rate after the Bankart repair was 6% of those with an on-track Hill–Sachs lesion and 33% of those with an off-track lesion. The odds ratio of recurrence of instability for the shoulder with off-track lesion was 8.3 (95% CI, 1.85–37.26) [73].

Table 22.1 How to determine whether Hill–Sachs lesion is "on-track" or "off-track" [5]

1. Measure the diameter (*D*) of the inferior glenoid, either by arthroscopy or from 3D CT scan
2. Determine the width of the anterior glenoid bone loss (*d*)
3. Calculate the width of the glenoid track (GT) by the following formula: GT = 0.83 *D* − *d*
4. Calculate the width of the HSI, which is the width of the Hill–Sachs lesion (HS) plus the width of the bone bridge (BB) between the rotator cuff attachments and the lateral aspect of the Hill–Sachs lesion: HSI = HS + BB
5. If HSI > GT, the HS is off-track or engaging. If HSI < GT, the HS is on-track or nonengaging

Shaha et al. through another study reported that the recurrence rate was 8% of on-track patients and 75% of off-track patients. The positive predictive value of 75% using the on-/off-track concept was significantly higher than using glenoid bone loss size (exceeding 20%). They concluded that the application of the glenoid track concept was superior to using glenoid bone loss alone [74].

Mook et al. used the on-/off-track concept to analyze surgical procedure outcomes. They reported that patients with an off-track lesion after the Latarjet procedure were four times more likely to experience postoperative instability than those with a postoperative on-track lesion [75].

22.6.3 Imaging Techniques

The CT is recognized, with limitations, as the most reliable method to assess shoulder bony defects on the glenoid side [45–47, 76] and the humeral side [60, 63]. Still, Schneider et al.

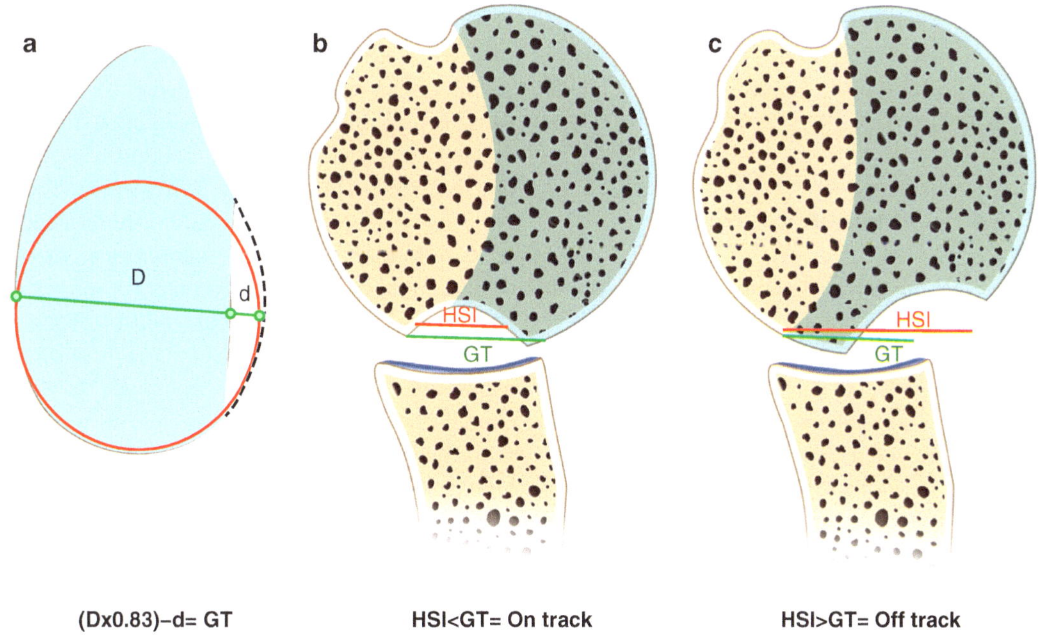

Fig. 22.6 (**a**) The glenoid track (GT) in an injured glenoid corresponds to the difference between the glenoid track of the healthy glenoid (83% of the glenoid width, *D*) and the width of the missing glenoid (*d*). The Hill–Sachs interval (HSI) is the distance from the medial margin of the footprint to the medial margin of the Hill–Sachs lesion. If HSI<GT, the lesion is "on-track" (**b**). If HIS>GT, the lesion is "off-track" (**c**)

reported limited reliability for the on-/off-track method, with an interobserver concordance of 71.8% and intraobserver concordance from 80.3% to 90.1%. While they found good reliability for glenoid defect measurement, the assessment of Hill–Sachs lesions presented a high variability, affecting the evaluation with on-/off-track method [62]. Gowd et al., by a revision of literature, recommended the use of a combination of Ozaki et al. [63] and Di Giacomo et al.'s [5] techniques to measure bipolar bone loss and assess the engagement and risk of instability, reporting good interrater reliability [60].

Applying the on-/off-track method on MR images, Gyftopoulos et al. calculated accuracy of 84.2% with a positive predictive value of 65.0% and a negative predictive value of 91.1% in their study. They concluded that the on-/off-track method can be used on MR imaging to accurately assess the bipolar bone and for predicting the presence of off-track lesions. They found that 2D MR images to be accurate without 3D reconstructions. MR facilitates the evaluation of the associated soft-tissue injuries and the location of the footprint, better estimating the HSI. Moreover, MR spares the patient from radiation exposure [77]. However, insertion of the infraspinatus remains difficult to evaluate for its oblique orientation.

22.6.4 Treatment Algorithms

Using the on-/off-track concept, Di Giacomo et al. proposed an algorithm for the treatment of shoulder instability with bipolar bone loss, as reported in Table 22.2 [5]. Maybe, these cutoff values have to be lowered [11, 60]. As mentioned before, Shaha et al. reported a clinically significant decrease in the WOSI score in the shoulder with a glenoid bone loss above 13.5% and judged it an unacceptable outcome in an active population [11]. Gowd et al. suggested that the threshold for a surgeon to perform a bone block procedure has to be lowered in the presence of a Hill–Sachs lesion [60].

22.6.5 Evaluating Bipolar Bone Defects by Size

Nakagawa et al. proposed a scoring system for bipolar bone loss based on the combined size of lesions [78]. They classified the size of both the glenoid defect and the Hill–Sachs lesion into five categories separately. The score ranges from 0 to 4, where 0 corresponds to the absence of lesions and 4 to a very large lesion. They used the cutoffs described in a previous study [68]. Subsequently, they summed the two scores to obtain a total score of the bipolar lesion and classified it in five classes: class 1 (0–1 point), 2 (2 points), 3 (3 points), 4 (4 points), and 5 (5 or >5 points). The main objective was to correlate the score to the recurrence of instability after Bankart repair. They found a progressive increasing of recurrence from class 3 to class 5, suggesting that Bankart repair for class-3 lesions and higher cannot guarantee stability, thus alternatives techniques have to be used [78]. Their results were consistent with other previous studies based on the combined evaluation of bipolar lesions size [70, 79–81]. They compared this scoring system to the on-/off-track method. In their series, they found no significant difference between the recurrence of on-track lesions and off-track lesions. Most off-track lesions were classified as class 5 and were often responsible for postoperative recurrence, but frequently the presence of on-track lesions was not protective. Indeed, their series was composed of high demanding athletes and recurrence was seen to be consistent also with the type of sport played.

Table 22.2 Treatment algorithm based on the assessment of bipolar bone loss and on-/off-track concepts [5]

Glenoid defect	Hill–Sachs lesion	Treatment
<25% of width	Small (on-track)	Arthroscopic Bankart repair
<25% of width	Medium (off-track)	Arthroscopic Bankart repair + remplissage
≥25% of width	Small (on-track)	Latarjet procedure/bone augmentation
≥25% of width	Medium/large (off-track)	Latarjet procedure + remplissage/HH bone graft

It was found a higher recurrence in athletes playing rugby and American football with lower bipolar lesions classes [78]. For these reasons, the authors suggested that such a method could be more predictive of recurrence in athletes than on-/off-track method.

References

1. Yamamoto N, Itoi E, Abe H, et al. Contact between the glenoid and the humeral head in abduction, external rotation, and horizontal extension: a new concept of glenoid track. J Shoulder Elbow Surg. 2007;16(5):649–56. https://doi.org/10.1016/j.jse.2006.12.012.
2. Burkhart SS, De Beer JF. Traumatic glenohumeral bone defects and their relationship to failure of arthroscopic Bankart repairs: significance of the inverted-pear glenoid and the humeral engaging Hill-Sachs lesion. Arthroscopy. 2000;16(7):677–94. https://doi.org/10.1053/jars.2000.17715.
3. Itoi E. 'On-track' and 'off-track' shoulder lesions. EFORT Open Rev. 2017;2(8):343–51. https://doi.org/10.1302/2058-5241.2.170007.
4. Omori Y, Yamamoto N, Koishi H, et al. Measurement of the glenoid track in vivo as investigated by 3-dimensional motion analysis using open MRI. Am J Sports Med. 2014;42(6):1290–5. https://doi.org/10.1177/0363546514527406.
5. Di Giacomo G, Itoi E, Burkhart SS. Evolving concept of bipolar bone loss and the Hill-Sachs lesion: from "engaging/non-engaging" lesion to "on-track/off-track" lesion. Arthroscopy. 2014;30(1):90–8. https://doi.org/10.1016/j.arthro.2013.10.004.
6. Sugaya H, Moriishi J, Dohi M, Kon Y, Tsuchiya A. Glenoid rim morphology in recurrent anterior glenohumeral instability. J Bone Jt Surg Am. 2003;85(5):878–84. https://doi.org/10.2106/00004623-200305000-00016.
7. Edwards TB, Boulahia A, Walch G. Radiographic analysis of bone defects in chronic anterior shoulder instability. Arthroscopy. 2003;19(7):732–9. https://doi.org/10.1016/S0749-8063(03)00684-4.
8. Griffith JF, Antonio GE, Yung PSH, et al. Prevalence, pattern, and spectrum of glenoid bone loss in anterior shoulder dislocation: CT analysis of 218 patients. Am J Roentgenol. 2008;190(5):1247–54. https://doi.org/10.2214/AJR.07.3009.
9. Boileau P, Villalba M, Héry JY, Balg F, Ahrens P, Neyton L. Risk factors for recurrence of shoulder instability after arthroscopic Bankart repair. J Bone Jt Surg Ser A. 2006;88(8):1755–63. https://doi.org/10.2106/JBJS.E.00817.
10. Milano G, Grasso A, Russo A, et al. Analysis of risk factors for glenoid bone defect in anterior shoulder instability. Am J Sports Med. 2011;39(9):1870–6. https://doi.org/10.1177/0363546511411699.
11. Shaha JS, Cook JB, Song DJ, et al. Redefining "critical" bone loss in shoulder instability. Am J Sports Med. 2015;43(7):1719–25. https://doi.org/10.1177/0363546515578250.
12. Kurokawa D, Yamamoto N, Nagamoto H, et al. The prevalence of a large Hill-Sachs lesion that needs to be treated. J Shoulder Elbow Surg. 2013;22(9):1285–9. https://doi.org/10.1016/j.jse.2012.12.033.
13. Nakagawa S, Mizuno N, Hiramatsu K, Tachibana Y, Mae T. Absorption of the bone fragment in shoulders with bony Bankart lesions caused by recurrent anterior dislocations or subluxations: when does it occur? Am J Sports Med. 2013;41(6):1380–6. https://doi.org/10.1177/0363546513483087.
14. Porcellini G, Campi F, Pegreffi F, Castagna A, Paladini P. Predisposing factors for recurrent shoulder dislocation after arthroscopic treatment. J Bone Jt Surg Ser A. 2009;91(11):2537–42. https://doi.org/10.2106/JBJS.H.01126.
15. Flinkkilä T, Hyvönen P, Ohtonen P, Leppilahti J. Arthroscopic Bankart repair: results and risk factors of recurrence of instability. Knee Surg Sport Traumatol Arthrosc. 2010;18(12):1752–8. https://doi.org/10.1007/s00167-010-1105-5.
16. Olds M, Ellis R, Donaldson K, Parmar P, Kersten P. Risk factors which predispose first-time traumatic anterior shoulder dislocations to recurrent instability in adults: a systematic review and meta-analysis. Br J Sports Med. 2015;49(14):913–22. https://doi.org/10.1136/bjsports-2014-094342.
17. Greis PE, Scuderi MG, Mohr A, Bachus KN, Burks RT. Glenohumeral articular contact areas and pressures following labral and osseous injury to the anteroinferior quadrant of the glenoid. J Shoulder Elbow Surg. 2002;11(5):442–51. https://doi.org/10.1067/mse.2002.124526.
18. Saito H, Itoi E, Sugaya H, Minagawa H, Yamamoto N, Tuoheti Y. Location of the glenoid defect in shoulders with recurrent anterior dislocation. Am J Sports Med. 2005;33(6):889–93. https://doi.org/10.1177/0363546504271521.
19. Yamamoto N, Itoi E, Abe H, et al. Effect of an anterior glenoid defect on anterior shoulder stability: a cadaveric study. Am J Sports Med. 2009;37(5):949–54. https://doi.org/10.1177/0363546508330139.
20. Yamamoto N, Muraki T, Sperling JW, et al. Stabilizing mechanism in bone-grafting of a large glenoid defect. J Bone Jt Surg Ser A. 2010;92(11):2059–66. https://doi.org/10.2106/JBJS.I.00261.
21. Barchilon VS, Kotz E, Barchilon Ben-Av M, Glazer E, Nyska M. A simple method for quantitative evaluation of the missing area of the anterior glenoid in anterior instability of the glenohumeral joint. Skeletal Radiol. 2008;37(8):731–6. https://doi.org/10.1007/s00256-008-0506-8.
22. Dickens JF, Owens BD, Cameron KL, et al. The effect of subcritical bone loss and exposure on recurrent instability after arthroscopic Bankart repair in Intercollegiate American Football. Am J Sports Med. 2017;45(8):1769–75. https://doi.org/10.1177/0363546517704184.

23. Itoi E, Nobuyuk Y, Taku H, Jun K. Overview of evaluation and management of the unstable shoulder with and without bone loss: definition, measurement, and guidelines on treatment. In: Imhoff AB, Savoie III FH, editors. Shoulder instability across the life span. Berlin: Springer; 2017. p. 83–91. https://doi.org/10.1007/978-3-662-54077-0_11.
24. Baudi P, Righi P, Rossi Urtoler E, Milano G. Shoulder instability: glenoid and humeral-head bone defect. In: Di Giacomo G, Costantini A, De Vita A, de Gasperis N, editors. Shoulder instability. Berlin: Springer; 2011. p. 19–33.
25. Shi L, Griffith JF, Huang J, Wang D. Excellent side-to-side symmetry in glenoid size and shape. Skeletal Radiol. 2013;42(12):1711–5. https://doi.org/10.1007/s00256-013-1728-y.
26. Griffith JF, Antonio GE, Tong CWC, Ming CK. Anterior shoulder dislocation: quantification of glenoid bone loss with CT. Am J Roentgenol. 2003;180(5):1423–30. https://doi.org/10.2214/ajr.180.5.1801423.
27. Chuang TY, Adams CR, Burkhart SS. Use of preoperative three-dimensional computed tomography to quantify glenoid bone loss in shoulder instability. Arthroscopy. 2008;24(4):376–82. https://doi.org/10.1016/j.arthro.2007.10.008.
28. Lacheta L, Herbst E, Voss A, et al. Insufficient consensus regarding circle size and bone loss width using the ratio—"best fit circle"—method even with three-dimensional computed tomography. Knee Surg Sport Traumatol Arthrosc. 2019;27(10):3222–9. https://doi.org/10.1007/s00167-019-05391-9.
29. Sugaya H, Moriishi J, Kanisawa I, Tsuchiya A. Arthroscopic osseous Bankart repair for chronic recurrent traumatic anterior glenohumeral instability. Surgical technique. J Bone Joint Surg Am. 2005;88(Suppl 1):159–69. https://doi.org/10.2106/JBJS.F.00319.
30. Burkhart SS, DeBeer JF, Tehrany AM, Parten PM. Quantifying glenoid bone loss arthroscopically in shoulder instability. Arthroscopy. 2002;18(5):488–91. https://doi.org/10.1053/jars.2002.32212.
31. Aigner F, Longato S, Fritsch H, Kralinger F. Anatomical considerations regarding the "bare spot" of the glenoid cavity. Surg Radiol Anat. 2004;26(4):308–11. https://doi.org/10.1007/s00276-003-0217-8.
32. Kralinger F, Aigner F, Longato S, Rieger M, Wambacher M. Is the bare spot a consistent landmark for shoulder arthroscopy? A study of 20 embalmed glenoids with 3-dimensional computed tomographic reconstruction. Arthroscopy. 2006;22(4):428–32. https://doi.org/10.1016/j.arthro.2005.12.006.
33. Barcia AM, Rowles DJ, Bottoni CR, Dekker TJ, Tokish JM. Glenoid bare area: arthroscopic characterization and its implications on measurement of bone loss. Arthroscopy. 2013;29(10):1671–5. https://doi.org/10.1016/j.arthro.2013.06.019.
34. Provencher MT, Detterline AJ, Ghodadra N, et al. Measurement of glenoid bone loss: a comparison of measurement error between 45° and 0° bone loss models and with different posterior arthroscopy portal locations. Am J Sports Med. 2008;36(6):1132–8. https://doi.org/10.1177/0363546508316041.
35. Bakshi NK, Patel I, Jacobson JA, Debski RE, Sekiya JK. Comparison of 3-dimensional computed tomography-based measurement of glenoid bone loss with arthroscopic defect size estimation in patients with anterior shoulder instability. Arthroscopy. 2015;31(10):1880–5. https://doi.org/10.1016/j.arthro.2015.03.024.
36. Baudi P, Righi P, Bolognesi D, et al. How to identify and calculate glenoid bone deficit. Chir Organ Mov. 2005;90(2):145–52. http://www.ncbi.nlm.nih.gov/pubmed/16422240.
37. Magarelli N, Milano G, Sergio P, Santagada DA, Fabbriciani C, Bonomo L. Intra-observer and interobserver reliability of the "Pico" computed tomography method for quantification of glenoid bone defect in anterior shoulder instability. Skeletal Radiol. 2009;38(11):1071–5. https://doi.org/10.1007/s00256-009-0719-5.
38. Magarelli N, Milano G, Baudi P, et al. Comparison between 2D and 3D computed tomography evaluation of glenoid bone defect in unilateral anterior glenohumeral instability. Radiol Med. 2012;117(1):102–11. https://doi.org/10.1007/s11547-011-0712-7.
39. Stecco A, Guenzi E, Cascone T, et al. MRI can assess glenoid bone loss after shoulder luxation: inter- and intra-individual comparison with CT. Radiol Med. 2013;118(8):1335–43. https://doi.org/10.1007/s11547-013-0927-x.
40. Huijsmans PE, Haen PS, Kidd M, Dhert WJ, van der Hulst VPM, Willems WJ. Quantification of a glenoid defect with three-dimensional computed tomography and magnetic resonance imaging: a cadaveric study. J Shoulder Elbow Surg. 2007;16(6):803–9. https://doi.org/10.1016/j.jse.2007.02.115.
41. Lee HJ, Kim NR, Moon SG, Ko SM, Park JY. Multidirectional instability of the shoulder: rotator interval dimension and capsular laxity evaluation using MR arthrography. Skeletal Radiol. 2013;42(2):231–8. https://doi.org/10.1007/s00256-012-1441-2.
42. E Souza PM, Brandão BL, Brown E, Motta G, Monteiro M, Marchiori E. Recurrent anterior glenohumeral instability: the quantification of glenoid bone loss using magnetic resonance imaging. Skeletal Radiol. 2014;43(8):1085–92. https://doi.org/10.1007/s00256-014-1894-6.
43. Gyftopoulos S, Beltran LS, Yemin A, et al. Use of 3D MR reconstructions in the evaluation of glenoid bone loss: a clinical study. Skeletal Radiol. 2014;43(2):213–8. https://doi.org/10.1007/s00256-013-1774-5.
44. Tian CY, Shang Y, Zheng ZZ. Glenoid bone lesions: comparison between 3D VIBE images in MR arthrography and nonarthrographic MSCT. J Magn Reson Imaging. 2012;36(1):231–6. https://doi.org/10.1002/jmri.23622.
45. Bishop JY, Jones GL, Rerko MA, Donaldson C. 3-D CT is the most reliable imaging modality when quan-

tifying glenoid bone loss. Clin Orthop Relat Res. 2013;471(4):1251–6. https://doi.org/10.1007/s11999-012-2607-x.

46. Sugaya H. Techniques to evaluate glenoid bone loss. Curr Rev Musculoskelet Med. 2014;7(1):1–5. https://doi.org/10.1007/s12178-013-9198-3.
47. Nacca CR, Owens BD. Editorial commentary: bone loss in shoulder instability occurs in 3 dimensions. Arthroscopy. 2018;34(8):2324–5. https://doi.org/10.1016/j.arthro.2018.05.002.
48. Moroder P, Plachel F, Huettner A, et al. The effect of scapula tilt and best-fit circle placement when measuring glenoid bone loss in shoulder instability patients. Arthroscopy. 2018;34(2):398–404. https://doi.org/10.1016/j.arthro.2017.08.234.
49. Hill HA, Sachs MD. The grooved defect of the humeral head. Radiology. 1940;35(6):690–700. https://doi.org/10.1148/35.6.690.
50. Calandra JJ, Baker CL, Uribe J. The incidence of Hill-Sachs lesions in initial anterior shoulder dislocations. Arthroscopy. 1989;5(4):254–7.
51. Hovelius L, Augustini BG, Fredin H, Johansson O, Norlin R, Thorling J. Primary anterior dislocation of the shoulder in young patients. A ten-year prospective study. J Bone Joint Surg Am. 1996;78(11):1677–84. https://doi.org/10.2106/00004623-199611000-00006.
52. Taylor DC, Arciero RA. Pathologic changes associated with shoulder dislocations. Am J Sports Med. 1997;25(3):306–11. https://doi.org/10.1177/036354659702500306.
53. Nakagawa S, Iuchi R, Hanai H, Hirose T, Mae T. The development process of bipolar bone defects from primary to recurrent instability in shoulders with traumatic anterior instability. Am J Sports Med. 2019;47(3):695–703. https://doi.org/10.1177/0363546518819471.
54. Rowe CR, Zarins B, Ciullo JV. Recurrent anterior dislocation of the shoulder after surgical repair. Apparent causes of failure and treatment. J Bone Joint Surg Am. 1984;66(2):159–68.
55. Chen AL, Hunt SA, Hawkins RJ, Zuckerman JD. Management of bone loss associated with recurrent anterior glenohumeral instability. Am J Sports Med. 2005;33(6):912–25. https://doi.org/10.1177/0363546505277074.
56. Millett PJ, Clavert P, Warner JJP. Open operative treatment for anterior shoulder instability. J Bone Jt Surg. 2005;87(2):419–32. https://doi.org/10.2106/JBJS.D.01921.
57. Raiss P, Aldinger PR, Kasten P, Rickert M, Loew M. Humeral head resurfacing for fixed anterior glenohumeral dislocation. Int Orthop. 2009;33(2):451–6.https://doi.org/10.1007/s00264-007-0487-6.
58. Sekiya JK, Wickwire AC, Stehle JH, Debski RE. Hill-Sachs defects and repair using osteoarticular allograft transplantation: biomechanical analysis using a joint compression model. Am J Sports Med. 2009;37(12):2459–66. https://doi.org/10.1177/0363546509341576.
59. Kaar SG, Fening SD, Jones MH, Colbrunn RW, Miniaci A. Effect of humeral head defect size on glenohumeral stability: a cadaveric study of simulated Hill-Sachs defects. Am J Sports Med. 2010;38(3):594–9. https://doi.org/10.1177/0363546509350295.
60. Gowd AK, Liu JN, Cabarcas BC, et al. Management of recurrent anterior shoulder instability with bipolar bone loss: a systematic review to assess critical bone loss amounts. Am J Sports Med. 2019;47(10):2484–93. https://doi.org/10.1177/0363546518791555.
61. Cho SH, Cho NS, Rhee YG. Preoperative analysis of the Hill-Sachs lesion in anterior shoulder instability: how to predict engagement of the lesion. Am J Sports Med. 2011;39(11):2389–95. https://doi.org/10.1177/0363546511398644.
62. Schneider AK, Hoy GA, Ek ET, et al. Interobserver and intraobserver variability of glenoid track measurements. J Shoulder Elbow Surg. 2017;26(4):573–9. https://doi.org/10.1016/j.jse.2016.09.058.
63. Ozaki R, Nakagawa S, Mizuno N, Mae T, Yoneda M. Hill-Sachs lesions in shoulders with traumatic anterior instability. Am J Sports Med. 2014;42(11):2597–605. https://doi.org/10.1177/0363546514549543.
64. Ho A, Kurdziel MD, Koueiter DM, Wiater JM. Three-dimensional computed tomography measurement accuracy of varying Hill-Sachs lesion size. J Shoulder Elbow Surg. 2018;27(2):350–6. https://doi.org/10.1016/j.jse.2017.09.007.
65. Di Giacomo G, Golijanin P, Sanchez G, Provencher MT. Radiographic analysis of the Hill-Sachs lesion in anteroinferior shoulder instability after first-time dislocations. Arthroscopy. 2016;32(8):1509–14. https://doi.org/10.1016/j.arthro.2016.01.022.
66. Itoi E, Yamamoto N. Shoulder instability: treating bone loss. Curr Orthop Pract. 2012;23(6):609–15. https://doi.org/10.1097/BCO.0b013e318265e0a1.
67. Itoi E, Yamamoto N, Kurokawa D, Sano H. Bone loss in anterior instability. Curr Rev Musculoskelet Med. 2013;6(1):88–94. https://doi.org/10.1007/s12178-012-9154-7.
68. Nakagawa S, Ozaki R, Take Y, Iuchi R, Mae T. Relationship between glenoid defects and Hill-Sachs lesions in shoulders with traumatic anterior instability. Am J Sports Med. 2015;43(11):2763–73. https://doi.org/10.1177/0363546515597668.
69. Lau BC, Conway D, Curran PF, Feeley BT, Pandya NK. Bipolar bone loss in patients with anterior shoulder dislocation: a comparison of adolescents versus adult patients. Arthroscopy. 2017;33(10):1755–61. https://doi.org/10.1016/j.arthro.2017.04.004.
70. Arciero RA, Parrino A, Bernhardson AS, et al. The effect of a combined glenoid and Hill-Sachs defect on glenohumeral stability: a biomechanical cadaveric study using 3-dimensional modeling of 142 patients. Am J Sports Med. 2015;43(6):1422–9. https://doi.org/10.1177/0363546515574677.
71. Gottschalk LJ, Walia P, Patel RM, et al. Stability of the glenohumeral joint with combined humeral head and glenoid defects. Am J Sports Med. 2016;44(4):933–40. https://doi.org/10.1177/0363546515624914.

72. Patel RM, Walia P, Gottschalk L, et al. The effects of Latarjet reconstruction on glenohumeral kinematics in the presence of combined bony defects. Am J Sports Med. 2016;44(7):1818–24. https://doi.org/10.1177/0363546516635651.
73. Locher J, Wilken F, Beitzel K, et al. Hill-Sachs off-track lesions as risk factor for recurrence of instability after arthroscopic Bankart repair. Arthroscopy. 2016;32(10):1993–9. https://doi.org/10.1016/j.arthro.2016.03.005.
74. Shaha JS, Cook JB, Rowles DJ, Bottoni CR, Shaha SH, Tokish JM. Clinical validation of the glenoid track concept in anterior glenohumeral instability. J Bone Jt Surg Am. 2016;98(22):1918–23. https://doi.org/10.2106/JBJS.15.01099.
75. Mook WR, Petri M, Greenspoon JA, Horan MP, Dornan GJ, Millett PJ. Clinical and anatomic predictors of outcomes after the Latarjet procedure for the treatment of anterior glenohumeral instability with combined glenoid and humeral bone defects. Am J Sports Med. 2016;44(6):1407–16. https://doi.org/10.1177/0363546516634089.
76. Rerko MA, Pan X, Donaldson C, Jones GL, Bishop JY. Comparison of various imaging techniques to quantify glenoid bone loss in shoulder instability. J Shoulder Elbow Surg. 2013;22(4):528–34. https://doi.org/10.1016/j.jse.2012.05.034.
77. Gyftopoulos S, Beltran LS, Bookman J, Rokito A. MRI evaluation of bipolar bone loss using the on-track off-track method: a feasibility study. Am J Roentgenol. 2015;205(4):848–52. https://doi.org/10.2214/AJR.14.14266.
78. Nakagawa S, Hanai H, Mae T, Hayashida K, Yoneda M. Bipolar bone loss in male athletes with traumatic anterior shoulder instability: an evaluation using a new scoring system. Orthop J Sports Med. 2018;6(7):1–9. https://doi.org/10.1177/2325967118782420.
79. Walia P, Miniaci A, Jones MH, Fening SD. Theoretical model of the effect of combined glenohumeral bone defects on anterior shoulder instability: a finite element approach. J Orthop Res. 2013;31(4):601–7. https://doi.org/10.1002/jor.22267.
80. Walia P, Miniaci A, Jones MH, Fening SD. Influence of combined Hill-Sachs and bony Bankart defects on range of motion in anterior instability of the shoulder in a finite element model. Arthroscopy. 2015;31(11):2119–27. https://doi.org/10.1016/j.arthro.2015.04.099.
81. Walia P, Patel RM, Gottschalk L, et al. The reduction in stability from combined humeral head and glenoid bony defects is influenced by arm position. Am J Sports Med. 2016;44(3):715–22. https://doi.org/10.1177/0363546515620588.

23 Remplissage Technique

Mikolaj Podsiadlo, Hubert Laprus, Adrian Błasiak, and Roman Brzóska

23.1 Introduction

In the past, many researchers diagnosed and then struggled with the high occurrence of bony Bankart lesions in many cases regarding shoulder instability. Moreover, much attention was paid to the role of such defects according to their size in increase of revision rate following stabilization procedures. In contrast, much less is focused on the role of the so-called Hill–Sachs lesion (HS), as well as its real impact on generating recurrent dislocations. The issue was first discussed in the article by Broca and Hartman in 1894 [1] over 100 years from now.

Patients suffering because of a combination of glenoid rim loss and HS (engaging Hill–Sachs lesion) have proven to be a challenge for anyone concerned about treatment despite the use of a variety of open and arthroscopic approaches (Fig. 23.1).

The story reflects in numerous papers, which all together lead to a conclusion that "in the presence of the combination of a glenoid defect and HS, the Latarjet [2] procedure is recommended" [3]. Nowadays, we also more precisely know that the borderline loss of glenoid area that should convince us to use the bony procedure [2] totals 20–25% [4, 5] (Fig. 23.2).

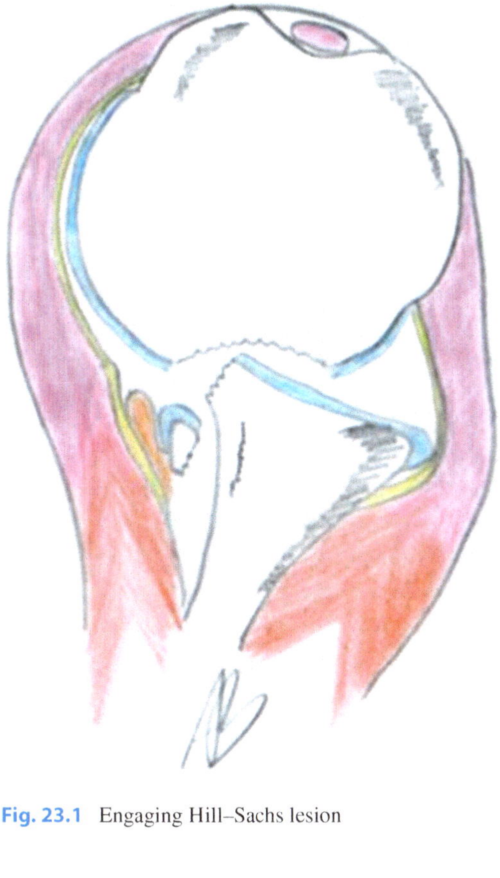

Fig. 23.1 Engaging Hill–Sachs lesion

The first arthroscopic technique introduced in 2004 by Wolf et al. [3] called Remplissage (Fr.: to fill in, or to fill up) evolved from being a shy but promising attempt into almost a routine pro-

M. Podsiadlo (✉) · H. Laprus · A. Błasiak · R. Brzóska
Shoulder and Upper Limb Department, St. Luke's Hospital, Bielsko-Biala, Poland
e-mail: podsiadlo@lukasza.pl; laprus@lukasza.pl; blasiak@lukasza.pl

R. Brzóska et al. (eds.), *360° Around Shoulder Instability*,
https://doi.org/10.1007/978-3-662-61074-9_23

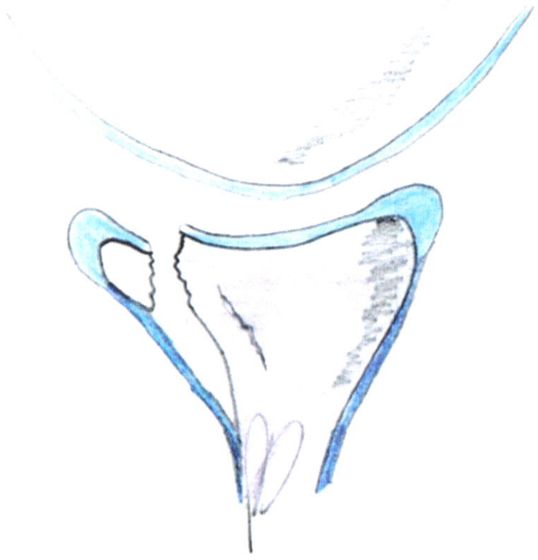

Fig. 23.2 Large bony Bankart lesion

cedure in cases were both Bankart lesion and a large engaging Hill–Sachs defect are involved.

HS is a common complication of anterior shoulder dislocation. According to available data, 80–93% of patients with persistent anterior dislocation have humeral head defects. The purpose of this chapter is to present arthroscopic treatment of HS and correlation between size or localization of HS and severity of anterior instability. The results of anterior instability treatment with BLS (Bankart repair with sutures between glenohumeral ligaments and subscapularis tendon) combined with remplissage procedure performed by authors on 100 cases and published recently [6] are presented as well.

23.2 Anatomical Highlights

The glenoid comprises scapular fossa, which is slightly concave and pear shaped with sagittal dimension larger in its lower part. The upper part is approximately 20% bigger compared to the lower one and its mean transverse length is around 25 mm, in contrary to 35 mm of mean lower part length. The glenoid alignment toward scapular plane is called the scapular version. Seventy-five percent of the whole population have their glenoids set in 7° of retroversion. The residual 25% is set in anteversion ranging from 2° to 10°. Meanwhile, the articular surface is headed slightly upward (the so-called glenoid tilt) around 5°. To maintain contact with the surface, the humeral head is most commonly 20° retroverted.

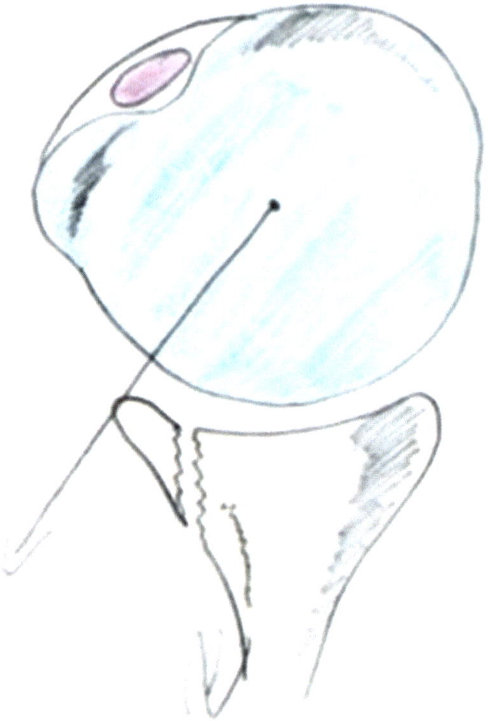

Fig. 23.3 Humeral head being a "golf ball on a stand"

The glenohumeral joint is distinctive for unusually disproportionate glenoid when compared with the whole humeral articular surface covered with cartilage—the problem of congruency is depicted below. Humeral head when looked at in transverse plane resembles a golf ball on a stand, where only one fourth of its total surface contacts with its glenoid while in motion (Fig. 23.3).

23.3 Measurements of Hill–Sachs Lesion and Anterior Glenoid Rim Loss

Among different ways to assess HS (Kaar [7], Kralinger [8]), Hardy's index [9] is a useful tool for measurement of humeral defect volume.

The lesion's volume correlates directly with anterior instability recurrence. The measurements needed to determine the ratio of HS volume to the humeral head are based on arthro-CT scans. Another indicator of HS that correlates with the treatment effect is the ratio of HS depth to the radius of humeral head, measured on X-ray of shoulder in internal rotation. Studies revealed that for Hill–Sachs lesions larger than 16% of the humeral head volume, treatment results in 61% were fair and bad. It fits the new presented concept of on-track and off-track lesion.

In supplement to the ways of HS assessment, there is a practical method of estimating anterior glenoid bone loss, easy to use during arthroscopic examination. The concept called "bare spot method" first described by Burkhard in 2002 [10] is based on the measurement of distances with the use of arthroscopic probe as shown below.

$$\frac{BC - AB}{2 * BC} * 100\%$$

The loss of glenoid over 20–25%, seen most commonly in arthroscopy as a "straight line sign," should be an indication to rather use Latarjet procedure [2].

23.4 Remplissage Procedure

Remplissage. The procedure of arthroscopic capsulotenodesis of the infraspinatus tendon can be applied as an efficient treatment of moderate- and large-sized Hill–Sachs lesions. This arthroscopic transfer of the posterior capsule and infraspinatus tendon into the HS effectively converts the lesion into an extra-articular one and prevents it from engaging the glenoid rim. According to Wolf [3], it is analogous to an arthroscopic repair of a partial-thickness rotator cuff repair. The principle standing behind the attempt is the change of force vector as shown on the picture. During external rotation, the humeral head after remplissage is pulled medially and backward instead of being subluxed at the anterior glenoid rim (Figs. 23.4 and 23.5).

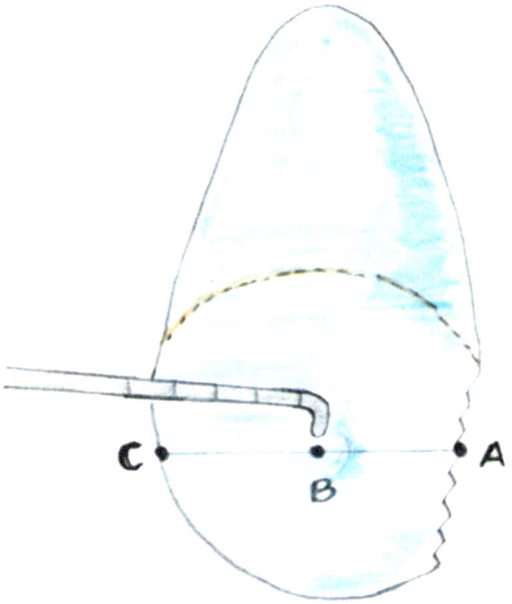

Fig. 23.4 Bare spot method: $\frac{BC - AB}{2 * BC} * 100\%$

The technique in addition diminishes the posteroanterior translation of the humeral head instead of its rotation.

Operative Technique. The first and major step is to scarify the surface of HS debriding it from connective and residual chondral tissue. The same must be done on the inner surface of the infraspinatus tendon to prepare conditions for proper tendon-to-bone healing.

The second step is the anchor placement. In the original work by Wolf [3], two anchors were used, but based on the work by Brzoska and Blasiak et al. [6], a single anchor with two sutures is as much effective, thus significantly reducing procedure time and costs.

The third step is then to place the sutures in a figure of four placing one of them from medial to lateral direction and the second from above to the bottom. This increases the area of tendon-to-bone adhesion, increasing the chance of successful tenodesis.

The last step is finally tying the sutures extracapsulary as to avoid glenoid irritation with knots and threads (Figs. 23.6 and 23.7).

Rehabilitation. For 6 weeks postoperatively, the patient is asked to wear orthosis and to per-

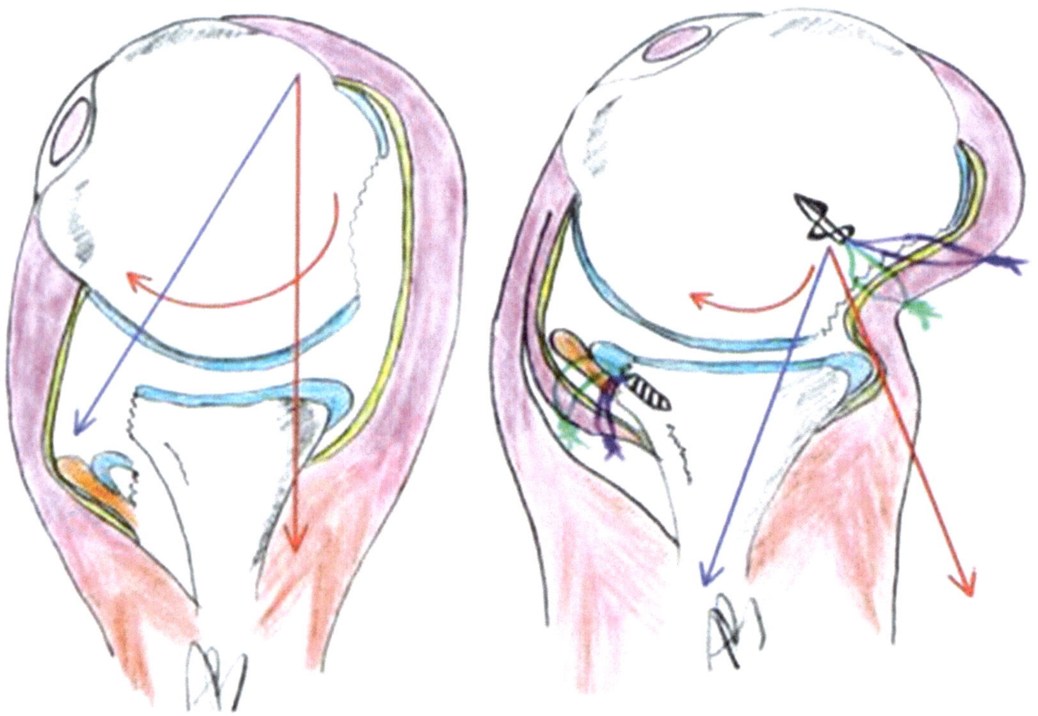

Fig. 23.5 Forces vectors

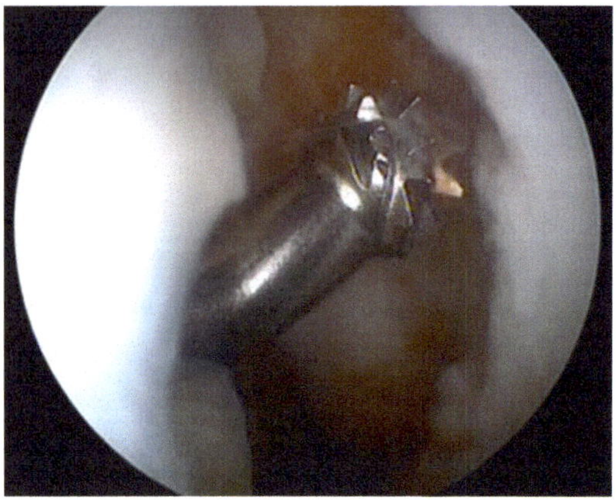

Fig. 23.6 Refreshing the HS surface

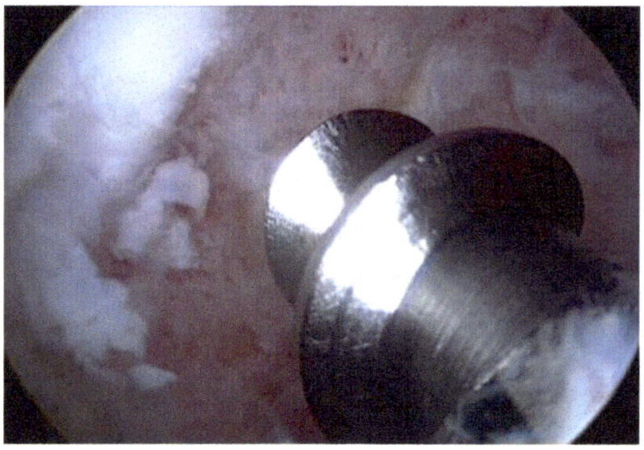

Fig. 23.7 Anchor placement

form passive exercises with the use of the healthy arm or another person to an extend the pain permits. This comprises slight external rotation and gravity-based passive motion.

From sixth week on, active exercises are used under the supervision of physiotherapist to increase the range of motion, scapular stabilization, and deltoid muscle tension.

From 12th week on, active resistance training can be introduced until the patient gradually fully recovers.

Challenges Ahead. Large lesions of humeral head with the size of 20–25% and more can in addition be treated with sandwich technique. In this procedure, a bone autograft or allograft is used to fill HS, and remplissage procedure is performed afterward in spot where bone graft had been implanted.

Some authors have presented case reports concerning treatment of very large HS with open humeral head allograft transplantation. As a result of this procedure, the defect of humeral head can be effectively filled, but the rate of graft resorption and final results consequently are difficult to predict. In addition, humeral head replacement remains a solution in the most severe cases.

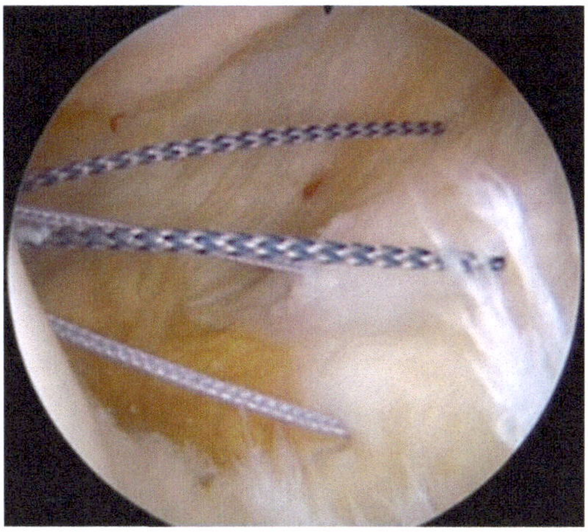

Fig. 23.8 Suture passage

23.5 Conditions Associated with Positive Outcome Score

There are several factors that contribute to the revision rate first summed up and published by Bigliani in 1998 [4]. Its feasibility found its way in the analysis by Leroux [11]. Among features, combined to form the so-called ISIS score, one may find age, involvement in contact or high-risk sports, hyperlaxity, anterior glenoid rim deficit visible on plain CR AP-view scan as well as HS lesion visible on CR in external rotation and sclerotic inferior glenoid contour. Nourissat in 2011 [12] suggested using Latarjet initially if the ISIS score exceeds or equals 3 points. He also noticed that the remplissage can, in fact, reduce ISIS score by 2 points defining more precisely the limits of operative treatment that are based on soft tissues. The procedure allows to eliminate one of the major factors that contributes to the risk of subsequent failure in terms of redislocation. It reduces the risk from previously described by Burkhart [5] and Provencher [13] and evaluated as being 5–67% to 3,4% described by Leroux [11]. Eighty-six percent positive outcomes with restoration of full joint stability were noted by Brzoska et al. [6], where BLS plus remplissage was the method of choice (Figs. 23.8, 23.9, 23.10 and 23.11).

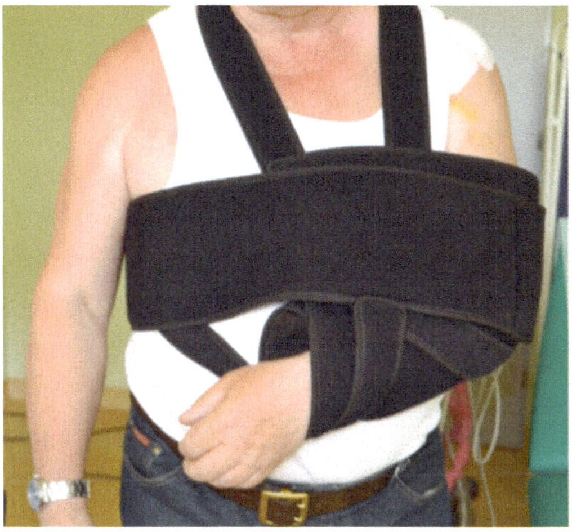

Fig. 23.9 Postoperative orthosis

23.6 Conclusions and Results

There exist various complications that one might be afraid of, among which recurrent dislocation or subluxation, a feeling of instability or persistent apprehension, adhesive capsulitis, and moreover persistent external rotation limitation more than 20°. None of them, however, was proven to be a major issue in most of cases. The problem that lies ahead, however, is omarthrosis that seems to be the last barrier to be broken. Harris et al. [14] estimated the level of arthrosis following arthroscopic stabilization procedures at 26% as opposed to open approaches 33% according to Samilson and Prieto classification [15]. All in all, the scientific results [6] state that the remplissage procedure is a mini-invasive (additional graft material not required) and efficient treatment of moderate- and medium-sized HS without significant glenoid bone loss.

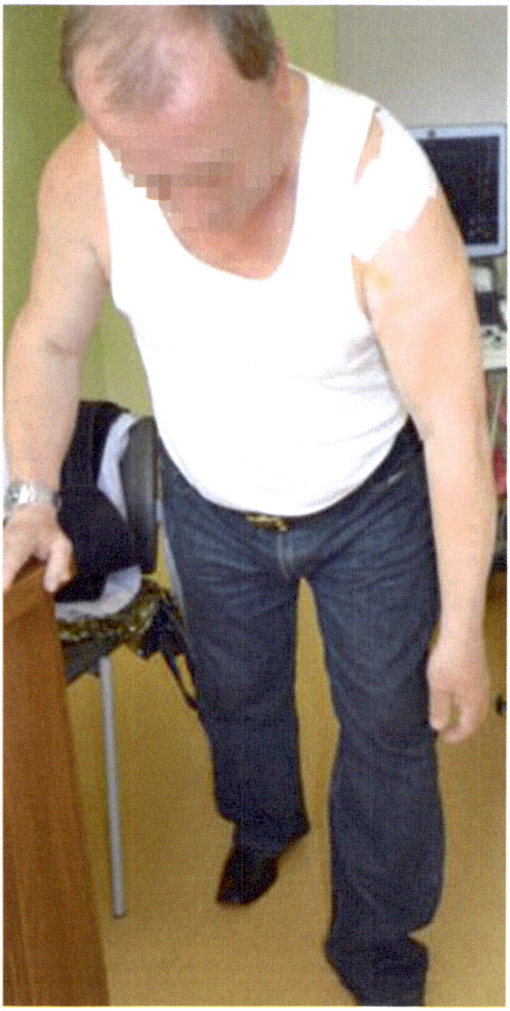

Fig. 23.10 Postoperative rehabilitation protocol

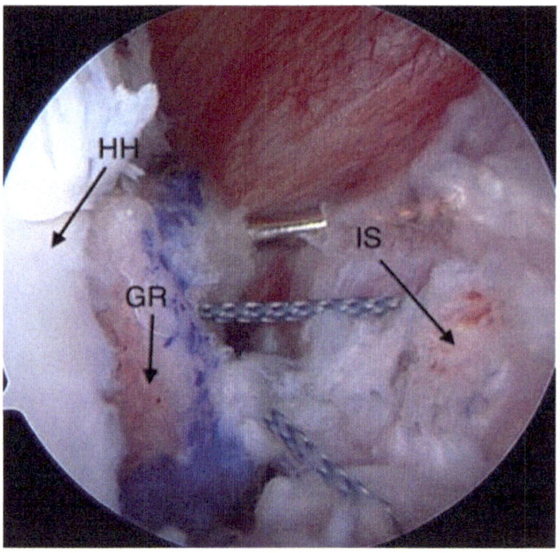

Fig. 23.11 Sandwich technique. *HH* humeral head, *IS* infraspinatus, *GR* bone graft

Acknowledgments The authors would hereby like to thank Dr Brzoska and his coworkers for giving an insight into the literature and for the experience that was gained around the topic for the past 15 years. The work by Dr Brzoska and his colleagues who contributed to the development of glenohumeral instability treatment gave proof that the firstly doubtful way of coping with HS became gradually a standard procedure in certain cases.

References

1. Broca A. Contribution à l'étude des luxations de l'épaule. Impr. Lemale et Cie. 1890.
2. Latarjet M. Technic of coracoid preglenoid arthroereisis in the treatment of recurrent dislocation of the shoulder. Lyon Chir. 1958;54(4):604–7. ISSN 0024-7782.
3. Wolf EM, Pollack ME. Hill-Sachs "Remplissage": an arthroscopic solution for the engaging Hill-Sachs lesion (SS-32). Arthroscopy. 2004;20:e14–5. https://doi.org/10.1016/j.arthro.2004.02.033. ISSN 07498063.
4. Bigliani LU, Newton PM, Steinmann SP, Connor PM, McIlveen SJ. Glenoid rim lesions associated with recurrent anterior dislocation of the shoulder. Am J Sports Med. 1998;26(1):41–5. https://doi.org/10.1177/03635465980260012301. ISSN 0363-5465.
5. Burkhart SS, De Beer JF. Traumatic glenohumeral bone defects and their relationship to failure of arthroscopic Bankart repairs. Arthroscopy. 2000;16(7):677–94. https://doi.org/10.1053/jars.2000.17715. ISSN 07498063.
6. Brzóska R, Laprus H, Michniowski P, Solecki W, Klon W, Błasiak A. Novel and effective arthroscopic extracapsular stabilization technique for anterior shoulder instability-BLS. Knee Surg Sports Traumatol Arthrosc. 2019;27(12):3897–904. https://doi.org/10.1007/s00167-019-05496-1. ISSN 0942-2056.
7. Kaar SG, Fening SD, Jones MH, Colbrunn RW, Miniaci A. Effect of humeral head defect size on glenohumeral stability: a cadaveric study of simulated Hill-Sachs defects. Am J Sports Med. 2010;38(3):594–9. https://doi.org/10.1177/0363546509350295. ISSN 1552-3365.
8. Kralinger FS, Golser K, Wischatta R, Wambacher M, Sperner G. Predicting recurrence after primary anterior shoulder dislocation. Am J Sports Med. 2002;30(1):116–20. https://doi.org/10.1177/03635465020300010501. ISSN 0363-5465.
9. Hardy P, Lopes R, Bauer T, Conso C, Gaudin P, Sanghavi S. New quantitative measurement of the Hill–Sachs lesion: a prognostic factor for clinical results of arthroscopic glenohumeral stabilization. Eur J Orthop Surg Traumatol. 2012;22(7):541–7. https://doi.org/10.1007/s00590-011-0883-x. ISSN 1633-8065.
10. Burkhart SS, DeBeer JF, Tehrany AM, Parten PM. Quantifying glenoid bone loss arthroscopically in shoulder instability. Arthroscopy. 2002;18(5):488–91. https://doi.org/10.1053/jars.2002.32212. ISSN 07498063.

11. Leroux T, Bhatti A, Khoshbin A, Wasserstein D, Henry P, Marks P, Takhar K, Veillette C, Theodoropolous J, Chahal J. Combined arthroscopic Bankart repair and remplissage for recurrent shoulder instability. Arthroscopy. 2013;29(10):1693–701. https://doi.org/10.1016/j.arthro.2013.06.007. ISSN 1526-3231.
12. Nourissat G, Kilinc AS, Werther JR, Doursounian L. A prospective, comparative, radiological, and clinical study of the influence of the "Remplissage" procedure on shoulder range of motion after stabilization by arthroscopic Bankart repair. Am J Sports Med. 2011;39(10):2147–52. https://doi.org/10.1177/0363546511416315. ISSN 0363-5465.
13. Provencher MT, Ghodadra N, Romeo AA. Arthroscopic management of anterior instability: pearls, pitfalls, and lessons learned. Orthop Clin North Am. 2010;41(3):325–37. https://doi.org/10.1016/j.ocl.2010.02.007. ISSN 00305898.
14. Harris JD, Gupta AK, Mall NA, Abrams GD, McCormick FM, Cole BJ, Bach BR, Romeo AA, Verma NN. Long-term outcomes after Bankart shoulder stabilization. Arthroscopy. 2013;29(5):920–33. https://doi.org/10.1016/j.arthro.2012.11.010. ISSN 07498063.
15. Samilson RL, Prieto V. Dislocation arthropathy of the shoulder. J Bone Joint Surg Am. 1983;65(4):456–60. ISSN 0021-9355.

Management of the Deep Hill–Sachs Lesion

24

Hubert Laprus and Joanna Wałecka

24.1 Introduction

The Hill–Sachs lesion is an osseous defect typically associated with anterior shoulder instability. It presents as a compression fracture that occurs during an anterior instability event as the result of compression of the posterosuperior part of the humeral head on the anterior glenoid rim (Fig. 24.1). This lesion was first described by Hill and Sachs in 1940 [1], when a defect of the humeral head in patients after an anterior shoulder dislocation episode was noticed on the internal rotation shoulder radiograph.

The clinical importance of the humeral head bony defects and their influence on recurrent glenohumeral instability were underlined and supported by many authors in recent years, especially in the glenoid track concept [2–4]. The articular-arc deficit that occurs in cases of deep Hill–Sachs lesion results in an engaging symptom when the arm is positioned in abduction and external rotation. This kind of lesion remains a severe risk factor for instability recurrence even after Bankart repair. Besides the well-known posterosuperior humeral head defect associated with anterior glenohumeral instability, injury of the anterior part of the humeral head associated with posterior instability and called a reverse Hill–Sachs is also described. However, posterior dislocation episodes are rather uncommon, and the impact of the reverse Hill–Sachs lesion on recurrent posterior dislocation has not been well described.

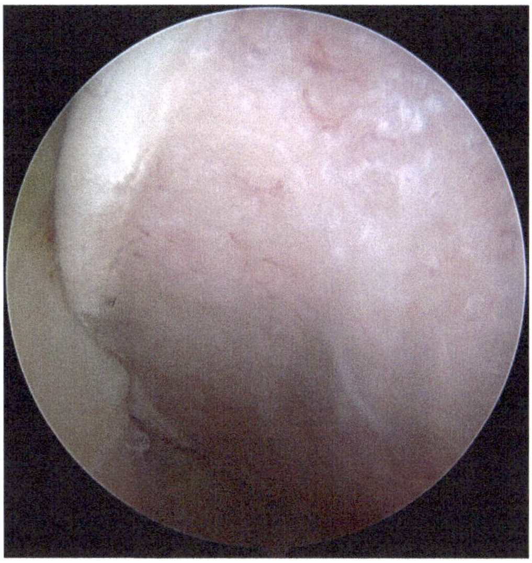

Fig. 24.1 Hill–Sachs lesion after anterior shoulder dislocation

The incidence of the Hill–Sachs lesion is high, starting from about 50% to 90% of all first-time anterior instability events [5–8] to approach perhaps 100% of persons with recurrent anterior shoulder instability [5]. Injury of the humeral head is typically associated with anterior capsu-

H. Laprus (✉)
Department of Orthopaedic Surgery, St. Luke's Hospital, Bielsko-Biała, Poland

J. Wałecka
Rehasport Clinic, Pozań, Poland

R. Brzóska et al. (eds.), *360° Around Shoulder Instability*,
https://doi.org/10.1007/978-3-662-61074-9_24

lolabral lesion, glenohumeral ligament injury, or anterior glenoid bone loss (GBL). Proper diagnosis of either the Hill–Sachs lesion or concomitant injuries is crucial to introduce adequate treatment. The incidence of the reverse Hill–Sachs lesion in magnetic resonance imaging (MRI) findings after posterior shoulder episodes was estimated by Saupe et al. [9] to be 86%.

Currently, there is a substantial amount of literature describing proper management of glenohumeral instability in the case of GBL or capsulolabral injury. Unfortunately, there is still a paucity of literature summarizing the imaging, classification, and management of a deep Hill–Sachs lesion.

24.2 Imaging

A number of imaging examinations can be used to diagnose and assess humeral head lesions. X-ray radiograms in true anteroposterior (AP) and internal or external rotation are typically obtained. Several other, more specific, X-ray views are dedicated to assess either a Hill–Sachs lesion or the presence of GBL. Among these, the Stryker view is specific to evaluate a humeral head defect, and the Bernageu (Fig. 24.2) view is the most popular when evaluating the GBL. However, X-ray views that are sufficient to find large bony lesions are not sufficiently precise to predict the shape, orientation, and dimensions of the bony lesion, which is crucial in the decision-making process and preoperative planning [10].

Computed tomography (CT) is the examination of choice in assessing defects after dislocation episodes as well as in the case of a presumed bony lesion that is not visible on the standard radiographs performed after an instability episode. CT imaging with three-dimensional (3D) osseous reconstruction technology has become the gold standard when determining the severity of Hill–Sachs lesions [11] (Fig. 24.3). Two-dimensional (2D)-CT is useful as well, especially in cases of a bipolar lesion, to analyze precisely all the small bony fragments that sometimes remain after dislocation episodes. On 2D imaging, the surgeon is able to analyze anatomic relationships between a Hill–Sachs lesion and a GBL, which is very useful in prediction of risk factors leading to further dislocations. However, Bokor et al. showed that 3D imaging in the hands of an orthopedic surgeon is a more precise and reproducible tool than 2D-CT and provides better measurement capabilities [12]. Further, CT with humeral head subtraction is the gold standard

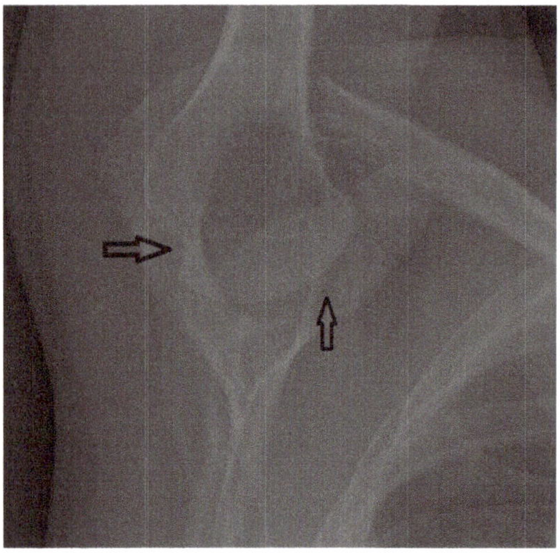

Fig. 24.2 Hill–Sachs lesion in Stryker view, X-ray examination

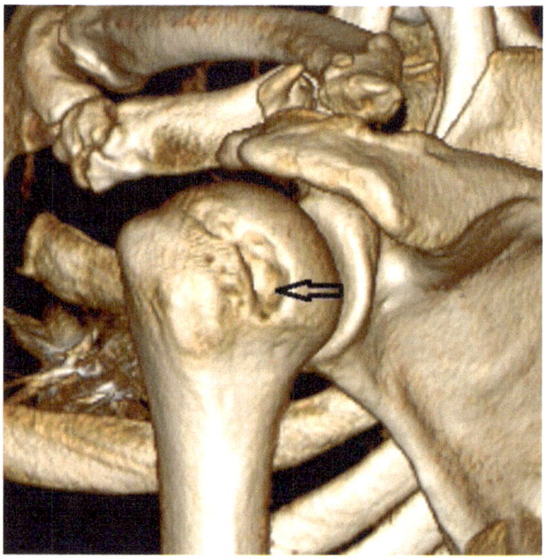

Fig. 24.3 Computed tomography (CT) imaging with 3D osseous reconstruction

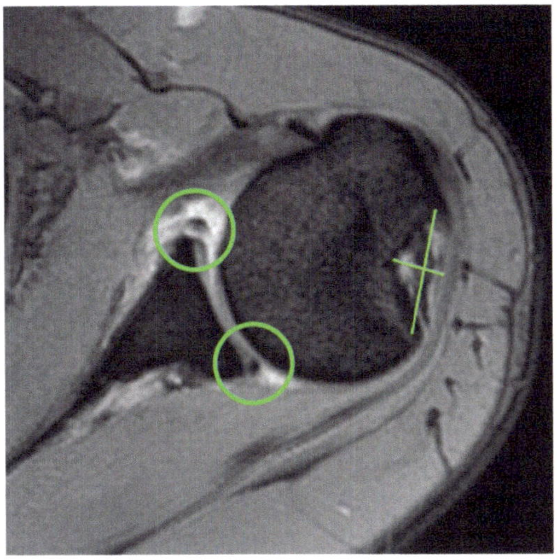

Fig. 24.4 Hill–Sachs lesion and concomitant pathologies (anterior labrum lesion and posterior labrum lesion, *circles*) in magnetic resonance imaging

method to measure GBL. In the glenoid track concept introduced by Di Giacomo et al. [4], the relationship between the position and dimensions of the Hill–Sachs and the size of the GBL observed in CT is used to predict the risk of further dislocations for an unstable patient with bony lesions.

The popularity of the MRI method has grown in recent years. For assessing soft-tissue anatomy after an instability episode, MRI has become the imaging method of choice [13]. Owens et al., by analyzing numerous patient MRIs after glenohumeral instability, prove that assessing GBL size is also possible and reproducible in MRI [14]. This finding is very useful, because the surgeon is able to assess a Hill–Sachs lesion, GBL, chondral lesions, fluid collections, soft-tissue injuries, and several other pathological conditions with one imaging examination, while avoiding the use of harmful CT radiation in preoperative diagnosis, which is especially important considering the typically young age of patients with glenohumeral instability (Fig. 24.4).

Despite the significant progress that has been made since the early 2000s in our imaging knowledge, there is still a need for further investigation to determine the best imaging modality for quantifying Hill–Sachs lesions [15, 16].

24.3 Classification and Decision-Making Process

Numerous classification systems have been already described to assess and grade the Hill–Sachs lesion. Most of them are very useful in diagnostic and clinical decision-making processes. The most common definition of Hill–Sachs size, although not universally accepted, is a lesion that covers more than 25% of the articular surface of the humeral head [17]. Lesions covering less than 25% of the humeral head surface are typically insignificant. Traditionally, classification systems are based on preoperative imaging or direct visualization during surgery. Among radiologic classifications, the most popular are the Rowe 3 steps grading system based on axillary radiograph imaging [18] and the Hall system based on notch view radiographs [19]. Among direct visualization classifications, typically the Calandra [6], Franceschi [20], or Flatow and Warner [21] grading systems are used. In the Calandra and Franceschi systems, the depth of the Hill–Sachs lesion is underlined as most relevant factor. The Flatow and Warner classifications separate the lesions according to surface: clinically insignificant, less than 20%; of variable significance, 20% to 40%; and clinically significant, more than 40%. The classifications and grading systems can be useful in clinical decision making, especially with larger lesions, but they have not yet proved helpful in determining successful management strategies because even a small Hill–Sachs lesion concomitant with GBL can become clinically significant [22]. Biomechanical studies performed by Taylor and Arciero proved that a clinically insignificant Hill–Sachs lesion compared with the 2-mm glenoid defect resulted in a 25% reduction of stability. When pairing a 6-mm glenoid defect with that same insignificant Hill–Sachs lesion, they found a 50% reduction of stability. This study supports the glenoid track concept introduced first by Yamamoto and subsequently by Di Giacomo. The glenoid track is defined as an area of the glenoid that is covered as the arm shifts during a movement of abduction and external rotation from the inferomedial to the superolateral portion of the humeral head. The size of this area is about 84% of the glenoid width. If the Hill–Sachs lesion is located closer than the size of the contact area, it becomes at high risk for engagement and, therefore, recurrent instability, thus requiring treatment [3, 4].

24.4 Nonsurgical Treatment

Nonsurgical treatment in the case of a large Hill–Sachs fracture is not traditionally considered as the treatment of choice. Large defects of the humeral head usually result in an engagement phenomenon and become an important risk factor of instability recurrence. However, for certain cases, such as elderly persons, with the presence of severe chronic diseases or other contraindications to surgery, conservative management has to be implemented. In such situations a physiotherapeutic protocol for shoulder instability performed by an experienced physiotherapist should be considered. The rehabilitation program should be focused on scapular stabilizing exercises and strengthening rotator cuff, pectoralis, deltoideus, and latissimus dorsi muscles. Exercises focused on control of the humeral head balance relative to the glenoid position should be also included. However, it should be emphasized that in the case of a deep Hill–Sachs fracture, conservative treatment is burdened with a high risk of failure, especially with uncontrolled arm movements, such as during sleep.

24.5 Surgical Treatment

24.5.1 Soft-Tissue Procedures

Among the soft-tissue procedures, currently only the remplissage procedure is likely to be used in a case of a large Hill–Sachs lesion. Historically, capsular tightening created by capsular shift has been also used. A capsular shift results in limitation of the shoulder range of motion and glenoid track modifications that can be effective in enhancing shoulder stability. Although this technique can be successfully used in posterior or multidirectional instability treatment, unfortunately, the loss of external rotation typically observed after capsular plication may be problematic for young active patients. Also, in cases of significant Hill–Sachs lesions, capsular plication alone may not be adequate for regaining shoulder stability.

The remplissage technique, originally described as open, was subsequently adapted by Wolf et al. for arthroscopic surgery [23]. Wolf's technique relies on fixation, into the surface of the Hill–Sachs lesion, capsulotendinous tissue of the infraspinatus muscle (Fig. 24.5). Wolf's technique was modified subsequently by Koo by using two anchors and double-pulley sutures. This modification should result in better healing properties and less tissue morbidity. The aim of the remplissage technique is to convert an intraarticular defect to an extraarticular one by transfer capsule insertion. The second consequence of this procedure is changing the force vector during arm movements, which results in higher humeral head pressure against the glenoid during external rotation. The main advantage of this technique is that it is a completely arthroscopic approach which allows performing concomitant procedures on the anterior wall soft tissue. Also, this technique is quite repetitive and not very demanding surgically, which permits predicting the post-

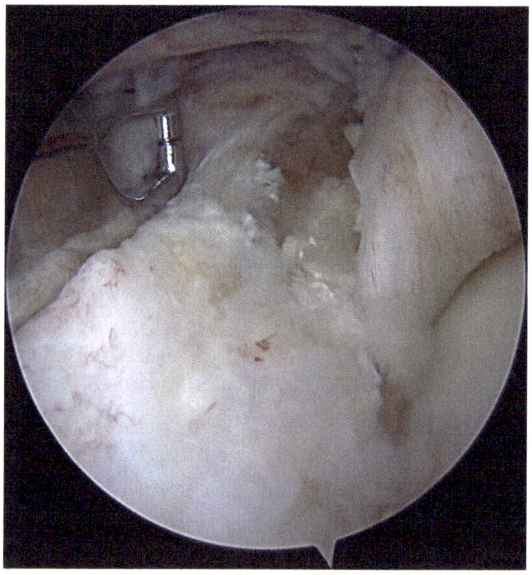

Fig. 24.5 Remplissage technique: view after anchor and sutures placement before knot tying

operative results. The arthroscopic approach usually is characterized by less tissue morbidity and a faster recovery time than open procedures.

The disadvantage of this method is, unfortunately, the commonly occurring limitation of external rotation, as was already proven by Kroll [24]. The following disadvantages are restrictions of this method. Remplissage can be a successful method of management of deep and not very broad defects because the conditions are adequate for tendon healing conditions. Patients with wide, shallow lesions or lesions with concomitant large GBL may require a Latarjet procedure or other Hill–Sachs reconstruction methods.

24.5.2 Bony Procedures

Bony procedures can be traditionally separated into glenoid augmentation procedures and techniques directly addressed to the Hill–Sachs lesion called humeral head augmentation procedures. Among glenoid augmentation techniques, the principal choices are iliac crest bone grafting and the Latarjet procedure, which remain the most efficient methods [25]. Glenoid augmentation procedures are utilized for significant Hill–Sachs lesions and concomitant GBL or anterior wall soft-tissue insufficiency that leads to recurrent glenohumeral instability. Latarjet and bone block techniques are described precisely elsewhere in this book.

Bony procedures that directly address the Hill–Sachs lesion are reserved for relatively rare cases of significant humeral head defect without concomitant GBL. The intent with these procedures is to fill the defect and restore native anatomy by effectively increasing the articular arc of the humerus as it rotates on the glenoid, thereby preventing engagement and instability [22]. These techniques can be divided, by the material used, into autograft procedures (usually grafts from the iliac crest), allografts (with size-matched humeral head fresh-frozen allografts), and synthetic materials (e.g., a metallic cap). Fresh-frozen allografts are currently a popular way to fill many osteochondral defects, especially in the U.S. and Japan. There are a few studies of the shoulder joint in a small group of patients that prove safety and good outcomes [26, 27]. The main advantage of a fresh-frozen humeral head allograft is that there is currently only one technique that provides the possibility of anatomic reconstruction. Thus, the surgeon is able to restore the native congruence of the shoulder joint without decreasing the range of motion and biomechanical joint properties. Unfortunately, allograft techniques are still at high risk of complications. The most serious of these is the relatively rarely occurring necrosis of the humeral head or infections. However, more likely complications observed are partial or total graft osteolysis, persistent pain, swelling, and arthritis [26, 27]. Also, fresh-frozen allografts are not available in every country. First, the high cost of allograft harvesting and its preparation restrict this method to wealthy countries. Second, legal regulations, especially in European countries, make fresh-frozen allografts hard to obtain and implant.

Meeting the expectations of treating a large and deep Hill–Sachs fracture, the authors of this chapter have proposed a sandwich technique in one single case. The patient was a young man, a mountain climbing enthusiast with a massive Hill–Sachs fracture with concomitant anterior labrum lesion without GBL. The deep and not greatly extended Hill–Sachs fracture was found by computed tomography (CT). The authors decided to treat this patient by labrum repair and remplissage technique. Because of the sporting activity of the patient, the authors decided to fill the defect previously with an iliac crest bone block and perform infraspinatus muscle tenodesis by a titanium anchor into the lesion filled by this graft (Fig. 24.6). The authors believed that previously fulfilling the defect by graft could minimize the risk of external rotation being decreased by a shortened tendon. After surgery, full stabilization of the joint was obtained. In the control CT, an adequate rebuild of graft was found, and the patient returned to full activity without limitation of arm range of motion. This technique requires confirmation of its effectiveness on a larger number of patients. However, it seems to be an interesting alternative for fresh-

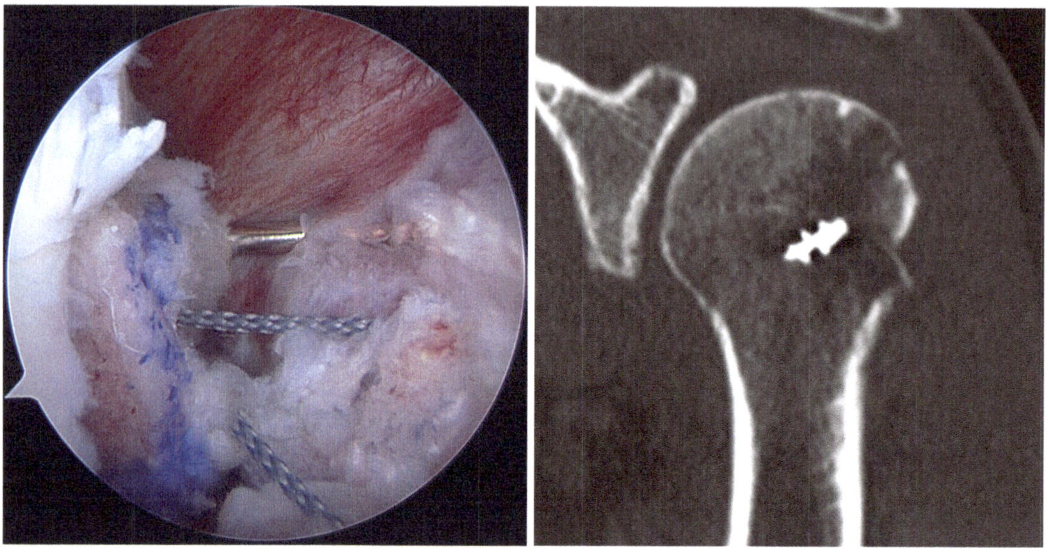

Fig. 24.6 Sandwich technique for deep Hill–Sachs lesion reconstruction

frozen allograft in cases of deep Hill–Sachs fractures. Another interesting and new possibility of management of a fresh and deep humeral head lesion is disimpaction. This new technique relies on elevating the impaction fracture and supporting it with bone graft, to allow the closest to native restoration of humeral head geometry without internal fixation [28]. Currently, there are few case series of patients treated by this method with any outcome.

24.5.3 Prosthesis and Resurfacing

Among humeral head surface replacement methods, complete or partial resurfacing can be distinguished. Partial reconstruction of the humeral head can be performed by metal implant (i.e., a humeral cap) in cases without an extended Hill–Sachs defect. Unfortunately, there are few reports in the literature of a large group of patients with long-term follow-up; only a few case series have been published so far with good short-term outcome after this method [29]. Taking under consideration that the shoulder is characterized by the greatest range of motion among all the joints, it seems that the nonanatomic covering of the humeral head with a metal cap can be a relevant risk factor of arthritis. Uncountable arm movements during the day means that any chondral replacement or chondral reconstructions methods in the shoulder are burdened with a much greater risk of failure compared to the knee, for example.

Complete humeral head resurfacing, called hemiarthroplasty, or total shoulder arthroplasty (TSA) are controversial methods of treatment in the deep Hill–Sachs lesion. First, the survival rates of TSA in younger patients are not as good as in older, less active patients. Cole et al. [30] reported survivorship of TSA in a group of young patients (33 patients with mean age of 46 years) to be as low as 61% at 10 years of follow-up, which supports joint-preserving techniques for deep Hill–Sachs lesion management for young active patients. Also, as there is a lack of clearly defined indications for such irreversible procedures, these should it be reserved for older or less active patients with widespread defects or with significant arthritis.

24.6 Reverse Hill–Sachs Management

Management of a reverse Hill–Sachs fracture in cases of chronic posterior shoulder instability similar to the typical deep lesion of the posterosuperior humeral head relies on filling the defect

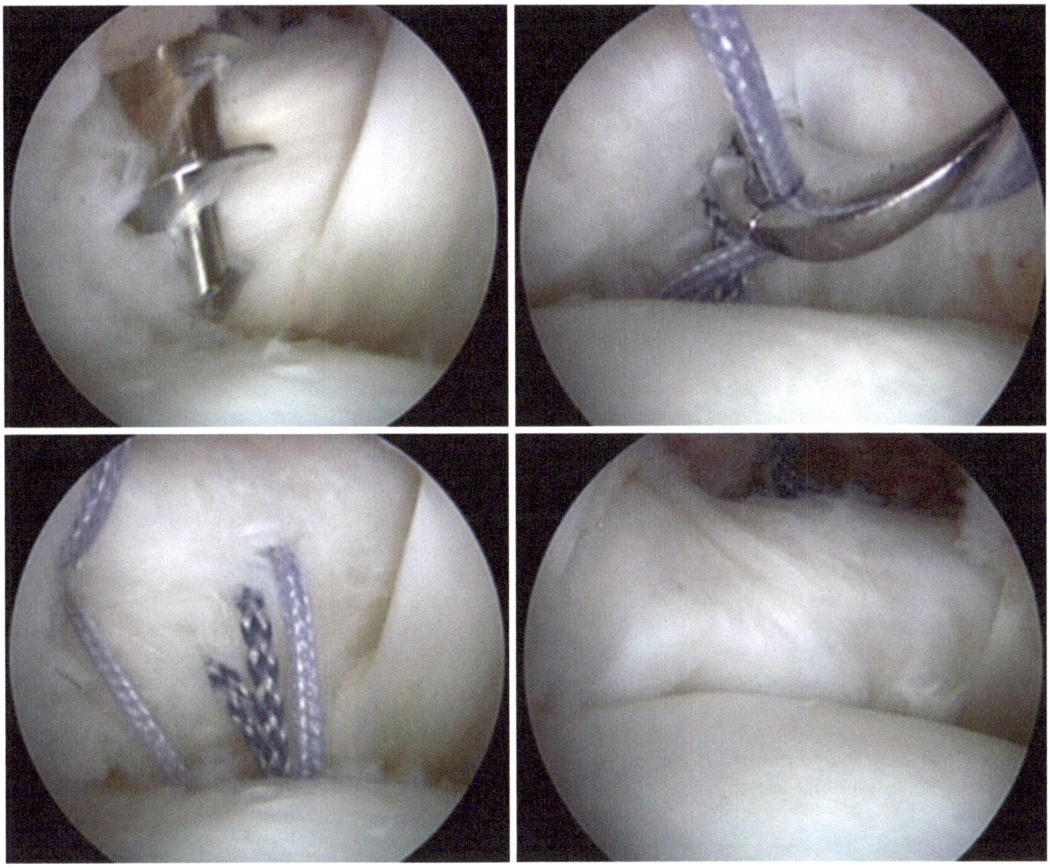

Fig. 24.7 McLaughlin procedure

by bone or tendon transfer. In contrast to a traditional Hill–Sachs fracture, lesions in the anterior part of humeral head typically are associated with wide cartilage injury and lead to shoulder joint arthritis [22].

The well-described and predictable procedure for treatment of reverse Hill–Sachs lesion is the McLaughlin procedure, which relies on tenodesis of the subscapularis muscle tendon into the humeral head lesion [31] (Fig. 24.7). Modification of the McLaughlin procedure involves lesser tuberosity transfer with footprint of the subscapularis tendon. That modification allows treatment of the larger lesions, but traditionally is burdened with restrictions of strength and range of internal rotation. An arthroscopic adaptation of the McLaughlin procedure was described by Krackhardt et al. [32] in a small case series without any serious complications.

Among bony procedures, fresh-frozen humeral head allografts are also useful. The first case report of successful treatment of a reverse, massive Hill–Sachs lesion by fresh-frozen graft was described by Gerber in 1994 [33].

References

1. Hill HA, Sachs MD. The grooved defect of the humeral head: a frequently unrecognized complication of dislocations of the shoulder joint. Radiology. 1940;35:690–700.
2. Burkhart SS, De Beer JF. Traumatic glenohumeral bone defects and their relationship to failure of arthroscopic Bankart repairs: significance of the inverted-pear glenoid and the humeral engaging Hill–Sachs lesion. Arthroscopy. 2000;16(7):677–94.
3. Yamamoto N, Itoi E, Abe H, et al. Contact between the glenoid and the humeral head in abduction, external rotation, and horizontal extension: a new

concept of glenoid track. J Shoulder Elbow Surg. 2007;16(5):649–56.
4. Di Giacomo G, Itoi E, Burkhart SS. Evolving concept of bipolar bone loss and the Hill–Sachs lesion: from "engaging/non-engaging" lesion to "on-track/off-track" lesion. Arthroscopy. 2014;30(1):90–8.
5. Taylor DC, Arciero RA. Pathologic changes associated with shoulder dislocations: arthroscopic and physical examination findings in first-time, traumatic anterior dislocations. Am J Sports Med. 1997;25(3):306–11.
6. Calandra JJ, Baker CL, Uribe J. The incidence of Hill–Sachs lesions in initial anterior shoulder dislocations. Arthroscopy. 1989;5(4):254–7.
7. Yiannakopoulos CK, Mataragas E, Antonogiannakis E. A comparison of the spectrum of intra-articular lesions in acute and chronic anterior shoulder instability. Arthroscopy. 2007;23(9):985–90.
8. Hovelius L. Anterior dislocation of the shoulder in teen-agers and young adults. J Bone Joint Surg. 1987;69A:393–9.
9. Saupe N, White LM, Bleakney R, et al. Acute traumatic posterior shoulder dislocation: MR findings. Radiology. 2008;248(1):185–93.
10. Griffith JF, Yung PS, Antonio GE, Tsang PH, Ahuja AT, Chan KM. CT compared with arthroscopy in quantifying glenoid bone loss. Am J Roentgenol. 2007;189(6):1490–3.
11. Kwon YW, Powell KA, Yum JK, Brems JJ, Iannotti JP. Use of three-dimensional computed tomography for the analysis of the glenoid anatomy. J Shoulder Elbow Surg. 2005;14(1):85–90.
12. Bokor DJ, O'Sullivan MD, Hazan GJ. Variability of measurement of glenoid version on computed tomography scan. J Shoulder Elbow Surg. 1999;8(6):595–8.
13. Gyftopoulos S, Yemin A, Mulholland T, et al. 3DMR osseous reconstructions of the shoulder using a gradient-echo based two-point Dixon reconstruction: a feasibility study. Skeletal Radiol. 2013;42(3):347–52.
14. Owens BD, Burns TC, Campbell SE, et al. Simple method of glenoid bone loss calculation using ipsilateral magnetic resonance imaging. Am J Sports Med. 2013;41:622–4.
15. Saliken DJ, Bornes TD, Bouliane MJ, Sheps DM, Beaupre LA. Imaging methods for quantifying glenoid and Hill–Sachs bone loss in traumatic instability of the shoulder: a scoping review. BMC Musculoskelet Disord. 2015;16:164.
16. Fox JA, Sanchez A, Zajac TJ, Provencher MT. Understanding the Hill–Sachs lesion in its role in patients with recurrent anterior shoulder instability. Curr Rev Musculoskelet Med. 2017;10(4):469–79.
17. Sekiya JK, Wickwire AC, Stehle JH, Debski RE. Hill–Sachs defects and repair using osteoarticular allograft transplantation: biomechanical analysis using a joint compression model. Am J Sports Med. 2009;37(12):2459–66. https://doi.org/10.1177/0363546509341576.
18. Rowe CR, Zarins B, Ciullo JV. Recurrent anterior dislocation of the shoulder after surgical repair: apparent causes of failure and treatment. J Bone Joint Surg Am. 1984;66(2):159–68.
19. Hall RH, Isaac F, Booth CR. Dislocations of the shoulder with special reference to accompanying small fractures. J Bone Joint Surg Am. 1959;41(3):489–94.
20. Franceschi F, Longo UG, Ruzzini L, Rizzello G, Maffulli N, Denaro V. Arthroscopic salvage of failed arthroscopic Bankart repair: a prospective study with a minimum follow-up of 4 years. Am J Sports Med. 2008;36(7):1330–6.
21. Flatow EL, Warner JI. Instability of the shoulder: complex problems and failed repairs. Part I. Relevant biomechanics, multidirectional instability, and severe glenoid loss. Instr Course Lect. 1998;47:9–112.
22. Frank RM. The Hill–Sachs lesion: diagnosis, classification, and management. J Am Acad Orthop Surg. 2012;20:242–52.
23. Wolf EM, Pollock ME, Smalley CC. Hill–Sachs "remplissage": an arthroscopic solution for the engaging Hill–Sachs lesion. Arthroscopy. 2007;23(6):e1–2.
24. Deutsch AA, Kroll DG. Decreased range of motion following arthroscopic remplissage. Orthopedics. 2008;31(5):492.
25. Shaha JS, Cook JB, Song DJ, Rowles DJ, Bottoni CR, Shaha SH, Tokish JM. Redefining "critical" bone loss in shoulder instability: functional outcomes worsen with "subcritical" bone loss. Am J Sports Med. 2015;43:1719–25. Epub 2015 Apr 16
26. Diklic ID, Ganic ZD, Blagojevic ZD, Nho SJ, Romeo AA. Treatment of locked chronic posterior dislocation of the shoulder by reconstruction of the defect in the humeral head with an allograft. J Bone Joint Surg Br. 2010;92(1):71–6.
27. Miniaci A, Gish MW. Management of anterior glenohumeral instability associated with large Hill–Sachs defects. Tech Shoulder Elbow Surg. 2004;5(3):170–5.
28. Kazel MD, Sekiya JK, Greene JA, Bruker CT. Percutaneous correction (humeroplasty) of humeral head defects (Hill–Sachs) associated with anterior shoulder instability: a cadaveric study. Arthroscopy. 2005;21(12):1473–8.
29. Bollier MJ, Arciero R. Management of glenoid and humeral bone loss. Sports Med Arthrosc. 2010;18(3):140–8.
30. Cole BJ, Yanke A, Provencher MT. Nonarthroplasty alternatives for the treatment of glenohumeral arthritis. J Shoulder Elbow Surg. 2007;16:S231–40.
31. McLaughlin H. Posterior dislocation of the shoulder. J Bone Joint Surg Am. 1952;24(3):584–90.
32. Krackhardt T, Schewe B, Albrecht D, et al. Arthroscopic fixation of the subscapularis tendon in the reverse Hill-Sachs lesion for traumatic unidirectional posterior dislocation of the shoulder. Arthroscopy. 22(2):227.el–227.e6.
33. Gerber C, Lambert SM. Allograft reconstruction of segmental defects of the humeral head for the treatment of chronic locked posterior dislocation of the shoulder. J Bone Joint Surg Am. 1996;78:376–82.

Part II

Posterior Shoulder Instability

25 History of Posterior Shoulder Instability

Shahbaz S. Malik, Sheraz S. Malik, Lennard Funk, and Peter B. MacDonald

25.1 Introduction

Posterior shoulder instability (PSI) is an uncommon disorder. The presenting clinical features can be vague, and its management remains challenging despite evolution of surgical treatment over decades. As the understanding of PSI aetiology and incidence has increased, so has the successful outcome of treatment. This chapter provides a summary of traditional and contemporary management options for the condition.

25.2 Posterior Shoulder Dislocation

Whereas the earliest written description of glenohumeral joint dislocation dates back to the ancient Egyptian era [1], White had reported the treatment of chronic posterior dislocations in 1741 [2] and later published a book in 1770 where he described reduction of the dislocation [3]. However, posterior shoulder dislocation (Fig. 25.1) first appeared in medical literature in 1822 [4]. Sir Astley Cooper

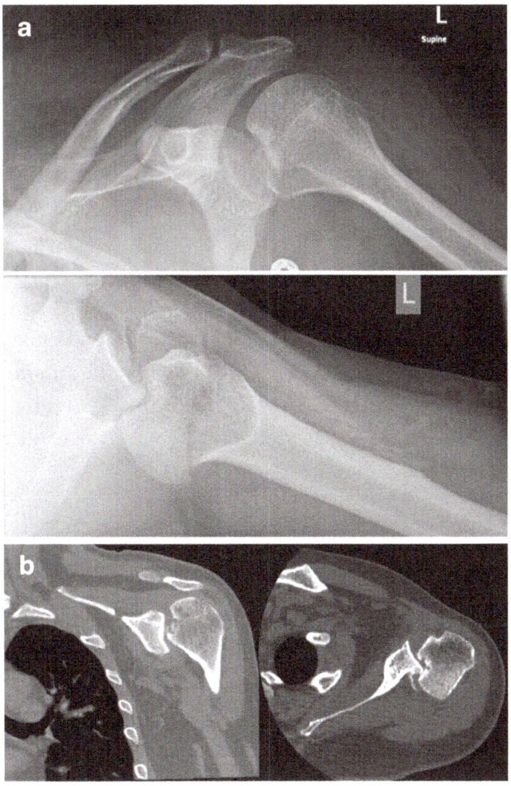

Fig. 25.1 (**a**) Radiographs of a locked posterior shoulder dislocation in 37-year-old male patient AP (top) and axillary view (bottom). Reverse Hill-Sachs lesion can be seen on both views. (Courtesy Jarret Woodmass, MD). (**b**) CT scan of patient in (**a**) showing locked posterior shoulder dislocation, coronal view (left) and axial view (right). (Courtesy Jarret Woodmass, MD)

S. S. Malik (✉) · P. B. MacDonald
Pan Am Clinic, University of Manitoba, Winnipeg, MB, Canada

S. S. Malik
Ashford and St Peters Hospitals NHS Foundation Trust, Chertsey, UK

L. Funk
Wrightington Hospital, Lancashire, UK

R. Brzóska et al. (eds.), *360° Around Shoulder Instability*,
https://doi.org/10.1007/978-3-662-61074-9_25

reported that a patient sustained a posterior shoulder dislocation from an epileptic seizure, which could not be reduced despite several attempts. A post-mortem performed some 7 years later revealed a detached subscapularis tendon and infraspinatus muscle stretched around the humeral head. The first case series of posterior shoulder dislocations was reported by Malgaignein in 1855. It consisted of 37 patients, with the diagnosis established clinically, as radiographs did not exist yet [5]. Souchon in 1898 published an account of 157 irreducible shoulder dislocations. There were 23 acute and 134 chronic dislocations, of which only 2 were dislocated backwards (posteriorly)—one acute and one chronic [6]. Both cases were managed with humeral head resection. At the time, operative treatment for irreducible dislocations, irrespective of anterior or posterior, carried significant mortality, due to various complications including haemorrhage, sepsis and pneumonia as well as tuberculosis and apoplexy.

The first detailed description of operative reduction for recurrent posterior shoulder dislocation appeared in 1907 [7]. The surgery was performed after 8 months of conservative treatment for recurrent dislocations. During the procedure, the biceps tendon was found dislocated over the centre of the glenoid.

25.3 Posterior Shoulder Instability

Posterior shoulder instability (PSI) was first described by Row and Yee in 1944 [8]. It is relatively uncommon, comprising approximately 10% of shoulder instability problems [9]. Acute posterior dislocation has an incidence of 1.1 per 100,000 person years [10]—this rate is almost 20 times less than the incidence of anterior shoulder dislocation [11, 12]. The terminology of PSI has traditionally been somewhat confusing and difficult because of the range of disorders covered by this term [13], i.e. traumatic/atraumatic, dislocations/subluxations or unidirectional/multidirectional. PSI could result from three types of pathologies: traumatic, atraumatic and cumulative microtrauma [14].

In *traumatic* PSI, an injury causes the shoulder to sublux or dislocate, and the instability persists after the acute episode. *Atraumatic* posterior dislocation is associated with generalised soft tissue laxity with no prior history of an injury. Patients report a sensation of instability in provocative positions and on doing higher demand activities [13].

PSI from *repetitive microtrauma* is observed in a sportsperson, especially those engaged in collision pursuits which load the shoulder from the front [14, 15]. Repetitive microtrauma results in a torn posterior labrum and stretching of the posterior band of the infra-glenohumeral ligament and is the most common cause of PSI. The labral detachment is termed reverse Bankart lesion. A Kim lesion (Fig. 25.2) occurs when there is a tear between the labrum and posterior glenoid cartilage but without complete detachment of the labrum [16]. These defects in the posterior inferior static stabilisers are caused by rim loading when the shoulder is placed in flexion, adduction and internal rotation. PSI develops as the glenoid becomes more retroverted and the labrum undergoes fatigue failure [17, 18]. Additionally, just as labral detachment with bony fragments anteriorly results in bony Bankart lesions, this may also occur at the posterior glenoid, producing a reverse bony Bankart lesion which predisposes patients to an even greater risk of instability [19].

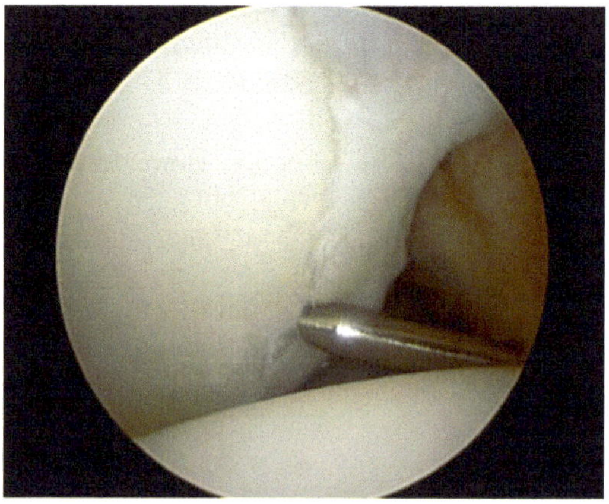

Fig. 25.2 Arthroscopic view of a Kim lesion. There is a tear between the labrum and posterior glenoid cartilage but without complete detachment of the labrum. (Courtesy Lennard Funk, MD)

25.4 Recurrent Posterior Shoulder Instability

Recurrent PSI is less common than anterior, but there is increasing incidence within the competitive athletic population. It can present with vague or non-specific symptoms, such as pain, discomfort, inability to perform certain actions and even recurrent subluxations [20]. In addition to the factors discussed earlier, PSI may also have an insidious onset, usually in athletes involved in throwing and sporting activities. This is seen in the pull through phase of swimming, follow through phase in golf, backhand shot in racket sports and baseball pitchers [21, 22]. These movements produce a gradual failure in the posterior capsule leading to laxity of capsule and passive stabilisers [22]. Other less common causes of recurrent PSI include epilepsy and electrocution or sporting activities such as riflery, archery or the use of a wheelchair, all of which involve a posterior directed vector force [23, 24].

25.5 Open Treatment

In the past, there has been an evolution of surgical techniques for addressing posterior shoulder instability. Current surgical intervention depends on the underlying pathology, i.e. whether it is soft tissue or a bony abnormality. The spectrum of operative procedures includes posterior bone block, soft tissue advancement, glenoid osteotomy and humerus derotation osteotomy.

25.5.1 Bone Block

25.5.1.1 Extracapsular

The use of a bone block to the posterior scapular neck was reported by Hidenbach in 1947 and subsequently by Jones in 1958 [25, 26]. The graft is attached outside the capsule so that it is a quarter to a third of an inch beyond the glenoid margin (Fig. 25.3). Both authors used an iliac crest autograft. The outcome in these two cases, as well as a later series, was reported to be successful, although complication of bone graft absorption leading to dislocation has also been documented [27–29]. Kouvalchouk et al. [30] were first to describe the use of acromial pediculated block with deltoid attached to the block in 1993. This was modified by Scapinelli [31] who suggested that inverting the posterior border of acromion would exert some pressure over the rotator cuff during PSI [32]. The results of early series using acromial bone block had found no recurrence [33]. In addition to the bone block procedure, further posterior capsulorrhaphy can be included as well [27].

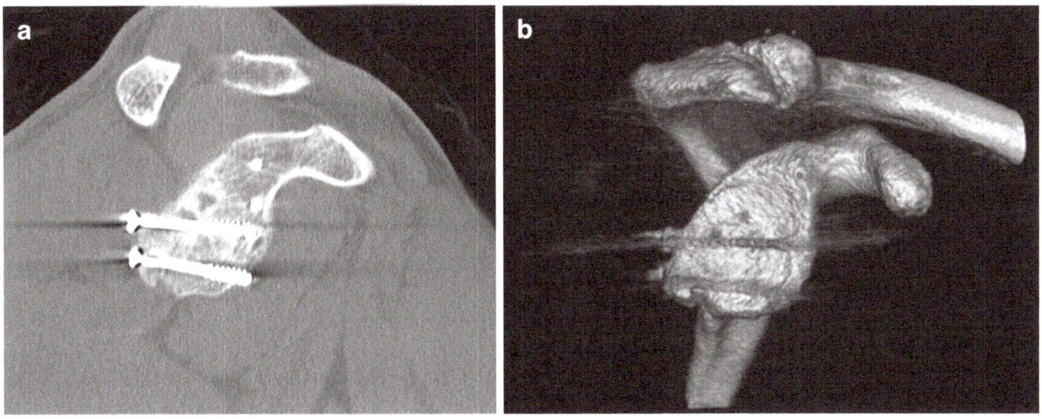

Fig. 25.3 (**a**) Sagittal view of CT scan of a patient who underwent a posterior bone augment procedure (Courtesy Lennard Funk, MD). (**b**) Three-dimensional CT scan of glenoid showing the posterior glenoid bone augment. (Courtesy Lennard Funk, MD)

25.5.1.2 Intracapsular

Over the last two decades, further novel techniques including arthroscopic bone block reconstruction have been developed [34, 35]. These utilise autograft and allografts to reconstruct posterior glenoid and include scapular spine [27, 36] or distal tibial allograft [37], distal clavicular autograft [34] and osteochondral glenoid allograft [38]. However, the rate of complications of recurrent instability and osteoarthritis is up to 36% [35, 39]. As such, focus has shifted to intracapsular techniques to address this issue with the use of distal tibial allograft for large posterior glenoid bone loss. Both Millet et al. [40] and Gupta et al. [37] published the technique using distal tibial allograft independently in 2013. Whilst Millet described an open approach, Gupta et al. described arthroscopic technique. In both reports, there was no recurrence of PSI.

25.5.2 Open Posterior Capsulorrhaphy

In 1980, Neer described the inferior capsular shift for treatment of PSI [41]. This technique eliminates the redundancy in the inferior capsule as the inferior flap is pulled superiorly and sutured to the superior capsular flap and to cuff of capsule on lateral humerus. Neer described this technique in patients with involuntary inferior and multidirectional subluxation and dislocation. Later studies reported of open posterior capsulorrhaphy in patients with PSI [42–44]. This procedure has also been combined with the posterior glenoid bone block procedure [27, 43, 45, 46]. The success rate of open posterior capsulorrhaphy is good to excellent in over 90% of cases [43, 44]. The outcome seems to be better in patients undergoing primary stabilisation than in those with previous surgeries. The rate of common complications has been reported up to 23% and includes post-operative stiffness and recurrence of instability [42, 43, 47].

Boyd and Sisk described a transfer of the long head of biceps tendon as a treatment for PSI. In this technique, the biceps tendon is transferred subdeltoid so it passes lateral to the humeral head and inserts on the posterior glenoid [48]. The authors reported no recurrence of PSI when this procedure was combined with posterior capsulorrhaphy. However, Hawkins found 33% recurrence of instability with the same procedure [49].

25.5.3 Glenoid Osteotomy

The aetiology of PSI is more commonly atraumatic than traumatic and usually as a consequence of generalised ligamentous laxity [21]. One of the risk factors in atraumatic recurrent PSI is developmental disruption of the glenohumeral anatomy, especially the shape of glenoid [50–52]. Studies have shown that patients with posterior instability have a higher incidence of a retroverted glenoid (Fig. 25.4) [53–55]. Furthermore, these patients often also have posterior instability of the contralateral shoulder [53].

For the retroverted glenoid, Scott, in 1967, described glenoplasty for attempted correction of glenoid version [56]. This involved an opening wedge osteotomy of scapular neck. Whilst Scott is acknowledged for the opening wedge glenoid osteotomy, Kretzler [57] 2 years earlier in 1965 reported the same procedure in patients with cere-

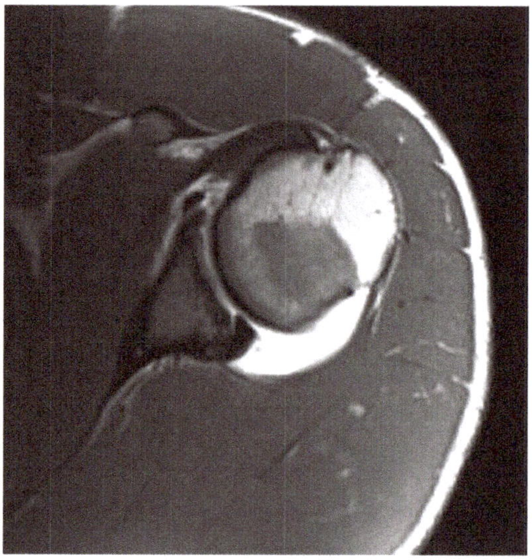

Fig. 25.4 MRI (axial) image showing a retroverted glenoid with chronic posterior chronic labral tear. (Courtesy Lennard Funk, MD)

bral palsy and PSI. Both, working independently, based their principles on acetabuloplasty for patients with developmental hip dysplasia. The outcome of no recurrent instability following glenoid osteotomy has been reported between 31 and 100% [54, 58–60]. Metcalf MH et al. reviewed 251 cases of glenoid osteotomy in the literature until 1999, of which post-operative stability was documented in 236 (94%) cases. At follow-up, 187 (79%) of patients reported a stable shoulder [52]. Graichen et al. reported one of the largest series which included 17 patients and found good or excellent results in 81% of patients although osteoarthritis was found in 25% of patients [61]. A more recent series of 12 patients in 2019 reported no recurrent dislocations, although one patient had signs of instability and four patients had glenoid neck fractures [62].

25.5.4 Proximal Humerus Derotational Osteotomy

The earliest report of humerus osteotomy was documented in 1974 by Chaudhuri and Saha [63]. They described rotation osteotomy of the shaft of humerus for both anterior and posterior recurrent dislocations of the shoulder. In their case series, only 1 of 16 cases had recurrent posterior dislocation. In all the cases, a transverse osteotomy of humerus was made. For recurrent anterior dislocation, the distal humeral fragment was rotated internally; for recurrent posterior dislocation, the distal fragment was rotated externally.

In 1990, Surin et al. described external rotational osteotomy (ERO) of humerus for patients with painful PSI [64]. This procedure was derived from the fact that patients could provoke instability by internal rotation of the arm. Therefore, performing ERO of the humeral head would restrict active internal rotation of the humeral head and contribute to stability. Successful outcome was achieved in ten (83%) patients. Only one patient had recurrence of instability, and one patient had a non-union of the osteotomy. ERO of proximal humerus has also been described for treatment of locked posterior dislocation [65, 66]. Keppler et al. [65] described the procedure in 1990 in a case series of ten patients with locked posterior dislocation with 20–40% reverse Hill-Sachs lesions. Only six (60%) patients had good to excellent outcome.

25.5.5 McLaughlin Procedure

In the mid-twentieth century, Harrison L. McLaughlin described the cause of recurrent posterior shoulder instability to be an anterior humeral bone defect (Fig. 25.1). This is known as the 'McLaughlin lesion' or otherwise as a 'reverse Hills-Sachs' defect [67]. The McLaughlin technique, described in 1952, involved reattachment of the subscapularis tendon in the defect with mattress sutures passed via holes drilled in the depth of the defect. A modification of this technique was described by Hawkins and Neer in 1987, in which the lesser tuberosity is osteotomised and used to fill the humeral head defect (Fig. 25.5) [68].

25.5.6 Reverse Putti-Platt Procedure

As a protege of Sir Harry Platt, Osmond-Clarke was the first to publish the Putti-Platt capsulorrhaphy in 1948 [69]. The reverse Putti-Platt procedure is an infraspinatus tenodesis to treat PSI originally described by Severin [70]. Whilst Severin shortened the infraspinatus, DePalma shortened both infraspinatus and teres minor together [71]. The procedure has been associated with high rate of recurrence [49, 72].

25.5.7 Reverse Bankart Procedure

One open soft tissue repair procedure is posterior Bankart repair, described by Rowe and Yee [8]. They noted posterior inferior labral detachment in two shoulders with posterior instability. The procedure involves securing the capsular flap with mattress sutures in drill holes placed through the glenoid rim to the medial bone. There have been few reports on the outcome of this procedure, but results have been satisfactory [49, 73].

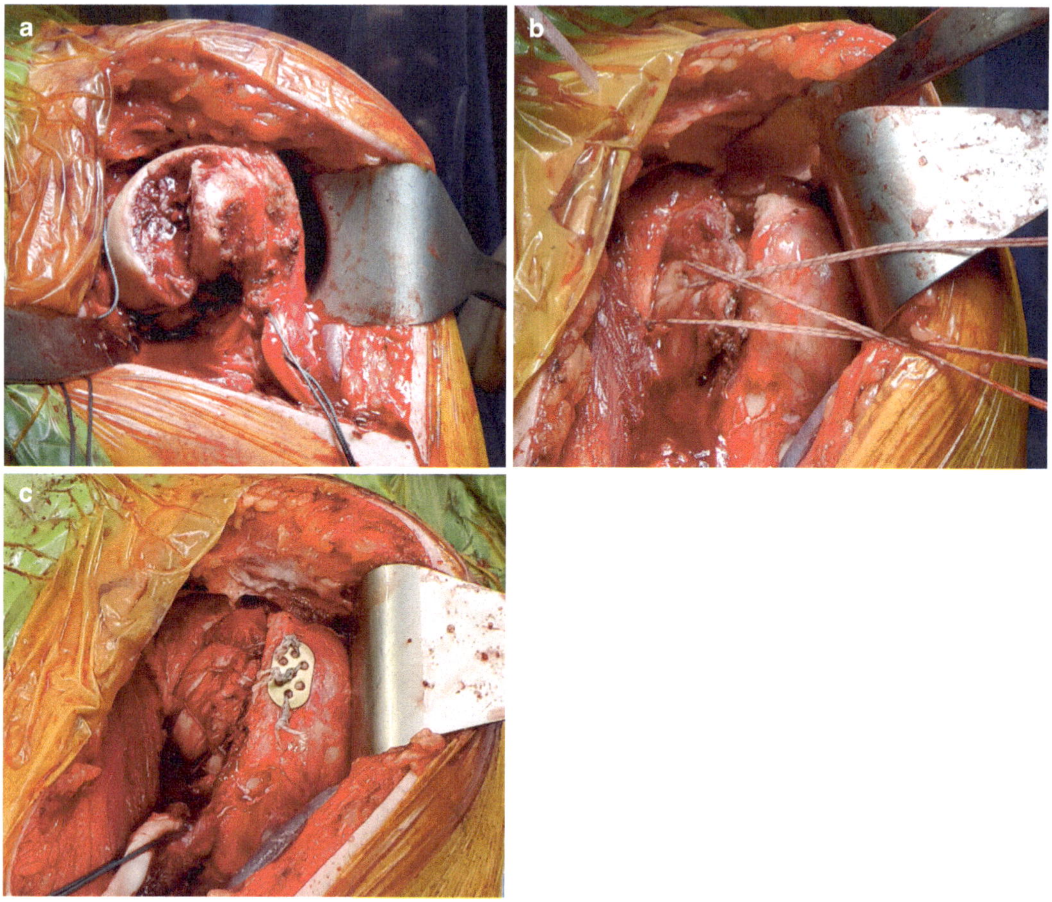

Fig. 25.5 (**a**) Intra-operative photo of patient in Fig. 25.1a showing the reverse Hill-Sachs defect after lesser tubercle osteotomy was performed (Courtesy Jarret Woodmass, MD). (**b**) Shows repair of osteotomy with No. 5 FiberWire (Arthrex, Inc., Naples, FL, USA) using a mattress backpack technique using a small metal plate as in (**c**). (Courtesy Jarret Woodmass, MD)

25.6 Arthroscopic Treatment

In the late twentieth century, the use of diagnostic arthroscopy in PSI had been described by some authors [74, 75]. Since then, treatment of recurrent PSI has shifted from open surgery to arthroscopic surgery with rapid technological advances. The modern arthroscopic techniques allow better assessment of pathology and direct minimally invasive treatment. Arthroscopy involves less dissection of tissue, with easier posterior capsulolabral complex access and identification of any concomitant intra-articular pathology.

Wolf presented outcomes of arthroscopic suture anchor techniques at the AANA annual meeting in 1996 [76], with 88% success rate. The success rate with bioabsorbable tracks in another study for traumatic posterior labral tears was greater than 90% [77]. McIntyre et al. [78] performed arthroscopic capsular shift with suture capsulorrhaphies for PSI. Their failure rate was 25%. Over the years, the outcome of arthroscopic management of PSI has continued to be good to excellent in 85–90% of patients [16, 79–81]. In the athletic population, the outcome of arthroscopic management of PSI has resulted in 90% of patients returning to their sport [79, 80]. A meta-analysis from 2015 looking at the clinical outcomes in the management of PSI found recurrence rate for patients undergoing open surgery to be more than double compared to arthroscopic surgery (19.4% vs. 8.1%, respectively) [20]. They concluded arthroscopic procedures are effective and reliable option in the treatment of unidirectional PSI. Furthermore, suture anchors instead of knotless techniques were associated with fewer recurrences [20].

A review evaluating modern arthroscopic techniques between 2003 and 2010 for treatment of PSI found a mean recurrence rate of 5.3%. The same review found the mean recurrence rate of open posterior capsular shift to be 15% for studies between 1989 and 2005 [82].

25.7 Conclusion

Our understanding of PSI has evolved in the last 100 years, with improved understanding of the aetiologies and pathologies. Operative treatment has similarly evolved from open bony procedures to arthroscopic procedures, resulting in overall low recurrence rates. Some open procedures have fallen out of favour over the years, whilst others continue to offer an option where bony abnormalities exist. As the number of patients with this condition is less than anterior, there are no compatible large series. Our understanding and treatments will continue to evolve, leading to improvements in outcomes for these patients.

References

1. Hussein MK. Kocher's method is 3,000 years old. J Bone Joint Surg Br. 1968;50:669–71.
2. Loebenberg MI, Cuomo F. The treatment of chronic anterior and posterior dislocations of the glenohumeral joint and associated articular surface defects. Orthop Clin North Am. 2000;31:23–34.
3. Tan CK, Guisasola I, Machani B, et al. Arthroscopic stabilization of the shoulder: a prospective randomized study of absorbable versus nonabsorbable suture anchors. Arthroscopy. 2006;22:716–20. https://doi.org/10.1016/j.arthro.2006.03.017.
4. Cooper A. A treatise on dislocations and fractures of the joints. London: Longman, Hurst, Rees, Orme and Brown; 1822.
5. Malgaigne J-F. Traité des fractures et des luxations. Baillière. 1847.
6. Souchon E. Operative treatment of irreducible dislocations of the shoulder joint, recent or old, simple or complicated. JAMA. 1898;XXX:1091. https://doi.org/10.1001/jama.1898.72440710023001f.
7. Sheldon JG. XIV. Old unreduced posterior dislocations of the shoulder. Ann Surg. 1907;46:623–7. https://doi.org/10.1097/00000658-190710000-00014.
8. Rowe CR, Yee LBK. A posterior approach to the shoulder joint. JBJS. 1944;26:580–4.
9. Owens BD, Duffey ML, Nelson BJ, et al. The incidence and characteristics of shoulder instability at the United States Military Academy. Am J Sports Med. 2007;35:1168–73. https://doi.org/10.1177/0363546506295179.
10. Robinson CM, Seah M, Akhtar MA. The epidemiology, risk of recurrence, and functional outcome after an acute traumatic posterior dislocation of the shoulder. J Bone Joint Surg Am. 2011;93:1605–13. https://doi.org/10.2106/JBJS.J.00973.
11. Zacchilli MA, Owens BD. Epidemiology of shoulder dislocations presenting to emergency departments in the United States. J Bone Joint Surg Am. 2010;92:542–9. https://doi.org/10.2106/JBJS.I.00450.
12. Simonet WT, Cofield RH. Prognosis in anterior shoulder dislocation. Am J Sports Med. 1984;12:19–24. https://doi.org/10.1177/036354658401200103.
13. Kovacic L, Funk L, Gleyze P. Posterior shoulder instability. In: Randelli P, Dejour D, van Dijk CN, et al., editors. Arthroscopy. Berlin: Springer; 2016. p. 483–98.
14. Provencher MT, Bhatia S, Ghodadra NS, et al. Recurrent shoulder instability: current concepts for evaluation and management of glenoid bone loss. J Bone Joint Surg Am. 2010;92(Suppl 2):133–51. https://doi.org/10.2106/JBJS.J.00906.
15. DeLong JM. Posterior shoulder instability in the athletic population: variations in assessment, clinical outcomes, and return to sport. World J Orthop. 2015;6:927. https://doi.org/10.5312/wjo.v6.i11.927.
16. Kim S-H, Ha K-I, Park J-H, et al. Arthroscopic posterior labral repair and capsular shift for traumatic unidirectional recurrent posterior subluxation of the shoulder. J Bone Joint Surg Am. 2003;85:1479–87. https://doi.org/10.2106/00004623-200308000-00008.
17. Kim S-H. Multidirectional instability of the shoulder—current concept. Sports Med Arthrosc Rehabil Ther Technol. 2009;1:12. https://doi.org/10.1186/1758-2555-1-12.
18. Kim S-H, Ha K-I, Yoo J-C, Noh K-C. Kim's lesion: an incomplete and concealed avulsion of the posteroinferior labrum in posterior or multidirectional posteroinferior instability of the shoulder. Arthroscopy. 2004;20:712–20. https://doi.org/10.1016/j.arthro.2004.06.012.
19. Owens BD, Campbell SE, Cameron KL. Risk factors for posterior shoulder instability in young athletes. Am J Sports Med. 2013;41:2645–9. https://doi.org/10.1177/0363546513501508.

20. DeLong JM, Jiang K, Bradley JP. Posterior instability of the shoulder: a systematic review and meta-analysis of clinical outcomes. Am J Sports Med. 2015;43:1805–17. https://doi.org/10.1177/0363546515577622.
21. Millett PJ, Clavert P, Hatch GFR, Warner JJP. Recurrent posterior shoulder instability. J Am Acad Orthop Surg. 2006;14:464–76.
22. Wanich T, Dines J, Dines D, et al. "Batter's shoulder": can athletes return to play at the same level after operative treatment? Clin Orthop. 2012;470:1565–70. https://doi.org/10.1007/s11999-012-2264-0.
23. Cho J-H, Chung N-S, Song H-K, Lee D-H. Recurrent posterior shoulder instability after rifle shooting. Orthopedics. 2012;35:e1677–9. https://doi.org/10.3928/01477447-20121023-32.
24. Fukuda H, Neer CS. Archer's shoulder. Recurrent posterior subluxation and dislocation of the shoulder in two archers. Orthopedics. 1988;11:171–4.
25. Hindenach JCR. Recurrent posterior dislocation of the shoulder. J Bone Joint Surg Am. 1947;29:582–6.
26. Jones V. Recurrent posterior dislocation of the shoulder; report of a case treated by posterior bone block. J Bone Joint Surg Br. 1958;40-B:203–7.
27. Fronek J, Warren RF, Bowen M. Posterior subluxation of the glenohumeral joint. J Bone Joint Surg Am. 1989;71:205–16.
28. Mowery CA, Garfin SR, Booth RE, Rothman RH. Recurrent posterior dislocation of the shoulder: treatment using a bone block. J Bone Joint Surg Am. 1985;67:777–81.
29. Fried A. Habitual posterior dislocation of the shoulder-joint; a report on five operated cases. Acta Orthop Scand. 1948;18:329–45. https://doi.org/10.3109/17453674908988979.
30. Kouvalchouk JF, Coudert X, Augouard LW, et al. Le traitement des instabilités postérieures de l'épaule par butée acromiale pédiculée à un lambeau deltoïdien. Rev Chir Orthop Réparatr Appar Mot. 1993;79:661–5.
31. Scapinelli R. Posterior addition acromioplasty in the treatment of recurrent posterior instability of the shoulder. J Shoulder Elb Surg. 2006;15:424–31. https://doi.org/10.1016/j.jse.2005.10.012.
32. DiMaria S, Bokshan SL, Nacca C, Owens B. History of surgical stabilization for posterior shoulder instability. JSES Open Access. 2019;3:350–6. https://doi.org/10.1016/j.jses.2019.08.008.
33. Sirveaux F, Leroux J, Roche O, et al. Surgical treatment of posterior instability of the shoulder joint using an iliac bone block or an acromial pediculated bone block: outcome in eighteen patients. Rev Chir Orthop Reparatrice Appar Mot. 2004;90:411–9.
34. Tokish JM, Fitzpatrick K, Cook JB, Mallon WJ. Arthroscopic distal clavicular autograft for treating shoulder instability with glenoid bone loss. Arthrosc Tech. 2014;3:e475–81.
35. Schwartz DG, Goebel S, Piper K, et al. Arthroscopic posterior bone block augmentation in posterior shoulder instability. J Shoulder Elb Surg. 2013;22:1092–101.
36. Struck M, Wellmann M, Becher C, et al. Results of an open posterior bone block procedure for recurrent posterior shoulder instability after a short- and long-time follow-up. Knee Surg Sports Traumatol Arthrosc. 2016;24:618–24. https://doi.org/10.1007/s00167-014-3495-2.
37. Gupta AK, Chalmers PN, Klosterman E, et al. Arthroscopic distal tibial allograft augmentation for posterior shoulder instability with glenoid bone loss. Arthrosc Tech. 2013;2:e405–11.
38. Petrera M, Veillette CJ, Taylor DW, et al. Use of fresh osteochondral glenoid allograft to treat posteroinferior bone loss in chronic posterior shoulder instability. Am J Orthop (Belle Mead NJ). 2013;42:78–82.
39. Meuffels DE, Schuit H, Van Biezen FC, et al. The posterior bone block procedure in posterior shoulder instability: a long-term follow-up study. J Bone Joint Surg Br. 2010;92:651–5.
40. Millett PJ, Schoenahl J-Y, Register B, et al. Reconstruction of posterior glenoid deficiency using distal tibial osteoarticular allograft. Knee Surg Sports Traumatol Arthrosc. 2013;21:445–9. https://doi.org/10.1007/s00167-012-2254-5.
41. Neer CS, Foster CR. Inferior capsular shift for involuntary inferior and multidirectional instability of the shoulder. A preliminary report. J Bone Joint Surg Am. 1980;62:897–908.
42. Bigliani LU, Pollock RG, McIlveen SJ, et al. Shift of the posteroinferior aspect of the capsule for recurrent posterior glenohumeral instability. J Bone Joint Surg Am. 1995;77:1011–20. https://doi.org/10.2106/00004623-199507000-00006.
43. Fuchs B, Jost B, Gerber C. Posterior-inferior capsular shift for the treatment of recurrent, voluntary posterior subluxation of the shoulder. JBJS. 2000;82:16–25.
44. Misamore GW, Facibene WA. Posterior capsulorrhaphy for the treatment of traumatic recurrent posterior subluxations of the shoulder in athletes. J Shoulder Elb Surg. 2000;9:403–8.
45. Bigliani LU, Endrizzi DP, McIlveon SJ. Operative management of posterior shoulder instability. Orthop Trans. 1989;13:232.
46. Ahlgren SA, Hedlund T, Nistor L. Idiopathic posterior instability of the shoulder joint. Results of operation with posterior bone graft. Acta Orthop Scand. 1978;49:600–3. https://doi.org/10.3109/17453677808993245.
47. Baumgarten KM, Altchek DW. Treatment options for recurrent posterior shoulder instability. Tech Shoulder Elb Surg. 2005;6:160–70.
48. Boyd HB, Sisk TD. Recurrent posterior dislocation of the shoulder. JBJS. 1972;54:779–86.
49. Hawkins RJ, Koppert G, Johnston G. Recurrent posterior instability (subluxation) of the shoulder. J Bone Joint Surg Am. 1984;66:169–74.
50. Lippitt SB, Vanderhooft JE, Harris SL, et al. Glenohumeral stability from concavity-compression: a quantitative analysis. J Shoulder Elb Surg. 1993;2:27–35. https://doi.org/10.1016/S1058-2746(09)80134-1.
51. Lazarus MD, Sidles JA, Harryman DT, Matsen FA. Effect of a chondral-labral defect on glenoid concavity and glenohumeral stability. A cadaveric model.

J Bone Joint Surg Am. 1996;78:94–102. https://doi.org/10.2106/00004623-199601000-00013.
52. Metcalf MH, Duckworth DG, Lee SB, et al. Posteroinferior glenoplasty can change glenoid shape and increase the mechanical stability of the shoulder. J Shoulder Elb Surg. 1999;8:205–13.
53. Gottschalk MB, Ghasem A, Todd D, et al. Posterior shoulder instability: does glenoid retroversion predict recurrence and contralateral instability? Arthroscopy. 2015;31:488–93. https://doi.org/10.1016/j.arthro.2014.10.009.
54. English E, Macnab I. Recurrent posterior dislocation of the shoulder. Can J Surg. 1974;17:147–51.
55. Brewer BJ, Wubben RC, Carrera GF. Excessive retroversion of the glenoid cavity. A cause of non-traumatic posterior instability of the shoulder. J Bone Joint Surg Am. 1986;68:724–31.
56. Scott DJ. Treatment of recurrent posterior dislocations of the shoulder by glenoplasty. Report of three cases. J Bone Joint Surg Am. 1967;49:471–6.
57. Kretzler HJ. Recurrent posterior dislocation of the shoulder in cerebral palsy. J Bone Joint Surg. 1966;48:1221.
58. Bestard EA. Glenoplasty: a simple, reliable method of correcting recurrent posterior dislocation of the shoulder. Orthop Rev. 1976;5:29–34.
59. Vegter, J, Marti, RK. Treatment of posterior dislocation of the shoulder by osteotomy of the neck of the scapula [abstract]. J Bone Joint Surg. 1981;63B:288.
60. Smith, KL, Seltzer, DG, Rockwood, CA Jr. Posterior glenoid osteotomy: complications and long-term follow-up. in: American Academy of Orthopedic Surgeons, New Orleans; 1994 Feb 26 (61st annual).
61. Graichen H, Koydl P, Zichner L. Effectiveness of glenoid osteotomy in atraumatic posterior instability of the shoulder associated with excessive retroversion and flatness of the glenoid. Int Orthop. 1999;23:95–9.
62. Lacheta L, Singh TSP, Hovsepian JM, et al. Posterior open wedge glenoid osteotomy provides reliable results in young patients with increased glenoid retroversion and posterior shoulder instability. Knee Surg Sports Traumatol Arthrosc. 2019;27:299–304. https://doi.org/10.1007/s00167-018-5223-9.
63. Chaudhuri GK, Sengupta A, Saha AK. Rotation osteotomy of the shaft of the humerus for recurrent dislocation of the shoulder: anterior and posterior. Acta Orthop Scand. 1974;45:193–8. https://doi.org/10.3109/17453677408989139.
64. Surin V, Blåder S, Markhede G, Sundholm K. Rotational osteotomy of the humerus for posterior instability of the shoulder. J Bone Joint Surg Am. 1990;72:181–6.
65. Keppler P, Holz U, Thielemann FW, Meinig R. Locked posterior dislocation of the shoulder: treatment using rotational osteotomy of the humerus. J Orthop Trauma. 1994;8:286–92. https://doi.org/10.1097/00005131-199408000-00003.
66. Ziran B, Nourbakhsh A. Proximal humerus derotational osteotomy for internal rotation instability after locked posterior shoulder dislocation: early experience in four patients. Patient Saf Surg. 2015;9:15. https://doi.org/10.1186/s13037-015-0062-9.
67. McLaughlin HL. Posterior dislocation of the shoulder. J Bone Joint Surg Am. 1952;24 A:584–90.
68. Hawkins RJ, Neer CS, Pianta RM, Mendoza FX. Locked posterior dislocation of the shoulder. J Bone Joint Surg Am. 1987;69:9–18.
69. Osmond-Clarke H. Habitual dislocation of the shoulder; the Putti-Platt operation. J Bone Joint Surg Br. 1948;30B:19–25.
70. Severin E. Anterior and posterior recurrent dislocation of the shoulder: the Putti-Platt operation. Acta Orthop Scand. 1953;23:14–22. https://doi.org/10.3109/17453675308991195.
71. DePalma AF. Unstable glenohumeral joint. In: Surgery of the shoulder. Philadelphia: Lippincott; 1983. p. 530–2.
72. Hurley JA, Anderson TE, Dear W, et al. Posterior shoulder instability: surgical versus conservative results with evaluation of glenoid version. Am J Sports Med. 1992;20:396–400.
73. Dugas RW, Scerpella TA, Clancy WG. Surgical treatment of symptomatic posterior shoulder instability. Orthop Trans. 1990;14:245.
74. Schwartz E, Warren RF, O'Brien SJ, Fronek J. Posterior shoulder instability. Orthop Clin North Am. 1987;18:409–19.
75. Tibone, JE, Bradley, JP. The treatment of posterior subluxation in athletes. Clin Orthop. 1993;291:124–137.
76. Wolf EM. Arthroscopic shoulder stabilization using suture anchors: technique and results. Paper presented at AANA Annual Meeting, April 11–14, 1996; Washington, D.C.
77. Mair SD, Zarzour RH, Speer KP. Posterior labral injury in contact athletes. Am J Sports Med. 1998;26:753–8. https://doi.org/10.1177/03635465980260060301.
78. McIntyre LF, Caspari RB, Savoie FH. The arthroscopic treatment of posterior shoulder instability: two-year results of a multiple suture technique. Arthroscopy. 1997;13:426–32. https://doi.org/10.1016/s0749-8063(97)90119-5.
79. Wolf EM, Eakin CL. Arthroscopic capsular plication for posterior shoulder instability. Arthroscopy. 1998;14:153–63. https://doi.org/10.1016/s0749-8063(98)70034-9.
80. Bradley JP, Baker CL, Kline AJ, et al. Arthroscopic capsulolabral reconstruction for posterior instability of the shoulder: a prospective study of 100 shoulders. Am J Sports Med. 2006;34:1061–71. https://doi.org/10.1177/0363546505285585.
81. Antoniou J, Duckworth DT, Harryman DT. Capsulolabral augmentation for the management of posteroinferior instability of the shoulder. J Bone Joint Surg Am. 2000;82:1220–30. https://doi.org/10.2106/00004623-200009000-00002.
82. Tjoumakaris FP, Bradley JP. The rationale for an arthroscopic approach to shoulder stabilization. Arthroscopy. 2011;27:1422–33. https://doi.org/10.1016/j.arthro.2011.06.006.

Influencing Factors of Posterior Instability

26

Robert Pełka and Wojciech Marek

Historically, the first description of a posterior dislocation and the manoeuvre was attributed to Hippocrates. Before the introduction of the medical radiology, Malgaigne described a series of 37 patients with posterior instability in 1855.

It is difficult to establish the prevalence of posterior instability because of the absence of clear criteria to diagnose it. However, it can be established in about 5% of all the patients with instability.

The affected patients are predominantly men between 20 and 30 years of age with high level of sports activity [1, 2].

The diagnosis of the posterior instability, in comparison with anterior and multidirectional instability, can be delayed or even highly eluded.

The simplest way to understand the problem may be application of a classification regarding its origin: traumatic (called in Moroder/Scheibel classification as 'first time') or atraumatic [3].

The atraumatic posterior instability appears in a more frequent way than the traumatic one and it is often observed in the context of a multidirectional instability by episodes of subluxations.

We can conclude that the posterior instability can be considered to be a syndrome in which the pathological processes are not completely clear and in which many predisposed factors can be influenced.

26.1 Wilfulness

Among the different predisposed factors, we emphasize:

Wilfulness—we define it as the demonstration of the aptitude to cause subluxations and dislocations under conscious control. It usually depends on psychiatric alterations [4, 5].

26.2 Position

Some patients present episodes of involuntary subluxation when their shoulders are situated in a position of flexion, adduction and internal rotation (Figs. 26.1). The shoulder can be relocated in a visible and sometimes audible form [6].

R. Pełka (✉) · W. Marek
NZOZ Ortopedia Opole/Głuchołazy, Opole, Poland

R. Brzóska et al. (eds.), *360° Around Shoulder Instability*,
https://doi.org/10.1007/978-3-662-61074-9_26

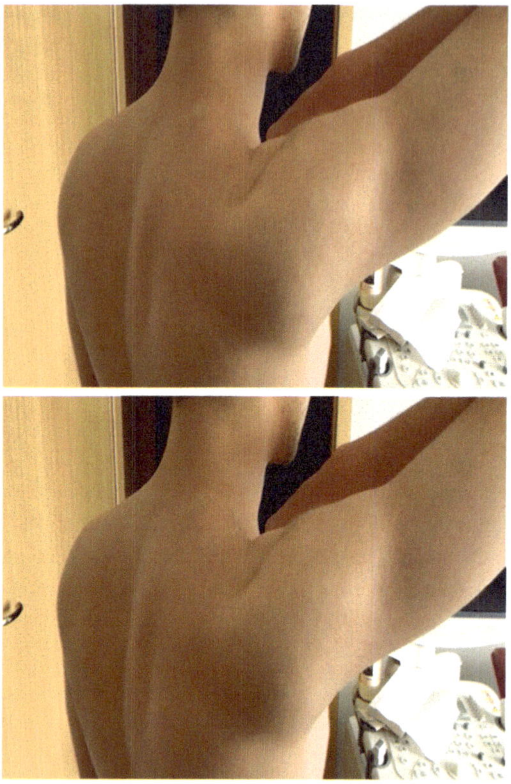

Fig. 26.1 Subluxation when shoulders are situated in a position of flexion

26.3 Muscular Alterations

This situation can admit exemplary mechanism: simple above-the-head position of the arm during sports activity, violent muscle contraction in case of neurological convulsion or electric shock (don't miss epileptic patients) and, for example, involuntary muscle contraction when the combination of the potency of internal rotators (latissimus dorsi, pectoralis major and subscapularis muscles) simply exceeds the potency of external rotators (infraspinatus and teres minor muscles) [7].

In patients with posterior instability, an existence of an alteration in the normal coordination of the glenohumeral and scapulothoracic rhythm can appear, but this theory is still little known [1].

The scapulothoracic dysfunction can be associated with fatigue of the serratus anterior, particularly in golf and swimming [8].

The most powerful element, which is opposed to the mechanism of posterior dislocation, is the subscapularis muscle, and its dysfunction can be an important influencing factor (Figs. 26.2) [9].

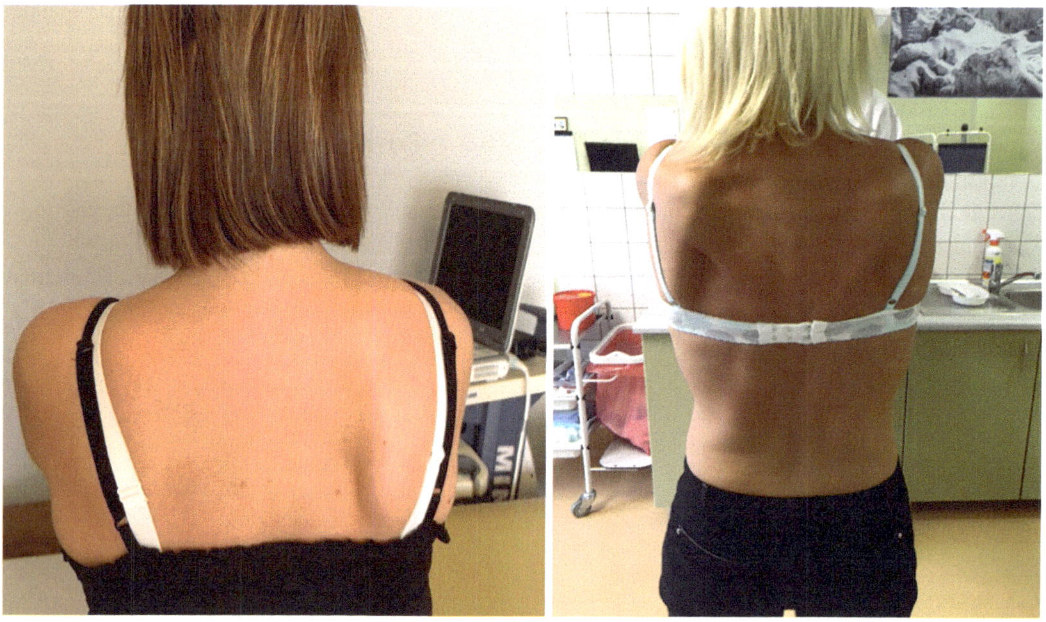

Fig. 26.2 The alteration in the normal coordination of the glenohumeral and scapulothoracic rythm

26.4 Injuries

Injuries with high energy cause complete dislocations, but first of all repetitive microtraumas can develop alterations from subluxation episodes to true dislocations (Fig. 26.3).

26.5 Sports Activity

High-level sports activity, typical movement of the arm over the head in swimming, golf, launching and contact sports create higher risk of suffering from this type of pathology [10, 11].

26.6 Soft Tissue Changes and Their Effects

The posterior joint capsule and the posterior band of the inferior glenohumeral ligament are structures involved in the posterior shoulder stability. The posterior labrum is anatomically different than the anterior, but plays a more important role by increasing the congruence of the joint (Fig. 26.4).

The interval rotator is also related to the phenomena of the posterior–inferior displacement of the humeral head (it is usually a concomitant pathology) [12, 13].

Successive subluxations can possibly cause a plastic deformation of the capsule.

Besides, other injuries can be associated with the posterior glenohumeral instability, such as the humeral avulsion of the posterior glenohumeral ligament injuries, posterior labrocapsular periosteal sleeve avulsion lesions or a Reverse Bony Bankart (Fig. 26.5) [14–16].

26.7 Bone Changes

The posterior instability can be caused by the increased glenoid retroversion, the hypoplasia of the postero-inferior glenoid or an increased humeral head retrotorsion (Fig. 26.6) [17, 18].

The previously originated bony leasions after the first subluxation or dislocation are erosion in the posterior glenoid and anterior humeral head bony defects called Reverse Hill–Sachs or McLaughlin sign are also secondary predisposed factors of posterior instability (Figs. 26.7) [19].

Calvo, Terol and Zurita elaborated in 2010 for ESSKA Upper Limb Committee a classification including all known influencing anatomical and functional factors and their complicated relations [20].

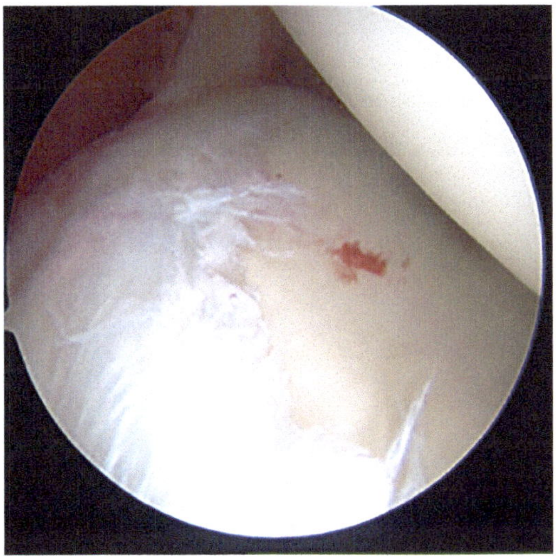

Fig. 26.3 Posterior labrum microtrauma lesions

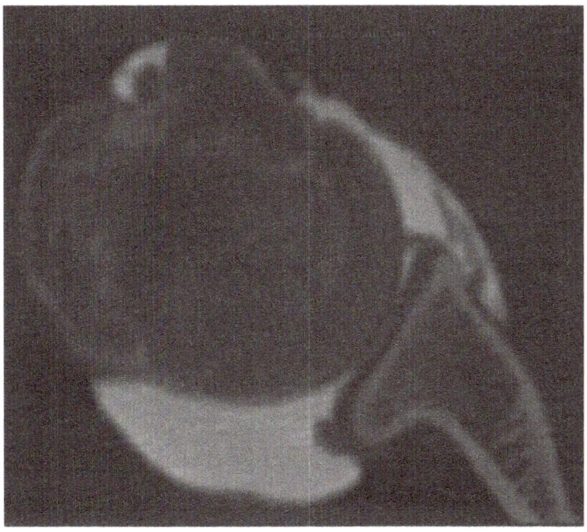

Fig. 26.4 The increased capacity of shoulder joint as a factor of posterior instability

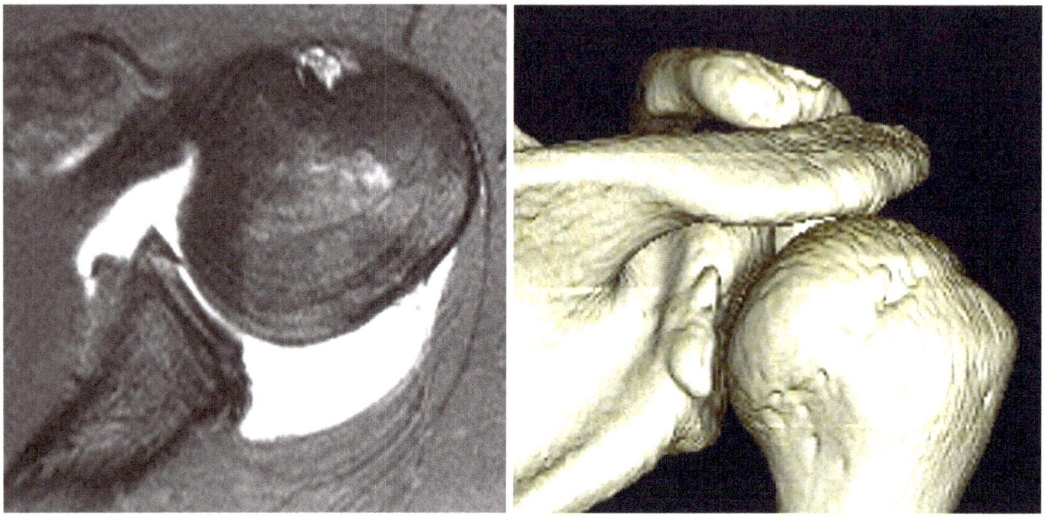

Fig. 26.5 The plastic deformation of the capsule and Reversed Bony Bankart lesion

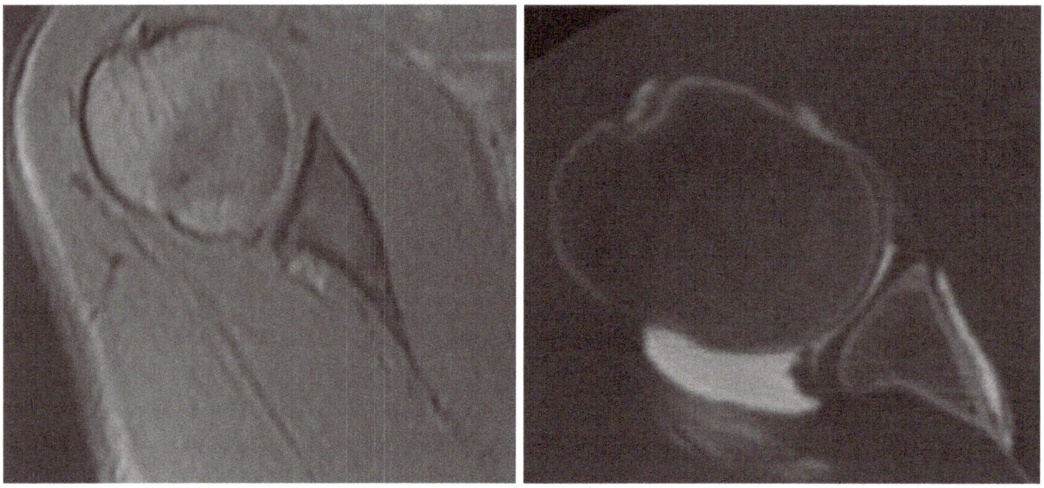

Fig. 26.6 The increased glenoid retroversion and the hypoplasia of the postero-inferior glenoid

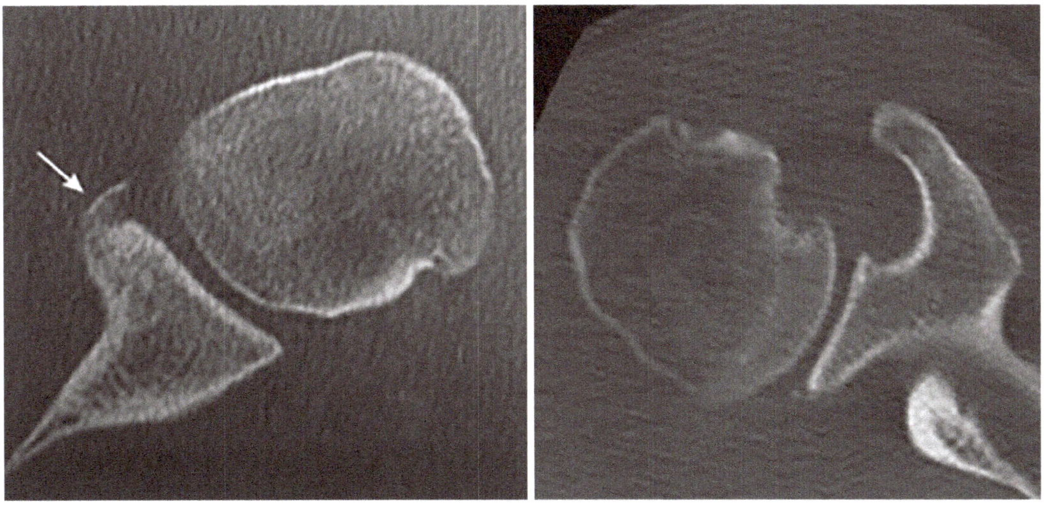

Fig. 26.7 The anterior humeral head bony defect (Reverse Hill-Sachs's/McLaughlin's lesion) and the erosion in the posteriori glenoid

26.8 Conclusions

The posterior shoulder instability can be caused by many predisposed and influencing factors coming out of wilfulness, anatomical changes in a soft tissue or bone, alterations in functional patterns, types of injury and sports activity and secondary changes in shoulder structures.

Many patients with posterior instability in fact have a multidirectional instability, but their symptoms refer principally to the posterior direction.

The orientation and the shape of the glenoid cavity are fundamental in interpreting the posterior shoulder instabilities, especially atraumatic ones.

Many of the influencing factors are still not well known and need further research.

References

1. Robinson CM, Aderinto J. Recurrent posterior shoulder instability. J Bone Joint Surg Am. 2005;87:883–92.
2. Wolf EM, Eakin CL. Arthroscopic capsular application for posterior shoulder instability. Arthroscopy. 1998;14:153–63.
3. Moroder P, Scheibel M. ABC classification of posterior shoulder instability. Obere Extrem. 2017;12(2):66–74.
4. McFarland EG. Voluntary glenohumeral instability. In: Jobe FW, editor. Operative techniques in upper extremity sports injuries. St. Louis: Mosby-Year Book; 1996. p. 285–94.
5. Ramsay ML, Klimkiewicz JJ. Posterior instability: diagnosis and management. In: Iannotti JP, Williams GR, editors. Disorders of the shoulder: diagnosis and management. Philadelphia: Lippincott Williams and Wilkins; 1999. p. 295–319.
6. Hawkins RJ, Belle RM. Posterior instability of the shoulder. Instr Course Lect. 1989;38:211–5.
7. Kao JT, Pink M, Jobe FW, Perry J. Electromyographic analysis of the scapular muscles during a golf swing. Am J Sports Med. 1995;23:19–23.
8. Hovis WD, Dean MT, Mallon WJ, Hawkins RJ. Posterior instability of the shoulder with secondary impingement in elite golfers. Am J Sports Med. 2002;30:886–90.
9. Pollock RG, Bigliani LU. Recurrent posterior shoulder instability. Diagnosis and treatment. Clin Orthop. 1993;291:85–96.
10. Jobe FW, Tibone JE, Pink MM, Jobe CM, Kvitne RS. The shoulder in sports. In: Rockwood Jr CA, Matsen 3rd FA, editors. The shoulder. 2nd ed. Philadelphia: WB Saunders; 2004. p. 1214–38.
11. McFarland EG, Campbell G, McDowell J. Posterior shoulder laxity in asymptomatic athletes. Am J Sports Med. 1996;24:468–71.
12. Harryman DT, Sidles JA, Harris SL, et al. The role of the rotator interval capsule in passive motion and stability of the shoulder. J Bone Joint Surg Am. 1992;74:53–66.
13. Robinson M, Akhtar A, Mitchell M, et al. Complex posterior fracture-dislocation of the shoulder, epidemiology, injury patterns and results of operative treatment. J Bone Joint Surg Am. 2007;89:1454–66.

14. Abrams JS. Arthroscopic repair of posterior instability and reverse humeral ligament avulsion lesions. Orthop Clin North Am. 2003;34:475–83.
15. Weinberg J, McFarland EG. Posterior capsular avulsion in a college football player. Am J Sports Med. 1999;27:235–7.
16. Yu JS, Ashman CJ, Jones G. The POLPSA lesion: MR imaging findings with arthroscopic correlation in patients with posterior instability. Skelet Radiol. 2002;31:396–9.
17. Wirth MA, Lyuons FR, Rockwood CA Jr. Hypoplasia of the glenoid. A review of sixteen patients. J Bone Joint Surg Am. 1993;75:1175–84.
18. Wirth MA, Seitzer DG, Rockwood CA Jr. Recurrent posterior glenohumeral dislocation associated with increased retroversion of the glenoid. A case report. Clin Orthop. 1994;308:98–101.
19. Sanders TG, Morrison WB, Miller MD. Imaging techniques for the evaluation of glenohumeral instability. Am J Sports Med. 2000;28:414–34.
20. Calvo A, Terol P, Zurita N. Shoulder instability. Posterior Instability: Clinical evaluation and treatment. ESSKA Upper Limb Committee; 2010. p. 87–108.

27 Traumatic Versus Voluntary Posterior Instability: Diagnostic Process

Antoon Van Raebroeckx

27.1 Introduction

The big challenge in the diagnostic process for posterior instability is in determining if the posterior findings are or will be responsible for the clinical presentation or complaints of the patient. In traumatic posterior instability, the key to diagnosis will be to judge if the lesion will cause problems in the future. In voluntary posterior instability, the main goal will be to look for the main reason for the instability. In both settings, we have to evaluate the history of the injury, the clinical and technical findings and the type of patient with a different purpose.

27.2 Traumatic Posterior Instability

In the acute setting, a posterior shoulder dislocation is one of the most missed pathologies at the emergency department. The history of a direct shoulder trauma with anterior impact should trigger the possibility of a posterior dislocation as well as shoulder pain after an epileptic insult. In most cases, the patient presents with the hand on the belly. Clinical neurological investigation must rule out any nerve injuries. The absence of active and passive external rotation is the most significant sign during the first clinical examination.

The diagnosis can be confirmed on a standard X-ray but should be followed by a computed tomography (CT) scan. The main reason for the immediate scan is not to miss a fracture dislocation before reduction manoeuvres are performed. On this scan, the risk for future instability or recurrence can be judged by the bony lesion of the dislocation on the glenoid and humeral side.

In case 1, the proper diagnosis was made by clinical investigation, confirmed on X-ray and CT scan.

A. Van Raebroeckx (✉)
Orthopaedic Department, Shoulder Unit, AZ Nikolaas Hospital, Sint Niklaas, Belgium

R. Brzóska et al. (eds.), *360° Around Shoulder Instability*,
https://doi.org/10.1007/978-3-662-61074-9_27

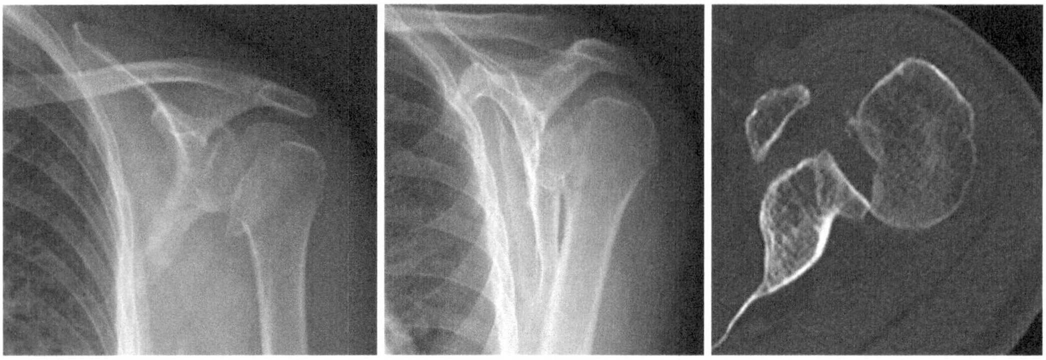

In case 2, the dislocation was missed due to an improper clinical investigation and X-rays. Only 3 days later in the outpatient clinic after correct clinical examination with a fixed internal rotation, a CT scan confirmed the diagnosis.

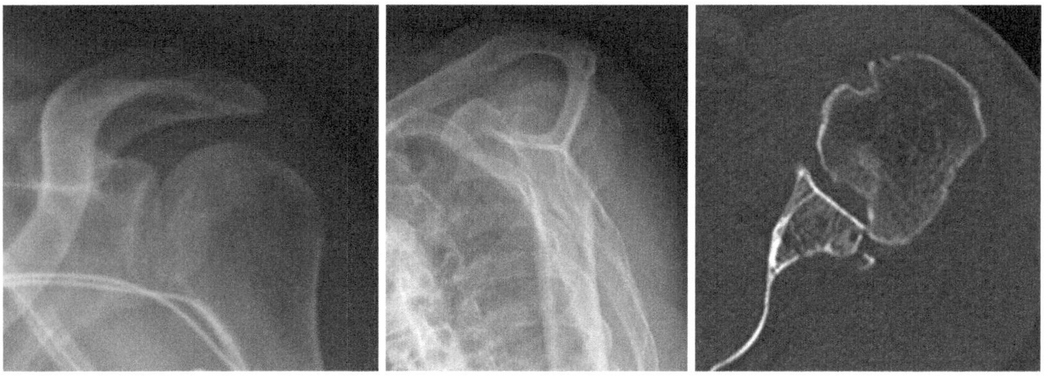

In the traumatic setting, the clinical suspicion of a posterior shoulder dislocation should always be confirmed by X-ray and CT scan. The diagnostic setup will serve to determine if the lesions will be a problem after the reduction on longer term.

In case 3, no dislocation was diagnosed but the CT scan showed a posterior fracture of the glenoid.

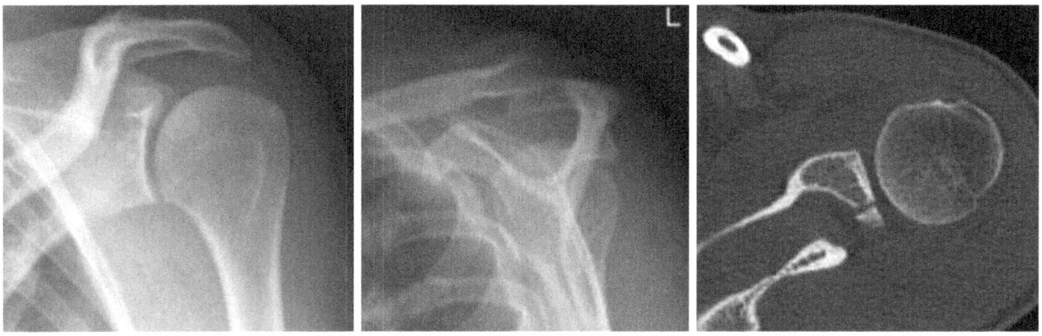

In case 4, no CT scan was made and a fracture dislocation was missed before reduction with disastrous consequences.

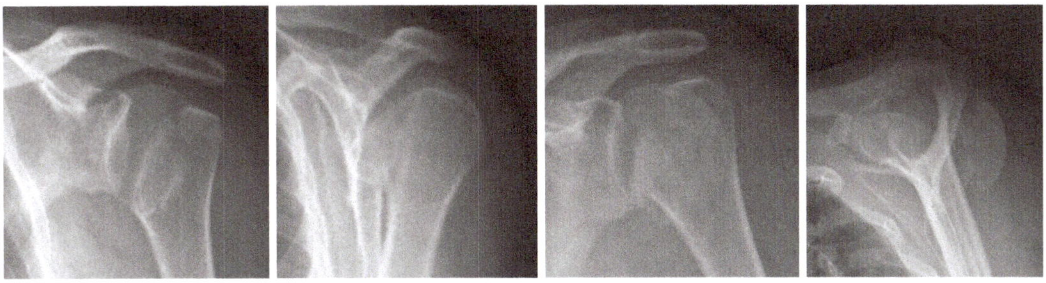

27.3 Voluntary Posterior Dislocation

The history of a voluntary posterior instability is completely different. These patients are seen at the outpatient clinic with a long story of shoulder problems starting mostly during childhood.

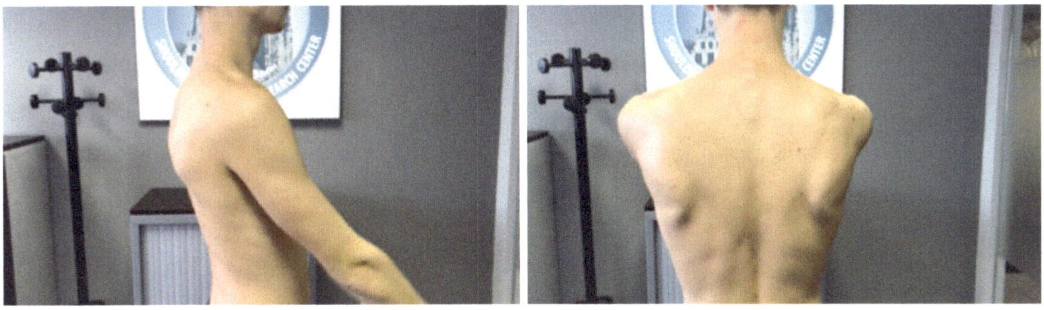

In many cases, patients will demonstrate the instability by a certain manoeuvre with a very bad dyskinesia. It is not uncommon that with anterior elevation palm down, the shoulder dislocates automatically and that the manoeuvre that the patient does is a voluntary relocation and not a dislocation.

Most of the time, if the patient focuses well or with some help from the investigator stabilizing the scapula, he or she will be able to show a normal scapulothoracic kinesia. It is up to the investigator to assess the psychological impact or mental status of the patient. At younger age, a psychological testing may be necessary if the dislocation becomes disabling. The most difficult situation is the voluntary dislocator who becomes really unstable at later age.

The classical sulcus sign and a positive Gagey test indicate an increased laxity. A general laxity will make the diagnosis of isolated posterior instability more difficult.

A posterior drawer test, posterior stress test and jerk test may confirm the posterior aspect of the problem. Apprehension during resistance in a 90° anterior elevation position palm down indicates a posterior instability.

27.4 Technical Investigations

The technical investigations may show the impact that the posterior instability has had on the posterior structures. A standard X-ray will show any congenital deformities. An arthro-CT or arthro-MRI (magnetic resonance imaging) will show the pathology of the posterior labrum with or without bony deficiencies. The patients history will help to differentiate between acute and chronic labrum lesions. This differentiation is mostly important as both pathologies needs different approaches in treatment. A reversed Hill–Sachs lesion may be present. Retroversion of the glenoid and translation of the humeral head can be judged on a standard CT- or MR-scan.

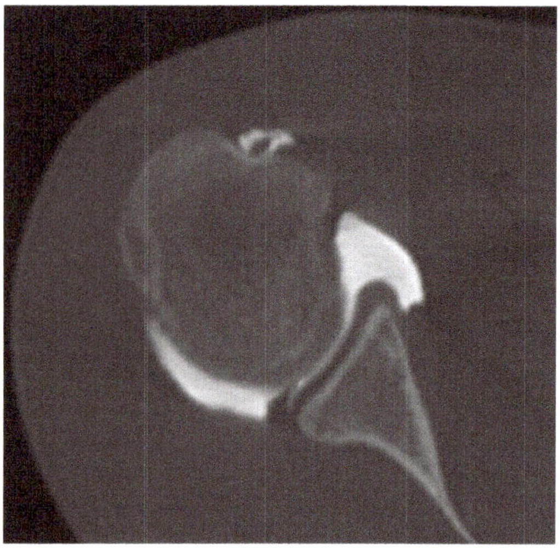

Posterior labrum lesion

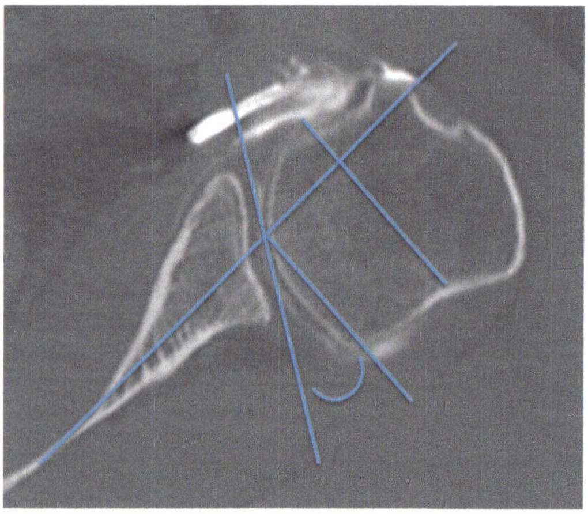

A congenital dysplastic glenoid as well as a static posterior subluxation may be pre-existing and the angulation can be measured.

To complete the diagnostic setup, an isokinetic shoulder measurement may be performed to judge the possibility of improving the scapulothoracic movement and the muscle balance. Insufficient control over the scapula may be corrected by proper rehabilitation if the weak muscle link is detected and there is space for improvement compared with the contralateral side or with the general population.

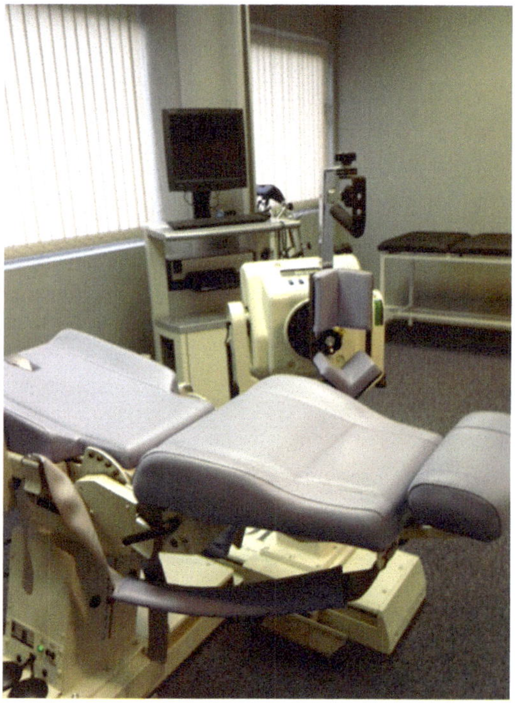

Isokinec Biodex 3 at our institution

In this chronic setting, the diagnostic setup will serve to see if the anatomic problems or the neuromuscular dyskinesia are the most important factors and to determine if the problem can be solved dynamically or surgically.

These days, a diagnostic arthroscopy is rare but still may add some information. The lesions will be confirmed but most of the time the arthroscopy is part of the treatment and not the diagnostic setup.

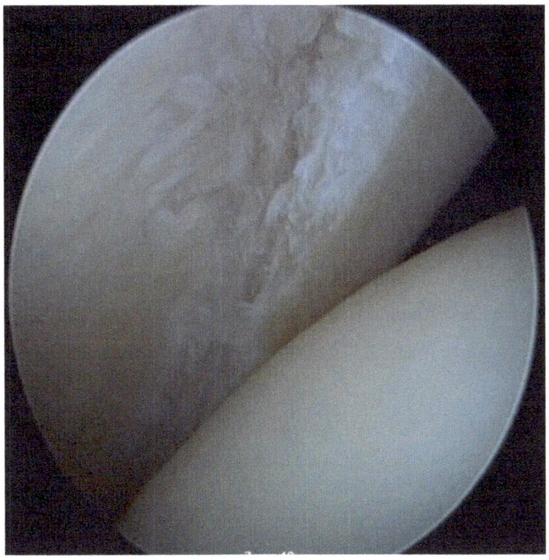

Posterior labrum lesion

27.5 Conclusion

In the acute posttraumatic posterior instability, X-ray and CT investigation will complete the history and clinical investigation. The purpose of the diagnostic setup is to determine if the anatomic injuries will be a problem in the short- and long term.

In the voluntary diagnostic setup, the goal is to determine the main underlying problem for the instability. History, clinical examination and arthro-scan will try do differentiate between psychology, dyskinesia problems, hyperlaxity, or the combination with anatomic lesions. If lesions are diagnosed, an isokinetic measurement of the shoulder muscles may help to judge the impact of the muscle imbalance and motivate the patient to go for a non-operative rehabilitation treatment. We should be aware that posterior labrum lesion on technical investigations might be of degenerative nature and not take them for acute lesions. Repairing a degenerative lesion posterior in the shoulder will lead to faster degeneration of the joint and needs to be avoided at any time.

Posterior Shoulder Instability and Sport Activities

28

Ladislav Kovačič and Benjamin Marjanovič

28.1 Introduction

Because of the lack of bony constraints, the shoulder is one of the most mobile and therefore one of the most vulnerable joints of our body. Static stabilizers such as bone constraints, the glenoid labrum, the glenohumeral ligaments, and negative intraarticular pressure are very important. Strong dynamic stabilizers, such as the rotator cuff and other muscular structures around the shoulder, provide additional stability. However, the high range of joint mobility frequently results in instability events, especially in the sports-active population. Shoulder dislocations as traumatic events represent up to 45% of all the dislocations in the human body [1]. Of all shoulder dislocations, those posterior are very rare, occurring in less than 10% [2, 3]. Besides traumatic posterior dislocations, a variety of pathological conditions have been recognized in the setting of posterior shoulder instability. In addition to traumatic events, repetitive microtraumas and atraumatic lesions in ligamentous laxity might be the cause of this condition. Complete dislocation does not always occur, and the signs of instability are often non-specific. Patients might present with a variety of symptoms. Frequently, generalized pain and pain in the posterior part of the shoulder is the main symptom of posterior shoulder instability, especially with the arm in posterior apprehension position.

Extreme range of motion (ROM), an extreme force generated in the shoulder joint, and excessive repetitions are the reasons for injuries and disorders in the athlete's shoulder. It is documented that more than 40% of elite athletes experience shoulder pain at least at some point of their career [4–6]. Shoulder pain is frequently the sign of overuse injury and decompensated shoulder function. Sometimes, the pain is caused by functional muscle disbalance, but more often it is the result of an advanced shoulder disorder with a underlying structural lesion. In the athletic population, shoulder structures are especially at risk in contact and overhead sports (Table 28.1). Posterior instability in this setting is discussed further here.

L. Kovačič (✉)
Department of Traumatology, University Medical Centre Ljubljana, Ljubljana, Slovenia

B. Marjanovič
Orthopedic Hospital Valdoltra, Ankaran, Slovenia
e-mail: benjamin.marjanovic@ob-valdoltra.si

Table 28.1 Characteristics of posterior shoulder instability in athletes regarding the sports specifics

Contact sport	Overhead sport
Traumatic event	Microinstability
Low number of true dislocations	Repetitive shear stresses
High number of subluxations	No complaint of subluxation or instability
Underlying posterior labral tear	Excessive translation and rotation cause pain

R. Brzóska et al. (eds.), *360° Around Shoulder Instability*,
https://doi.org/10.1007/978-3-662-61074-9_28

28.2 Contact Athletes

Posterior instability in contact and collision athletes is usually the result of overload to the posterior part of the shoulder joint with the arm position in 90° of forward elevation, adduction, and internal rotation [7, 8]. It might be caused by a single traumatic event or even repetitive microtrauma. Force applied in the posterior direction leads to injury of the posterior shoulder restraints, which are the posterior capsule, labrum, and the shape and orientation of the glenoid cavity.

Static stabilizers of the posterior part of the shoulder differ considerably from those of the anterior part. In contrast to the thick ligamentous composition of the anterior structures, the posterior capsule is relatively thin. Ligamentous components are not so well defined [9]. Posterior thickening of the capsule contains the posterior band of the inferior glenohumeral ligament (PIGHL), which is the main restraint in posterior loading position [10].

28.2.1 Traumatic Origin

In some contact sports, the posterior instability frequently has a traumatic origin. Patients might experience true dislocation or only a subluxation. The traumatic event is sometimes minor with low energy. We have to be aware that even true posterior shoulder dislocation is frequently misdiagnosed. The proper assessment of the injured patient is crucial. Pain, restricted external rotation, and deformation in the shoulder region with flattening of the anterior part should raise suspicion for that injury (Fig. 28.1).

Glenoid detachment of the posterior labrum together with its articular capsule and the PIGHL (posterior Bankart lesion) is the typical presentation after posterior glenohumeral dislocation. Corresponding to this, a reversed Hill–Sachs lesion is frequently found on the anterior part of the humeral head. As a consequence, patients after such an injury may develop recurrent episodes of posterior dislocations. Less frequently, pathological changes such as posterior bony Bankart lesion, reverse humeral avulsion of the glenohumeral ligament (RHAGL), and mid-capsule tear can be present [11].

28.2.2 Repetitive Microtraumas and Injury of the Posterior Capsulolabral Complex

Repetitive microtrauma of the posterior shoulder complex is the most frequent cause of posterior shoulder instability. When patients are involved in sports activities with loading of the shoulder in front of the body, the shoulder is placed in flexion, adduction, and internal rotation. Posterior loading on the structures results in the injury to the posterior shoulder static restraints.

The importance of the posterior labrum as a static stabilizer in the posterior direction has been neglected in the past. Progress in arthroscopic surgery has revealed the importance of identifying and treating posterior labral lesions. The so-called Kim lesion, an isolated posteroinferior labral lesion, is an incomplete and concealed avulsion of the posteroinferior labrum [12, 13]. Arthroscopically, this condition is associated with an apparently small dissociation of articular cartilage and posterior labrum. When using a probe, the lesion appears as a detachment of the deep portion of the posteroinferior labrum.

With repetitive loading of the shoulder in the posterior direction, further pathoanatomic changes develop on the posterior capsulolabral complex (Fig. 28.2). Cumulative posterior rim loading leads to loss of chondrolabral containment, subsequent development of posterior labral marginal cracks, or partial avulsion of the glenoid labrum [14]. Loss of chondrolabral containment results in both an increase in glenoid retroversion and a loss of the appropriate concavity of the glenoid because of decreased posterolabral height [15]. Further posterior loading of the shoulder results also in a stretch of the PIGHL. The condition is often associated with a dynamic dysfunction of the shoulder kinematics or capsular laxity.

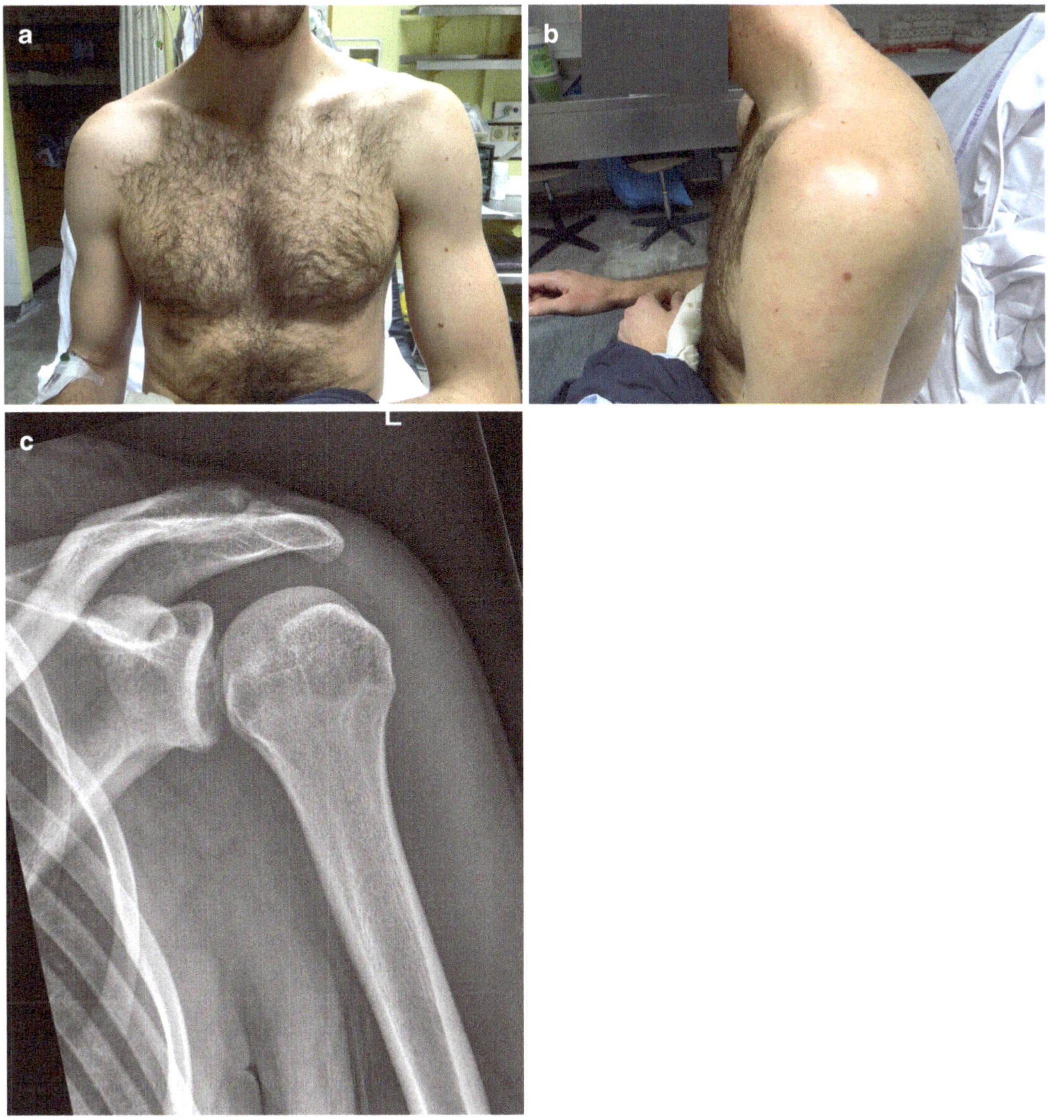

Fig. 28.1 Posterior shoulder dislocation of the left shoulder in athlete injured while playing basketball and receiving the hit from anterior to posteroanterior aspect (**a**). Lateral aspect of the left shoulder with posterior shoulder dislocation (**b**). X-ray of the same patient showing posterior shoulder dislocation (**c**)

28.3 Overhead Athletes

The biomechanical model of throwing consists of several phases: the wind-up, cocking, acceleration, and follow-through phases. This model is well described and has been studied often [16, 17]. The late cocking phase and follow-through phase with extreme deceleration are the two points at which the shoulder is most exposed. It was shown that the arm can reach a velocity of 140 km/h and angular velocity as high as 7000°/s (degrees per second) [18]. In the deceleration phase, compressive forces on the shoulder joint can be as much as 1090 N and posterior shear forces as much as 400 N [19]. These forces are all at the limits of natural tissue resistance, which in the anterior capsule, for example, is 800–1200 N [20]. The athlete is able to achieve such energy

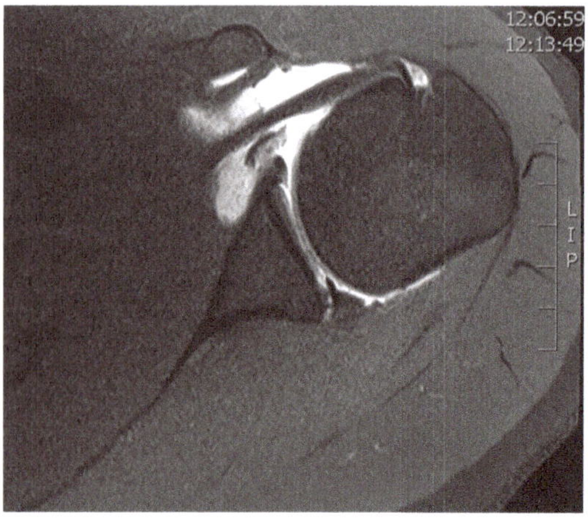

Fig. 28.2 Loss of posterior chondrolabral containment as seen on transverse plane of computed tomography (CT) scan with arthrography of the left shoulder

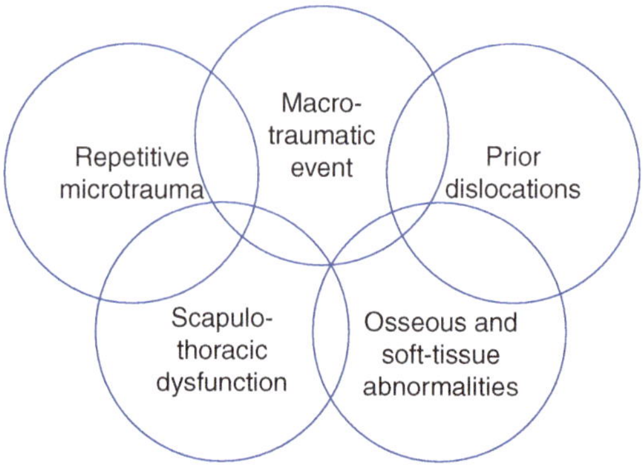

Fig. 28.3 Assessment of the patient with posterior shoulder instability should include assessment of possible macrotraumatic event, prior dislocations, repetitive microtrauma, scapulothoracic dysfunction, and osseous and soft-tissue abnormalities

when throwing or striking a ball only by activation of the entire kinematic chain. The coordinated delivery of muscle power to generate and transmit energy from leg to trunk toward shoulder and arm includes the body as a whole. High energy can be achieved also in sports other than baseball. The velocity of the objects transmitted by the overhead athlete to the ball can be as high as 160 km/h in baseball and, in some types of sport popular in Europe, as great as 250 km/h in tennis and 130 km/h in volleyball and handball [21].

A posterior shoulder problem in overhead athletes, if present, is rarely in isolation. Concomitant injuries or pathological findings are common. According to Bradley, associated pathologies were found in as many as 40% of surgical patients [8, 22, 23]. The patient's history and clinical examination are essential. It is crucial to determine the correct pathogenesis, possible underlying lesion, concomitant pathology, and other factors that can influence shoulder stability. In this aspect, we have to check for history of repetitive microtraumas, a possible traumatic event with clear onset of the problem, presence of prior dislocations, osseous and soft-tissue abnormalities, and signs of scapulothoracic dysfunction (Fig. 28.3). The clinical examination must be comprehensive. All the aspects of shoulder function have to be evaluated as they might have an influence on the posterior shoulder instability presentation. Thus, five elements of the shoulder should be addressed in the examination: shoulder stability, scapular dyskinesia, total range of motion (TROM) and presence of glenohumeral internal rotation deficit (GIRD), superior labral anteroposterior lesions (SLAP), together with long head of biceps, and finally rotator cuff problems. All these findings have to be compared to the opposite shoulder.

One of the important risk factors for posterior shoulder instability is scapular dyskinesia. Especially in the athletic population, control of the scapula position has to be examined during the clinical workup. The scapula has a complex interplay between stability and mobility of the shoulder. Scapular dyskinesia is one of the possible causes of shoulder disability on the one hand, and on the other hand, scapular dyskinesia increases the risk of injury.

28.4 Shoulder Laxity and Posterior Instability

In many athletes, laxity of the shoulder is advantageous in sports activity. In these individuals, there is a fine line between high performance and disability. Some adaptive changes of the shoulder joint are present in overhead athletes to accommodate appropriate ROM, such as capsular laxity or increased humeral retroversion.

There is a need for equilibrium between adaptive laxity and sufficient stability, which inhibits subluxation or even frank instability of the shoulder joint. Patients with general ligamentous laxity are prone to shoulder instability [24]. In these atraumatic cases of posterior shoulder instability, patients gradually develop pain and a sensation of unstable shoulder. In the beginning, the symptoms are present in highly demanding activities, but progression may lead to the symptoms being present during the activities of daily living. In this setting, adaptations make the diagnosis difficult, as the surgeon has to differentiate between adaptive capsular laxity and pathological instability.

A connection between labral lesion, dynamic shoulder dysfunction, and capsular laxity has been suggested [25]. All three factors are important in the development and presentation of posterior shoulder instability (Fig. 28.4). The labral lesion in the patient's shoulder may lead to dynamic shoulder dysfunction. Complex coordination of the many muscles around the shoulder joint and scapula is necessary to oppose biomechanical stresses on the structures at risk. Extremes of motion, generated forces, and the speed with which the motion occurs further influence the shoulder capsule. Protection of the stabilizing structures with a deficit in dynamic shoulder function is insufficient, leading to progression of the capsular laxity. Microinstability events in the decompensated shoulder with excessive laxity lead to further worsening of the labral lesion. This process continues, with the influence on shoulder function, and a vicious circle develops.

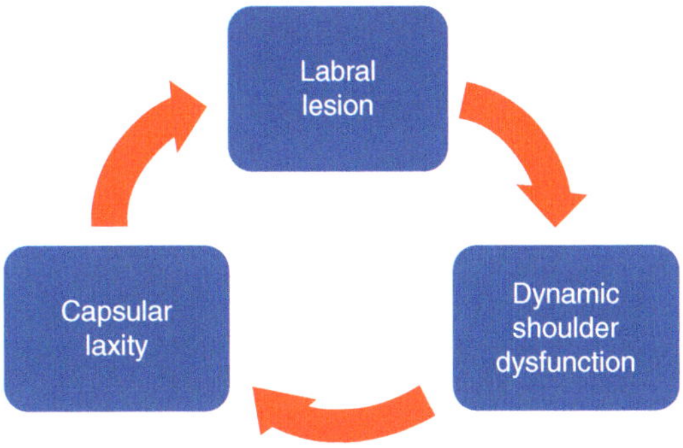

Fig. 28.4 The vicious cycle in the development and presentation of posterior shoulder instability. A labral lesion may lead to dynamic shoulder dysfunction, which influences the capsular laxity. Then, this may further worsen the labral lesion

28.5 Treatment of Posterior Shoulder Instability in Athletes

The initial treatment for patients with posterior shoulder instability is a period of nonoperative rehabilitation. If this is not successful and there is an underlying structural lesion, surgical treatment is indicated. The treatment of choice in patients without significant bony injury is arthroscopic repair. The key elements necessary to successfully treat posterior shoulder instability are to increase the glenohumeral stability ratio by restoring the glenoid concavity, to reduce the capsular redundancy, to reset capsular tension for proprioceptive feedback, and to rehabilitate the scapulohumeral and scapulothoracic musculature [26].

A large meta-analysis including 815 shoulders that compared arthroscopic and open procedures for posterior instability of the shoulder showed that arthroscopic repair has superior outcomes. A lower recurrence rate, higher percentage to return to sport, higher patient satisfaction, and higher subjective stability rate were seen with arthroscopic treatment [23, 27]. Arthroscopic treatment results in less tissue dissection, easier access to the posterior capsulolabral complex, easier identification of the pathology, and ability to address concomitant injuries.

Some studies show no difference in outcome after arthroscopic repair of posterior shoulder instability between contact athletes and the entire cohort of patients [28, 29]. There was also no difference in the outcome between traumatic and atraumatic injuries. A difference in outcomes was seen when comparing the results of throwing and nonthrowing athletes, indicating that throwing athletes are much more difficult to treat. Results were comparable regarding pain, stability, shoulder function, range of motion, strength, and ASES score, but there was a significant difference regarding return to pre-injury sports level. Nonthrowing athletes achieve much better results; 71% of nonthrowing athletes were able to return to the sport compared to 55% of throwing athletes [29].

28.6 Conclusion

Posterior shoulder instability is a complex and rare pathology compared to anterior shoulder instability. The most common cause in athletes is repetitive microtrauma to the posterior capsulolabral complex. Injuries in overhead athletes are different from those in contact sport athletes. Throwing athletes have more dynamic glenohumeral demands, and good results are more difficult to achieve with surgical treatment. Overhead athletes may develop specific adaptive mechanisms such as capsular laxity. This adaptation makes the diagnosis challenging as the examiner must differentiate between adaptive capsular laxity and pathological instability. Conservative approach and prevention of further instability events must be the first treatment option. The rehabilitation program is equally important after surgical treatment to decrease the risk of reinjury. In cases of traumatic posterior shoulder instability with structural pathological changes to the posterior capsulolabral complex, surgical treatment provides the best chance to return to sports activities.

References

1. Khiami F, Gérometta A, Loriaut P. Management of recent first-time anterior shoulder dislocations. Orthop Traumatol Surg Res. 2015;101:S51–7.
2. Bäcker HC, Galle SE, Maniglio M, Rosenwasser MP. Biomechanics of posterior shoulder instability: current knowledge and literature review. World J Orthop. 2018;9:245–54.
3. Steinmann SP. Posterior shoulder instability. Arthroscopy. 2003;19(Suppl 1):102–5.
4. Oberlander M, Chisar MA, Campbell B. Epidemiology of shoulder injuries in throwing and overhead athletes. Sports Med Arthrosc Rev. 2000;8:115–23.
5. Speed C, Wallace A. Injuries to the shoulder. In: Hutson M, Speed C, editors. Sports injuries. Oxford: Oxford University Press; 2011.
6. Myklebust G, Hasslan L, Bahr R, Steffen K. High prevalence of shoulder pain among elite Norwegian female handball players. Scand J Med Sci Sports. 2013;23(3):288–94.
7. Ovesen J, Nielsen S. Anterior and posterior shoulder instability. A cadaver study. Acta Orthop Scand. 1986;57:324–7.
8. Savoie FH 3rd, Holt MS, Field LD, Ramsey JR. Arthroscopic management of posterior instability: evolution of technique and results. Arthroscopy. 2008;24:389–96.
9. Bey MJ, Hunter SA, Kilambi N, Butler DL, Lindenfeld TN. Structural and mechanical properties of the glenohumeral joint posterior capsule. J Shoulder Elb Surg. 2005;14:201–6.
10. Blasier R, Soslowsky L, Malicky D, Palmer M. Posterior glenohumeral subluxation: active and passive stabilization in a biomechanical model. J Bone Joint Surg Am. 1997;79:433–40.
11. Kovacic L, Funk L, Pascal G. Posterior shoulder instability. In: Randelli P, Dejour D, van Dijk CN, Denti M, Seil R, editors. Arthroscopy: basic to advanced. New York: ESSKA, Springer; 2016. p. 483–98.
12. Kim S, Ha K, Park J, Kim Y, Lee Y, Lee J, Yoo J. Arthroscopic posterior labral repair and capsular shift for traumatic unidirectional recurrent posterior subluxation of the shoulder. J Bone Joint Surg Am. 2003;85:1479–87.
13. Seung HK, Kwon IH. Kim's lesion: an incomplete and concealed avulsion of the posteroinferior labrum in posterior or multidirectional posteroinferior instability of the shoulder. Arthroscopy. 2004;20:712–20.
14. Kim S, Ha K, Yoo J, Noh K. Kim's lesion: an incomplete and concealed avulsion of the posteroinferior labrum in posterior or multidirectional posteroinferior instability of the shoulder. Arthroscopy. 2004;20:712–20.
15. Kim S, Noh K, Park J, et al. Loss of chondrolabral containment of the glenohumeral joint in atraumatic posteroinferior multidirectional instability. J Bone Joint Surg Am. 2005;87:92–8.
16. Meister K. Injuries to the shoulder in the throwing athlete. Part one: biomechanics/pathophysiology/classification of injury. Am J Sports Med. 2000;28:265–75.
17. Perry J. Anatomy and biomechanics of the shoulder in throwing, swimming, gymnastics, and tennis. Clin Sports Med. 1983;2:247–70.
18. Wagner H, Buchecker M, von Duvillard SP, et al. Kinematic description of elite vs. low level players in team-handball jump throw. J Sports Sci Med. 2010;9:15–23.
19. Fleisig GS, Andrews JR, Dillman CJ, et al. Kinetics of baseball pitching with implication about injury mechanism. Am J Sports Med. 1995;23:233–9.
20. Blasier RB, Guldberg RE, Rothman ED. Anterior shoulder stability: contributions of rotator cuff forces and the capsular ligaments in a cadaver model. J Shoulder Elb Surg. 1992;1:140–50.

21. Reeser JC, Fleisig GS, Bolt B, Ruan M. Upper limb biomechanics during the volleyball serve and spike. Sports Health. 2010;2:368–74.
22. Bahk MS, Karzel RP, Snyder SJ. Arthroscopic posterior stabilization and anterior capsular plication for recurrent posterior glenohumeral instability. Arthroscopy. 2010;26:1172–80.
23. DeLong JM, Jiang K, Bradley JP. Posterior instability of the shoulder: a systematic review and meta-analysis of clinical outcomes. Am J Sports Med. 2015;43:1805–17.
24. Gaskill TR, Taylor DC, Millett PJ. Management of multidirectional instability of the shoulder. J Am Acad Orthop Surg. 2011;19:758–67.
25. Itoi E, Hsu HC, An KN. Biomechanical investigation of the glenohumeral joint. J Shoulder Elb Surg. 1996;5:407–24.
26. Antoniou J, Harryman DT 2nd. Posterior instability. Orthop Clin N Am. 2001;32:463–73.
27. DeLong JM, Bradley JP. Posterior shoulder instability in the athletic population: variations in assessment, clinical outcomes, and return to sport. World J Orthop. 2015;6:927–34.
28. Bradley JP, McClincy MP, Arner JW, Tejwani SG. Arthroscopic capsulolabral reconstruction for posterior instability of the shoulder: a prospective study of 200 shoulders. Am J Sports Med. 2013;41:2005–14.
29. Radkowski CA, Chhabra A, Iii CLB, et al. Arthroscopic capsulolabral repair for posterior shoulder instability in throwing athletes compared with nonthrowing athletes. Am J Sports Med. 2008;36:693–9.

29 Conservative Treatment in Posterior Dislocation

Paweł H. Surdziel

29.1 Introduction

This chapter describes the general approach to the patients with first-time shoulder trauma resulting in posterior dislocation or temporary posterior dislocation (subluxation) of the shoulder. Fracture dislocation or MDI is not considered. Clinical picture, examination diagnosis, and conservative treatment of posterior dislocation (PSD) are presented.

Full posterior dislocation of the shoulder joint (PSD) without fracture of the humeral head or glenoid is an extremely sparse case. Much more often in our practice, we deal with patients after an episode of sprain or subluxation and spontaneous reposition of dislocated humeral head. Posterior dislocation is usually associated with a fractured head of the inverted Hill–Sacks type [1] (McLaughlin lesion), some with subscapularis insertion lesion, and damage to the posterior–inferior acetabular labrum. Concomitant neurovascular or rotator cuff lesions are much less common after posterior dislocation compared to anterior dislocation [2, 3].

The spectrum of dislocation varies from acute to chronic traumatic dislocation, irreducible dislocation and in conjunction with proximal fractures of the humerus.

P. H. Surdziel (✉)
Katedra i Klinika Traumatologii, Ortopedii i Chirurgii Ręki, Uniwersytet Medyczny im. Karola Marcinkowskiego w Poznaniu, Poznań, Poland

R. Brzóska et al. (eds.), *360° Around Shoulder Instability*, https://doi.org/10.1007/978-3-662-61074-9_29

Usually, the cause of a posterior dislocation of the shoulder is a direct or indirect trauma to the anterior side of the shoulder, for example, in contact sports or falls on the adducted and extended arm in internal rotation. Electric shock or epilepsy may also create extreme muscle contraction with flexion, adduction, and internal rotation of the affected arm. These are pathognomonic factors of the posterior shoulder dislocation.

Considering the above, we will decrease the probability of overlooking the shoulder joint damage, which may lead to subsequent posterior instability and early degenerative changes.

29.2 Initial Assessment

Anamnesis:

- High-energy direct or indirect trauma to the anterior side of the shoulder (e.g., contact sports) or.
- fall on the adducted and extended arm in internal rotation (e.g., cycling or skiing accidents),
- shoulder cluck or "out-of-the-socket experience",
- electric shock or epilepsy seizures, usually bilateral,

These are pathognomonic factors of the posterior shoulder dislocation.

Clinical picture of a patient with *existing posterior dislocation* of the shoulder joint:

- very painful,
- the shoulder may be swollen (hematoma) and its shape has changed,
- the shoulder is put forward and high,
- the scapula usually is rotated and leans forward to decrease pain and tension,
- the humeral head may be visible posteriorly in skinny patients,
- the coracoid is more prominent,
- the arm in characteristic internal rotation (10–60°) and adduction,
- the arm seems to be fixed in above-described position,
- no active nor passive motion, especially external rotation is possible,
- no ability to supinate the forearm when the arm is in flexion,

Clinical picture of a patient *without existing posterior dislocation* of the shoulder joint (after subluxation or dislocation with subsequent reposition):

- less pain,
- the shoulder may be swollen (hematoma) and its shape has changed,
- the shoulder is leveled,
- the scapula in normal position on the ribcage,
- the humeral head in place,
- the coracoid normal,
- the arm in neutral rotation and some abduction,
- the arm may be moved whilst hanging freely by doctor on examination,
- active or passive motion is possible to some extent,
- supination the forearm is possible with arm in flexion.

The main symptom is loss of movement of the affected shoulder, particularly external rotation.

29.3 Emergency

Immediate immobilization with simple, Velpeau or Desoult sling and painkillers.

29.4 Imaging

The cause of overlooking PSD by the physician is a failure to suspect the diagnosis and insufficient radiographic investigation. The key to diagnosis of this injury is to obtain proper X-ray. Diagnosis must be confirmed by two orthogonal X-rays of the affected shoulder joint, for example, antero-posterior (AP) and axial views. If the axial view is difficult to obtain due to abduction limitations and pain, the Y scapular or Velpeau view should be taken. I recommend an a–p view in internal rotation, which may reveal flattening of the humeral head at the subscapularis insertion (Fig. 29.1).

According to Wu Xu, only 11.4% cases of PSD were confirmed by AP radiographs only, but if axillary or Y view radiographs were taken at the initial investigation, the diagnosis was confirmed in all patients [4]. Ultrasound, CT, or MRI should also be considered if available.

Closed reduction of the dislocation should be attempted immediately under sedation, often successful, or under general analgesia with muscle relaxants [5]. The method of lateralization and ventralization of the humeral head, using the surgeon's arm as a fulcrum is most commonly used. Alternatively an elevation of the internally rotated arm with longitudinal traction, is applied [6].

If closed reduction is not possible, additional imaging should be performed.

CT scan allows to asses the size of osteochondral impression fracture of the ventromedial articular surface of the humeral head (reversed Hill–Sacks lesion) and a state of the labrum or the bony glenoid rim [2, 7].

If PSD is not locked and reposition of the humeral head have been achived and stable, with defect of no more then 25% of the articular surface of the humeral head, patient can be treated by conservative methods.

An imperative condition to decide of nonoperative treatment is a stable joint after closed reduction. Patient has to be informed of long-term results, possible instability, or reconstructive surgery if necessary in case conservative management fails.

It is recommended to perform magnetic resonance imaging (MRI) after reposition of the joint, as it allows the assessment of soft tissues, with

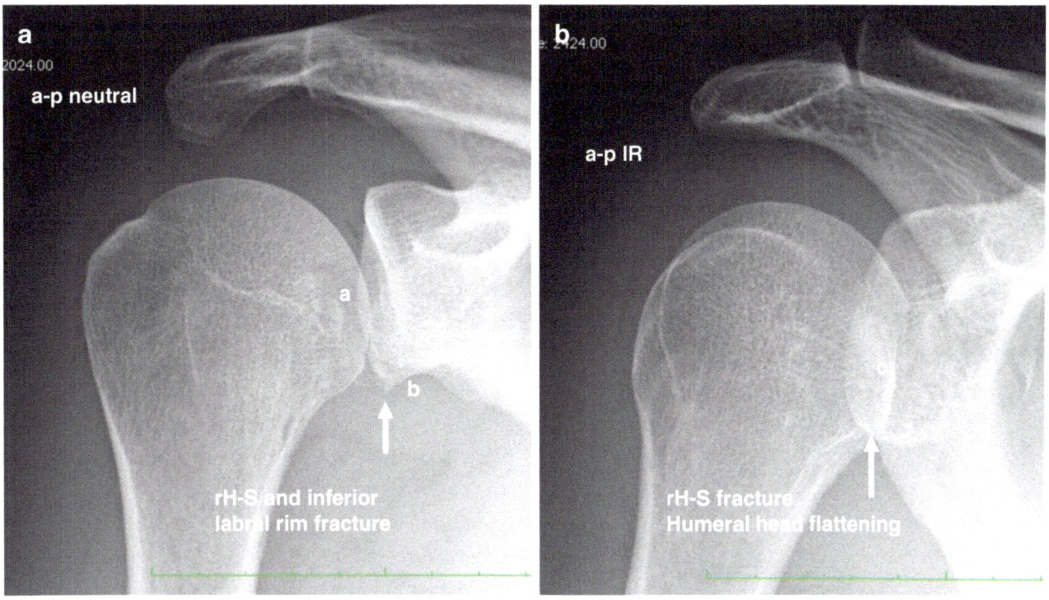

Fig. 29.1 An a-p view in neutral (**a**) and internal rotation (**b**) after spontaneous PSD relocation reveling: *a*—reversed Hill–Sacks fracture, *b*—inferior labral rim fracture, *c*—flattening of the humeral head at rH-S Fx

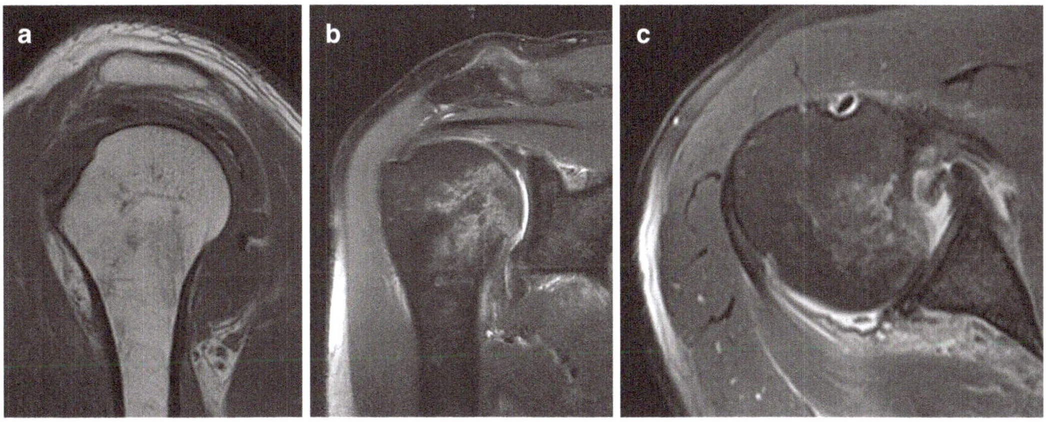

Fig. 29.2 Reversed H-G lesion in shoulder. RC intact. (**a**) Inferior glenoid rim fracture. Observe hematoma as a natural "artroMRI" contrast (**b**, **c**)

hematoma serving as a natural "contrast," just like in artroMRI (Fig. 29.2).

This examination may unveil labral and chondral lesions, small fragment avulsion fractures of the subscapularis muscle tendon insertion, LHBT instability, or other rotator cuff pathology.

CT or MRI also may give important clues for possible residual posterior shoulder instability due to existing dysplasia, retroversion, or inclination of the glenoid (Figs. 29.3 and 29.4).

Coexisting neurovascular injuries or lesions of the rotator cuff occur much rarely after posterior dislocation. However, high-energy trauma to the shoulder often involves traction injury to the brachial plexus, which may be not seen at the initial examination.

This may be recognized later as a scapular dyskinesis, limb weakness, or proprioceptive position disorder, and thus compromise and extend the improvement process of rehabilitation up to the time of full brachial plexus recovery.

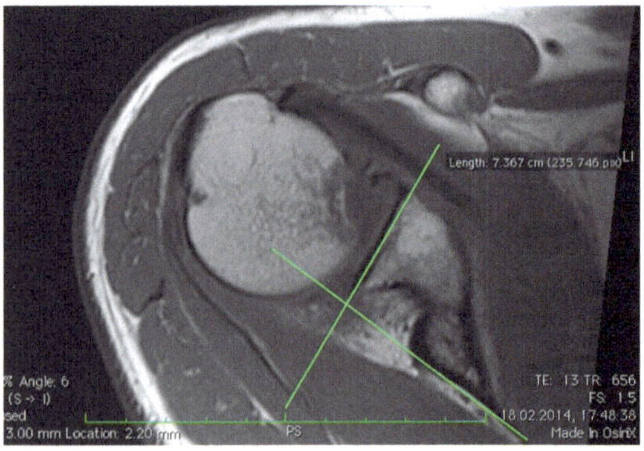

Fig. 29.3 Reversed H-G lesion in shoulder with neutral glenoid version. Conservative treatment with no instability, full recovery. Did not require any surgery

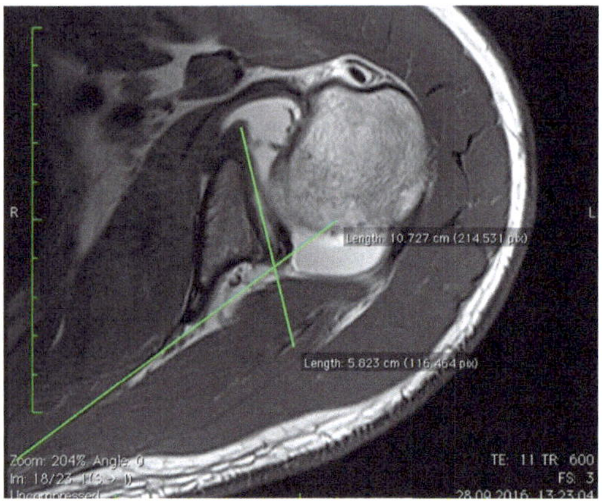

Fig. 29.4 Reversed H-G lesion in shoulder with glenoid retroversion. Conservative treatment failed with development of posterior instability. Arthroscopic posteroinferior labral reconstruction required at 15 months after injury

29.5 Aftercare

The arm should be immobilized for 6 weeks in neutral to 20° of internal rotation in abduction ER orthosis. This position ensures optimal healing conditions for the attachment of the subscapular muscle tendon and also is probably the best for healing damaged posterior capsule and labrum.

In case of patients with confirmed retroversion of the glenoid (CT or MRI), adequate correction of external rotation should be considered.

29.6 Rehabilitation

General rules of shoulder rehab apply. Rehabilitation plays a crucial role in maximizing the functional outcome. In the early phases of rehabilitation, it is necessary to protect the joint to allow healing. Pendulum movements of the shoulder to certain ranges of motion in sagittal plane are allowed. Orthosis/sling is removed only for rehabilitation exercises.

Isometric RC and scapular stabilizers strengthening exercises are introduced as soon as possible with pain settlement. Elbow, forearm, wrist and scapular active ROM exercise program, with emphasis on postural exercises, is introduced despite the use of an orthosis. Here, PowerBall and Swing Stick may be implemented, as these devices that allow muscle strengthening and proprioceptive training without changing position of the shoulder itself.

No shoulder internal rotation past neutral for 6 weeks and no shoulder internal rotation with abduction for 8 weeks.

Cardiovascular fitness has to be preserved: walking, stationary bike, avoid running and jumping until at least 8 weeks. Swimming breaststroke at 3–4 months.

Stretching of the posterior capsule (by internal rotation) avoided for 4 months.

Return to full activities is allowed at 6–8 months.

References

1. McLaughlin HL. Posterior dislocation of the shoulder. J Bone Joint Surg Am. 1952;24(3):584–90.
2. Roberts A, Wickstrom J. Prognosis of posterior dislocation of the shoulder. Acta Orthop Scand. 1971;42(4):328–37.

3. Mestdagh H, Maynou C, Delobelle JM, Urvoy P, Butin E. Traumatic posterior dislocation of the shoulder in adults. Apropos of 25 cases. Ann Chir. 1994;48(4):355–63.
4. Wu X, et al. Neglected posterior dislocation of the shoulder: a systematic literature review. J Orthop Translat. 2015;3(2):89–94.
5. Cicak N. Posterior dislocation of the shoulder. J Bone Joint Surg Br. 2004;86-B:324–32.
6. Benedikt S. Locked posterior shoulder dislocation: treatment options and clinical outcomes. Arch Orthop Trauma Surg. 2011;131:1127–34. https://doi.org/10.1007/s00402-011-1310-9.
7. Ovesen J, Söjbjerg JO. Posterior shoulder dislocation. Muscle and capsular lesions in cadaver experiments. Acta Orthop Scand. 1986;57(6):535–6.

Soft-Tissue Procedures: *Indications, Algorithm from Imaging to Decision-Making*

30

Selim Ergün, Umut Akgün, and Mustafa Karahan

30.1 Introduction

The glenohumeral joint is often likened to a golf ball on a tee, which provides a functional benefit of a large arc of motion. In return, predisposition to an inherent instability is present, which can result in traumatic anterior shoulder dislocation. In the general population, the incidence of traumatic shoulder instability has been reported to be 1.7% [1, 2]. Anterior is the most common direction of glenohumeral joint dislocations, accounting for over 90% of all shoulder dislocations. As a common complication after an anterior shoulder dislocation, Bankart lesions can be seen specifically at the anteroinferior aspect of the glenoid labral complex.

In 1923, Bankart reported that capsulolabral soft-tissue detachment of inferior glenohumeral ligament (IGHL) cannot heal on fibrous cartilage tissue [3], and treated the "Bankart" lesion by an open surgical method. Then, in 1987, Morgan ve Bodenstab [4] introduced the first arthroscopic management, "transglenoid suture method."

Usage of suture anchors in arthroscopic surgeries, the basis of modern fixation methods, was first introduced by Wolf [5] and has gained gradual popularity in recent years. Recurrence is one of the most important and undesired complications of Bankart repair. Recently, it has been shown in a meta-analysis study that there is no significant difference in between "open Bankart repair" and "arthroscopic Bankart repair with suture anchors" regarding frank redislocation and revision surgery due to recurrence [6]. However, subluxation and apprehension were significantly higher in arthroscopic repairs than in open repairs.

Smaller skin incisions, more complete glenohumeral joint inspection, less soft-tissue dissection, and maximal preservation of external rotation are the advantages of arthroscopic management. Furthermore, recent technical advances resulting in improved ability to diagnose and manage coexisting intraarticular lesions allowed arthroscopic soft-tissue repair to become the standard technique for Bankart lesions.

30.2 Spectrum of Intraarticular Lesions Treatable with Soft-Tissue Procedures in Anterior Instability *(Common Indications)*

In the presence of an acute or recurrent anterior instability, multiple soft-tissue damages are often encountered [7].

1. **Avulsion of the anterior labrum and anterior inferior glenohumeral ligament (AIGHL)** is the Bankart lesion, which is 90%

S. Ergün · U. Akgün · M. Karahan (✉)
Orthopedics and Traumaology, School of Medicine, Acıbadem Mehmet Ali Aydınlar University, İstanbul, Turkey

R. Brzóska et al. (eds.), *360° Around Shoulder Instability*, https://doi.org/10.1007/978-3-662-61074-9_30

present with a traumatic anterior shoulder dislocation.
2. **Humeral avulsion of glenohumeral ligaments (HAGL)** may be present particularly in the elderly. It may cause recurrent instability if not recognized and repaired.
3. **Detachment of the superior glenoid labrum** (Superior labrum anterior posterior—SLAP lesion) may accompany a Bankart lesion, which is detrimental to anterior shoulder stability [8].
4. **Capsular lesions** are usually present in patients with traumatic shoulder dislocations. It is shown that only translation of the humeral head on the glenoid can occur with a Bankart lesion alone, accompanying capsular stretch or elongation is necessary for dislocation [9].
5. **Anterior labral periosteal sleeve avulsion (ALPSA)** is labral avulsion from the anterior glenoid rim, displacing and healing in a medial and inferior position underneath an avulsed but intact periosteum. ALPSA lesions may impede restoring the normal anatomy.
6. **Subscapularis and posterosuperior rotator cuff injuries** might be encountered after acute anterior dislocations. Subscapularis tendon tears are associated with severe instability events, and generally seen in patients older than 40 years.
7. **Glenoid bone loss and/or Hill–Sachs lesions** are not rare after an anterior shoulder dislocation. Different soft-tissue (remplissage) and bone-grafting procedures might be necessary according to the size of the defect.

The principle of arthroscopic soft-tissue repair is to identify and repair all diagnosed lesions that contribute to glenohumeral instability. This involves debridement, repair of labral and ligamentous tears, capsular tensioning, repair of coexisting biceps and rotator cuff pathologies, remplissage, and closure of the rotator interval if necessary. All pathologies in this spectrum must be cleared by physical examination, imaging methods, and peroperative assessment; next should be the decision-making process to choose the optimum treatment for the right patient. The preoperative decision will be crosschecked with the operative assessment.

30.3 Decision-Making

The final decision regarding the surgical treatment for anterior shoulder instability with soft-tissue procedures is a topic of debate. It must be linked to multiple factors, not only the diagnostic spectrum listed above. First, a detailed patient history, physical examination, and review of appropriate imaging studies should be done. Then, a discussion should take place between the patient and the treating surgeon, which will be concluded in the operating room. As the shoulder joint has many variations, surgeons should be ready for procedural changes during the surgery.

30.3.1 Preoperative Decision-Making

Multiple factors must be considered prior to surgical treatment. These include the patient's age, present and desired activity levels, dislocation history, duration since the first dislocation episode, and radiologic findings regarding accompanying lesions, particularly bone defects at the glenoid and humeral head. The indication for surgical stabilization should be established by analyzing risk factors and the implications of recurrence.

1. **Age and Sex:** Young age and male sex are strong risk factors for either progression to recurrent anterior instability, or postoperative failure and poor outcome after arthroscopic Bankart repairs [10]. Instability surgery is advised for younger patients (with coexisting other factors; male sex and competitive or contact sports) [11]. But, high failure risk in young patients should be kept in mind and the patient should be informed about that. Calvo et al. found that patients younger than 28 years of age had increased risk of failure after arthroscopic soft-tissue management [12]. Vermeulen et al. looked for long-term outcomes (mean 6.3 years) after arthroscopic

Bankart repair and observed good results in patients "older" than 20 years age, and asked the question "whether the arthroscopic soft-tissue procedures might not be the optimal treatment for patients aged younger than 20 years," inquiring the necessity of a Laterjat procedure [13]. A systemic review comparing surgical versus nonoperative treatment in instability patients up to 18 years old found that recurrence rate was significantly lower in the surgical group [14]. All these studies unite in a common point that younger age has an increased risk of poor outcome and recurrence risk whether treated surgically or conservatively, but better clinical results are found in patients treated surgically compared to conservative management.

2. **First Time vs. Recurrent Dislocations:** How to manage a Bankart lesion seen on Magnetic Resonance Imaging (MRI) after the first dislocation, repair it or wait and see if it dislocates again. This is still a question of debate. Actually, the answer to this question depends on other factors like age, gender, and activity level of the patients. Imhoff et al. found that patients with a single preoperative dislocation had a significantly lower rate of postoperative recurrence than did patients who had more than one dislocation prior to arthroscopic surgery [15]. Crall et al. more specifically evaluated this factor and compared the cost-effectiveness of initial observation versus primary surgery for the first-time anterior shoulder dislocation, and found that primary surgery was less costly and more effective (regarding clinical outcomes, recurrence, and complication rates) for 15-year-old boys, 15-year-old girls, and 25-year-old men. However, for 25-year-old women and 35-year-old men and women, surgery was more effective but more costly [16]. Recently, Rugg et al. analyzed databases for surgical trends in the treatment of patients with a single shoulder instability by a multicenter study, and they found that when compared with recurrent dislocators, first time dislocators were less likely to have bone loss or biceps pathology [17].
3. **Time From the First Dislocation:** Recurrent instability after arthroscopic Bankart repair is an undesired complication for both the patient and the surgeon. To assess the factors which increase the risk, Porcellini et al. found that patients who were surgically managed for more than 6 months after the first dislocation were 2.6 times more likely to have a redislocation in comparison with those who were operated within 6 months [18]. The most important finding in the study of Lee et al. was that increased recurrent shoulder anterior instability in patients below 30 years of age was strongly associated with surgical delay after the first dislocation and they suggested that arthroscopic Bankart repair within 6 months of the first dislocation should be considered, especially in young patients [19].
4. **Activity Level and Expectations**: It is very well known that athletes should be evaluated separately from non-athlete patients. Especially in-season athletes are initially managed with nonsurgical rehabilitation and planned for surgery during the off-season. However, early surgery might be necessary in athletes with high-risk branches (American football, rock climbing, etc.). Buss et al. reported that 30 "competitive in-season athletes" experienced an anterior shoulder instability in an in-season period and initially treated nonoperatively with rehabilitation and bracing; 26 of the 30 (87%) were able to return to play and complete the season after approximately 10 days of missed time; however, 37% of these experienced at least one more instability episode at the same season; 16 of the 30 required surgical intervention following their competitive season [20].
5. **Imaging Workup:** Imaging workup begins with conventional X-rays including anteroposterior (AP), scapular–Y, and axillary views. The West Point view is a specialized view to assess glenoid bone loss and the Stryker Notch view to assess Hill–Sachs lesions.

   Patients might have a variety of co-pathologies in addition to the Bankart lesion. MRI is the gold standard to evaluate capsulolabral structures and other soft-tissue structures in patients with shoulder instability. On the other hand, Computed Tomography (CT) provides a useful measurement method for glenoid and humeral head bone losses. There are many different measurement methods for these bone defects.

(a) **For the glenoid bone loss,** the distance between the glenoid bare spot and the anterior rim (*A*) and the distance between the bare spot and posterior rim are measured in millimeters (*B*) [21]. Glenoid bone loss ratio is calculated by the formula: $((B - A)/2B) \times 100\%$ (Fig. 30.1). However, in some cases, it may not be possible to find or estimate the bare spot; therefore, using the size of the contralateral shoulder as a template would be a useful method (Fig. 30.1). Several studies are present in literature that quantify the amount of anterior glenoid bone loss leading to glenohumeral instability and making bone grafting necessary. Critical bone loss amounts for bone grafting range from 20 to 36% [22–24]; however, greater than 15% is identified as a risk factor for failed arthroscopic soft-tissue procedures by some authors, especially in the presence of a Hill–Sachs lesion [12, 18].

(b) **Humeral head bone loss** due to a Hill–Sachs lesion can be measured by edge-to-edge distances and depth of the defect in each axial, sagittal, and coronal planes [25]. Among those, edge-to-edge measurements of defective areas on three different planes of the affected humerus seem to be a reproducible way to calculate the size of a Hill–Sachs lesion [25] (Fig. 30.2). Unfortunately, there is no perfect method to calculate the exact volume of bone loss on the humeral surface. Provencher et al. proposed to use computer software capable of digital subtraction in order to achieve correct volumetric data in these cases [21]. It is shown that ligamentous laxity and an accompanying Hill–Sachs lesion greater than 250 mm^3 is a risk factor for failure after arthroscopic Bankart repairs [26].

(c) **Bipolar Bone Defects:** Hill–Sachs lesions and glenoid bone loss are both present in bipolar defects.

(d) **Engagement Concept:** Because a Hill–Sachs lesion is located away from the glenoid contact surface of the humeral head, it is related to end-range stability, rather than mid-range stability. With the abduction and external rotation of the arm, the Hill–Sachs lesion and the glenoid come closer. At this posterior end range, it is important to assess the risk of engagement of the lesion on the glenoid. This risk can be assessed at the time of surgery, and should be tested after the Bankart repair. Arthroscopically, the relative relationship

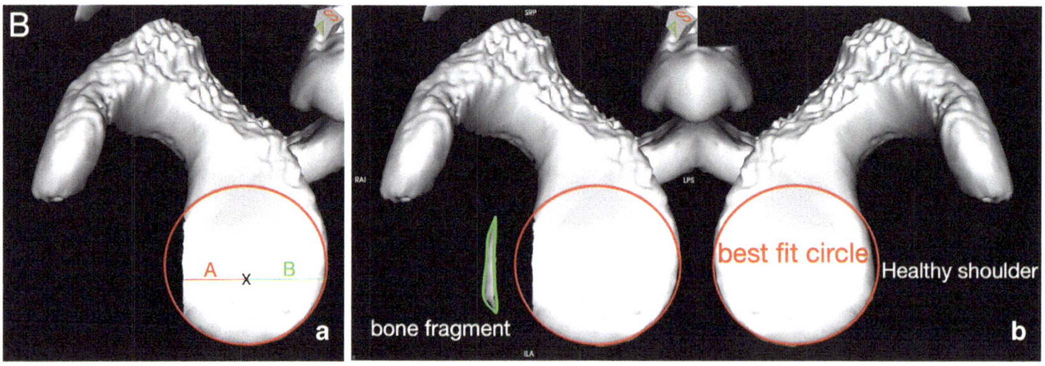

Fig. 30.1 (**a**) Using a bare spot to measure the radius of the healthy glenoid <B> on the posterior to compare to the defective anterior glenoid <A> side. (**b**) Pico method to calculate glenoid bone loss by using a healthy shoulder as a template. A best-fit circle obtained from the healthy glenoid is applied on the defective side

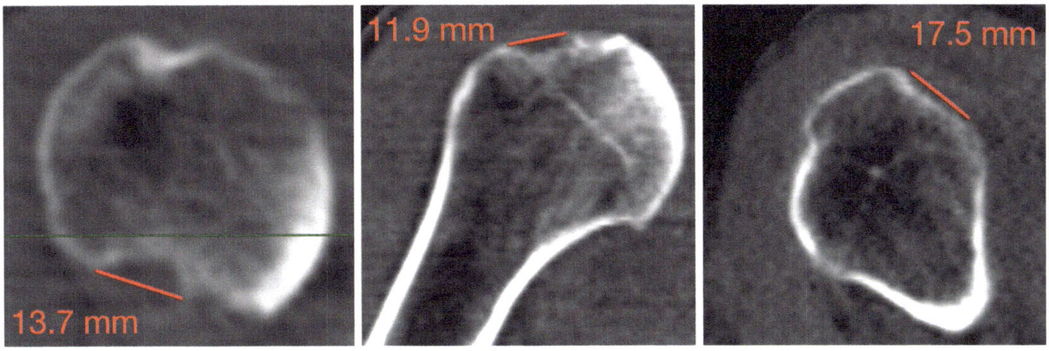

Fig. 30.2 Edge-to-edge measurement of a Hill–Sachs lesion on axial, coronal, and sagittal CT images

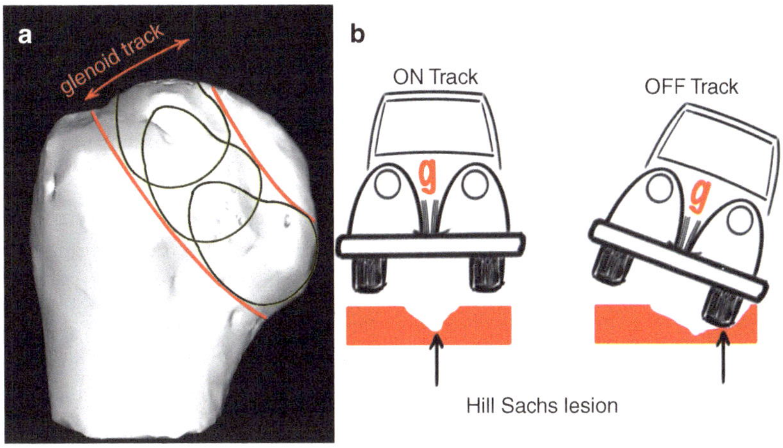

Fig. 30.3 (**a**) Red lines on the humeral head show the medial and lateral border of the glenoid track (the contact footprint of the glenoid on the posterior–superior aspect of humeral head during abduction and external rotation). (**b**) Concept of an on track–off track lesion, the car demonstrates the effective glenoid surface, the road is the humeral head, and the depression on the road is the Hill–Sachs lesion. If the depression is between the tyres, then the car will not fall down: On TRACK LESION = NON-ENGAGING HILL SACHS. If the depression is in line with the tyres, then the car will fall in it: Off-TRACK LESION = ENGAGING HILL SACHS

between the Hill–Sachs Lesion and the glenoid can be assessed dynamically. If the lesion is out of the glenoid coverage, then it may engage with the anterior rim of the glenoid and cause a dislocation.

The second way to assess the risk of engagement before surgery is the "glenoid track" concept. The glenoid track is a zone of contact between the glenoid rim and the humeral head (Fig. 30.3). It is calculated as 83% of the radiologically measured glenoid width (Table 30.1). If there is a bipolar bone defect, then the anterior glenoid bone loss is extracted from the calculated width (Table 30.1) [27].

If the size of the Hill–Sachs lesion is > the glenoid Track, then it will engage, and it is called "off-track concept" or "off-track Hill–Sachs Lesion" (Fig. 30.3), and addition of a remplissage procedure would be necessary. If the Hill–Sachs lesion is < the glenoid Track, then it will not engage, and is called "on-track concept" or "on-track Hill–Sachs Lesion" (Fig. 30.3) [27].

(e) **Soft-tissue co-pathologies associated with anterior instability** are capsulolabral lesions, rotator cuff and long head of biceps tendon pathologies, and they all can be detected on MR or MR arthrogram

Table 30.1 Formulas used to determine the effective glenoid track and risk of engagement

Glenoid track size = $(D \times 0.83) - d$	
Hill–Sachs size[a] < glenoid track = on Track	Non-ENGAGE!
Hill–Sachs size[a] > glenoid track = off Track	ENGAGE!

D glenoid diameter, *d* anterior glenoid bone loss (if none = 0)

[a]In cases with medially located Hill–Sachs lesion with a healthy bony bridge between the cuff foot print and the lesion, the concept will be changed as the Hill–Sachs interval and should be calculated as the Hill–Sachs size + healthy bony bridge size = Hill–Sachs Interval. If this is greater than the glenoid track, the lesion will ENGAGE

Table 30.2 Instability severity index score (ISIS) based on a preoperative questionnaire, clinical examination, and radiological findings [28]

Prognostic factors	Points
Age at surgery (year)	
≤20	2
>20	0
Degree of sport participation (preoperative)	
Competitive	2
Recreational or none	0
Type of sport (preoperative)	
Contact or forced overhead	1
Other	0
Shoulder hyperlaxity	
Shoulder hyperlaxity (anterior or inferior)	1
Normal laxity	0
Hill–Sachs on AP radiograph	
Visible in external rotation	2
Not visible in external rotation	0
Glenoid loss of contour on AP radiograph	
Loss of contour	2
No lesion	0
Total (points)	10

images. Preoperative awareness of these lesions is necessary, but intraoperative findings can change preoperative plans and add new strategies.

6. **Instability Severity Index Score (ISIS)**: As discussed above, age, activity level, and humeral and glenoidal bone defects are important prognostic factors. Boileau et al. developed the ISIS to help surgeons regarding the decision-making process in 2007 [28]. The ISIS is calculated by summing the values for each of these factors, with a possible total of 10 points (Table 30.2). Increase in total points shows increased risk of recurrence following arthroscopic stabilization, and Boileau emphasize that if the total score is ≥7, arthroscopic soft-tissue procedures may not be enough to prevent glenohumeral instability. Although the ISIS scoring system does not quantitatively evaluate glenoidal and humeral bone defects, also no criterion is present regarding the duration of symptoms or time from the first dislocation episode, and number of dislocations. Phadnis et al. confirmed that the ISIS is a useful preoperative tool, but advised to consider alternative forms of stabilization other than soft-tissue procedures in patients with ISIS score ≥ 4 [29].

30.3.2 Intraoperative Decision-Making

Before starting the operative management, physical examination under anesthesia is essential; anterior, inferior, or posterior translation of humeral head should be noted. Easy dislocation of the glenohumeral joint can be predictive of intensive capsular damage and/or any bony defect. The opposite shoulder must be also evaluated.

Diagnostic arthroscopy is essential for diagnosis of all co-pathologies. During arthroscopy, the diagnostic and therapeutic algorithm should follow the checklist in Fig. 30.4.

1. Labral pathologies should be diagnosed. Is there only a Bankart lesion, does it extend to the biceps anchor, is there an ALPSA or HAGL lesion present? Both sides of the anteroinferior ligamentous complex should be visualized. It is easier to see a medially displaced ALPSA lesion from an anterior portal (Fig. 30.5). Before fixing the torn labral tissues, a careful release and mobilization is needed to achieve good tension on the capsuloligamentous tissues (Fig. 30.5).

   Attachment of the superior labrum is quite variable, and a mobile superior labrum without evidence of trauma should not be classified as a SLAP lesion. If the superior glenoid is covered with cartilage, and the labrum shows no evidence of trauma, then it is possible to be a normal variant. Traumatic separation includes the signs of tears within the

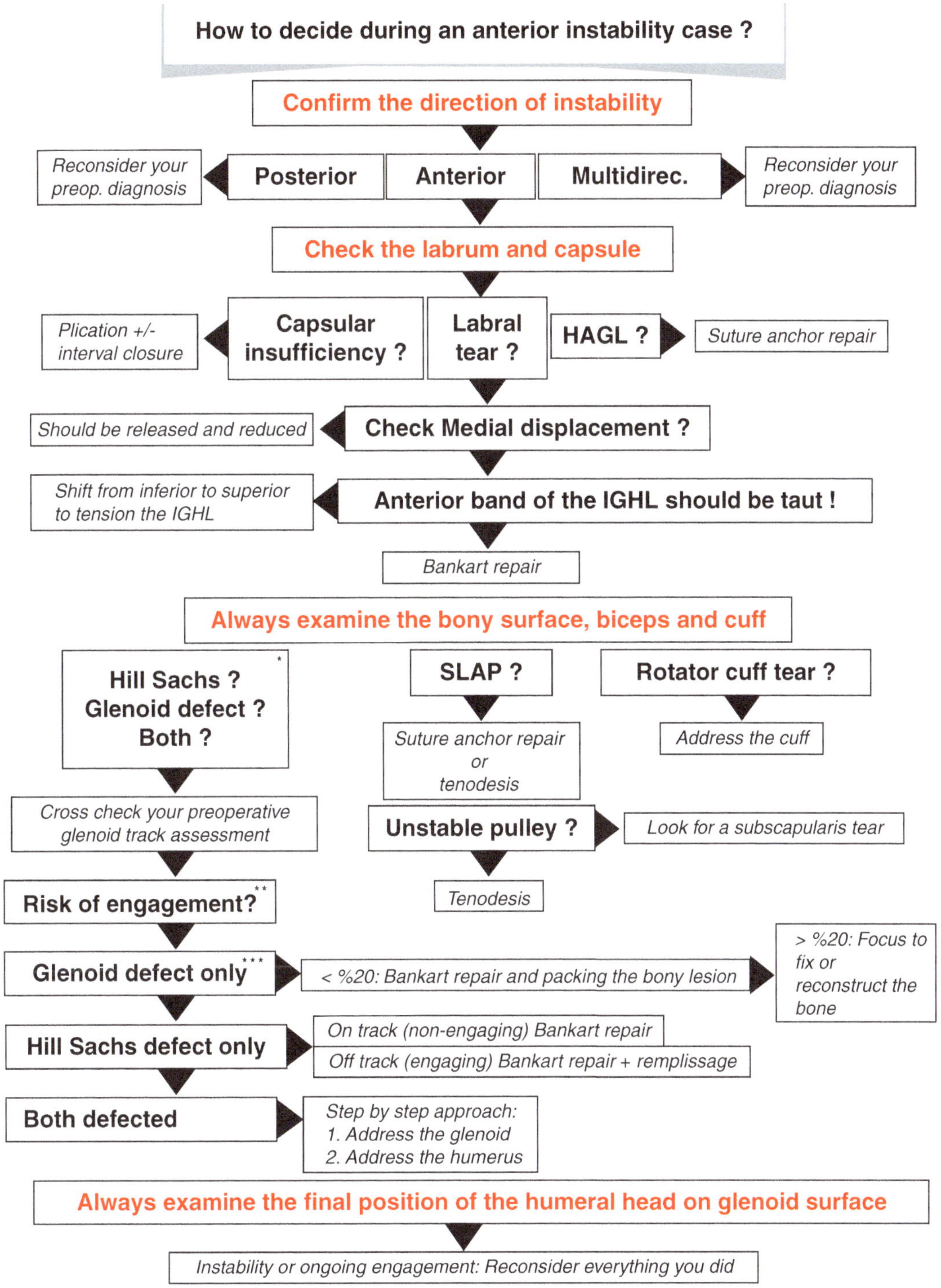

Fig. 30.4 Intraoperative decision-making in anterior glenohumeral instability. (Asterisk) Bony lesions should be measured before surgery. There is a small room for surprises. (Double asterisk) In case of an engagement, the size and location of the lesion will dictate the solution. Preoperative assessment is of utmost importance in these cases. Lesions exceeding the limits for soft-tissue repair should be treated with bone procedures. (Triple asterisk) Anterior glenoid defect would put too much pressure on the Bankart repair that may fail the construct. Twenty percent lesion size cut-off can be acceptable for glenoid defects alone. If there is an accompanying Hill–Sachs lesion, the cut-off will be reduced to 15%

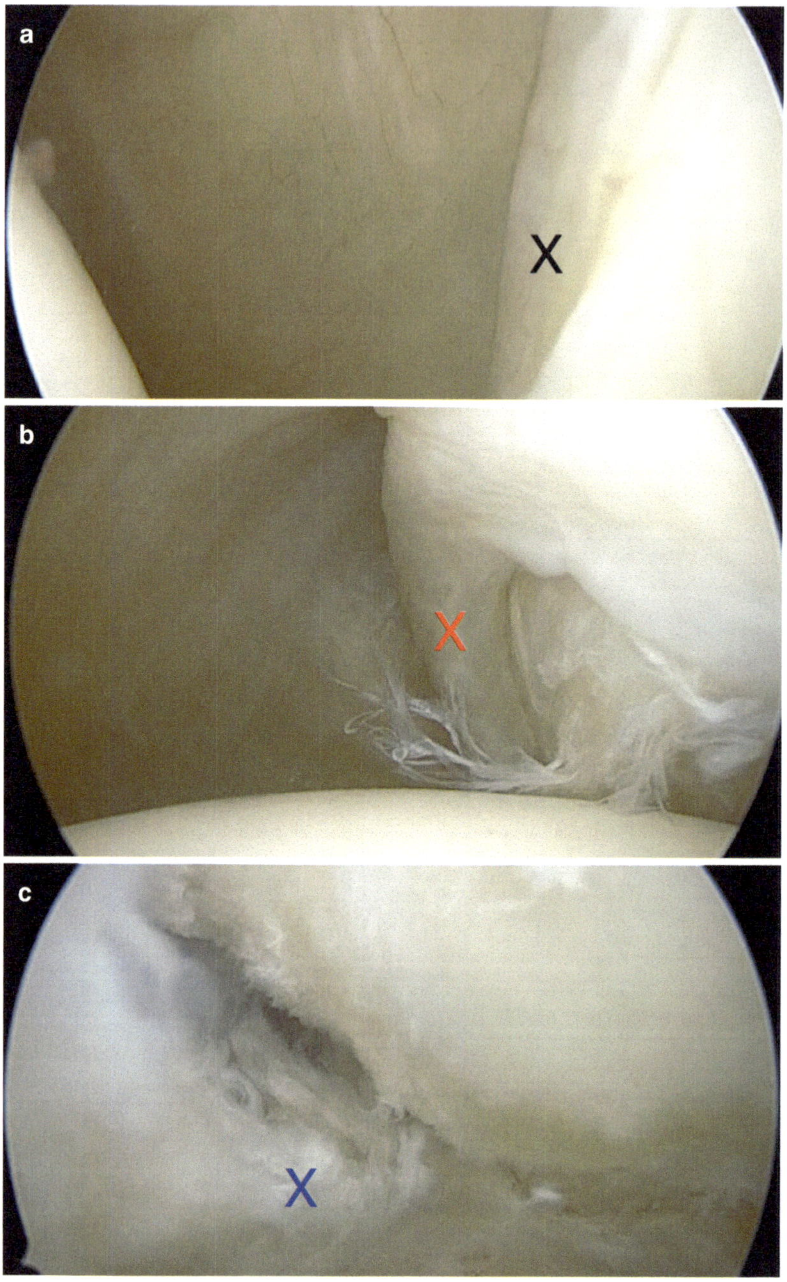

Fig. 30.5 (**a**) Medially displaced labral lesion (black X) viewed from posterior portal. (**b**) Same lesion (red X) that can be seen clearly from the anterior superior portal. (**c**) Displaced labrum (blue X) properly released from the glenoid neck and ready to be fixed

substance of the superior labrum, cartilage loss with exposed bone at the site of labrum attachment, and an increase in superior labrum separation with abduction and external rotation of the arm.

2. Glenoid bone loss can be calculated intraoperatively. The distance between the bare spot and the anterior glenoid rim is measured in millimeters (*A*) by an arthoscopic probe as is the distance between a bare spot and the posterior glenoid rim (*B*) [22]. Bone loss ratio = $((B - A)/2B) \times 100\%$. Small-sized cortical lesions on the glenoid edge can be managed by a labral repair that includes the bony lesion within the suture loop (Fig. 30.6). Hill–Sachs lesions are very important and should

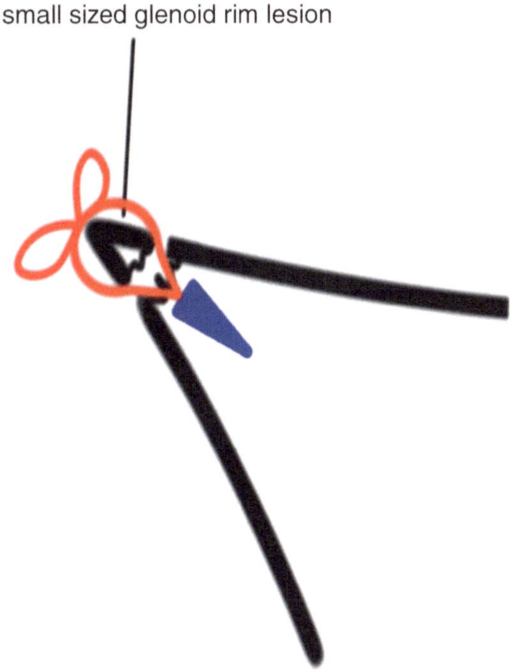

Fig. 30.6 Small-sized bony lesion can be packed within the soft-tissue repair by using a suture anchor

be carefully evaluated regarding engagement. In case of an engaging lesion, tenodesis of the infraspinatus tendon within the defective humeral area (Remplissage) is a useful technique with predictable outcomes.

3. Coexisting capsular tear and humeral HAGL lesions are not uncommon among patients with a Bankart lesion [30]. Injury to the capsule is often assumed to be present (30–70%). Older age, complete dislocation, and an associated Hill–Sachs lesion were significant risk factors for the occurrence of capsular lesions. If capsular stretching is present, anterior capsular plication may be necessary as well. After repairing the labrum and torn ligaments, humeral head translation should not exceed 25% of the glenoid diameter while moving the arm at different degrees of abduction and external rotation directions and viewing on arthroscopy, otherwise capsular plication should be the choice. Capsular plication can be done by stitching the capsule to the labrum. If the durability of the labrum were at risk then using a suture anchor would be more effective. The tensioning side should be decided according to the preoperative and peroperative direction of instability. In selected cases, multidirectional tensioning of the capsulolabral tissues is needed.
4. Sometimes, same direction and degree of translation may not be stabilized with Bankart repair and capsular plication, and may require a rotator interval repair. The effect of the rotator interval on shoulder instability is a topic of debate. A rotator interval closure is an option for patients with multidirectional instability, positive sulcus sign on an adducted and externally rotated shoulder, and persistent anterior–inferior instability after a Bankart repair.

The intraoperative decision-making is complex, but it accurately reflects the reality of the clinical situation.

30.4 Contraindications for Soft-Tissue Procedures

Patients able to cause glenohumeral instability with voluntary muscle contractions while the arm is in adduction position have commonly a poor postoperative outcome. Glenoid bone loss of more than 15–20%, engaging Hill–Sachs lesion, or bipolar bone defects that cannot be addressed by remplissage or anchor repair, brachial plexus and axillary nerve injuries, deltoid dysfunction, and infections are the contraindications for soft-tissue procedure in the management of anterior shoulder instability.

References

1. Simonet WT, Melton LJ, Cofield RH, Ilstrup DM. Incidence of anterior shoulder dislocation in Olmsted County, Minnesota. Clin Orthop Relat Res. 1984;(186):186–91.
2. Boone JL, Arciero RA. Management of failed instability surgery: how to get it right the next time. Orthop Clin North Am. 2010;41(3):367–79.
3. Bankart AS. Recurrent or habitual dislocation of the shoulder-joint. Br Med J. 1923;2(3285):1132–3.
4. Morgan CD, Bodenstab AB. Arthroscopic Bankart suture repair: technique and early results. Arthroscopy. 1987;3(2):111–22.

5. Wolf EM, Wilk RM, Richmond JC. Arthroscopic Bankart repair using suture anchors. Oper Tech Orthop A. 1991;1(2):184–91.
6. Miura K, Tsuda E, Tohyama H, Iwahori Y, Mae T, Mochizuki Y, Nakagawa K, Nakamae A, Nakamura T, Takao M, Uchida S, Muneta T, Ochi M. Can arthroscopic Bankart repairs using suture anchors restore equivalent stability to open repairs in the management of traumatic anterior shoulder dislocation? A meta-analysis. J Orthop Sci. 2018;23(6): 935–41.
7. Hintermann B, Gächter A. Arthroscopic findings after shoulder dislocation. Am J Sports Med. 1995;23:545–51.
8. Rodosky MW, Harner CD, Fu FH. The role of the long head of the biceps muscle and superior glenoid labrum in anterior stability of the shoulder. Am J Sports Med. 1994;22(1):121–30.
9. Speer KP, Deng X, Borrero S, Torzilli PA, Altchek DA, Warren RF. Biomechanical evaluation of a simulated Bankart lesion. J Bone Joint Surg Am. 1994;76(12):1819–26.
10. Wasserstein DN, Sheth U, Colbenson K, Henry PD, Chahal J, Dwyer T, Kuhn JE. The true recurrence rate and factors predicting recurrent instability after nonsurgical management of traumatic primary anterior shoulder dislocation: a systematic review. Arthroscopy. 2016;32(12):2616–25.
11. Streubel PN, Krych AJ, Simone JP, Dahm DL, Sperling JW, Steinmann SP, O'Driscoll SW, Sanchez-Sotelo J. Anterior glenohumeral instability: a pathology-based surgical treatment strategy. J Am Acad Orthop Surg. 2014;22(5):283–94.
12. Calvo E, Granizo JJ, Fernandez-Yruegas D. Criteri for arthroscopic treatment of anterior instability of the shoulder. A prospective study. J Bone Joint Surg Br. 2005;87(5):677–83.
13. Vermeulen AE, Landman EBM, Veen EJD, Nienhuis S, Koorevaar CT. Long-term clinical outcome of arthroscopic Bankart repair with suture anchors. J Shoulder Elbow Surg. 2019;28(5):e137–43. pii: S1058-2746(18)30717-1
14. Longo UG, van der Linde JA, Loppini M, Coco V, Poolman RW, Denaro V. surgical versus nonoperative treatment in patients up to 18 years old with traumatic shoulder instability: a systematic review and quantitative synthesis of the literature. Arthroscopy. 2016;32(5):944–52.
15. Imhoff AB, Ansah P, Tischer T, et al. Arthroscopic repair of anterior-inferior glenohumeral instability using a portal at the 5:30-o'clock position: analysis of the effects of age, fixation method, and concomitant shoulder injury on surgical outcomes. Am J Sports Med. 2010;38:1795–803.
16. Crall TS, Bishop JA, Guttman D, Kocher M, Bozic K, Lubowitz JH. Cost-effectiveness analysis of primary arthroscopic stabilization versus nonoperative treatment for first-time anterior glenohumeral dislocations. Arthroscopy. 2012;28(12):1755–65.
17. Rugg CM, Hettrich CM, Ortiz S, Wolf BR, MOON Shoulder Instability Group, Zhang AL. Surgical stabilization for first-time shoulder dislocators: a multicenter analysis. J Shoulder Elb Surg. 2018;27(4):674–85.
18. Porcellini G, Campi F, Pegreffi F, Castagna A, Paladini P. Predisposing factors for recurrent shoulder dislocation after arthroscopic treatment. J Bone Joint Surg Am. 2009;91(11):2537–42.
19. Lee SH, Lim KH, Kim JW. Risk factors for recurrence of anterior-inferior instability of the shoulder after arthroscopicbankart repair in patients younger than 30 years. Arthroscopy. 2018;34(9):2530–6.
20. Buss DD, Lynch GP, Meyer CP, Huber SM, Freehill MQ. Nonoperative management for in-season athletes with anterior shoulder instability. Am J Sports Med. 2004;32(6):1430–3.
21. Provencher MT, Bhatia S, Ghodadra NS. Recurrent shoulder instability: current concepts for evaluation and management of glenoid bone loss. J Bone Joint Surg Am. 2010;92(Suppl 2):133–51.
22. Lo IK, Parten PM, Burkhart SS. The inverted pear glenoid: an indicator of significant glenoid bone loss. Arthroscopy. 2004;20(2):169–74.
23. Itoi E, Lee SB, Berglund LJ, Berge LL, An KN. The effect of a glenoid defect on anteroinferior stability of the shoulder after Bankart repair: a cadaveric study. J Bone Joint Surg Am. 2000;82(1):35–46.
24. Yamamoto N, Muraki T, Sperling JW, et al. Stabilizing mechanism in bonegrafting of a large glenoid defect. J Bone Joint Surg Am. 2010;92(11):2059–66.
25. Kodali P, Jones MH, Polster J, Miniaci A, Fening SD. Accuracy of measurement of Hill-Sachs lesions with computed tomography. J Shoulder Elb Surg. 2011;20(8):1328–34.
26. Voos JE, Livermore RW, Feeley BT. Prospective evaluation of arthroscopic Bankart repairs for anterior instability. Am J Sports Med. 2010;38(2):302–7.
27. Di Giacomo G, Itoi E, Burkhart SS. Evolving concept of bipolar bone loss and the hill-sachs lesion: From 'engaging/non-engaging' lesion to 'on-track/off-track' lesion. Arthroscopy. 2014;30:90–8.
28. Balg F, Boileau P. The instability severity index score: a simple pre-operative score to select patients for arthroscopic or open shoulder stabilisation. J Bone Joint Surg Br. 2007;89(11):1470–7.
29. Phadnis J, Arnold C, Elmorsy A, Flannery M. Utility of the instability severity index score in predicting failure after arthroscopic anterior stabilization of the shoulder. Am J Sports Med. 2015;43(8):1983–8.
30. Nakagawa S, Iuchi R, Mae T, Mizuno N, Take Y. Clinical outcome of arthroscopic Bankart repair combined with simultaneous capsular repair. Am J Sports Med. 2017;45(6):1289–96. https://doi.org/10.1177/0363546516687752. Epub 2017 Jan 30.

Open and Arthroscopic Posterior Bankart Repair

31

Ángel Calvo Díaz, Pablo Carnero Martín de Soto, and Néstor Zurita Uroz

31.1 Introduction

Posterior shoulder instability is a relatively uncommon pathology that is increasingly recognized as a cause of pain and dysfunction. It accounts from 2% to 17% of all cases of shoulder instability and is more frequent in males after a high-energy trauma or as a result of a sport injury, specially throwing sports [1, 2].

Clinical presentation may differ from anterior instability, leading to delayed or even missed diagnosis. There is a wide variability in symptoms and clinical findings. Patients might refer to an initial traumatic event that originates recurrent dislocations since then, although this straightforward history is not found often. More frequently, instability is secondary to microtraumas or repetitive activities that cause progressive injury of the static stabilizers of the posterior part of the shoulder, producing mostly pain. In other cases, posterior instability can be present as a chronic locked posterior dislocation that was missed at early presentation. In some patients, posterior instability is part of a laxity pattern associated with multidirectional instability.

The spectrum of anatomical injuries found in posterior instability is large [3]. All the static stabilizers responsible of posterior glenohumeral stability are at risk when there is a loss of congruity of the joint or repetitive microtraumas. Besides the lesion of the capsulolabral complex, identifying associated injuries like bony deficiencies or ligament stretching is crucial to obtain favorable outcomes after surgery.

Injury of the posterior labrum is, most of the times, the prime lesion that predisposes to development of the instability. The goal of this chapter is to describe the characteristics of the injuries of the labrum in posterior shoulder instability and its treatment.

31.2 Pathophysiology

Labrum injuries vary depending on the etiology of the instability. In cases of atraumatic instability (i.e., hyperlaxity pattern with secondary posterior instability, multidirectional instability, or glenoid dysplasia), inspection of posterior labrum might not show a tear, as the cause of the pathology is not a labrum deficiency. In these cases, a redundant capsule or a determined bone morphology predisposes to the injury. Instead, the labrum often looks hypertrophic with strong attachment to the glenoid rim, in order to supply the function that another static stabilizer is not achieving.

When the origin of instability is considered to be traumatic, labrum tears appear. There are

Á. Calvo Díaz (✉) · P. Carnero Martín de Soto
Arthrosport Zaragoza, Zaragoza, Spain

N. Zurita Uroz
IMED Elche Hospital, Alicante, Spain

R. Brzóska et al. (eds.), *360° Around Shoulder Instability*,
https://doi.org/10.1007/978-3-662-61074-9_31

various degrees of trauma intensity that might cause labrum lesion. High-energy trauma, like car accidents or seizures, often produce complete glenohumeral dislocation with need of reduction by thirds. In these cases, complete displaced detachment of the capsulolabral complex and posterior glenoid periosteum disruption is more likely to happen. This injury is known as "reverse Bankart lesion" and mimics the anterior homonymous lesion. In the same manner, when there is a fracture of the posteroinferior glenoid rim border and the bone fragment keeps attached to the labrum causing bone loss on the articular glenoid surface, it is called a "reverse bony Bankart." These lesions can be accompanied of pathological stretching of the posterior bundle of the inferior glenohumeral ligament and the posterior capsule (Fig. 31.1). In other cases, the displaced labrum tear is scarred medial, over the posterior glenoid neck, and the labrum might look thinned at this area. This is the posterior labrocapsular periosteal sleeve avulsion (POLSPA), which has to be systematically assessed in cases of suspected labrum deficiencies after traumatic instability.

Minor traumas can also cause posteroinferior labrum tearing. Repetitive movements in flexion, adduction, and internal rotation of the arm induce pathologic load to the posterior labrum and capsular attachment. As a consequence, patients usually refer pain, loss of strength, dead-arm syndrome, and, occasionally, subluxation of the joint. This is frequently observed in overhead throwers, weightlifters, and contact-sports athletes. In these cases, complete detachment of posterior labrum is rare. In 2003, Kim et al. described four types of posterior labrum injuries in the setting of posterior instability [4]. Type I was described as an incomplete stripping of the posteroinferior aspect of the labrum, which was torn from its junction with the glenoid articular cartilage but not displaced. It was the most frequent lesion found in their series and was the equivalent to the reverse Bankart injury. Type II consisted on a "marginal crack," a superficial tear between the posterior aspect of the labrum and the glenoid articular cartilage.

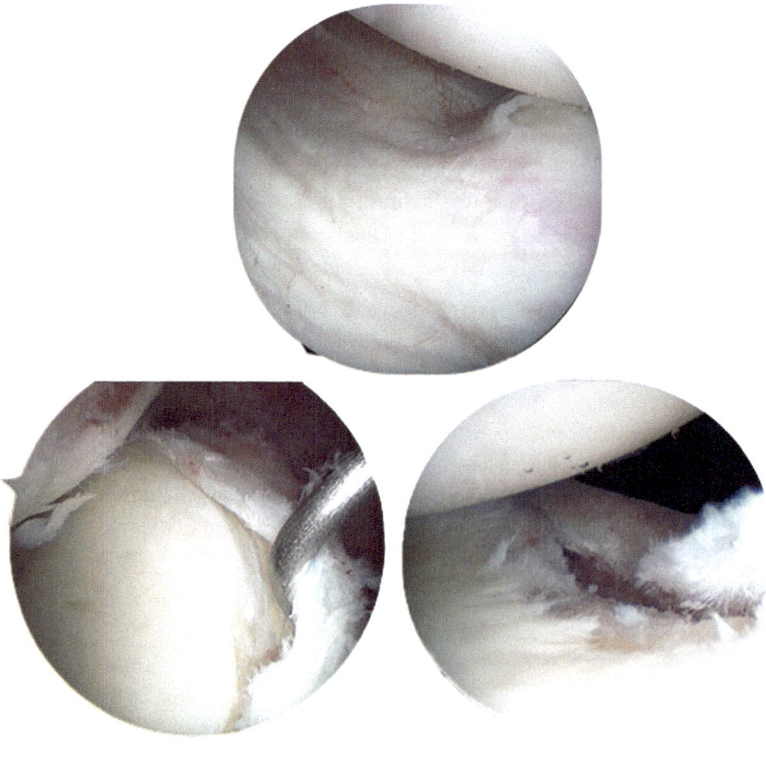

Fig. 31.1 (Up) Pathological stretching of the posterior bundle of the inferior glenohumeral ligament. (Down left) Extensive reverse Bankart lesion. (Down right) Reverse Bony Bankart injury

The posterior aspect of the labrum loses its normal height, and probing demonstrates detachment of the inner portion of the labrum from the medial surface of the glenoid. This injury has been widely named as the "Kim's lesion" and can be easily missed if not probed during arthroscopy. Type III was a chondrolabral erosion, similar to the glenolabral articular disruptions (GLAD injuries) described by Neviaser [5]. Type IV included a labral detachment with flap tear.

Other injuries like posterior humeral avulsion of glenohumeral ligaments (reverse HAGL), posterior glenoid bone losses, or reverse Hill-Sachs have to be identified and properly treated, as they might be the source of pain or recurrent instability and are not uncommon when a traumatic event is the origin.

31.3 Evaluation

Different clinical presentations can be found in the patient with posterior instability, so a high index of suspect is needed to diagnose it.

As said before, instability after the initial traumatic event is not the most frequent clinical form, and patients do not always complain about instability symptoms. Indeed, the most common finding is deep pain within the posterior aspect of the shoulder, usually related with worsening during athletic performance and endurance [4, 6]. If mechanical symptoms like popping, clicking, or apprehension are referred, articular loose bodies and displaced labral tears must be suspected.

During physical examination, signs of generalized ligamentous laxity, like sulcus sign or increased range of motion of other joints of the body, have to be looked for. In addition, complete examination including observation and assessment of range of motion in both shoulders has to be performed.

In contrast to anterior instability, the two main tests used for diagnosing posterior instability do not look for apprehension symptoms solely, as they can be considered positive whether pain is reported.

The Jerk test is performed by stabilizing the scapula with one hand, while the other hand holds the elbow with the arm in 90° of abduction and internal rotation. Then the arm is adducted while an axial compression is applied. A sudden pop and pain is considered positive, secondary to the relocation of the posteriorly subluxated humeral head on the glenoid fossa.

Kim test is a modification of Jerk test. It is performed with the patient in a sitting position and the arm in 90° of abduction. The examiner grasps the elbow and lateral aspect of the proximal arm. When elevating to 45°, axial load and posterior force are applied [7]. The test is positive if the patient complains of pain during this maneuver. The combination of a positive Kim and Jerk tests has a 97% sensitivity for posterior instability [8].

31.4 Surgical Treatment

31.4.1 Indications

Traditionally, posterior shoulder instability has been treated nonsurgically, probably due to the lack of knowledge about the natural history of the disease. However, recent research about this topic has shown that conservative treatment might not obtain good outcomes in all the situations.

Posterior instability in the setting of multidirectional instability or impaired muscular balance must follow conservative treatment as a first step. Activity modification added to physical therapy focused on strengthening the rotator cuff, posterior deltoid, and the scapular stabilizers, and proprioception training have shown to be effective in the majority of atraumatic instabilities [9]. In case of persistence of symptoms after 6 months of conservative treatment, surgery is recommended.

Surgical treatment is often indicated when a traumatic etiology is present. Preoperative assessment of labrum injury is crucial to determine surgical indication. Indeed, some authors advocate that, when traumatic posterior instability is suspected and Kim and Jerk test are positive, surgical stabilization should be performed even if image studies are negative [10], as 85% of patients following conservative treatment will not improve if Kim or Jerk tests are painful.

In the recent years, arthroscopic posterior capsulolabral repair has gained popularity compared to open procedures. A lesser surgical site morbidity, improved visualization of the entire labrum, possibility to address concomitant injuries, and progressive training by shoulder surgeons are the reasons of the predominancy of the arthroscopic technique. In addition, recent studies suggest that arthroscopic repair might obtain better clinical outcomes with lesser recurrence rates [11–13]. Therefore, we consider that arthroscopic capsulolabral repair should be the technique of choice when surgical treatment is chosen for posterior shoulder instability with no or minimal bone loss.

Open techniques are indicated whether there is significant glenoid bone loss or when a previous soft-tissue stabilization has failed. They account for posterior glenoid bony augmentation with bone graft, glenoid osteotomy, or rotational osteotomy of the humeral neck. Extrapolating from research of anterior glenoid bone loss, some authors advocate that posterior defects of 20% of the glenoid surface should be treated with augmentation [6]. However, arthroscopic bone-block procedures for posterior glenoid bone losses using several autografts or allografts have been published with good outcomes [14, 15]; therefore, even in the setting of posterior glenoid defects, arthroscopic techniques may be employed.

31.5 Arthroscopic Surgical Technique

31.5.1 Positioning

We use the lateral decubitus position, with the affected arm placed in a longitudinal traction device at 45° of abduction and approximately 15° of forward flexion. No more than 5 kg is used for traction, and axillary traction bandage is not routinely used. A combined anesthesia with general anesthesia and interscalene block is performed.

31.5.2 Surgical Steps

A posterior portal is located 2 cm medial and 2 cm inferior to the posterolateral border of the acromion. This first portal is used for initial visualization of the joint. Next, an anterior portal is placed at the rotator interval just upward the superior border of the subscapularis tendon and an 8-mm cannula is inserted through it. An anterosuperior portal is also used as a second portal at the rotator interval. It is located 1 cm lateral to the anterolateral border of the acromion, and should exit immediately anterior to the anterior border of the supraspinatus tendon. A 7-mm cannula is placed through it. Both anterior portals are done with an out-in technique using a spinal needle to set the portal position, according to surgeon's preference (Fig. 31.2).

First inspection of the joint includes visualization of the anterior structures from the posterior portal and palpation with a probe introduced from any of the anterior portals. Once finished, the scope is placed through the cannula of the anterosuperior portal which allows complete visualization of the posterior labrum, almost reaching the 6 o'clock position of the glenoid. An accessory posteroinferior portal, also called the 7 o'clock portal [16], is then done, and an 8-mm cannula is inserted through it. This portal is located 2 cm lateral and 1–2 cm anterior from the posterior portal and permits direct access to the posteroinferior labrum, the posterior bundle of the inferior glenohumeral ligament, the posterolateral aspect of the humeral head, and posterior glenoid neck (Fig. 31.3).

Probing posteroinferior labrum has to be done routinely not to miss hidden or incomplete lesions. Kim lesions may mimic superficial fraying but, when the probe is pushed deeper in the chondrolabral transition, absence of capsular and labral anchorage is noted. Other injuries like POLPSA and reverse HAGL are then visualized.

Once the labrum pathology is diagnosed, it has to be gently elevated and mobilized using a

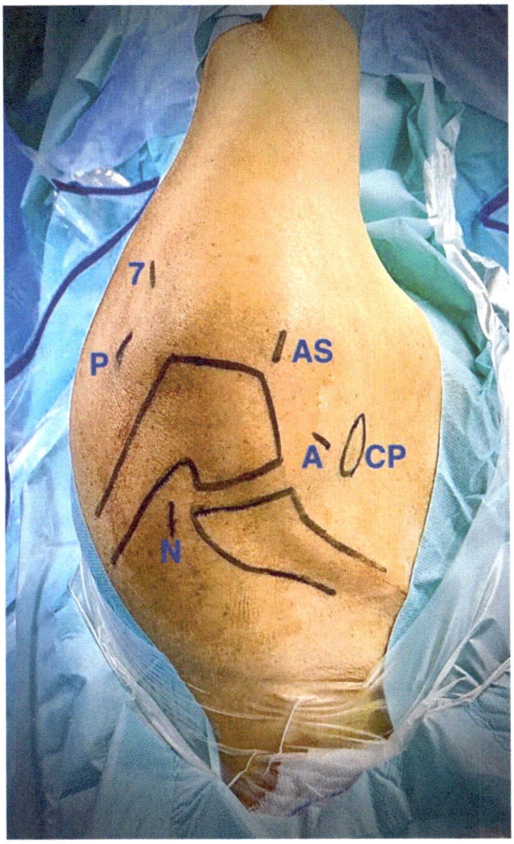

Fig. 31.2 Location of portals used in arthroscopic posterior labrum repair. *CP* coracoid process, *P* posterior portal, *A* anterior portal, *AS* anterosuperior portal, *7* 7 o'clock or accessory posteroinferior portal, *N* Neviaser portal (not routinely used)

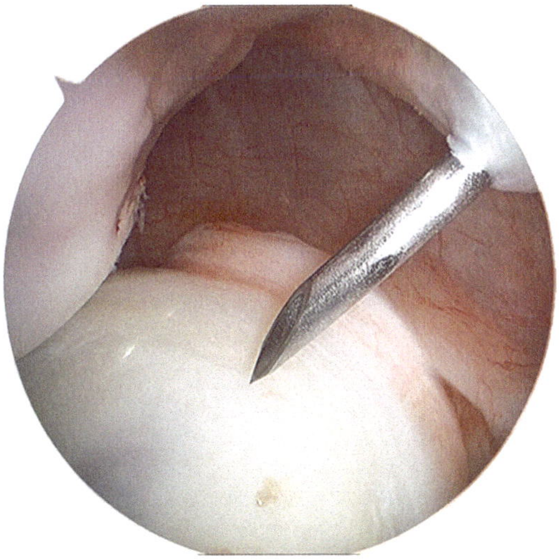

Fig. 31.3 Spinal needle used for out-in technique for 7 o'clock portal

periosteal elevator. The glenoid rim is debrided with the shaver to erase any scar or fibrous tissue in the healing area where the labrum will be reattached. In cases of scarring to the medial glenoid, a combination of the elevator, curette, and a shaver has to be used to obtain adequate labrum reduction to its anatomical attachment. When incomplete lesions are observed, direct repair should not be performed, as it could lead to firm attachment of the superficial portion of the labrum, but loose fixation of its deeper portion and the capsule. Instead, it should be entirely freed to allow suture passage through the whole labrum and the capsule.

We recommend using suture anchors to achieve firm fixation of the labrum to the glenoid. The number of anchors employed depends on the labrum injury's extension and surgeon's preferences. In case of using several anchors, the first inserted has to be the most inferior one, trying not to place it inferior to the 7 o'clock position on the glenoid. They should be separated at least 5 mm to avoid bone weakening. The accessory posteroinferior portal offers an ideal access to the posteroinferior glenoid rim for anchor placement, which should be angled at 45° with respect to the glenoid surface. This orientation is easily reached with this portal, and full access to the posterior rim is obtained to place all the anchors needed.

Once the anchors are inserted, sutures have to be passed through the labrum. Decision on associating a capsular plication has to be made on a case-by-case basis. Capsular redundancy and stretching of the posterior bundle of the inferior glenohumeral ligament is frequently observed when the instability is secondary to traumatic etiology, so capsular shift could be beneficial. However, the exact amount of tissue included on the suture passage is difficult to determine. Penetrating the capsule 1 cm inferior and 1 cm lateral to the anchor is often recommended on an inferior-to-superior and lateral-to-medial direction (Fig. 31.4). Axillary nerve injury during plication is avoided by not placing the anchor inferior to the 7 o'clock position and by not directing the suture passer anteriorly.

Overhead athletes often carry out shoulder movements that exceed the normal range of motion to obtain an optimal performance. In these cases, excessive plication should not be done in order to avoid any limitation of motion. Furthermore, capsular plication might be ignored in some situations, passing the sutures only through the torn labrum. Therefore, the amount of tissue included in capsular shift and its convenience on patients with physical high-demands are still controverted.

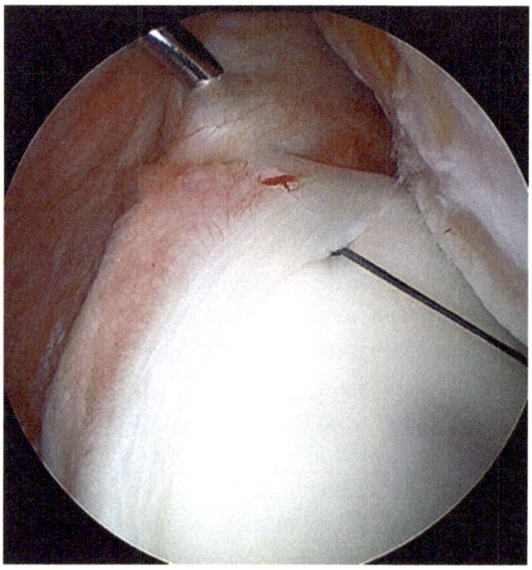

Fig. 31.4 Indirect suture passer penetrating the capsule and the labrum. Amount of capsular tissue included on the stitch varies depending on capsular redundancy

Depending on the soft-tissue quality, direct or indirect suture passer devices can be employed. We prefer using curved soft-tissue-penetrating graspers to capture directly one suture limb from the anchor through the 7 o'clock portal, after penetrating the capsule and the torn labrum (Fig. 31.5). When soft-tissues seem thin and weak, we use the spectrum hook suture passer (ConMed Linvatec, Largo, FL, USA) with polydioxanone (PDS; Ethicon Inc., Somerville, NJ) number 0 as a shuttle suture because its inferior diameter compared to the penetrating graspers allows less tissue damage. It is inserted through the 7 o'clock portal and, after penetrating the tissue, the shuttle suture is released. Then, the shuttle suture and one limb of the anchor suture are retrieved with a suture capturer from the anterior portal and tied together out of the joint. The suture limb from the anchor is passed through the tissue by pulling from the shuttle suture. Finally, both limbs of the anchor suture will end up located at the 7 o'clock portal, ready for knot tying (Fig. 31.6).

When labrum integrity is found, as in many cases of atraumatic instability, pathology may be related to an excessive capsular volume, so cap-

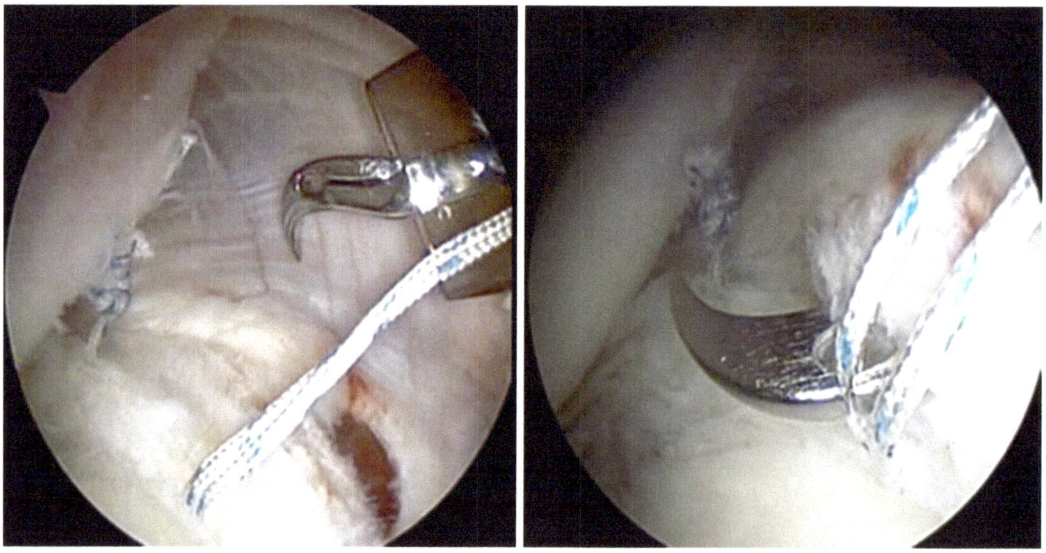

Fig. 31.5 (Left) curved soft-tissue penetrating grasper choosing entry point for capsular shift. (Right) Grasper holding a suture limb from the anchor

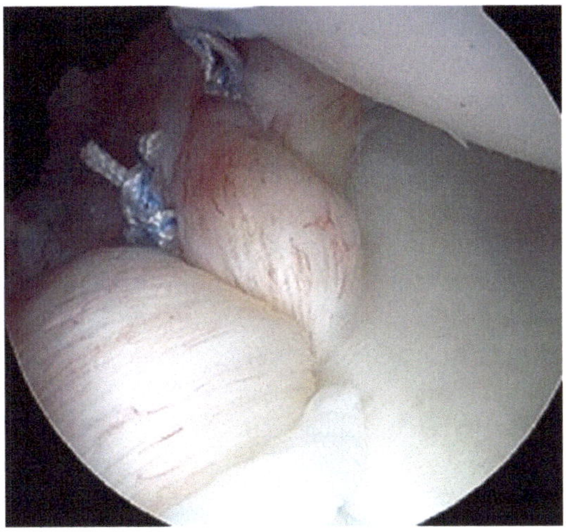

Fig. 31.6 Final look after the knot is tied

sular plications alone should be indicated. Decrease of the capsular redundancy can be done with suture anchors or isolated sutures. In both cases, after gentle abrasion of the capsule with the shaver to allow some bleeding, tissue penetrators perforate the capsule and exit through the chondrolabral joint, to use the labrum like an anchorage point when the knot is tied. Again the exact amount of tissue that has to be included on the plication to obtain an effective lowering of the humeral head translation is difficult to determine.

Once labrum fixation is finished, the concomitant articular injuries should be treated. The reverse Hill-Sachs lesion, also called McLaughlin lesion, is an impacted osteochondral fracture of the anterosuperior portion of the humeral head produced when it impacts against the posterior glenoid border. There is no consensus about the size of the defect that requires specific treatment. Some author advocate that injuries involving 10% of the humeral head should be treated because this lesions involve more articular surface than the conventional Hill-Sachs lesion [17, 18]; while other state that a clear relationship between the size of the defect and higher recurrence rates does not exist [19]. We believe that the decision on treating these bone defects has to be individualized based on patient characteristics. If during arthroscopy the McLaughlin lesion seems to be large enough to endanger the posterior labral repair, it must be treated. Surgical options depend on the size. Small injuries (10–30% of the humeral head approximately) can be treated with a soft-tissue procedure, in which the medium glenohumeral ligament [20] or the superior border of the subscapularis tendon [21] is sutured into the injury, similar to the *remplissage* technique used in posterior Hill-Sachs. Larger injuries (30–50%) require filling the defect with bone graft. In case of enormous injuries (>50%), arthroplasty should be considered.

31.5.3 Postoperative Protocol

After the arthroscopy, the operated arm is placed on a sling in neutral rotation for 6 weeks. Patients are encouraged to retire the sling 2–3 times a day to move actively the elbow, wrist, and fingers. Pendulums and gentle passive abduction (maximum 90°) are allowed from the beginning. At 4 weeks, patients are remitted to physical therapy to aid with passive exercises. At 6 weeks, the sling is discontinued and passive full range of motion is permitted. Once reached, active motion and strength exercises are allowed progressively. Special attention is paid to scapular stabilizers strengthening, which should be initiated at the second month postoperatively. Physical activities that include contact are never recommended before the fourth month.

31.6 Outcomes

A thorough evaluation of the results of posterior labrum repair in shoulder posterior instability is difficult to do due to the variability of the reports published. Different surgical techniques have been described and the spectrum of patients and lesions found during surgery is wide, as are the types of instability (unidirectional posterior, bidirectional posterior and anterior, multidirectional with posterior predominance, posteroinferior, etcetera).

While first reports showed unacceptable recurrence rates after open repair ranging from 30% to

50% [22, 23], DeLong et al. [11] published a systematic review and meta-analysis about outcomes of surgical treatment for posterior instability that probed that these rates decreased to 19.4% with open surgery and 8.1% with arthroscopic treatment. They also showed better results when repair was done with anchors.

Arthroscopic labral repair has consistently showed good clinical outcomes in terms of patient's satisfaction, recurrence rate, and return to play in athletes population. Leivadiotou [24] documented a mean postoperative ASES score of 91.3 and a mean UCLA score of 33 in their systematic review including 396 shoulders at a mean follow up of 44.4 months. Large case series also show this clinical improvement, with mean ASES values improving from 45 to 81 points [25] and good to excellent results ranging from 73% to 90% [6, 26].

Both persistent pain and recurrent instability are considered causes of failure. Recurrent instability is reported in 3.5–12% [11, 24, 27, 28] of cases, although in some isolated study the rate rises to 20% [29]. Persistent pain ranges from 6% to 15% [6, 10, 25, 29], and seems to be related with age over 35 at the time of surgery and concomitant osteochondral injuries [30].

Regarding return to sports, the majority of the reports communicate positive results in above 90% of cases [4, 24–26]. However, reaching pre-injury sport level is not so favorable and seems to depend on the sport played. Throwers have the lowest likelihood of returning to previous level, with rates of 55–68% [26, 31, 32].

31.7 Conclusion

Posterior shoulder instability might be present as diverse clinical presentations. In case of traumatic etiology, posterior labrum injuries are often found, and therefore arthroscopic reparation is usually needed to restore shoulder normal function, but it might not be the only surgical procedure necessary. Need of capsular plications and treatment of bone losses have to be assessed as well. Open procedures are limited to treatment of glenoid bone loss and recurrent instability after soft-tissue procedures and include posterior glenoid augmentation with bone grafts, glenoid osteotomies, and rotational proximal humerus osteotomies. However, some of these procedures can be already done arthroscopically, so open surgical techniques for posterior instability are being progressively abandoned.

Outcomes of arthroscopic labral repair for traumatic unidirectional posterior instability in general population are very satisfactory and surgical techniques described are safe and reproducible, although certain specific patients populations, like throwers athletes, might not obtain enough improvement to reach the same pre-injury level.

References

1. Lanzi JT Jr, Chandler PJ, Cameron KL, Bader JM, Owens BD. Epidemiology of posterior glenohumeral instability in a young athletic population. Am J Sports Med. 2017;45(14):3315–21.
2. Tannenbaum E, Sekiya JK. Evaluation and management of posterior shoulder instability. Sports Health. 2011;3(3):253–63.
3. Van Tongel A, Karelse A, Berghs B, Verdonk R, De Wilde L. Posterior shoulder instability: current concepts review. Knee Surg Sports Traumatol Arthrosc. 2011;19(9):1547–53.
4. Kim SH, Ha KI, Park JH, Kim YM, Lee YS, Lee JY, Yoo JC. Arthroscopic posterior labral repair and capsular shift for traumatic unidirectional recurrent posterior subluxation of the shoulder. J Bone Joint Surg Am. 2003;85-A(8):1479–87.
5. Neviaser TJ. The GLAD lesion: another cause of anterior shoulder pain. Arthroscopy. 1993;9(1):22–3.
6. Frank RM, Romeo AA, Provencher MT. Posterior glenohumeral instability: evidence-based treatment. J Am Acad Orthop Surg. 2017;25(9):610–23.
7. Kim SH, Ha KI, Yoo JC, Noh KC. Kim's lesion: an incomplete and concealed avulsion of the posteroinferior labrum in posterior or multidirectional posteroinferior instability of the shoulder. Arthroscopy. 2004;20(7):712–20.
8. Kim SH, Park JS, Jeong WK, Shin SK. The Kim test: a novel test for posteroinferior labral lesion of the shoulder—a comparison to the jerk test. Am J Sports Med. 2005;33(8):1188–92.
9. McIntyre K, Bélanger A, Dhir J, Somerville L, Watson L, Willis M, Sadi J. Evidence-based conservative rehabilitation for posterior glenohumeral instability: a systematic review. Phys Ther Sport. 2016;22:94–100.
10. Castagna A, Conti M, Garofalo R. Soft tissue-based surgical techniques for treatment of posterior shoulder instability. Obere Extrem. 2017;12(2):82–9.

11. DeLong JM, Jiang K, Bradley JP. Posterior instability of the shoulder: a systematic review and meta-analysis of clinical outcomes. Am J Sports Med. 2015;43(7):1805–17.
12. Provencher MT, LeClere LE, King S, McDonald LS, Frank RM, Mologne TS, Ghodadra NS, Romeo AA. Posterior instability of the shoulder: diagnosis and management. Am J Sports Med. 2011;39(4):874–86.
13. Bradley JP, Baker CL III, Kline AJ, Armfield DR, Chhabra A. Arthroscopic capsulolabral reconstruction for posterior instability of the shoulder: a prospective study of 100 shoulders. Am J Sports Med. 2006;34(7):1061–71.
14. Wellmann M, Pastor MF, Ettinger M, Koester K, Smith T. Arthroscopic posterior bone block stabilization-early results of an effective procedure for the recurrent posterior instability. Knee Surg Sports Traumatol Arthrosc. 2018;26(1):292–8.
15. Schwartz DG, Goebel S, Piper K, Kordasiewicz B, Boyle S, Lafosse L. Arthroscopic posterior bone block augmentation in posterior shoulder instability. J Shoulder Elb Surg. 2013;22(8):1092–101.
16. Davidson PA, Rivenburgh DW. The 7-o'clock posteroinferior portal for shoulder arthroscopy. Am J Sports Med. 2002;30(5):693–6.
17. Robinson CM, Seah M, Akhtar MA. The epidemiology, risk of recurrence, and functional outcome after an acute traumatic posterior dislocation of the shoulder. J Bone Joint Surg Am. 2011;93(17):1605–13.
18. Provencher MT, Frank RM, Leclere LE, Metzger PD, Ryu JJ, Bernhardson A, Romeo AA. The Hill-Sachs lesion: diagnosis, classification, and management. J Am Acad Orthop Surg. 2012;20(4):242–52.
19. Longo UG, Rizzello G, Locher J, Salvatore G, Florio P, Maffulli N, Denaro V. Bone loss in patients with posterior gleno-humeral instability: a systematic review. Knee Surg Sports Traumatol Arthrosc. 2016;24(2):612–7.
20. Duey RE, Burkhart SS. Arthroscopic treatment of a reverse Hill-Sachs lesion. Arthrosc Tech. 2013;2(2):e155–9.
21. Lavender CD, Hanzlik SR, Pearson SE, Caldwell PE III. Arthroscopic reverse remplissage for posterior instability. Arthrosc Tech. 2016;5(1):e43–7.
22. Tibone JE, Prietto C, Jobe FW, Kerlan RW, Carter VS, Shields CL Jr, Lombardo SJ, Collins HR, Yocum LA. Staple capsulorrhaphy for recurrent posterior shoulder dislocation. Am J Sports Med. 1981;9(3):135–9.
23. Hawkins RJ, Koppert G, Johnston G. Recurrent posterior instability (subluxation) of the shoulder. J Bone Joint Surg Am. 1984;66(2):169–74.
24. Leivadiotou D, Ahrens P. Arthroscopic treatment of posterior shoulder instability: a systematic review. Arthroscopy. 2015;31(3):555–60.
25. Bradley JP, McClincy MP, Arner JW, Tejwani SG. Arthroscopic capsulolabral reconstruction for posterior instability of the shoulder: a prospective study of 200 shoulders. Am J Sports Med. 2013;41(9):2005–14.
26. Radkowski CA, Chhabra A, Baker CL III, Tejwani SG, Bradley JP. Arthroscopic capsulolabral repair for posterior shoulder instability in throwing athletes compared with nonthrowing athletes. Am J Sports Med. 2008;36(4):693–9.
27. Arner JW, McClincy MP, Bradley JP. Arthroscopic stabilization of posterior shoulder instability is successful in American Football Players. Arthroscopy. 2015;31(8):1466–71.
28. Provencher MT, Bell SJ, Menzel KA, Mologne TS. Arthroscopic treatment of posterior shoulder instability: results in 33 patients. Am J Sports Med. 2005;33(10):1463–71.
29. Andrieu K, Barth J, Saffarini M, Clavert P, Godenèche A, Mansat P, French Arthroscopy Society. Outcomes of capsulolabral reconstruction for posterior shoulder instability. Orthop Traumatol Surg Res. 2017;103(8S):S189–92.
30. Bateman DK, Black EM, Lazarus MD, Abboud JA. Outcomes following arthroscopic repair of posterior labral tears in patients older than 35 years. Orthopedics. 2017;40(2):e305–11.
31. Bahk MS, Karzel RP, Snyder SJ. Arthroscopic posterior stabilization and anterior capsular plication for recurrent posterior glenohumeral instability. Arthroscopy. 2010;26(9):1172–80.
32. McClincy MP, Arner JW, Bradley JP. Posterior shoulder instability in throwing athletes: a case-matched comparison of throwers and non-throwers. Arthroscopy. 2015;31(6):1041–51.

Reverse Humeral Avulsion of Glenohumeral Ligaments (rHAGL)

32

Adrian Błasiak, Hubert Laprus, Wojciech Solecki, and Roman Brzóska

32.1 Introduction

The glenohumeral ligaments belong to a complex of primary static stabilizers of the shoulder. The ligament complex consists of the superior, middle, and inferior glenohumeral ligament (SGHL, MGHL, and IGHL). The latter one is composed of an anterior and posterior band along with a capsule of axillary pouch. Elasticity of that complex provides static stabilization in different positions, preventing anterior, posterior, and inferior translation of the humeral head [1, 2].

The humeral insertion of the IGHL is located close to the articular margin [1]. According to Bui-Mansfield, the anterior band (AIGHL) extends from 2 to 4 o'clock and the posterior band (PIGHL) from 7 to 9 o'clock [3]. The glenoid attachment of both bands originates from the labrum.

Bigliani et al., who assessed the tensile properties of the IGHL in a cadaveric model, indicated that the posterior band was the weakest of the complex [4].

Similarly, Ticker et al. showed in a cadaveric model that the posterior band was the weakest of the IGHL regions, with comparatively poor viscoelastic properties [5].

A. Błasiak (✉) · H. Laprus · W. Solecki · R. Brzóska
Shoulder and Upper Limb Department, St. Luke's Hospital, Bielsko-Biała, Poland
e-mail: blasiak@lukasza.pl

R. Brzóska et al. (eds.), *360° Around Shoulder Instability*,
https://doi.org/10.1007/978-3-662-61074-9_32

Traumatic anterior dislocation of the shoulder can result in disruption of the MGHL along with the labrum from the anterior glenoid and the IGHL either from the anteroinferior glenoid along with the labrum or at its humeral insertion. The first situation results in Bankart lesion and the latter one in HAGL lesion.

In 1942, Nicola first described an acute shoulder dislocation with avulsion of the IGHL from the scapular neck [6].

In 1995, Wolf et al. used the term HAGL (humeral avulsion of glenohumeral ligaments) as a cause of anterior shoulder instability following anterior dislocation [7].

Similarly posterior shoulder dislocation can result in reverse lesions such as a posterior Bankart lesion or posterior eventually reverse HAGL lesion [8].

In specific cases, a combination of these both lesions, so called floating PIGHL, can be observed and teres minor tendon tear has also been linked to bony posterior HAGL injury [9, 10].

32.2 Definition and Epidemiology

Various descriptions of that lesion exist in the literature. A few of them should be mentioned like in example "lateral capsular disruption of the posterior aspect of the shoulder" according to Laurencin et al., "humeral detachment along the posterior humeral head", called a reverse HAGL (rHAGL) lesion, and "posterior humeral avulsion of the posterior portion of the IGHL" [8, 11, 12].

Bokor et al., who described the largest series of treatment of such lesion so far, gave their own definitions [13]. They mentioned a reverse humeral avulsion of the glenohumeral ligament to be an avulsion of the posterior capsule of the glenohumeral joint above the level of the PIGHL, which may or may not extend into the posterior band of the IGHL and the posterior HAGL or avulsion of the posterior band of the inferior glenohumeral ligament.

However, in this chapter, the name reverse HAGL lesion is used for all lesions involving an avulsion of either the posterior band of the IGHL or posterior capsule from the humeral neck.

Typically the anterior HAGL lesion is more common than similar injuries of posterior aspect of humeral neck. Nevertheless, while rare, both of them have been shown to contribute to recurrent instability [9, 14].

Furthermore, rHAGL lesions can be often seen in combination with other pathologies like posterior Bankart or posterior bony Bankart lesions [9].

According to Bokor et al., the mechanism of injury differs from the more common overuse syndromes in throwing athletes [13]. The fall on a forward flexed arm is a common cause of posterior instability, but in their group almost half of patients (mostly rugby players) reported a violent, forced cross-body adduction force as the predominant injury mechanism.

The HAGL lesions incidence is rare but reported increasingly and is estimated around 10% in patients with shoulder instability, and even more frequent in patients needing revision procedures [7, 15].

The epidemiology of rHAGL lesion refers to patients with posterior instability and no strict data exist in the literature to date. However, the incidence of rHAGL lesions is assessed to be much less common than that of HAGL lesions [9, 13, 16].

32.3 Diagnosis

Crucial step in making diagnosis of the rHAGL is taking patient's meticulous history.

Nonspecific shoulder complaints with a typical history of shoulder instability (dislocations or subluxations) are often present. The mechanism of primary injury with the arm flexed and adducted can lead to humeral avulsion of posterior IGHL. Furthermore, in some cases, the anterior instability or even no episode of anterior or posterior dislocation or subluxation can be reported by patients with rHAGL [13, 17].

Therefore, particular attention should be paid to patients with recurrent instability who underwent surgery or patients with recurrent instability in the absence of characteristic glenoid-side lesions (Bankart or bony Bankart lesion). There is a strong likelihood of either HAGL or rHAGL lesion in those patients [18].

Castagna et al. described 16 consecutive patients who underwent an arthroscopic repair of an rHAGL lesion [17]. In 7 of those patients, the rHAGL lesion was found after a previous shoulder surgery, and 6 of them underwent previous anterior shoulder stabilization. One patient underwent thermal capsule shrinkage to treat multidirectional shoulder instability.

The examination of patient with suspected rHAGL lesion comprises all steps of complete examination of unstable shoulder. Therefore, a full active and passive range of motion and strength in forward flexion, abduction, adduction, external rotation, and internal rotation should be assessed.

Since either HAGL or rHAGL lesion can suggest hyperlaxity alone or together with multidirectional instability, evaluation of both shoulders is very important.

In daily practice, the author applies modified Beighton scoring system for the assessment of hyperlaxity [19]. According to it, one point for each side of the body for the paired tests and one for forward bend is given to the patient. The range of scoring is thus between 0 and 9, with high scores denoting greater joint laxity.

Then, the following provocative test should be performed: apprehension test, the anterior and posterior load and shift test, and Kim or jerk test.

All tests mentioned above are symptomatic for instability, but there is no specific test to detect rHAGL lesion.

Bokor et al. found symptoms of posterior instability in 15 of the 19 treated patient in preoperative assessment [13]. In three patients, they could not pinpoint the dominant direction, and one had no clinical evidence of instability.

In their research, Castagna et al. found test results compatible with a posterior apprehension in 7 patients representing 78% of their series [17]. In remaining two patients, who presented with an associated lesion of the anterior capsulolabral complex, the results of the anterior apprehension test were positive.

Both authors stated that there are no consistent, specific signs or symptoms to suggest an rHAGL. At the same time, they agreed that the most consistent symptom in majority of patients was posterior shoulder pain.

32.4 Imaging

Routinely performed diagnostic pattern in cases of shoulder instability comprises true AP and "Y" X-rays to exclude possible fractures either of the humeral tuberosities or glenoid rim. Axillary view may be helpful to identify Hill-Sachs lesion and any concomitant glenoid rim fractures as well.

Magnetic resonance imaging (MRI) with or without intraarticular contrast remains the recommended imaging of choice in cases of suspected HAGL or rHAGL lesions [3, 20].

Bui-Mansfield et al. reported that the inferior glenohumeral ligament is best visualized on coronal oblique or sagittal oblique T2-weighted fat-suppressed modality [3].

According to Rebolledo et al., the axial fast spin-echo images are most useful for identifying capsular injury, including subtle partial tears [20]. In their research, extracapsular soft tissue edema signal on fluid-sensitive sequences is another useful indicator of an acute posterior HAGL lesion.

Remarkable in MRI scans is a "U shape" axillary pouch which contains fluid, visible on the coronal or sagittal oblique views of normal shoulder joint. In cases of IGHL disruption the contrast, fluid or blood extravasation, in acute lesions, results in absence of that sign.

Chronic HAGL lesions are usually partially healed and difficult to visualize for that reason [21].

According to Castagna et al., precise arthroscopic evaluation of the joint, including viewing from the anterior portal, is crucial to make the diagnosis of an rHAGL lesion [17]. The intraoperative inspection reveals also many concomitant lesions.

Bokor et al. also advocate routine, systematic assessment of the posterior capsule at the time of surgery, which is achieved by viewing through the anterior portal, because failing to do so may result in incomplete visualization of the posterior capsule [13].

Rebolledo et al. found among 28 cases that additional shoulder injuries associated with the posterior HAGL lesion occurred in 93% of cases [20]. The most common concomitant injuries were reverse Hill-Sachs lesions (36%), anterior Bankart lesions (29%), and posterosuperior rotator cuff tears (25%). The presence of anterior labral or capsular injury was found in 50% of these patients, signifying bidirectional disruption of the capsule.

Similar observations were made by Bokor et al. Among 199 patients, in 58% labral tear was present, 32% a SLAP lesion, 26% a reverse Bankart lesion, 21% a chondral injury, and 21% rotator cuff injury [13].

These findings suggest meticulous analysis of the shoulder MRI is crucial to reveal various concomitant lesions associated with shoulder instability, especially in cases with suspected IGHL complex lesions.

32.5 Treatment

Conservative management is typically reserved for partial, intrasubstance lesions of the IGHL complex without any significant concomitant injuries. Such situations concern asymptomatic patients.

Immobilization followed by strengthening of the shoulder girdle muscles, physical therapy, and regaining of range of motion could be helpful to prevent development of recurrent instability.

Surgical treatment is applied for athletes, high-demanding individuals, in cases of persistent pain, shoulder dysfunction, or failed nonsurgical treatment with recurrent instability [21].

Although still limited, data with small case series and reports exist, and results of arthroscopy and open repair are satisfactory and seem to be comparable [13, 17].

32.6 Surgical Technique

The surgical treatment of rHAGL lesion can be performed either open or arthroscopically. However, the crucial issue whether the surgical treatment should be indicated is the proper diagnosis of the injury. The rHAGL lesion can imitate various associated intraarticular pathologies and can be missed in routine examination of the unstable shoulder. Furthermore, even the MRI offers no solid evidence of detection the lesion. Bokor et al. reported accurate identification of the posterior capsular injury in only 7/14 cases (50%). Exclusively on retrospective postoperative review, the rHAGL was apparent in 11/14 (78.6%) patients of this series [13].

For that reason, an arthroscopic approach is more desirable, at least as a first diagnostic stage of the entire procedure.

Subsequently, if an open procedure is selected for posterior repair, first a diagnostic arthroscopy through either standard posterior portal or anterolateral portal is performed and rHAGL lesion is confirmed or revealed.

The posterior capsule can only be fully visualized during diagnostic arthroscopy by using the anterolateral portal (Fig. 32.1).

Concomitant injuries are treated at this stage. In every case of suspected intraarticular shoulder pathologies, an exhaustive arthroscopic inspection is indicated as the last step of diagnostic process.

Then, the posterior portal is enlarged to 5–6 cm along the deltoid muscle fibers, followed by dissection between the infraspinatus and the teres minor. The posterior capsule is then exposed. The capsular avulsion can be identified through this interval. The ruptured capsule and underlying bone bed on the humeral neck are debrided and reattached with suture anchors.

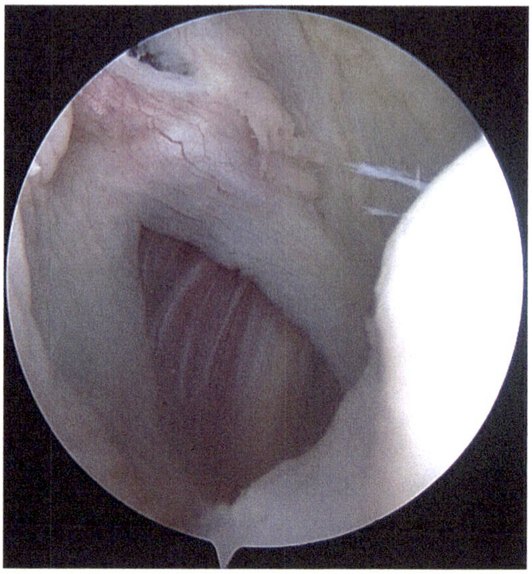

Fig. 32.1 rHAGL—anterior view

This technique has been reported uncommonly, but with successful results [22, 23].

The arthroscopic treatment of the rHAGL lesion is almost always accessible from an arthroscopic approach.

The arthroscopic surgical technique is similar to anterior HAGL lesion repair; however, an accessory posteroinferior portal for anchor placement is required.

Although extracapsular repairs can also be accomplished, intraarticular anchor placement, suture passage, and knot tying are relatively easier and more accessible. The clinical outcomes of arthroscopic treatment of the rHAGL lesion have been uniformly successful, as in the case of the anterior HAGL lesion repair [11, 13, 17, 24].

The operation can be performed in either a lateral decubitus or a beach-chair position. The author prefers the latter one.

The patient is placed in the beach chair position under general anesthesia following interscalene block, with the operated arm placed in traction of 1.5–2.0 kg, 30° of forward flexion, neutral rotation, and no abduction.

The standard posterior portal is established. Next an additional anterolateral portal is created.

The diagnostic arthroscopic examination starts with the arthroscope inserted into the posterior portal.

Precise inspection of the entire humeral head, glenoid surface, and glenohumeral ligament complex of the anterior compartment of the joint and axillary pouch is performed in order to detect concomitant lesions. It is critical to expose the entire attachment of the IGHL and posterior capsule to the humeral neck (Fig. 32.2).

At this point, the arthroscope is switched into anterolateral portal to complete the joint inspection by visualization of the posterior compartment and confirms the initial diagnosis.

In some cases, the rHAGL lesion (especially extensive one) can be exposed from the posterior portal by pushing the humeral head slightly anteriorly (Fig. 32.3).

Nonetheless, the visualization and repair is usually performed with scope in anterolateral portal. Full thickness tears enable to reveal posterior rotator cuff muscles through the ruptured capsule (Fig. 32.4).

At this point, an additional posteroinferior working portal should be established. This should be performed under direct scope visualization either form posterior or anterolateral portal. The entry point is located approximately 2–3 cm below the standard posterolateral portal, namely 5–6 cm inferiorly to the posterolateral corner of the acromion along with the fibers of the deltoid muscle (Fig. 32.5). Its position is equivalent to anteroinferior, so called 5

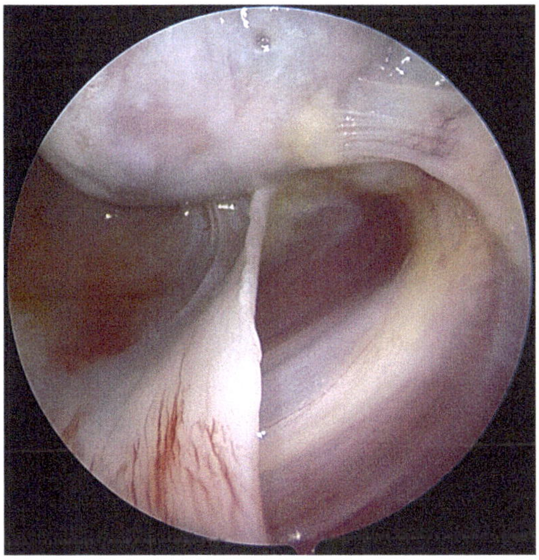

Fig. 32.2 rHAGL—posterior view

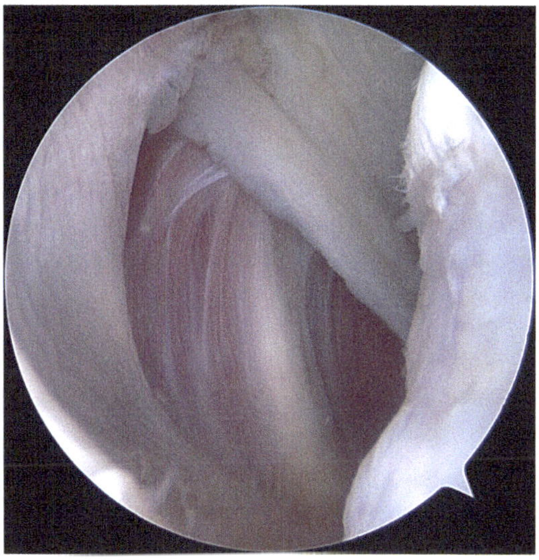

Fig. 32.4 rHAGL—anterior view with concomitant Hill-Sachs lesion

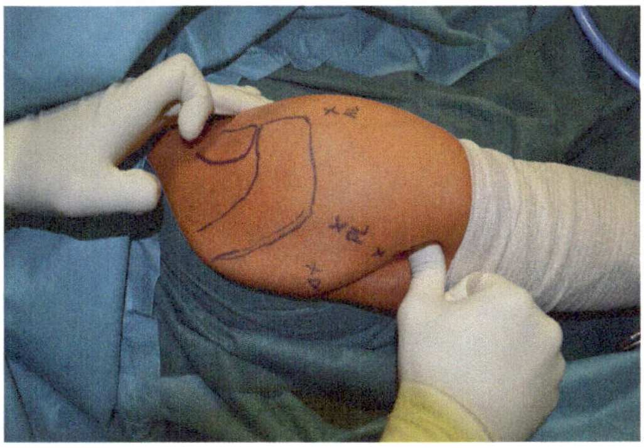

Fig. 32.3 Pushing the humeral neck anteriorly figure

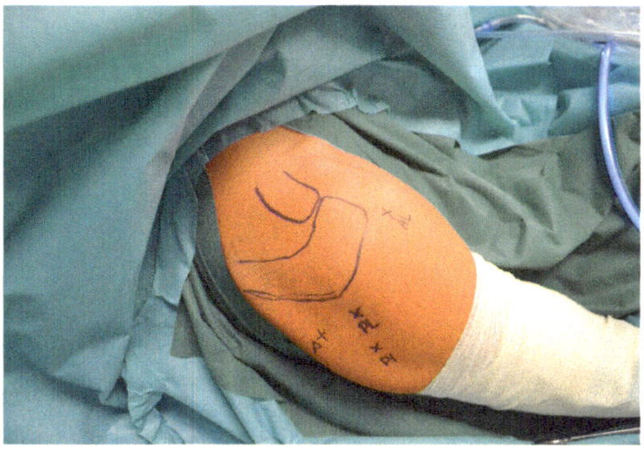

Fig. 32.5 Posteroinferior portal (PI)

o'clock portal. The best way for planning the portal is to use an 18 gauge needle.

The author doesn't use any cannulas; however, it is important to avoid further damage of the fragile posterior capsule while inserting a cannula.

Then, the posterior humeral neck is refreshed with an arthroscopic device (shaver, burr, or rasp) at the desired location of insertion of the posterior IGHL.

Then, usually one suture anchor is placed, through posteroinferior portal, at the humeral footprint of posterior IGHL (Fig. 32.6).

Since posterior capsule is a fragile structure, the mattress sutures should be passed with a very gentle and precise tool and the attention should be paid while knot tying (Fig. 32.7).

Too aggressive manipulations can lead to subsequent damage of the capsule and enlargement of the tear.

The reduction of the lesion to the humeral neck is performed in a neutral position of the arm to avoid overtightening of the posterior capsule resulting in postoperative limitation of range of motion.

The careful suture passing, limited only to the capsule, is important to prevent the injuries of axillary nerve and medial circumflex artery, which however is located more anteriorly.

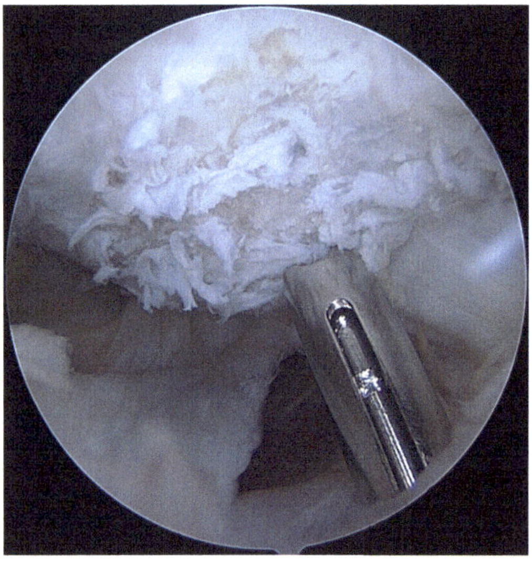

Fig. 32.6 rHAGL—posterior view anchor placement

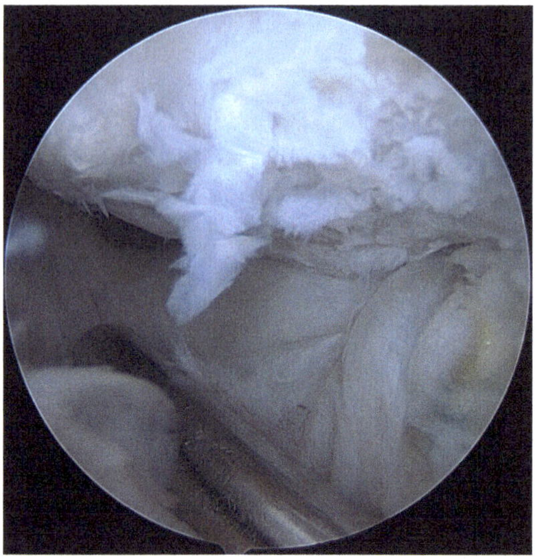

Fig. 32.7 rHAGL—posterior view after repair

Some casuistic cases of rHAGL lesion were also published.

Ames and Millett described a variant of floating posterior HAGL lesion with present concomitant posterior bony Bankart lesion, and Mitchell et al. found it together with a reverse Hill-Sachs lesion [9, 25].

In such cases, all pathologies should be addressed during surgery.

The postoperative protocol comprises shoulder brace in neutral position for 4–6 weeks with passive rotational movements within pain limits. Physical therapy begins 3–4 weeks after surgery. Active exercises start at 6 weeks after surgery followed by strengthening of shoulder girdle muscles and increasing of range of movement.

32.7 Conclusion

The rHAGL lesion is relatively a rare injury related to shoulder instability. There are only few reports regarding this pathology including small case series. Although its incidence is low, rHAGL lesion exceptionally occurs as an isolated pathology. It is frequently associated with a spectrum of pathologic intraarticular changes and if misdiagnosed can lead to improper diagnosis and incomplete surgical treatment followed by recurrent instability.

Furthermore, symptoms related to an rHAGL lesion can be concealed by concomitant injuries and could result in delayed diagnosis and exacerbate glenohumeral pathologic changes. Therefore, a high suspicion is indicated in the presence of atypical history and symptoms of anterior, posterior, or combined anteroposterior shoulder instability. Exact history taking, precise examination, and properly performed MRI do not guarantee proper diagnosis; therefore, meticulous arthroscopic joint evaluation from posterior and anterolateral portals is the best way not to overlook that lesion. Arthroscopic treatment of rHAGL lesion does not seem to be a technically demanding procedure and has shown to yield good clinical outcomes.

References

1. O'Brien SJ, Neves MC, Arnoczky SP, Rozbruck SR, Dicarlo EF, Warren RF, et al. The anatomy and histology of the inferior gleno-humeral ligament complex of the shoulder. Am J Sports Med. 1990;18:449–56.
2. Turkel SJ, Panio MW, Marshall JL, Girgis FG. Stabilizing mechanisms preventing anterior dislocation of the glenohumeral joint. J Bone Joint Surg. 1981;63A:1208–17.
3. Bui-Mansfield LT, Taylor DC, Uhorchak JM, Tenuta JJ. Humeral avulsions of the glenohumeral ligament: imaging features and a review of the literature. AJR Am J Roentgenol. 2002;179:649–55.
4. Bigliani LU, Pollock RG, Soslowsky LJ, et al. Tensile properties of the inferior glenohumeral ligament. J Orthop Res. 1992;10(2):187–97.
5. Ticker JB, Bigliani LU, Soslowsky LJ, et al. Inferior glenohumeral ligament: geometric and strain-rate dependent properties. J Shoulder Elb Surg. 1996;5(4):269–79.
6. Nicola T. Anterior dislocation of the shoulder: the role of the articular capsule. J Bone Joint Surg. 1942;25A:614–6.
7. Wolf EM, Cheng JC, Dickson K. Humeral avulsion of glenohumeral ligaments as a cause of anterior shoulder instability. Arthroscopy. 1995;11:600–7.
8. Laurencin CT, Paletta GA, Potter H, Wickiewicz TL. Disruption of the posterior-lateral shoulder capsule. J Shoulder Elb Surg. 1995;4:391–4.
9. Ames JB, Millett PJ. Combined posterior osseous Bankart lesion and posterior humeral avulsion of the glenohumeral ligaments: a case report and pathoanatomic subtyping of "floating" posterior inferior glenohumeral ligament lesions. J Bone Joint Surg. 2011;93A:e1181–4.
10. Smith PA, Nuelle CW, Bradley JP. Arthroscopic repair of a posterior bony humeral avulsion of the glenohumeral ligament with associated teres minor avulsion. Arthrosc Tech. 2014;3(1):e89–94.
11. Abrams JS. Arthroscopic repair of posterior instability and reverse humeral glenohumeral ligament avulsion lesions. Orthop Clin North Am. 2003;34:475–83.
12. Safran O, DeFranco M, Hatem S, Ianotti JP. Posterior humeral avulsion of the glenohumeral ligament as a cause of posterior shoulder instability: a case report. J Bone Joint Surg Am. 2004;86:2732–6.
13. Bokor DJ, Fritsch BA. Posterior shoulder instability secondary to reverse humeral avulsion of the glenohumeral ligament. J Shoulder Elb Surg. 2010;19:853–8.
14. Bui-Mansfield LT, Banks KP, Taylor DC. Humeral avulsion of the glenohumeral ligaments: the HAGL lesion. Am J Sports Med. 2007;35:1960–6.
15. Bokor DJ, Conboy VB, Olson C. Anterior instability of the gleno- humeral joint with humeral avulsion of the glenohumeral ligament. A review of 41 cases. J Bone Joint Surg. 1999;81B:93–6.
16. Hill JD, Lovejoy JF Jr, Kelly RA. Combined posterior Bankart lesion and posterior humeral avulsion of the glenohumeral ligaments associated with recurrent posterior shoulder instability. Arthroscopy. 2007;23:327e1–3.
17. Castagna A, Snyder SJ, Conti M, Borroni M, Massazza G, Garofalo R. Posterior humeral avulsion of the glenohumeral ligament: a clinical review of 9 cases. Arthroscopy. 2007;23:809–15.
18. Martetschläger F, Ames JB, Millett PJ. HAGL and reverse HAGL lesions. In: Milano G, Grasso A, editors. Shoulder arthroscopy. London: Springer-Verlag; 2014.
19. Beighton P, Solomon L, Soskolne CL. Articular mobility in an African population. Ann Rheum Dis. 1973;32:413–8.
20. Rebolledo BJ, Nwachukwu BU, Konin GP. Posterior humeral avulsion of the glenohumeral ligament and associated injuries: assessment using magnetic resonance imaging. Am J Sports Med. 2015;43:2913–7.
21. George MS, Khazzam M, Kuhn JE. Humeral avulsion of glenohumeral ligaments. J Am Acad Orthop Surg. 2011;19:127–33.
22. Hasan SS, Fleckenstein C, Albright J. Open treatment of posterior humeral avulsion of the glenohumeral ligaments: a case report and review of the literature. J Shoulder Elb Surg. 2007;16(4):e3–5.
23. Weinberg J, McFarland EG. Posterior capsular avulsion in a college football player. Am J Sports Med. 1999;27(2):235–7.
24. Chhabra A, Diduch DR, Anderson M. Arthroscopic repair of a posterior humeral avulsion of the inferior glenohumeral ligament (HAGL) lesion. Arthroscopy. 2004;20(Suppl 2):73–6.
25. Mitchell JJ, Vap AR, Sanchez G, et al. Concomitant reverse Hill-Sachs lesion and posterior humeral avulsion of the glenohumeral ligament: treatment with fresh talus osteochondral allograft and arthroscopic posterior humeral avulsion of the glenohumeral ligament and labrum repair. Arthrosc Tech. 2017;6(4):e987–95.

Revisions After Failed Posterior Instability

33

Achilleas Boutsiadis, John Swan, and Johannes Barth

33.1 Introduction

Posterior shoulder instability is a relatively rare clinical condition, with an incidence approximately 20 times lower than that of anterior shoulder instability in initial reports [1, 2]. It occurs in less than 10% of the patients with shoulder instability [3], is more frequent in athletes participating in contact or overhead sports, and is more common in the military population [4]. Typically, posterior instability is the result of repetitive microtrauma in flexion, adduction, and internal rotation of the humerus [5]. Respectively, an acute episode in the same position can lead to a traumatic posterior dislocation.

However, newer studies suggest that we initially underestimated the incidence, with posterior glenohumeral instability (PGHI) actually accounting for up to 24% of young and active patients [6, 7]. Recently, Andrieu et al. studied the outcomes of capsulolabral reconstruction for posterior shoulder instability and reported relatively high failure rates in both their retrospective (35%) and prospective (22%) cohort [8]. This large discrepancy in diagnosis and successful treatment results highlight the importance of precise clinical diagnosis and comprehensive understanding of underlying pathology.

Posterior instability is defined as a history of permanent or sudden loss of contact between the humeral and glenoid articular surfaces, potentially leaving passage lesions that could lead to symptoms such as apprehension or pain. The patient often has a positive apprehension and a simultaneous defensive muscular contraction during clinical examination provocative testing. This should be clarified from any other conditions that could mimic posterior instability, such as shoulder hyperlaxity, voluntary instability, muscle imbalance, and static posterior humeral head subluxation sometimes present in the early stages of degenerative arthritis with Walch B type glenoid morphologies.

Posterior instability presents a challenge to both patients and clinicians alike. Often, patients can themselves be unclear on the cause of their shoulder problem and will often present with vague and sometimes mild signs and symptoms, which is in contrast to classic anterior shoulder instability where patients clearly experience apprehension and instability. This, along with the myriad of pathoanatomies causing posterior instability, makes clinician diagnosis and management ever challenging. The purpose of this chapter is to present the multifaceted pathology,

A. Boutsiadis (✉)
2nd Orthopaedic Department, 401 Military Hospital of Athens, Athens, Greece

J. Swan · J. Barth
Department of Orthopaedic Surgery, Centre Osteoarticulaire des Cèdres, Grenoble, France

R. Brzóska et al. (eds.), *360° Around Shoulder Instability*,
https://doi.org/10.1007/978-3-662-61074-9_33

to outline the diagnostic difficulties, and to understand the reasons of a failed PGHI. Thereafter, the possible treatments (nonoperative or operative) will be discussed in order to help optimize management.

33.1.1 Understanding the Underlying Pathology

Several authors have attempted to understand and describe the patho-anatomy of PGHI. Literature reports that PGHI occurs on a spectrum, from subtle subluxation to frank dislocation and atraumatic to traumatic.

The different proposed injury mechanisms include:

(a) Acute trauma during posteriorly directed force and with the arm in adduction and forward flexion.
(b) Repetitive microtrauma leading progressively to posterior capsulular and posterior labral injury.
(c) Insidious laxity resulting in stretching of the posterior capsule and stabilizers [4, 9].

In most cases a reverse Bankart lesion (detachment of the posterior labrum), a Kim lesion (tear between the posteroinferior labrum and the cartilage without complete detachment) and/or a reverse Hill–Sachs lesion are usually present [1]. The reverse Hill–Sachs can result in <25%, 25% to 50% or to >50% humeral head bone loss that is important to evaluate in developing a treatment strategy and the type of operation [10]. Additionally, posterior glenoid defects can also be present in chronic cases and can cause recurrent dislocation. Recently, Nacca et al. proposed that the critical posterior glenoid bone loss in posterior shoulder instability is 20% [11], beyond which the shoulder still remains unstable after isolated reverse Bankart repair.

Apart from the aforementioned lesions, any abnormal underlying anatomy could also contribute significantly to the presence or recurrence of posterior instability of traumatic or atraumatic causes. On assessment of the scapula, the presence of glenoid dysplasia or increased retroversion should be looked for. Glenoid dysplasia is the condition characterized from osseous deficit mainly of the posteroinferior part of the glenoid with concomitant abnormalities of the labrum and/or the posterior capsule. Weishaupt et al. [12] and Edelson et al. [13] proposed a qualitative description of the glenoid hypoplasia as a rounded "lazy J form" and as a triangular osseous deficiency called "delta form" (Fig. 33.1). The authors supported that recurrent posterior shoulder instability should be considered in patients when this bony deficiency has a craniocaudal length of more than 12 mm [12]. Harper et al. further classified glenoid dysplasia in mild, moderate, and severe forms and found that the incidence of posteroinferior labral pathology increases with the severity of the glenoid deformity. Interestingly, authors using MRI arthrograms found that labral tears were prevalent in approximately 11% of mild cases of dysplasia, enhancing the potential clinical importance of this finding [14]. Furthermore, glenoid retroversion has also been described as a risk factor for the development of posterior instability. Radiological studies have shown that the "normal glenoid version" (orientation of the glenoid articular surface to the axis of the scapula) is generally 4–7° posteriorly oriented (retroversion) [15]. Also, the mean glenoid retroversion in patients with PGHI was found to be higher at 17.6° [16].

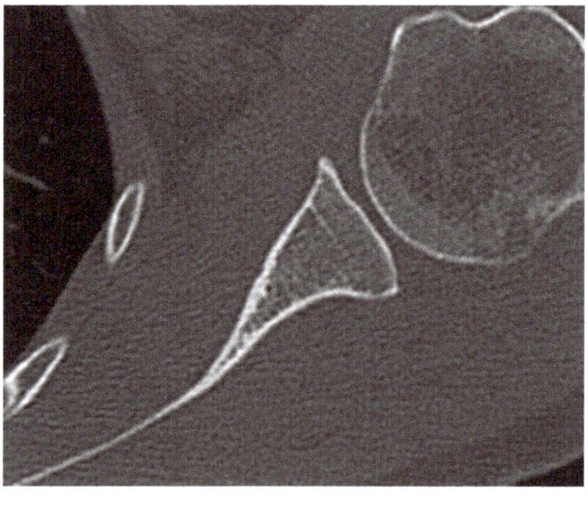

Fig. 33.1 Computed tomography of a patient with posterior instability and glenoid dysplasia

Finally, it is proposed that increased glenoid retroversion is a risk factor for failure of both surgical or conservative treatments [16, 17].

Assessment of the humerus shows the humeral head has an inclination of approximately 130° (relative to the shaft) and retroversion of 25–35° relative to the distal humeral condylar axis [18, 19]. Despite no cutoff values being proposed, it is thought that retroversion greater than 35° may predispose to posterior subluxation [18]. Additionally, in throwers, excessive humeral retroversion is correlated with increased incidence of posterior labral tears [20].

It is also proposed, but not yet studied in detail, that reduced development of posterior acromial curvature, and therefore reduced posterior humeral head coverage, could predispose patients to posterior instability.

33.1.2 Classification of Posterior Instability (Fig. 33.2)

From the aforementioned data, it is clear that the patho-anatomy of PGHI is multifactorial and the precise diagnosis and hence planning of treatment is challenging. In order to facilitate diagnosis and improve strategy, Moroder and Scheibel proposed the ABC classification of posterior shoulder instability which classifies cases into first time, dynamic and static instability [6]. *Group A* includes patients that had an acute traumatic posterior instability event that resulted in either a subluxation (A1—without humeral head engagement to the posterior glenoid rim) or a true locked posterior shoulder dislocation (A2).

In *Group B*, dynamic posterior shoulder instability is present. This could be functional (B1) as a result of deficiencies such as hyperlaxity, glenoid dysplasia, or increased glenoid retroversion. Usually in type B1, the development of instability is atraumatic. However, the type B2 is characterized as structural dynamic posterior instability and lesions such as reverse Bankart, posterior glenoid bone loss, and reverse Hills–Sachs are present. We should mention that this type of PGHI could be enhanced by the concomitant presence of the deficiencies found in Group B1.

Finally, in *Group C* the patients' have a chronic static PGHI. Subtype C1 is the least understood group, with patients having a constitutional static posterior subluxation. Usually, abnormalities like increased humeral head translation, congenital convex-shaped glenoids, increased retroversion, and muscular imbalance are present. However, in group C2 the clinical condition is clearer, where acquired severe lesions such as large reverse Hills–Sachs and glenoid bone defects result in a permanently subluxated or dislocated humeral head with or without secondary arthritic changes.

It is important to note that different subtypes can co-exist or even progress over time from one group to another. A first time dislocator can progress to dynamic structural multiple time dislocator and if still inadequately managed can worsen to a static dislocation with secondary arthritis.

33.1.3 Clinical Assessment of the Patient with Failed Posterior Instability

In order to ensure correct diagnosis, the history and the clinical examination is of ultimate importance in patients with failed surgery for PGHI. Details of the previous operations and the preoperative clinical condition should be acquired.

The clinician must distinguish the primary complaint and the precipitent for the new consultation: stiffness, pain, recurrent instability (new trauma), or a combination.

The examination should commence with inspection of both shoulders. Evaluate for asymmetry, muscle atrophy, previous scars, signs of swelling

	Type 1	Type 2
Type A (1st Time-Traumatic)	Subluxation	Dislocation
Type B (Dynamic)	Functional	Structural
Type C (Static-Chronic)	Constitutional	Acquired

Fig. 33.2 The ABC classification of posterior shoulder instability proposed by Moroder and Scheibel

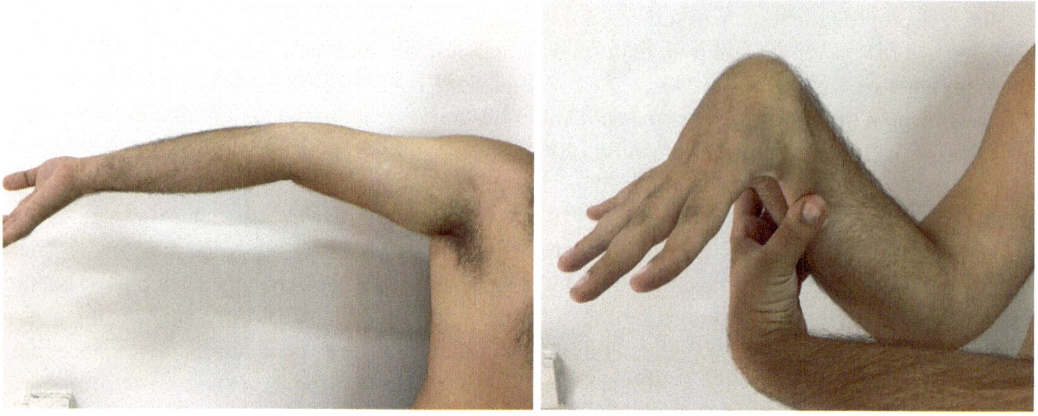

Fig. 33.3 Patient with voluntary posterior instability and concomitant hyperlaxity

or inflammation, any obvious dislocation or deformity, and also the position of the scapula (winging).

After gaining patient confidence, passive and active range of motion, including forward flexion, abduction, external, and internal rotation in positions 1 and 2, should be evaluated in both upright and lying positions. Comparisons with the contralateral healthy side are also mandatory. It is important to note any signs of shoulder or generalized hyperlaxity, and therefore, the Beighton score should be calculated in these cases [21] (Fig. 33.3).

In failed posterior instability the density, the characteristics and the location of any pain should be evaluated. In recurrence of instability the location of the pain is usually along the posterior joint line and it is provoked during examination maneuvers, especially with the arm in 90° forward flexion, adduction, and internal rotation. Discomfort is often caused by activities that load the posterior aspect of the joint such as bench press and push-ups. However, when there exists any concomitant long head of biceps pathology, rotator cuff lesions, static posterior subluxation, and/or arthritic changes, pain could be more severe and there can be limited function and sleep quality [22].

Furthermore, the specific tests for the diagnosis of posterior shoulder instability should be performed:

- The posterior drawer test [23]: The test is performed sitting or supine. The examiner stabilizes the shoulder joint with one hand while with the other applies a medially and posteriorly directed force on the humerus. The grade of the posterior translation is evaluated:

  - Grade 0: The head does not translate to the glenoid rim.
  - Grade I: The head translates to the glenoid rim and is greater than the contralateral shoulder
  - Grade II: The head translates over the rim and reduces spontaneously
  - Grade III: The head translates over the rim and does not reduce

- The Jerk test: The test is performed with the patient sitting and the limb in forward flexion, adduction, and internal rotation. The examiner applies a posteriorly directed force causing a posterior translation of the humeral head. Thereafter, the arm is brought gradually into extension and as the humeral head is reduced a painful clunk may be produced. This indicates a posterior labral tear and in many cases is an indication for surgical treatment [24, 25].
- The Kim test: The test is performed sitting with the shoulder in 90° abduction and internal rotation. The examiner holds the elbow, elevates the arm at 45°, and applies axial load posteriorly directed. By this manner, the humeral head is forced posteriorly out of the glenoid socket. The examination is positive when pain and/or a clunk are reproduced [26].

In some cases of PGHI, the O'Brien test can also be positive. To complete the examination, shoulder hypermobility should be assessed via the Sulcus sign and the Hyperabduction-Gagey test [22, 27].

33.2 Imaging

Radiographic assessment should include antero-posterior views in neutral-external and internal rotation, Y-views, and a glenoid profile view of Bernageau [28]. Importantly, the position of any implants from previous surgery, any arthritic changes, posterior subluxation, any glenoid bone loss, or glenoid dysplasia should be noted.

In multiply operated cases, the use of intra-articular contrast and the use of magnetic resonance arthrography are particularly useful. The condition of the labrum, the presence of any posterior labral cysts, the condition and the position of any materials used, and any arthritic changes can be more easily diagnosed.

In many cases, a computed tomography (CT) scan including three-dimensional reconstructions should be ordered, which enables the measurement and assessment of glenoid retroversion, the presence of glenoid dysplasia or any posterior bony Bankart lesion (Fig. 33.4).

33.3 Revisions of the PGHI According to the Failure Type

33.3.1 Recurrence of Instability

33.3.1.1 Conservative Treatment

Before considering surgical treatment, the clinician should clarify if there is any place for conservative treatment for patients that have previously been operated on or not. It is also critically important to distinguish which patients are unlikely to benefit from further surgical intervention. Unfortunately, patients with shoulder hyperlaxity or voluntary posterior subluxation have poor surgical prognoses [29]. Furthermore, the static posterior humeral head subluxation is characterized as a Walch B0 glenoid, and it is a pre-osteoarthritic condition of the shoulder joint [30]. In many cases, any surgical intervention not only did not alter the natural history of the condition, but instead it accelerated progression to osteoarthritis [30].

In some cases of functional dynamic posterior instability, underactivity of the rotator cuff and periscapular muscles exists. This can lead to subluxation during shoulder movements [31]. Any surgical intervention could aggravate pain and further diminish shoulder function. Classic conservative treatment has been proven to be also

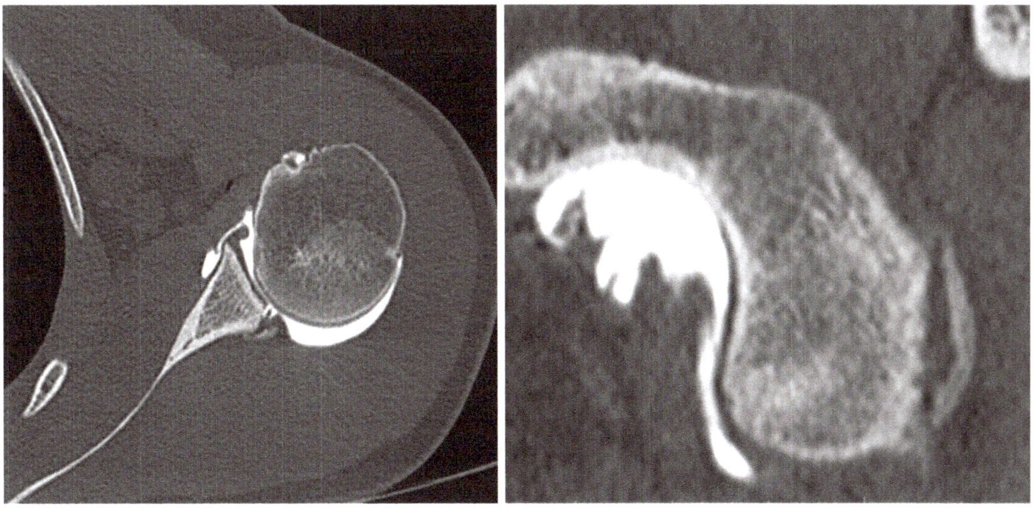

Fig. 33.4 Computed tomography of a patient with posterior bony Bankart lesion. In this patient, the conservative treatment for posterior instability failed

ineffective in such cases. In these cases, Moroder et al. propose the use of the "shoulder pacemaker," which is an external device that stimulates the external rotators of the shoulder and retractors of the scapula [32]. This solution appears promising and the authors reported that all the patients that have used this device were able to move their arms freely without pain, discomfort, free of subjective or objective signs of instability [32].

33.3.1.2 Operative Treatment

Arthroscopic Posterior Capsulolabral Repair

This type of procedure can be proposed in cases of failed initial conservative treatment, without excessive glenoid bone loss [8, 11]. The posterior labrum should be progressively detached and the glenoid bed gently decorticated. The labrum should be reattached with the use of three or four suture anchors. The authors' preferred technique is the use of knotless anchors with the combination of suture tape or all suture soft anchors that can minimize postoperative complications (Fig. 33.5). The most critical step of this operation is accurate establishment of the arthroscopic portals. It is very important while establishing the Wilmington portal to not cut the infraspinatus tendon transversely, which may result in iatrogenic tendon rupture. Furthermore, the use of an arthroscopic cannula should be avoided in this portal.

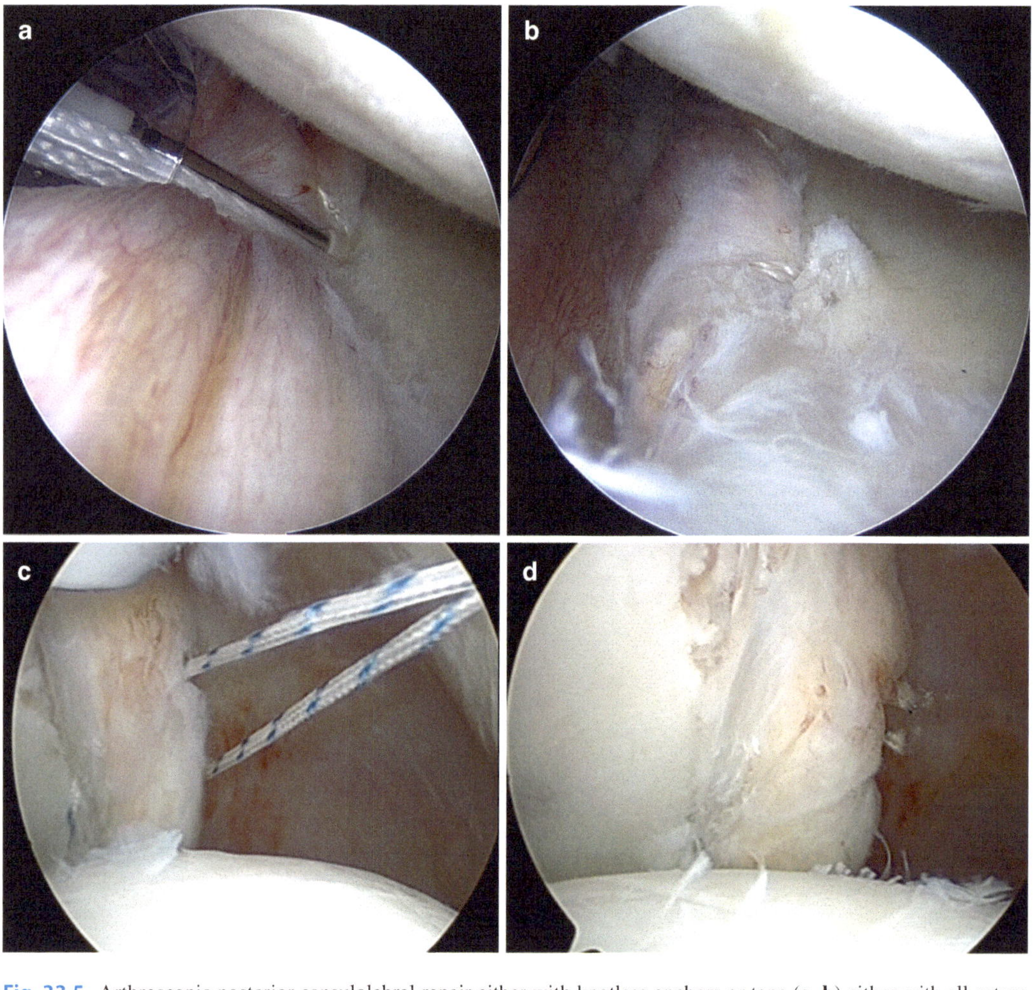

Fig. 33.5 Arthroscopic posterior capsulolabral repair either with knotless anchors or tape (**a**, **b**) either with all suture anchors or fixation with mattress configuration (**c**, **d**)

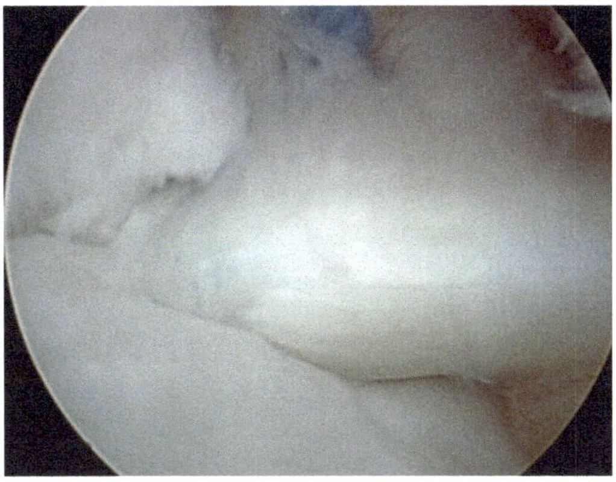

Fig. 33.6 Arthroscopic anterior remplissage in a reverse Hill–Sachs lesion (Left shoulder)

In cases with a reverse Hill–Sachs lesion of 10–25% humeral head bone loss, a second arthroscopic technique similar to "reverse remplissage" [33] should be performed to fill the defect. By using suture anchors, the medial glenohumeral ligament or the distal subscapularis tendon is fixed into the humeral head defect [34] (Fig. 33.6).

Bone Procedures

Glenoid Bone Loss

Recent systematic reviews highlighted the lack of precise guidelines regarding which bone defects should be treated with bony procedures and the correlation between the extent of bone loss and the risk of recurrent dislocation [10, 33]. Only Nacca et al. in a recent cadaveric study showed that the critical bone loss of the posterior glenoid is probably >20% [11].

With regard to the type of bone graft used, iliac crest bone block is the most frequently used [33]. Several open or arthroscopic techniques have been described [33]. The authors' preferred technique is the arthroscopic posterior bone graft passed through the transrotator interval and fixed with screws [35]. With this technique, a 25 mm long, 15 mm large, and 10 mm thick bone block is harvested from the iliac crest. The graft is shuttled into the joint via the rotator interval in order to minimize any iatrogenic injury to the rotator cuff muscles. Finally, it is fixed onto the glenoid with two percutanous screws (Fig. 33.7). Thereafter, the labrum can be repaired with suture anchors on the glenoid.

Sirveaux et al. and Metais et al. have recently described the technique of Kouvalchouk performing an arthroscopically assisted acromial pediculated bone block transfer [36, 37]. The authors support that this is an alternative to iliac bone block, enabling triple shoulder locking by the blocking effect, the retention hammock provided by the deltoid flap and posterior capsule repair. The results presented are promising, but the technique is technically demanding [37].

Studies show that posterior bone block procedures are effective with good subjective and objective outcomes. However, a relatively high complication rate has been described. A partial or considerable osteolysis of the graft has been found in about 64% of the cases [38]. Furthermore, some authors reported recurrence of instability in 36–70% of cases. We should not ignore also the possibility of development of persistent pain and secondary osteoarthritis of the glenohumeral joint. These complications show that posterior bone block procedures are sometimes less than ideal for patients and technically demanding and the surgeon should be very careful during final graft placement and fixation.

Glenoid Deformity

An identified risk factor for failures of PGHI, especially in atraumatic cases, is increased glenoid retroversion. Recently, Lacheta et al. proposed the posterior opening wedge osteotomy in patients with failed prior nonoperative treatment or soft-tissue interventions [39]. However, the high procedural technical demands are evidenced by the reported four asymptomatic complications that did not affect the final outcome, three non-displaced intra-articular osteotomy extensions, and one non-displaced extra-articular osteotomy extension (anterior cortical breach). At this stage, only short-term clinical outcomes are reported and longer follow-up is, therefore, still necessary [39].

Humeral Side

An important reason for revision surgery in patients with recurrent posterior instability is

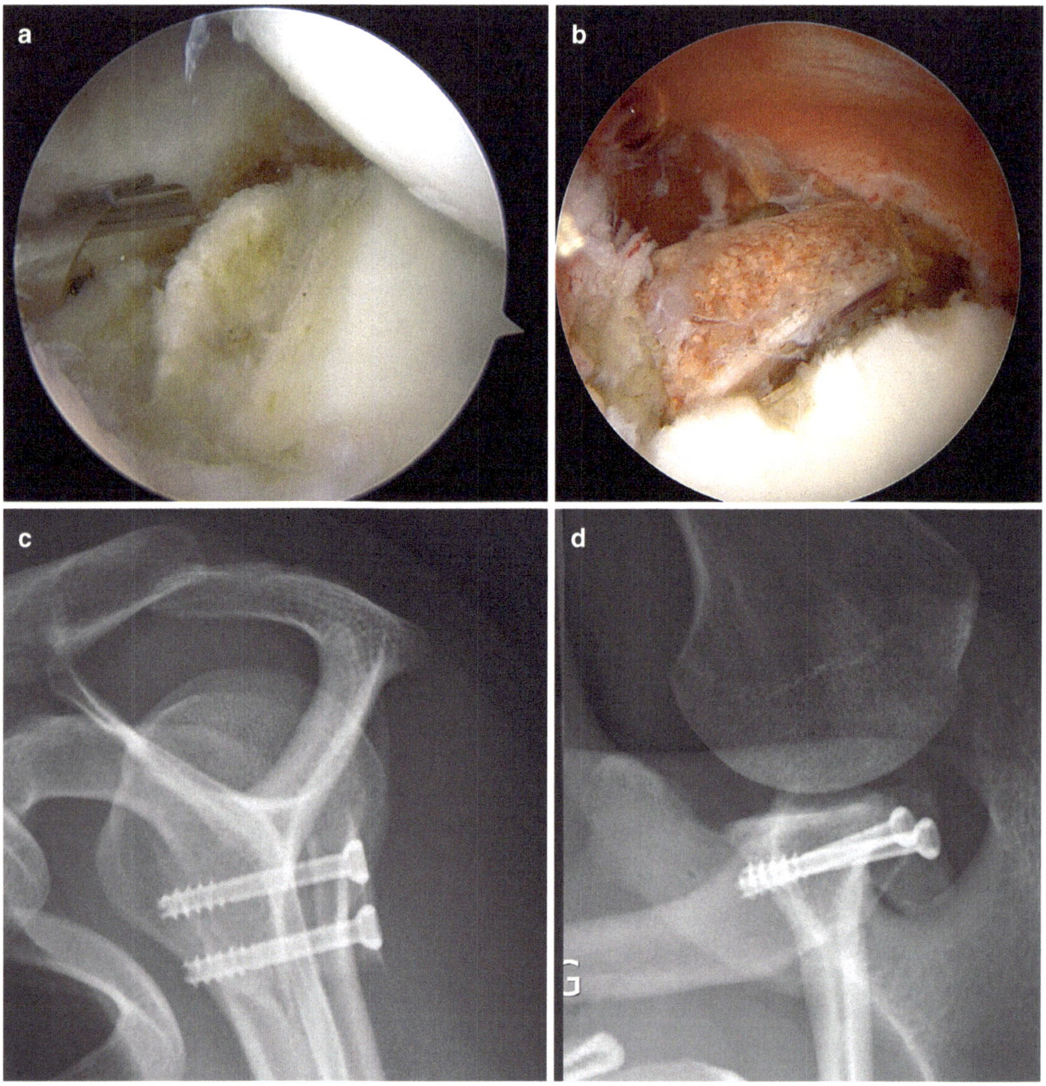

Fig. 33.7 Malunited posterior bony Bankart (**a**) treated with posterior bone block arthroscopically placed (**b**). Postoperative radiographs show the final position of the iliac bone autograft (**c**, **d**)

the untreated reverse Hill–Sachs lesion and the underestimated humeral bone loss. This leads to the development of different methods for the evaluation of the reverse Hill–Sachs lesion. Moroder et al. proposed a best-fit circle technique in the axial and coronal CT images in order to estimate the size and location of the Hill–Sachs lesion. This assessment method appears to have the highest intra and inter observer reliability [40].

However, the decision making process for the management of humeral bone loss should also take into account other patient factors. Paul et al. have proposed an algorithm regarding the treatment of such defects [41] that takes into account the size of the lesion, the patient's age, patient demands, and the presence of osteoarthritis (Fig. 33.8).

Several open or arthroscopic modified McLaughlin procedures with or without additional bone block have been described. Despite the relatively small case series reported, the improvement of functional scores and clinical results show that this nonanatomic procedure is a reliable solution for defects of <40% of the humeral articular surface [42]. For larger defects,

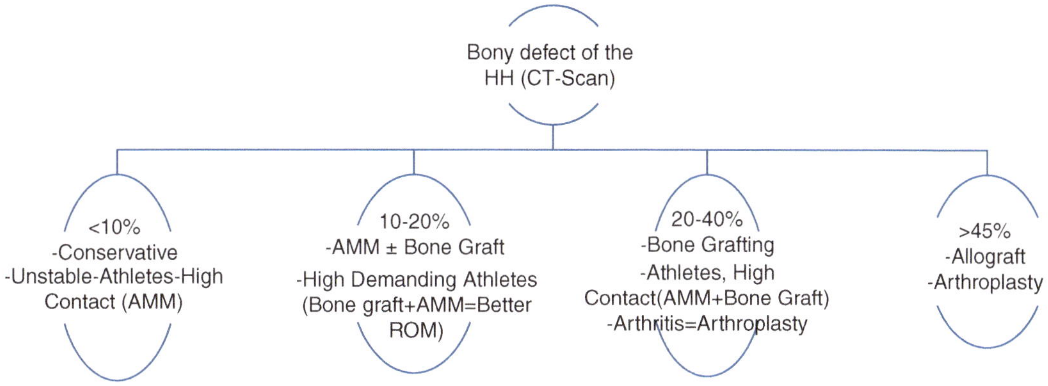

Fig. 33.8 Algorithm for the management of humeral bone loss according to Paul et al.

Gerber et al. proposed open anatomical reconstruction using allograft [43]. The long-term results of defect reconstruction using segmental femoral or humeral head allograft were excellent in 95% of cases [44].

33.3.2 Pain and Stiffness Related to the Previous Operations

33.3.2.1 The Role of the Rotator Interval

A possible cause for revision is the presence of persistent postoperative stiffness. Prolonged immobilization, open procedures, excessive postoperative bleeding, McLaughlin-type procedures, and aggressive rotator interval closure may result in significant postoperative stiffness. The initial treatment approach should include corticosteroid injections combined with hydrotherapy. In cases of failed conservative treatment, arthroscopic release can be considered. This could include release of the rotator interval, the anterior joint capsule, any adhesions between the coracoid process and conjoined tendon, and the subscapularis tendon to potentially improve external rotation range. Increase of the subscapularis excursion by 1 cm can provide additional external rotation by 20° [22].

33.3.2.2 Painful Hardware

Arthroscopic posterior capsulolabral repair is a technically demanding procedure and accurate placement of the suture anchors is important in order to avoid hardware related complications. Malposition, loosening, or migration of the implants can cause serious cartilage damage with painfully restricted range of motion and sometimes audible crepitus. For this reason, implants used for glenohumeral soft-tissue fixation have evolved over time. Bioabsorbable materials have replaced metallic anchors and recently all suture soft anchors have gained popularity for this type of procedure.

MRA or CT should be obtained preoperatively. Open or arthroscopic hardware removal is mandatory in order to prevent further chondral injury (Fig. 33.9). Rarely the placement of the suture knots towards the articular surface can also cause chondral lesions and should be removed [22].

33.3.2.3 Advanced Osteoarthritis

Unfortunately, the nonabsorbable hardware of failed soft-tissue procedures, the prominent bone or hardware of posterior bone block procedures, and the chronically locked posterior dislocation can all result in advanced osteoarthritis of the glenohumeral joint [4, 22]. Humeral head resurfacing procedures, interposition of a pyrocarbon sphere, hemiarthroplasty, or total shoulder arthroplasty could be reliable salvage solutions [22, 45]. However, reverse total shoulder arthroplasty can be considered in cases of bone deformity in posterior static humeral head subluxation and cases of significant glenoid retroversion.

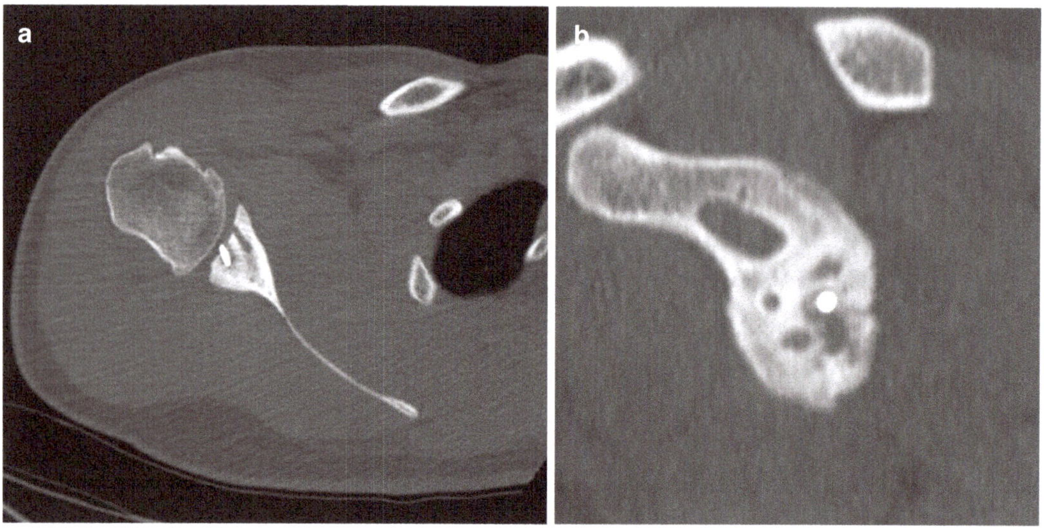

Fig. 33.9 Computed tomography showing the wrong position of a metal anchor and the postoperative arthritis of the glenohumeral joint (**a**) transverse and (**b**) sagittal view

33.4 Conclusion

Before any surgical intervention or revision, the surgeon should evaluate the underlying pathology and take time to understand the aetiology. The surgeon should also consider, in patients with failed management, if the original management was appropriate for a correct diagnosis, or if in fact the patient's condition was initially misdiagnosed or poorly understood. Patients with predominant posterior instability, positive apprehension, and defensive muscular contraction can have a good surgical prognosis (either soft tissue or bone procedure). However, in cases with hyperlaxity, voluntary instability, muscle imbalance, and static posterior humeral head subluxation, the clinician should exercise caution and optimize nonsurgical treatment options primarily. Finally, the presence of pain and stiffness are likely secondary to hardware failure, and development of arthritis and soft-tissue contracture. Most importantly, as orthopaedic understanding and experience of treatment of the various groups of posterior instability types evolves, successful patient outcomes will be become more common.

References

1. Brelin A, Dickens JF. Posterior shoulder instability. Sports Med Arthrosc Rev. 2017;25(3):136–43.
2. Zacchilli MA, Owens BD. Epidemiology of shoulder dislocations presenting to emergency departments in the United States. J Bone Joint Surg Am. 2010;92(3):542–9.
3. Owens BD, Duffey ML, Nelson BJ, DeBerardino TM, Taylor DC, Mountcastle SB. The incidence and characteristics of shoulder instability at the United States Military Academy. Am J Sports Med. 2007;35(7):1168–73.
4. Antosh IJ, Tokish JM, Owens BD. Posterior shoulder instability. Sports Health. 2016;8(6):520–6.
5. Robinson CM, Aderinto J. Recurrent posterior shoulder instability. J Bone Joint Surg Am. 2005;87(4):883–92.
6. Moroder P, Scheibel M. ABC classification of posterior shoulder instability. Obere Extrem. 2017;12(2):66–74.
7. Song DJ, Cook JB, Krul KP, Bottoni CR, Rowles DJ, Shaha SH, et al. High frequency of posterior and combined shoulder instability in young active patients. J Shoulder Elb Surg. 2015;24(2):186–90.
8. Andrieu K, Barth J, Saffarini M, Clavert P, Godenèche A, Mansat P. Outcomes of capsulolabral reconstruction for posterior shoulder instability. Orthop Traumatol Surg Res. 2017;103(8 Suppl):S189–92.

9. DeLong JM, Bradley JP. Posterior shoulder instability in the athletic population: variations in assessment, clinical outcomes, and return to sport. World J Orthop. 2015;6(11):927–34.
10. Longo UG, Rizzello G, Locher J, Salvatore G, Florio P, Maffulli N, et al. Bone loss in patients with posterior gleno-humeral instability: a systematic review. Knee Surg Sports Traumatol Arthrosc. 2016;24(2):612–7.
11. Nacca C, Gil JA, Badida R, Crisco JJ, Owens BD. Critical glenoid bone loss in posterior shoulder instability. Am J Sports Med. 2018;46(5):1058–63.
12. Weishaupt D, Zanetti M, Nyffeler RW, Gerber C, Hodler J. Posterior glenoid rim deficiency in recurrent (atraumatic) posterior shoulder instability. Skelet Radiol. 2000;29(4):204–10.
13. Edelson JG. Localized glenoid hypoplasia. An anatomic variation of possible clinical significance. Clin Orthop Relat Res. 1995;321:189–95.
14. Harper KW, Helms CA, Haystead CM, Higgins LD. Glenoid dysplasia: incidence and association with posterior labral tears as evaluated on MRI. Am J Roentgenol. 2005;184(3):984–8.
15. Eichinger JK, Galvin JW, Grassbaugh JA, Parada SA, Li X. Glenoid dysplasia: pathophysiology, diagnosis, and management. J Bone Joint Surg Am. 2016;98(11):958–68.
16. Owens BD, Campbell SE, Cameron KL. Risk factors for posterior shoulder instability in young athletes. Am J Sports Med. 2013;41(11):2645–9.
17. Hurley JA, Anderson TE, Dear W, Andrish JT, Bergfeld JA, Weiker GG. Posterior shoulder instability: surgical versus conservative results with evaluation of glenoid version. Am J Sports Med. 1992;20(4):396–400.
18. Bäcker HC, Galle SE, Maniglio M, Rosenwasser MP. Biomechanics of posterior shoulder instability—current knowledge and literature review. World J Orthop. 2018;9(11):245–54.
19. Barth J, Garret J, Boutsiadis A, Sautier E, Geais L, Bothorel H, et al. Is global humeral head offset related to intramedullary canal width? A computer tomography morphometric study. J Exp Orthop [Internet]. 2018 Sep 12 [cited 2019 Jan 6]; 5. Available from https://www.ncbi.nlm.nih.gov/pmc/articles/PMC6135727/.
20. Gelber JD, Soloff L, Schickendantz MS. The Thrower's shoulder. J Am Acad Orthop Surg. 2018;26(6):204–13.
21. Juul-Kristensen B, Røgind H, Jensen DV, Remvig L. Inter-examiner reproducibility of tests and criteria for generalized joint hypermobility and benign joint hypermobility syndrome. Rheumatology (Oxford). 2007;46(12):1835–41.
22. Forsythe B, Ghodadra N, Romeo AA, Provencher MT. Management of the failed posterior/multidirectional instability patient. Sports Med Arthrosc Rev. 2010;18(3):149–61.
23. Gerber C, Ganz R. Clinical assessment of instability of the shoulder. With special reference to anterior and posterior drawer tests. J Bone Joint Surg Br. 1984;66(4):551–6.
24. Cofield RH, Irving JF. Evaluation and classification of shoulder instability. With special reference to examination under anesthesia. Clin Orthop Relat Res. 1987;(223):32–43.
25. Kim S-H, Park J-C, Park J-S, Oh I. Painful jerk test: a predictor of success in nonoperative treatment of posteroinferior instability of the shoulder. Am J Sports Med. 2004;32(8):1849–55.
26. Kim S-H, Park J-S, Jeong W-K, Shin S-K. The Kim test: a novel test for posteroinferior labral lesion of the shoulder—a comparison to the jerk test. Am J Sports Med. 2005;33(8):1188–92.
27. Gagey OJ, Gagey N. The hyperabduction test. J Bone Joint Surg Br. 2001;83(1):69–74.
28. Bernageau J, Patte D, Debeyre J, Ferrane J. [Value of the glenoid profile in recurrent luxations of the shoulder]. Rev Chir Orthop Reparatrice Appar Mot. 1976;62(2 Suppl):142–7.
29. Levigne C, Garret J, Walch G. Posterior bone block for posterior instability. Tech Should Elbow Surg. 2005;6(1):26.
30. Domos P, Checchia CS, Walch G. Walch B0 glenoid: pre-osteoarthritic posterior subluxation of the humeral head. J Shoulder Elb Surg. 2018;27(1):181–8.
31. Jaggi A, Lambert S. Rehabilitation for shoulder instability. Br J Sports Med. 2010;44(5):333–40.
32. Moroder P, Minkus M, Böhm E, Danzinger V, Gerhardt C, Scheibel M. Use of shoulder pacemaker for treatment of functional shoulder instability. Obere Extrem. 2017;12(2):103–8.
33. Cerciello S, Visonà E, Morris BJ, Corona K. Bone block procedures in posterior shoulder instability. Knee Surg Sports Traumatol Arthrosc. 2015;24:1–8.
34. Castagna A, Conti M, Garofalo R. Soft tissue-based surgical techniques for treatment of posterior shoulder instability. Obere Extrem. 2017;12(2):82–9.
35. Barth J, Grosclaude S, Lädermann A, Denard PJ, Graveleau N, Walch G. Arthroscopic posterior bone graft for posterior instability: the transrotator interval sparing cuff technique. Tech Should Elbow Surg. 2011;12(3):67–71.
36. Métais P, Grimberg J, Clavert P, Kouvalchouk J-F, Sirveaux F, Nourissat G, et al. Posterior shoulder instability managed by arthroscopic acromial pediculated bone-block. Technique. Orthop Traumatol Surg Res. 2017;103(8 Suppl):S203–6.
37. Sirveaux F, Leroux J, Roche O, Gosselin O, De Gasperi M, Molé D. Traitement de l'instabilité postérieure de l'épaule par butée iliaque ou acromiale: À propos d'une série de 18 cas. Rev Chir Orthop Reparatrice Appar Mot. 2004;90(5):411–9.
38. Clavert P, Furioli E, Andieu K, Sirveaux F, Hardy MB, Nourissat G, et al. Clinical outcomes of posterior bone block procedures for posterior shoulder instability: multicenter retrospective study of 66 cases. Orthop Traumatol Surg Res. 2017;103(8 Suppl):S193–7.
39. Lacheta L, Singh TSP, Hovsepian JM, Braun S, Imhoff AB, Pogorzelski J. Posterior open wedge glenoid osteotomy provides reliable results in young patients

with increased glenoid retroversion and posterior shoulder instability. Knee Surg Sports Traumatol Arthrosc [Internet]. 2018 [cited 2019 Jan 5]. https://doi.org/10.1007/s00167-018-5223-9.
40. Moroder P, Tauber M, Hoffelner T, Auffarth A, Korn G, Bogner R, et al. Reliability of a new standardized measurement technique for reverse Hill–Sachs lesions in posterior shoulder dislocations. Arthroscopy. 2013;29(3):478–84.
41. Paul J, Buchmann S, Beitzel K, Solovyova O, Imhoff AB. Posterior shoulder dislocation: systematic review and treatment algorithm. Arthroscopy. 2011;27(11):1562–72.
42. Alepuz ES, Pérez-Barquero JA, Jorge NJ, García FL, Baixauli VC. Treatment of the posterior unstable shoulder. Open Orthop J. 2017;11:826–47.
43. Gerber C, Lambert SM. Allograft reconstruction of segmental defects of the humeral head for the treatment of chronic locked posterior dislocation of the shoulder. J Bone Joint Surg Am. 1996;78(3):376–82.
44. Gerber C, Catanzaro S, Jundt-Ecker M, Farshad M. Long-term outcome of segmental reconstruction of the humeral head for the treatment of locked posterior dislocation of the shoulder. J Shoulder Elb Surg. 2014;23(11):1682–90.
45. Garret J, Godeneche A, Boileau P, Molé D, Etzner M, Favard L, et al. Pyrocarbon interposition shoulder arthroplasty: preliminary results from a prospective multicenter study at 2 years of follow-up. J Shoulder Elb Surg. 2017;26(7):1143–51.

Open Bone Block Procedures for Posterior Shoulder Instability

34

Birol Aktas, Yiğit Umur Cirdi, and Mustafa Karahan

Shoulder joint is a complex and highly dynamic mechanism which holds together with the forces generated by both dynamic and static stabilizers. Pathoanatomy of the posterior shoulder instability includes capsule, rotator interval, labrum, bones, and many other stabilizing ligaments. Consequently, diagnosis and treatment would be challenging for physicians. Discrimination of instability and laxity is crucial for modeling the treatment program for each individual. It must be kept in mind that laxity is a nonpathologic finding, whereas it may vary widely between individuals and affected by many variables such as age, gender, musculature, and genetic factors. On the other hand, instability is a pathologic process that results in excessive translation of the humeral head on the glenoid that results in pain, weakness, or performance degradation [1]. Examination of the contralateral side and comparison of dynamics are crucial for interpreting the symptoms.

Glenohumeral instability is relatively a common pathology affecting 2% of general population [2], especially in young and highly active athletes. However, only 2–5% of those with glenohumeral instability develop posterior instability [3]. Although posterior dislocations cover only small percentage of shoulder dislocations, complications related to posterior dislocations should be screened by physician. Otherwise, misdiagnose of posterior instability is likely. In a review, only 50% of patients with posterior instability symptoms had discrete injury that initiated symptoms [4]. Consequently, the onset of symptoms might be elusive.

Joint congruency, glenoid version, and labrum contribute to joint stability. Structural damages or irregularities in these anatomic structures may cause posterior instability. Posterior capsule, inferior glenohumeral ligament, and posterior labrum support the posterior side mainly. Therefore, even an isolated lesion in any of these structures carry high possibility of causing posterior instability [5]. In other words, if sum of forces pushing shoulder joint posteriorly cannot be countepoised by posterior stabilizing structures, generation of instability syndromes is likely to occur. Increased glenoid version is another predisposing factor, and it directly affects the force required to subluxation. However, the stability of the joint is provided by both bone and soft tissue stabilizers.

B. Aktas (✉)
Department of Orthopedic Surgery and Traumatology, Acıbadem Atasehir Surgical Center, Istanbul, Turkey

Y. U. Cirdi
Department of Orthopedic Surgery and Traumatology, Erciyes University School of Medicine, Kayseri, Turkey
e-mail: yigitcirdi@erciyes.edu.tr

M. Karahan
Department of Orthopedic Surgery and Traumatology, Acıbadem Kerem Ali Aydınlar University School of Medicine, Istanbul, Turkey

R. Brzóska et al. (eds.), *360° Around Shoulder Instability*,
https://doi.org/10.1007/978-3-662-61074-9_34

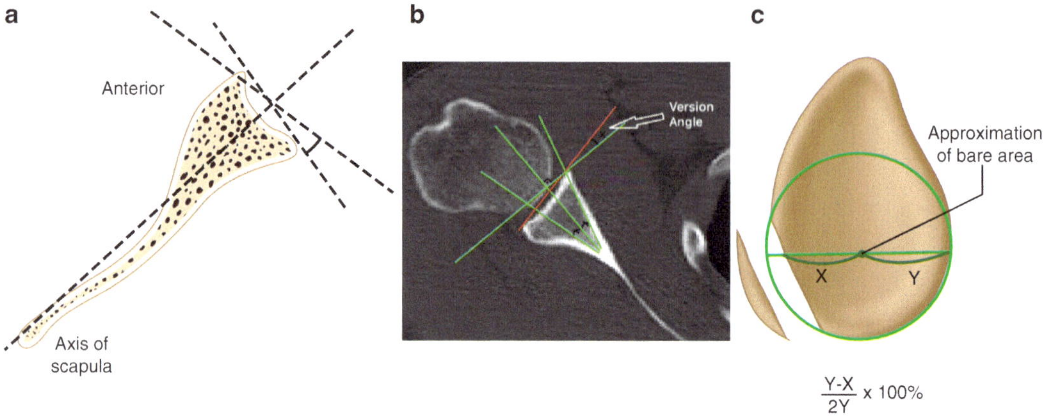

Fig. 34.1 (a) Conventional method for the measurement of glenoid version which uses the line passing through medial edge of the scapula. (b) Glenoid vault method for the measurement of glenoid version which uses endosteal vault of the glenoid as landmark. (c) Measurement method of glenoid bone loss using perfect circle and distance from bare spot to posterior edge

Average glenoid is retroverted between 4° and 7°. More than 7° is called abnormal [6, 7]. However, normal glenoid retroversion range may be wider depending on the different glenoid morphology [8]. In another study, Weishaupt et al. demonstrated that all patients with posterior recurrent shoulder instability had a retroverted glenoid mean (7.8°) [9]. Increased retroversion of glenoid is associated with not only posterior instability, but it also enhances the chance of instability in contralateral side [10]. However, etiology of the posterior instability should not be evaluated by assessing the glenoid version only. For instance, professional basketball pitchers show increased retroversion especially in their dominant shoulder as a mechanical adaptation without showing any instability sign and symptoms such as posterior laxity and sulcus sign [11].

34.1 How to Measure Glenoid Version?

Conventional method for measurement of glenoid version was described by Friedmen et al. in 1992 [12]. Measurements were made on axial planes of CT scans. Line starting from medial edge of the scapula to the mid-point of glenoid cavity was drawn. Another line perpendicular to the previous line was drawn which shows neutral version (Fig. 34.1a). Second line was drawn between the anterior edge and posterior edge of the glenoid. Angle between those lines corresponds to glenoid version. On the other hand, glenoid version is highly affected by the position of the scapula, and glenoid must be perpendicular to the axial slices. Recent review showed that internal rotation, external rotation, and even abduction and adduction of the scapula influence the glenoid version measurement [8]. Based on this problem, Poon and Thing offered another measurement technique which does not depend on the position of scapula [13]. In this technique, measurement is based on endosteal vault of the glenoid instead of the medial edge of the scapula and showed more precise measurements (Fig. 34.1b). Yet, the average measurement values are slightly greater than the conventional method. In other words, with this technique, glenoid retroversion tends to be more retroverted, so interpretation should be made by considering increased baseline value.

34.2 How to Assess Glenoid Bone Loss and Humeral Head Defects

Quantitative measurement of the glenoid bone loss is an important step for the evaluation of the glenoid condition. Even there are several methods described for the visualization of the glenoid rim via plain radiography, these techniques offer limited diagnostic value. For better understanding of the glenoid defect, the current preferred method is computed tomography with 3D reconstruction. Digital subtraction of the humeral head provides perfect visualization of the glenoid for measurement. Many different measurement techniques have been designated for calculation. Surface area method is a simple and useful option to use [14]. With this method, a perfect fit circle is placed on the lower two-third of the glenoid, centering the bare area. Then, proportion of the defect surface area to the imaginary perfect circle surface area was measured [15] (Fig. 34.1c). This technique resembles the arthroscopic measurement of the bone loss via arthroscopy probe. Percentage of the glenoid bone loss is obtained. Comparison of the glenoid rim distances can also predict the glenoid bone loss. With this technique, CT slice with largest anteroposterior length is obtained. Then, a perfect fit circle centering the bare spot of the glenoid has been drawn fitting the two-third inferior of the glenoid. The percentage of the bone loss is calculated [16]. With this quantitative information, surgeon is now able to choose between different reconstruction or repair techniques depending on morphology of the bone loss. It has to be kept in mind that management of the posterior glenoid defects may be challenging.

In a recent systematic review by Longo et al., bony glenoid defect was present in 9% and humeral head defect was present in 39% of shoulders with posterior instability [17]. Presence of the humeral head defect (reverse Hill-Sachs lesion) is much more common than the glenoid rim defects as mentioned. In addition, Paul et al. advanced the idea that the size of the humeral head defect is a crucial landmark to determine the treatment plan and decisive information for the surgery [18]. Moroder et al. described a standardized technique with high reliability. This technique aims to calculate the ratio of surface area of the defect size to the entire articular surface of the humeral head. These calculations are made on axial and coronal slices of CT scan to estimate the percentage of the impacted area. Measurements are also based on simple perfect-fit circle technique [19].

In summary, according to the treatment algorithm presented by Paul et al., the treatment modality for each individual highly depends on patients' need and athletic demand. This is why patients with low activity level and uncontrolled epilepsy are recommended to be treated conservatively.

34.3 Humeral Head Pathologies

The fracture of the humeral head is one of the important parts of the injury pattern, and anatomical procedures are more favorable than nonanatomic procedures. The choice of the surgical technique depends on the size of the bone defect, and it is evaluated in computed tomography (CT). If the defect is less than 25% of the humeral head, closed reduction with posterior capsular repair is mostly adequate without any surgical intervention on humeral head. When the defect is greater than 50%, it is recommended to consider shoulder arthroplasty. Controversies still present in defects including 25–50% of the humeral head. Each surgical intervention has its individual advantage and disadvantages. McLaughlin technique, modified McLaughlin technique, rotational osteotomy of the humerus, and reconstruction with allograft or autograft are commonly preferred techniques for the humeral head defects [17].

34.3.1 Reconstruction with Allograft

The deltopectoral approach is mostly preferred. Subscapularis tendon and surrounding capsule are dissected carefully. After capsulotomy, the size of the defect is identified. Then the graft is shaped to fix the humeral lesion. The graft is then fixed with one or two compression screws. C-arm is used to confirm the fixation. Capsule and subscapularis tendon are repaired anatomically [20] (Fig. 34.2a).

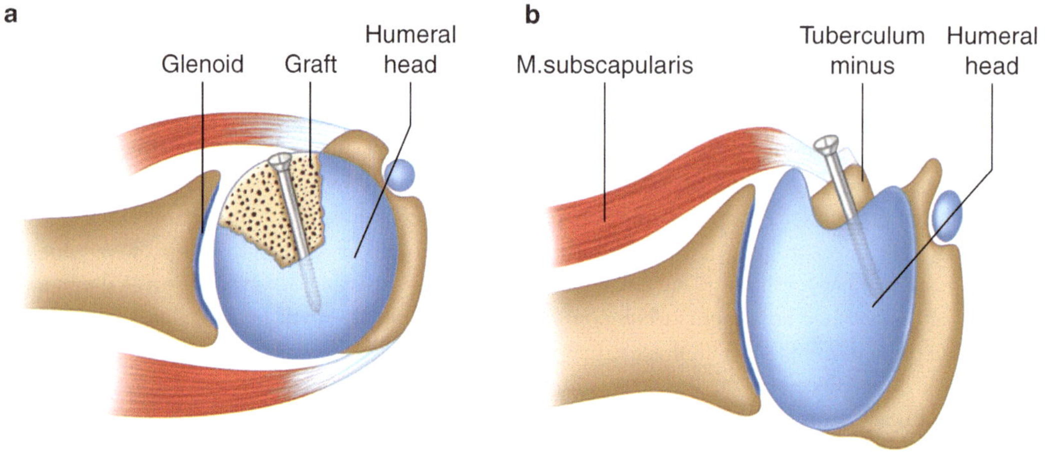

Fig. 34.2 (**a**) Reconstruction with allograft in reverse Hill-Sachs. (**b**) Transferring tuberculum minus into the humeral head cavity

34.3.2 Disimpaction and Filling with Bone Graft

This technique is used in acute lesions (<14 days) when the lesions do not exceed more than 50% of the articular surface. The condition of the cartilage is important. The surgical technique is applied through deltopectoral approach. Then the subscapularis is detached. After capsulotomy, the lesion occurs and the cartilage quality is evaluated. If the cartilage is in good condition, the humerus is rotated internally and a hole on the opposite side of the humeral head is opened for the impactor. Fracture is disimpacted carefully. The bone graft is inserted through the hole to fill the existing gap. Two parallel cortical screws can be used for fixation to avoid the graft getting loose [21].

34.3.3 Nonanatomical Techniques

Transfer of subscapularis tendon to reverse Hill-Sachs lesion was first described by McLaughlin in 1952 [22]. The aim of this intervention is to limit the maximum internal rotation. Thereby, the humeral defect is prevented to engage with posterior part of the glenoid. Thereafter, Neer et al. described modified McLaughlin technique for the transferring subscapularis tendon with the lesser tuberosity which promotes better healing capacity, as well as providing a bone-bone fixation [23] (Fig. 34.2b).

Rotational osteotomy of the humerus is an another seldomly preferred non- anatomical technique but it is not recommended by most of authors, due to its association with severe complications such as humeral head necrosis and ostoarthritis [4].

34.4 Glenoid Pathologies

The decision making on bony procedures of the glenoid dysplasia and version are important. Significant posterior glenoid defects are mostly restored with a bone block or reconstruction of the bony glenoid. Positive result on the Jerk test with >25% glenoid bone loss also require glenoid intervention. In some series, corrective humeral rotational osteotomies are described, but they were not used widely. When retroversion angle is >20°, an opening wedge osteotomy for the glenoid is indicated. Essentially, bone reconstruction surgeries have to be kept in mind especially following the failed soft tissue procedures.

34.4.1 Opening Wedge Glenoid Osteotomy

We prefer the lateral decubitus position and incision on posterior axillary fold. The deltoid

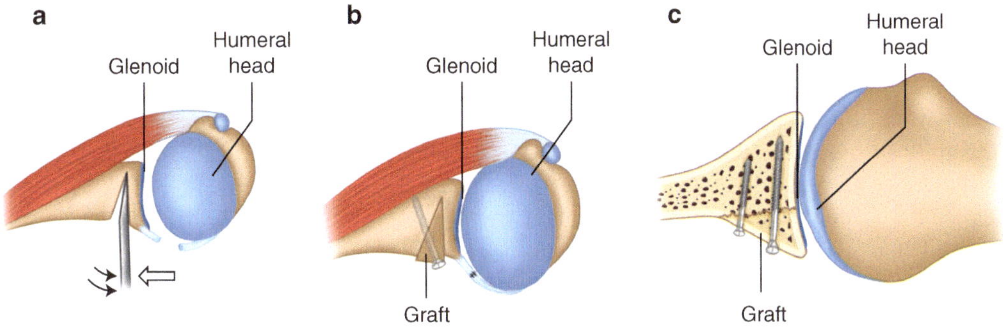

Fig. 34.3 (**a**) Correcting the version angle of the glenoid with using the osteotome. (**b**) Fixation of the graft after correcting the retroversion angle. (**c**) Posterior bone block technique, using two screws for fixation to prevent the rotation of the graft

muscle is split longitudinally. Then the infraspinatus is split to expose the joint capsule. Care must be taken to avoid dividing no more than 1.5 cm medial to the glenoid in order to protect the branches of suprascapular nerve. The capsule is incised from medial to lateral. In addition, capsulotomy can be done by using the technique of T-plasty. Then the posteromedial neck of the glenoid is exposed. An autologous tricortical graft which is usually harvested from iliac crest can be used. The width of the graft (usually 10–25 mm) is determined depending on the desired degree of the correction (Fig. 34.3). Anterior glenoid cortex should be intact during the osteotomy. A C-arm can be used to check and confirm that hinge-type osteotomy is achieved. Then the harvested graft is applied to the osteotomy site to restore the desired version of the glenoid. Fixation of the graft is provided with single screw (Fig. 34.3b). Numerous complications have been reported such as nerve injury, intra-articular fracture, hardware problems, and malreduction [3].

34.4.2 Posterior Bone Block Procedure

Preoperative preparation was made as described previously. After capsulotomy, the posterior glenoid is exposed and abraded in preparation for the bone graft. Afterwards, a tricortical bone graft harvested from iliac spine is shaped for conformity. The graft is expected to be at least 20–30 mm long and 10 mm wide. Care must be taken while positioning the graft at the same level with the glenoid cartilage. Two 3.5-mm cannulated screws (3.2 mm drill) are used for the fixation (Fig. 34.3c). Fluoroscopy guidance is helpful for determining the place of the graft and the fixation.

Posterior focal glenoid defects can be reconstructed with an intra- or extra-articular bone graft. The autograft can be obtained from either iliac crest, distal clavicle, scapular spine, distal tibia, or acromion. Extra-articular bone graft, which is mostly preferred, serves as a buttress for the humeral head. It should be kept in mind that excessive medially placed graft may result in inadequate compression force, and excess lateralization of the graft may cause impingement symptoms. Hardware problems and graft lysis are the other undesired complications defined [14].

34.5 Postoperative Rehabilitation

An orthosis should be used following the surgery to maintain abduction, neutral rotation, and external rotation of the shoulder. Immobilization period varies between 4 and 6 weeks, depending on the stability of the surgery. Passive mobilization of shoulder abduction and flexion can be applied. Active range-of-motion exercises are started at 6 weeks. Strengthening exercises are avoided for 3 months. Contact sports can be allowed after 6 months.

34.6 Complications

Recurrence is the most common complication which may be due to a new lesion, reabsorption of the graft, or inadequate treatment. Estimated recurrence rate is around 10%. Avascular necrosis can occur as a result of a fracture dislocation or delayed treatment in posterior inveterate dislocations. Immediate reduction and stabilization are important for the revascularization.

After the use of bone block, radiographic degenerative changes can be identified. Osteoarthritis treatment is based on patient's symptoms. Initially, patients benefit from nonsurgical treatment. Total shoulder arthroplasty should be indicated in advanced stage [24].

Stiffness is common following delayed treatment with deformities of the humeral head. Following the posterior instability surgery, stiffness is described as a loss of 10° of internal rotation. This does not affect the patients' daily activities but might be a problem especially in overhead athletes, tennis players, and swimmers [25].

References

1. Owens BD, Burns TC, DeBerardino TM. Examination and classification of Instability. In: Romeo AA, Provencher MT, editors. Shoulder instability: a comprehensive approach. Saunders Elsevier Inc.; 2012. p. 20.
2. Hovelius L. Incidence of shoulder dislocation in Sweden. Clin Orthop Relat Res. 1982;166:127–31.
3. Millett PJ, et al. Recurrent posterior shoulder instability. JAAOS - J Am Acad Orthop Surg. 2006;14(8):464–76.
4. Robinson CM, Aderinto J. Recurrent posterior shoulder instability. J Bone Joint Surg Am. 2005;87(4):883–92.
5. Tannenbaum E, Sekiya JK. Evaluation and management of posterior shoulder instability. Sports Health. 2011;3(3):253–63.
6. Brewer BJ, Wubben RC, Carrera GF. Excessive retroversion of the glenoid cavity. A cause of non-traumatic posterior instability of the shoulder. J Bone Joint Surg Am. 1986;68(5):724–31.
7. Hurley JA, et al. Posterior shoulder instability. Surgical versus conservative results with evaluation of glenoid version. Am J Sports Med. 1992;20(4):396–400.
8. Sabo MT, McBride T, Trail IA. A review of the use of imaging techniques for measurement of glenoid morphology and its application to computer-assisted surgery. Shoulder Elbow. 2013;5(1):19–23.
9. Weishaupt D, et al. Posterior glenoid rim deficiency in recurrent (atraumatic) posterior shoulder instability. Skelet Radiol. 2000;29(4):204–10.
10. Gottschalk MB, et al. Posterior shoulder instability: does glenoid retroversion predict recurrence and contralateral instability? Arthroscopy. 2015;31(3):488–93.
11. Crockett HC, et al. Osseous adaptation and range of motion at the glenohumeral joint in professional baseball pitchers. Am J Sports Med. 2002;30(1):20–6.
12. Friedman RJ, Hawthorne KB, Genez BM. The use of computerized tomography in the measurement of glenoid version. J Bone Joint Surg Am. 1992;74(7):1032–7.
13. Poon PC, Ting FS. A 2-dimensional glenoid vault method for measuring glenoid version on computed tomography. J Shoulder Elb Surg. 2012;21(3):329–35.
14. Provencher MT, et al. Recurrent shoulder instability: current concepts for evaluation and management of glenoid bone loss. J Bone Joint Surg Am. 2010;92(Suppl 2):133–51.
15. Sugaya H, et al. Glenoid rim morphology in recurrent anterior glenohumeral instability. J Bone Joint Surg Am. 2003;85-a(5):878–84.
16. Sugaya H, Kon Y, Tsuchiya A. Arthroscopic repair of glenoid fractures using suture anchors. Arthroscopy. 2005;21(5):635.
17. Longo UG, et al. Bone loss in patients with posterior gleno-humeral instability: a systematic review. Knee Surg Sports Traumatol Arthrosc. 2016;24(2):612–7.
18. Paul J, et al. Posterior shoulder dislocation: systematic review and treatment algorithm. Arthroscopy. 2011;27(11):1562–72.
19. Moroder P, et al. Reliability of a new standardized measurement technique for reverse Hill-Sachs lesions in posterior shoulder dislocations. Arthroscopy. 2013;29(3):478–84.
20. Alepuz ES, et al. Treatment of the posterior unstable shoulder. Open Orthop J. 2017;11:826–47.
21. Tannenbaum EP, Sekiya JK. Posterior shoulder instability in the contact athlete. Clin Sports Med. 2013;32(4):781–96.
22. McLaughlin LH. Posterior dislocation of the shoulder. J Bone Joint Surg Am. 1952;24 a(3):584–90.
23. Hawkins RJ, et al. Locked posterior dislocation of the shoulder. J Bone Joint Surg Am. 1987;69(1):9–18.
24. Meuffels DE, et al. The posterior bone block procedure in posterior shoulder instability. J Bone Joint Surg. 2010;92-B(5):651–5.
25. Robinson CM, Aderinto J. Posterior shoulder dislocations and fracture-dislocations. J Bone Joint Surg Am. 2005;87(3):639–50.

Arthroscopic Bone Block Procedures

35

Maciej Kiciński, Andrzej Boszczyk, and Bartłomiej Kordasiewicz

35.1 Anteroinferior Instability

35.1.1 Introduction

Anteroinferior shoulder instability represents 93–95% of all shoulder instabilities. It is due to a particular anatomy and physiology of a glenohumeral joint, which present us with advantageous range of motion (the largest in human body) but unfortunately by a cost of the joint stability. The dimensions and a shape of a glenoid result in 25% of humeral head articular surface being covered by a socket. This poor ratio (for instance, comparing to a ball and socket acetabulofemoral joint, covering 50% of an articulating head surface) makes any further bone deficiencies difficult to compensate [1]. Therefore, a bone deficiency is crucial in the development of a shoulder instability. Those may vary in shape and extent. It may have a form of a fractured fragment or an erosion-like deficiency in case of a glenoid, being a result of a humeral head impact during dislocation or reposition. For humeral head bone loss, known as a Hill–Sachs lesion (HSL), is a compression fracture of the humeral head caused by the anterior rim of the glenoid when the humeral head is dislocated anteriorly in front of the glenoid. Four out of five patients with recurrent anterior dislocation presents "bipolar" lesion, which is HSL combined with an anterior glenoid rim bone loss. An HLS position onto humeral head is important along with its dimensions (depth in particular). An HSL, which stays on the glenoid track (on-track lesion), cannot engage with the glenoid and cannot cause dislocation. On the other hand, an HSL, which is out of the glenoid track (off-track lesion), has a risk of engagement and dislocation. Figure 35.1 presents this concept published by Itoi [2].

35.1.2 Indications

Those bone deficiencies are a principal indication for a bone block, weather it is arthroscopic or open procedure. It is utmost difficult to stabilise a shoulder with soft tissue advancement, when anterior glenoid rim deficiency surpasses 25%, being itself a non-disputed indication. As well as engaging bipolar off-track lesion shall be addressed with a bone block procedure. Recently, an anatomical study performed by Sang-Jin Shin et al. expands bone block indications even further, down to 15% instead of traditional 20–25%

M. Kiciński (✉)
Trauma and Orthopaedics Department, SPSK im. A. Grucy, Otwock, Poland

A. Boszczyk · B. Kordasiewicz
Trauma and Orthopaedics Department, SPSK im. A. Grucy, Otwock, Poland

Centre of Postgraduate Medical Education, Warsaw, Poland

R. Brzóska et al. (eds.), *360° Around Shoulder Instability*,
https://doi.org/10.1007/978-3-662-61074-9_35

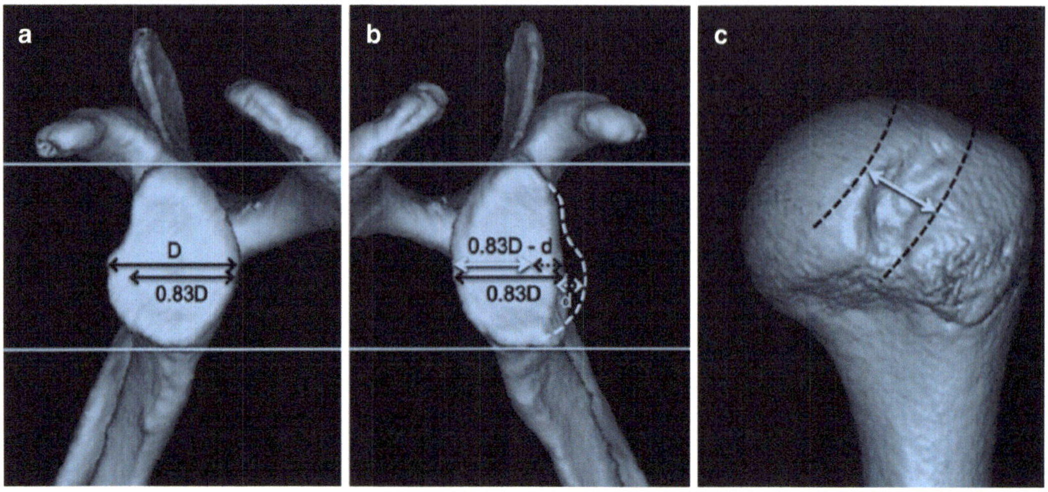

Fig. 35.1 Drawing of the glenoid track: (**a**) on the "en face" view of the intact glenoid, 83% of the glenoid width is obtained (0.83*D*); (**b**) on the involved side, there is a defect (*d*; white dotted double-headed arrow). The width of the glenoid track is obtained by subtracting '*d*' (black dotted double-headed arrow) from 83% value (0.83*D* – *d*; white double-headed arrow); (**c**) this glenoid track width (0.83*D* – *d*) is applied to the posterior view of the humeral head. In this case, the HSL stays in the glenoid track, making this lesion an "on-track" HSL [2]

Table 35.1 Simplified decision-making algorithm for anteroinferior shoulder instability

	Bone loss			
Hill–Sachs lesion		<15%	15–25%	>25%
	No H-S	Bankart	BLS/Bankart + capsular shift/bone block	Bone block
	H-S on track	Bankart ± R	Bankart + R/bone block	Bone block
	H-S off track	Bankart + R/HH bone block	Bone block	Bone block

R remplissage, *H-S* Hill–Sachs lesion, *BLS* between labrum and subscapularis procedure (LIT), *HH* humeral head

of anterior glenoid bone loss, proving in cadaveric study the soft tissue advancement insufficient in such cases [3]. A brief proposition of recurrent anterior shoulder instability management is presented in Table 35.1. Additional factors influencing the decision-making process in favour of bone block are poor anterior compartment soft tissue quality and revision surgery after failed soft tissue repair/advancement.

35.1.3 Surgical Procedures

Bone blocks can be divided in three subgroups: coracoid transfers, autografts (ileum mostly) and allografts (glenoid or tibia).

35.1.3.1 Coracoid Transfers

These techniques are by far the most popular of bone blocks around shoulder. Originally, Latarjet [4] described his technique of transferring the horizontal part of the coracoid onto the anteroinferior margin of the glenoid, fixing it with one screw, after partial subscapularis tenotomy. Since then the technique has evolved introducing subscapularis split and the second screw (Patte).

Arthroscopic Latarjet first described by Lafosse, has been performed since 2003 (first publication in 2007). It requires a specially designed arthroscopic instruments and high level of arthroscopic skills (Figs. 35.2 and 35.3). Since 2003, this technique has been constantly improved,

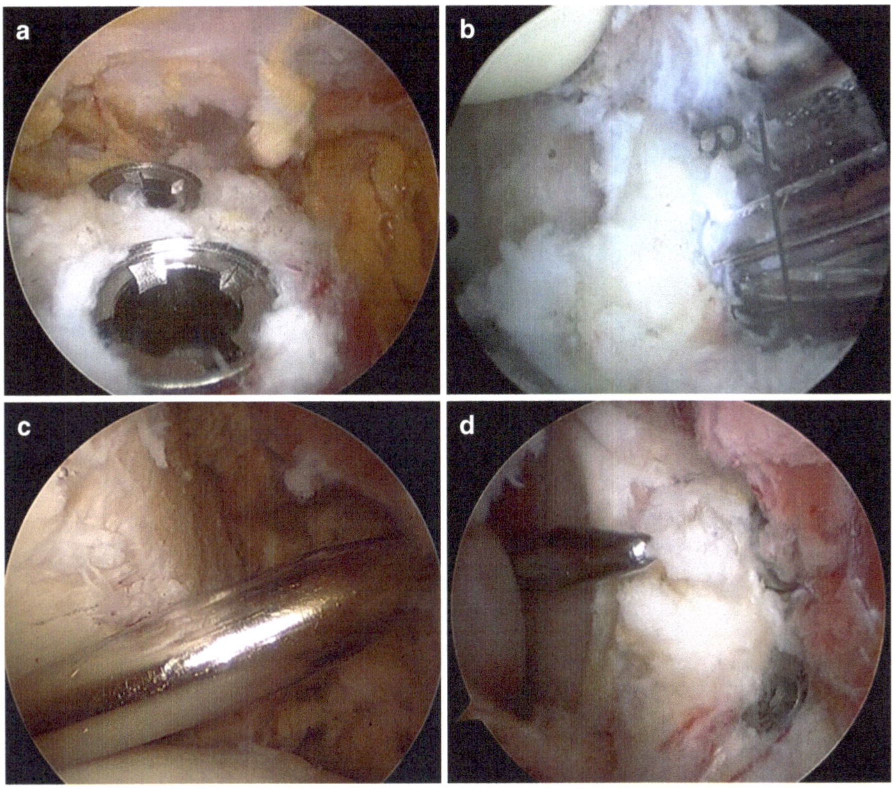

Fig. 35.2 Key steps of the procedure: (**a**) coracoid preparation, top hats in position; (**b**) graft handling with use of the coracoid canula; (**c**) subscapularis split level marked with switching stick; and (**d**) final coracoid fixation, flush position

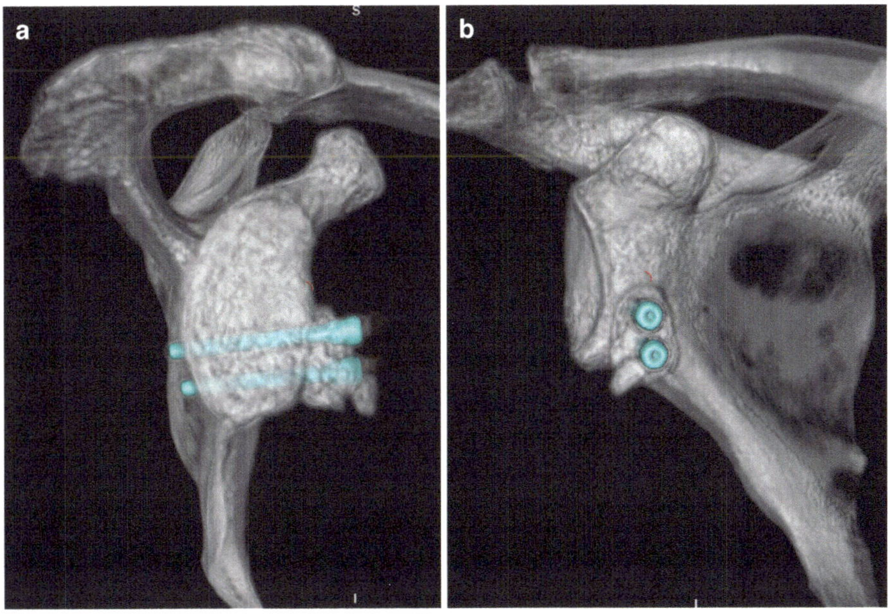

Fig. 35.3 Arthroscopic Latarjet postoperative computed tomography (CT) scans with 3D reconstruction: (**a**) sagittal view and (**b**) coronal view

evolving to the present form. Here are the main steps on the way to a successful arthroscopic Latarjet:

- Standard arthroscopy allowing to appreciate soft tissue lesions and soft tissue quality as well as the glenoid bone loss together with Hill–Sachs lesion—intraoperative tests such as H–S engagement confirms the indication for coracoid transfer.
- If necessary additional lesions repair (e.g., SLAP).
- Open the rotator interval and expose both sides of subscapularis.
- Coracoid soft-tissue preparation. The coracoacromial ligament and coracoid insertion of pectoralis minor muscle are released. Further liberation of fascia anterior to conjoint tendon down to the pectoralis major tendon.
- To define the H portal, two needles are placed locating the tip and the midpoint of the coracoid.
- With a specially designed guiding tool, two K wires are introduced marking the position of two screws to come.
- Insertion of the top hat.
- Harvesting the coracoid graft—osteotomy at the base of the acromion.
- Subscapularis split.
- An inferior K wire is being placed in position desired for an inferior screw.
- A tunnel with cannulated drill gives a way for another cannulated tubular wire overpassing (from posterior to anterior) previously introduced K wire.
- Coracoid graft is being captured onto arthroscopic Latarjet cannula, and fixed onto inferior K wire.
- Bear-based ventral coracoid surface and anterior glenoid rim preparation.
- Final fixation with two screws.
- Additional Bankart/capsular shift might be performed.

However, postoperative apprehension (up to 9.9%–Metais [5]) and loss of external rotation (up to 18°–Lafosse) deteriorate the final outcome, the arthroscopic Latarjet stabilisation procedure demonstrates satisfactory results upon clinical and radiographic evaluation in short-term follow-up. The recurrence rate varies from 0% to 4.5% and outcomes reach satisfying level: Rowe score: 90–95.4; Walch–Duplay score: 88–96; Constant score: 92.9–95; Western Ontario Shoulder Instability Index: 82.3–90.6 [6, 7], which has been presented in Table 35.2. Advantages of arthroscopy are mini-invasive approach, possibility to perform intra-operatively tests of provocation and precise evaluation of the anterior compartment, confirming indication for a bone block procedure. Concomitant lesions have been reported as well in 5–7% of cases (Zhu [10]), which could be addressed at the very same surgical procedure, benefiting from the shoulder arthroscopy.

Although initial results appear to be promising, one shall bear in mind a large amount of complications have been reported with this technique in some studies reaching a level of 29%. (Tables 35.2 and 35.3) The most severe of those complications are neurovascular lesions, osteoarthritis and graft healing problems. The resorption of proximal part of the grafted coracoid has been widely described as well. Overall revision rate reaches 16.7% [14].

Boileau et al. changed the fixation of the graft favouring transglenoid suture stabilisation instead of the screws (Fig. 35.4). This technique introduced different tools to control, prepare and position the coracoid graft [12, 13]. For instance, it utilises specific glenoid drill guide, ensuring that the cortical button suture tunnel is almost parallel (10° of angulation) and positioned 5 mm medial to the anterior glenoid rim. It allows also intra-articular drilling from posterior to anterior, limiting drilling by a drill stop to avoid neurovascular injury. Boileau introduced two low-profile mechanical subscapularis spreaders for gentle subscapularis split. But the principle remains true to the old Latarjet concept. The results of 76 patients published in 2016 reveal high incidence of non-unions (9%) with smoking being the only statistically significant risk factor and good overall outcome at 14 months of follow-up. No revision surgery was required and no true dislocation has been reported. One patient

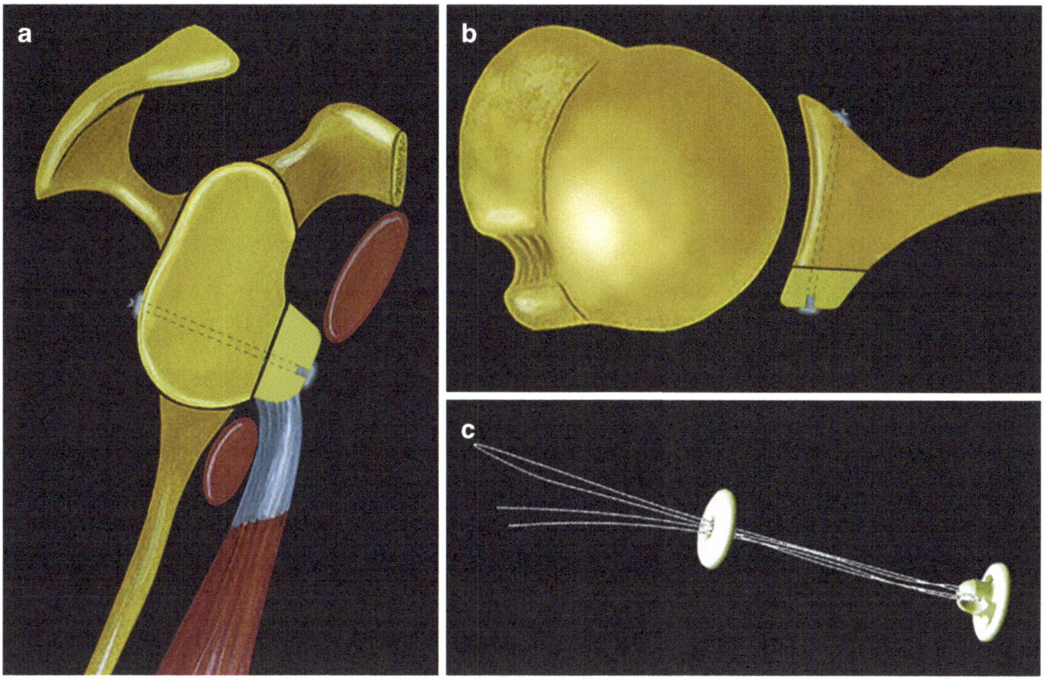

Fig. 35.4 Arthroscopic Latarjet procedure with cortical button fixation. (**a**) The coracoid process is transferred, passed through the subscapularis and fixed on the anterior neck of the scapula with two cortical buttons and a four-strand suture (Bone-Link). (**b**) The anterior (coracoid) button has a pegged eyelet (to avoid cutting the bone with the suture) and is placed first; the posterior (glenoid) button has a single hole and is placed after having pulled the suture in the back of the shoulder. (**c**) A sliding knot (Nice-Knot) is tied posteriorly, and the suture is tensioned to obtain bone-to-bone compression; three additional surgeon's knots are tied to definitively lock the construct. Boileau, P., Gendre, P., Baba, M., Thélu, C.-É., Baring, T., Gonzalez, J.-F., & Trojani, C. (2016). *A guided surgical approach and novel fixation method for arthroscopic Latarjet. Journal of Shoulder and Elbow Surgery, 25(1), 78–89.* https://doi.org/10.1016/j.jse.2015.06.001. (With Elsevier permission)

presented subluxation during trauma while playing rugby. In clinical findings, improvement in Rowe and Walch–Duplay scores were 95 (range: 84–100) and 96 (range: 86–100), respectively. In radiological findings, 96% of grafts were judged to be positioned correctly, congruent with the glenoid articular surface. Despite single-axis stabilisation (with no derotational effect of a second screw/endobutton) no secondary rotational displacement has been discovered. Ninety-three percent of patients had returned to their preinjury level of sports.

Tang raised an importance of preserving the coraco-acromial ligament (transected in Latarjet) for the shoulder girdle function, as he described similar suture-based coracoid graft stabilization in Bristow procedure with endobutton. In this technique, a 5-mm-high, 8- to 9-mm-wide pillar is fashioned on the proximal side of the coracoid tip. On an anterior glenoid rim, a 8–9 mm wide, 5 mm deep socket is reamed to receive the graft, improving its primary stability and bone-to-bone healing rate. Tang and Zhao technique remains arthroscopic-assisted mini-invasive procedure, requiring taking the coracoid outside the shoulder onto the skin through anterior portal for its preparation [17].

35.1.3.2 Autograft

Eden and Hybinnette (1918/1932) first described L-shape ilium autograft subperiosteal fixation. Shape and fixation of this bone block has changed

Table 35.2 Comparison of arthroscopic Latarjet outcome published in the literature

	Time of surgery (min)	Constant	Rowe	W-D	Complication (%)	Nerve palsy (%)	Recurrence (%)	Apprehension (%)	Revision	Delta ER
Lafosse [27]	45–240				13	1.6	0			18°
Cunningham [8]	146			88	29		3.6	5.5		
Ladermann,										
Zhu AJSM [9]	122.8	95	95.4		0		0	0		0
Zhu A [10]	119	92.9	92.2		0		0	0	0	2.2
Marion [6]	77								8.3%	
Athwal [11]	139–156				10	1.2	4		8.4%	
Metais [5]			93	91	6.3		4.5	9.9	4.8%	2.5
Boileau [12, 13]			95	96			1.3		0%	
Dumont [7]							1.6		15.6%	
Castricini [14]			90		10		0		16.7%	12°
Casabianca! [16]	161				10.5					
Kany [15]	103–76*					1			2.8%	

W–D Walch–Duplay score, *delta ER* loss of external rotation

Table 35.3 The radiological findings in patients treated with arthroscopic Latarjet

	Graft healing problems	Flush (%)	Lateralization (%)	Medialization (%)	Correct graft position sagittal	Screw angle	Screw removal	Arthrosis (%)	FU
Lafosse [27]	6.5%	80	12	8	78%	29°	4%	11	26
Cunni ngham [8]						11.5			6.6
Zhu AJSM [9]	0	100			91.3%	21.7°	0		26.9
Zhu A [10]	0	100			91.5%	22.6	0	1.7	28.4
Marion [6]	27.3% (3.3 months postop)		0	90.9	59.1%	28.6	5.3%		29.8
Athwal [11]							4%		17
Metais [5]							4.2%		22.7
Boileau [12, 13]	9%					20.2	0%		14
Dumont [7]							12.5%		76.4
Castricini [14]									13
Casabianca [16]	22%	94	0	6		19.9°			3.1
Kany [15]		68.4	24	7.4	91.5%	21°	1%	1	41

Review of the literature. *FU* follow-up (in months)

over time leading to tricortical graft fixed with screws to the anteroinferior margin of the glenoid. Scheibel et al. described such grafting in lateral decubitus position in 2008 as Taverna et al. in beach chair position [18, 19]. In addition, Taverna et al. proposed transglenoid suture fixation through rotator interval instead of the screw fixation being the first to do so. In 2016, the results of 15 patients treated by Scheibel have been issued with iliac crest arthroscopic bone grafting onto anterior glenoid rim (Fig. 35.5). At the final follow-up of 20.6 months in average, the mean active range of flexion and abduction was similar in both shoulder whereas external rotation has been restricted by 22° in the affected arm. No recurrent subluxations or dislocations were observed. Improvement in Constant, Rowe, Western Ontario Shoulder Instability Index and Subjective Shoulder Value was found, being statistically significant in all but Constant score. Radiological findings revealed graft union in all cases and osteoarthritis grade two in 1 patient and grade one in 2 patients.

35.1.3.3 Allograft

Iliac crest autografts have been criticised for a donor site morbidity as coracoid transfers for its non-anatomical aspect, leading to a shoulder dyskinesia. Allografts are not being a subject of such, though very limited reports on its use in shoulder instability do not permit to fully compare these techniques. Tjoumakaris and Sekiya achieved good short-term results using glenoid allograft with patient returning to former activities. Skendzel and Sekiya described an arthroscopic version of the technique (frozen iliac crest graft). Provencher et al. used fresh tibia grafts to restore anterior glenoid defects, reporting its good incorporation. Even more limited data is available on that techniques though, with no patient series for statistical analysis (3 patients). The literature review performed by Skendzel and Sekiya reveal bibliographic insufficiency in that matter—taking into consideration open and arthroscopic techniques 24 patients were described in four publications [20–22].

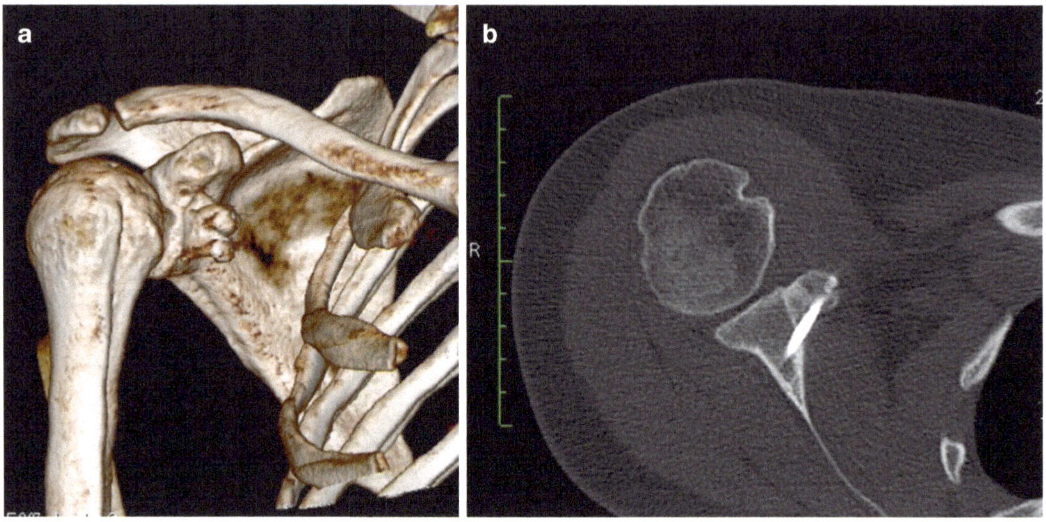

Fig. 35.5 An example of arthroscopic Eden–Hybinnette procedure (free iliac crest graft onto anteroinferior glenoid margin) performed with use of arthroscopic Latarjet instruments

35.2 Posterior Instability

Posterior instability associated with posterior glenoid rim deficiency has been treated with bone block procedure since 1947 [23]. Kouvalchouk et al. described 5 patients treated with an acromion-based bone block with excellent results (none redislocated, full range of movement has been achieved and all the patients returned to sport at a former level after 1.5 years' follow-up) [24]. Sirveaux et al. confirmed those good results in longer follow-up of 13.5 years in average. He reported the results of two groups of patients, 18 in total, treated with acromion-based graft and an iliac crest bone graft, favouring the technique described by Kouvalchouk. None redislocated though six of them had positive apprehension. As major complication, noticeable risk of osteoarthritis has been evoked [25].

Arthroscopic posterior bone block procedure has been introduced by Lafosse et al., using iliac crest grafting. This technique does not differ significantly from the anterior block, taking benefit from the very same surgical instruments. Care must be taken, though, not to damage neurovascular structures, anterior to scapula, while drilling K wires from the posterior to anterior. Nineteen cases were reported by Lafosse with a median follow-up of 20.5 months. A statistically significant improvement has been achieved in Rowe scale from 18.4 points to 82.1 points, and Walch–Duplay scores from 37.4 points to 82.9 points. Sixteen percent of patients were dissatisfied after the surgery for persistent instability and prominent iliac crest bone graft. Figure 35.6 presents the key steps of the procedure. Further in 2018, Haeni [26] and Lafosse reported simultaneous anterior and posterior arthroscopic block in seven cases. Improvement in Walch–Duplay and Rowe scores were reported from 30 (15–55) to 62.5 (15–90) and from 30 (15–50) to 62.5 (30–90), respectively, providing still good results, but worse outcome comparing to a posterior block simple. Only one patient returned to a former level of sport and three revision surgeries were required: three screw removals and one additional arthroscopic Eden–Hybinette procedure. Radiological findings confirmed excellent graft healing with correct screw angle and bone union in all patients. One grade 1 osteoarthritis was reported.

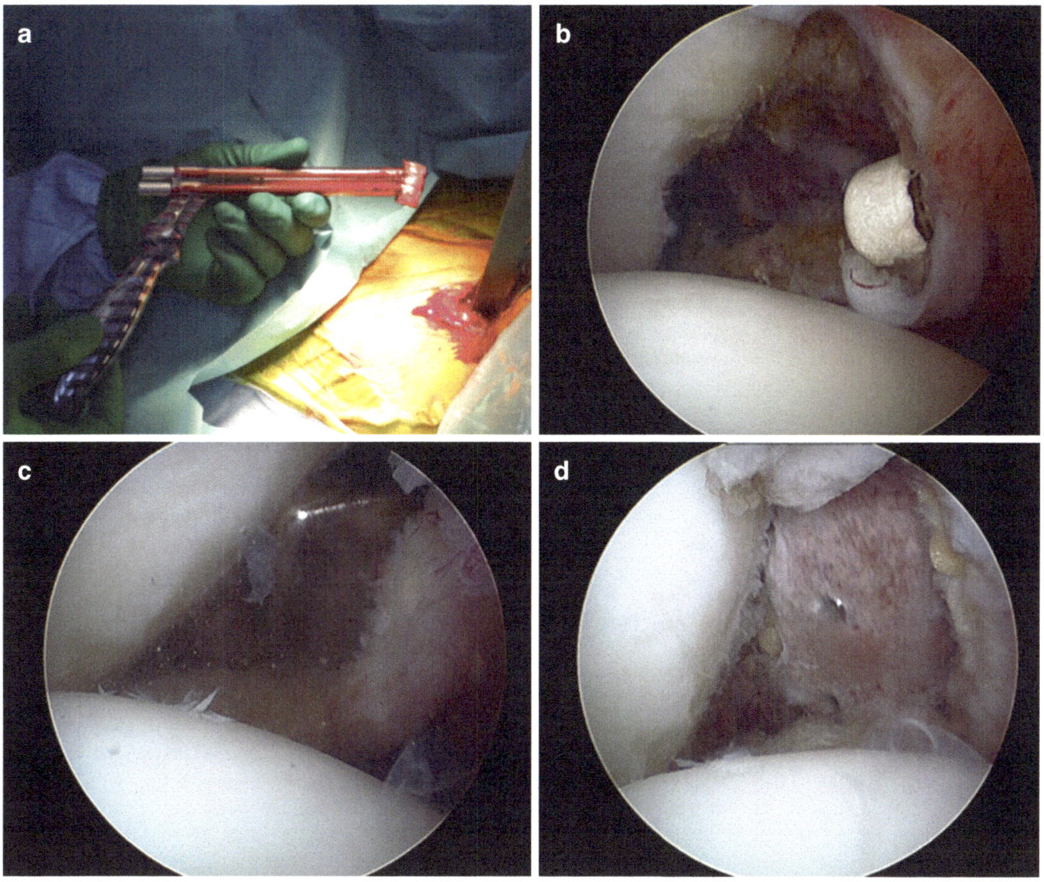

Fig. 35.6 (**a**) Graft attached to a handle (DePuy Mitek, Raynham, MA, USA) to facilitate graft insertion and positioning during arthroscopy. (**b**) Posterior capsule detachment through the "B" posterosuperior portal. (**c**) A blunt rectangle trocar is introduced through the "A" portal and inserted to create a channel for the graft. (**d**) Graft insertion into the joint through the infraspinatus muscle (posterior portal). Schwartz, D. G., Goebel, S., Piper, K., Kordasiewicz, B., Boyle, S., & Lafosse, L. (2013). *Arthroscopic posterior bone block augmentation in posterior shoulder instability. Journal of Shoulder and Elbow Surgery, 22(8), 1092–1101.* https://doi.org/10.1016/j.jse.2012.09.011. (With Elsevier permission)

35.2.1 Conclusion

Bone block procedures have been reliable and popular techniques addressing shoulder instability for decades. For 20 years, arthroscopic bone blocks incessantly gain popularity over open ones, providing similar results and offering all advantages of an arthroscopic surgery at the same time. It secures better stability comparing to a soft tissue procedure, but on the other hand it has been issue of a higher rate of severe complications. It shall remain a tool then, in the hands of experienced in arthroscopy surgeons.

The past 20 years have seen also a constant improvement of young arthroscopic techniques, arising hopes for the future to come.

References

1. Turkel SJ, Panio MW, Marshall JL, Girgis FG. Stabilizing mechanisms preventing anterior dislocation of the glenohumeral joint. J Bone Joint Surg. 1981;63A:1208–17.
2. E. Itoi. On-track' and 'off-track' shoulder lesions. EFORT Open Rev. 2017 Aug 1;2(8):343–351. https://doi.org/10.1302/2058-5241.2.170007. eCollection 2017 Aug.

3. Shin S-J, Koh YW, Bui C, Jeong WK, Akeda M, Cho NS, McGarry MH, Lee TQ. What is the critical value of glenoid bone loss at which soft tissue Bankart repair does not restore glenohumeral translation, restricts range of motion, and leads to abnormal humeral head position? Am J Sports Med. 2016;44(11):2784–91. https://doi.org/10.1177/0363546516656367.
4. Latarjet M. [Treatment of recurrent dislocation of the shoulder]. Lyon Chir. 1954;49:994–7.
5. Metais P, Clavert P, Barth J, et al. Preliminary clinical outcomes of Latarjet-Patte coracoid transfer by arthroscopy vs. open surgery: prospective multicentre study of 390 cases. Orthop Traumatol Surg Res. 2016;102:S271–6. https://doi.org/10.1016/j.otsr.2016.08.003.
6. Marion B, Klouche S, Deranlot J, et al. A prospective comparative study of arthroscopic versus mini-open Latarjet procedure with a minimum 2-year follow-up. Arthroscopy. 2017;33:269–77. https://doi.org/10.1016/j.arthro.2016.06.046.
7. Dumont GD, Fogerty S, Rosso C, Lafosse L. The arthroscopic Latarjet procedure for anterior shoulder instability: 5-year minimum follow-up. Am J Sports Med. 2014;42:2560–6. https://doi.org/10.1177/0363546514544682.
8. Cunningham G, Benchouk S, Kherad O, Lädermann A. Comparison of arthroscopic and open Latarjet with a learning curve analysis. Knee Surgery, Sports Traumatology, Arthroscopy. 2015;24(2):540–45. https://doi.org/10.1007/s00167-015-3910-3.
9. Zhu Y, Jiang C, Song G. Arthroscopic versus open latarjet in the treatment of recurrent anterior shoulder dislocation with marked glenoid bone loss: a prospective comparative study. Am J Sports Med. 2017;45(7):1645–53. https://doi.org/10.1177/0363546517693845. Epub 2017 Mar 28.
10. Zhu Y-M, Jiang C, Song G, et al. Arthroscopic Latarjet procedure with anterior capsular reconstruction: clinical outcome and radiologic evaluation with a minimum 2-year follow-up. Arthroscopy. 2017;33:2128–35. https://doi.org/10.1016/j.arthro.2017.06.014.
11. Athwal GS, Meislin R, Getz C, et al. Short-term complications of the arthroscopic Latarjet procedure: a north American experience. Arthroscopy. 2016;32:1965–70. https://doi.org/10.1016/j.arthro.2016.02.022.
12. Boileau P, Gendre P, Baba M, Thélu CÉ, Baring T, Gonzalez JF, Trojani C. A guided surgical approach and novel fixation method for arthroscopic Latarjet. J Shoulder Elb Surg. 2016;25(1):78–89. https://doi.org/10.1016/j.jse.2015.06.001. Epub 2015 Aug 7
13. Boileau P, Mercier N, Roussanne Y, et al. Arthroscopic Bankart-Bristow-Latarjet procedure: the development and early results of a safe and reproducible technique. Arthroscopy. 2010;26:1434–50. https://doi.org/10.1016/j.arthro.2010.07.011.
14. Castricini R, De Benedetto M, Orlando N, et al. Arthroscopic Latarjet procedure: analysis of the learning curve. Musculoskelet Surg. 2013;97(Suppl 1):93–8. https://doi.org/10.1007/s12306-013-0262-3.
15. Kany J, Flamand O, Grimberg J, et al. Arthroscopic Latarjet procedure: is optimal positioning of the bone block and screws possible? A prospective computed tomography scan analysis. J Shoulder Elb Surg. 2016;25:69–77. https://doi.org/10.1016/j.jse.2015.06.010.
16. Casabianca L, Gerometta A, Massein A, et al. Graft position and fusion rate following arthroscopic Latarjet. Knee Surg Sport Traumatol Arthrosc. 2016;24:507–12. https://doi.org/10.1007/s00167-015-3551-6.
17. Tang J, Zhao J. Arthroscopic transfer of the conjoined tendon-coracoid tip complex for anterior shoulder instability. Arthrosc Tech. 2017;7(1):e33–8. https://doi.org/10.1016/j.eats.2017.08.047. eCollection 2018 Jan
18. Scheibel M, Kraus N, Diederichs G, Haas NP. Arthroscopic reconstruction of chronic anteroinferior glenoid defect using an autologous tricortical iliac crest bone grafting technique. Arch Orthop Trauma Surg. 2008;128(11):1295–300. Epub 2007 Nov 22
19. Taverna E, D'Ambrosi R, Perfetti C, Garavaglia G. Arthroscopic bone graft procedure for anterior inferior glenohumeral instability. Arthrosc Tech. 2014;3(6):e653–60.
20. Tjoumakaris FP, Sekiya JK. Combined glenoid and humeral head allograft reconstruction for recurrent anterior glenohumeral instability. Orthopedics. 2008;31(5):497.
21. Skendzel JG, Sekiya JK. Arthroscopic glenoid osteochondral allograft reconstruction without subscapularis takedown: technique and literature review. Arthroscopy. 2011;27(1):129–35.
22. Provencher MT, Ghodadra N, LeClere L, Solomon DJ, Romeo AA. Anatomic osteochondral glenoid reconstruction for recurrent glenohumeral instability with glenoid deficiency using a distal tibia allograft. Arthroscopy. 2009;25(4):446–52.
23. Hindenach JC. Recurrent posterior dislocation of the shoulder. J Bone Joint Surg Am. 1947;29:582–6.
24. Kouvalchouk JF, Coudert X, Watin Augouard L, Da Silva RR, Paszkowski A. Treatment of posterior instability of the shoulder joint using an acromial stop with a pediculated deltoid flap [in French]. Rev Chir Orthop Reparatrice Appar Mot. 1993;79:661–5.
25. Sirveaux F, Leroux J, Roche O, Gosselin O, De Gasperi M, Mole D. Surgical treatment of posterior instability of the shoulder joint using an iliac bone block or an acromial pediculated bone block: outcome in eighteen patients [in French]. Rev Chir Orthop Reparatrice Appar Mot. 2004;90:411–9.
26. Haeni D, Sanchez M, Johannes P, Victoria L, Henderson D, Munji J, Petkin K, Lafosse L. Arthroscopic double bone block augmentation is a salvage procedure for anterior and posterior shoulder instability secondary to glenoid bone loss. Arthroscopy. 2018;26(8):2447–53. https://doi.org/10.1007/s00167-018-4975-6.
27. Lafosse L, Boyle S. Arthroscopic Latarjet procedure. J Shoulder Elb Surg. 2010;19(2 Suppl):2–12. https://doi.org/10.1016/j.jse.2009.12.010.

Surgical Treatment of Humeral Head Defect in Shoulder Posterior Instability

36

Riccardo Compagnoni, Matteo Lo Duca, and Pietro S. Randelli

36.1 Introduction

Posterior instability of glenohumeral joint represents 3% of all shoulder dislocations [1]. Posterior instability can be classified according to the grade, direction, mechanism of displacement and timing of the trauma (acute, chronic, locked or non-locked and recurrent posterior subluxation). McLaughlin described two main types of posterior instability: chronic posterior displacement and recurrent posterior subluxation [2]. Posterior dislocation is to be considered chronic after 3 weeks from the traumatic event; the recurrent form can be caused by a single traumatic posterior displacement, but usually less than 10% of such dislocations have a recurrence. Possible causes of recurrence include microtrauma due to repeated shoulder movements in a risky position, like in some athletes (rugby, bench press, swimming, etc.) or professionals. An enhanced laxity, generalized or localized to the shoulder girdle, has to be investigated in all cases of posterior shoulder dislocations.

Posterior dislocation can develop reverse capsule and labrum tears of anterior dislocation. Some patients with posterior instability display posterior glenoid labrum detachment, also known as posterior Bankart lesion with associated osteochondral damage of the anterior surface of the humeral articular surface secondary to impaction with glenoid, otherwise known as reverse Hill–Sachs lesion (Fig. 36.1).

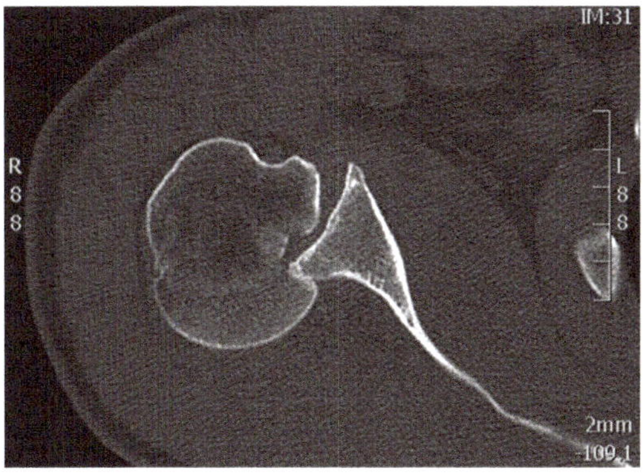

Fig. 36.1 Posterior dislocation with McLaughlin lesion of the humeral head

R. Compagnoni · P. S. Randelli (✉)
Laboratory of Applied Biomechanics, Department of Biomedical Sciences for Health, Università degli Studi di Milano, Milan, Italy

1° Clinica Ortopedica, ASST Centro Specialistico Ortopedico Traumatologico Gaetano Pini-CTO, Milan, Italy

Research Center for Adult and Pediatric Rheumatic Diseases (RECAP-RD), Department of Biomedical Sciences for Health, Università degli Studi di Milano, Via Mangiagalli 31, 20133, Milan, Italy
e-mail: pietro.randelli@unimi.it

M. Lo Duca
1° Clinica Ortopedica, ASST Centro Specialistico Ortopedico Traumatologico Gaetano Pini-CTO, Milan, Italy

R. Brzóska et al. (eds.), *360° Around Shoulder Instability*,
https://doi.org/10.1007/978-3-662-61074-9_36

Reverse Hill–Sachs lesion or McLaughlin lesion is an impaction fracture of the anteromedial part of the humeral head following posterior dislocation of the shoulder. This kind of lesion was first described in 1952 by the orthopaedic surgeon H. McLaughlin as a bony defect of the humeral head in patients who reported a previous posterior shoulder dislocation [2].

A recent study showed that after the first episode of posterior dislocation, 86% of patient had a reverse Hill–Sachs lesion [3]. Depending on its size, Hill–Sachs lesion can engage the posterior rim of glenoid during the internal rotation of the shoulder leading to pain and increased risk of recurrence.

Correct surgical treatment indication and choice is related to time lapse from trauma, humeral head, articular surface deficiency and the presence of degenerative joint lesions [4].

36.2 Clinical Evaluation

Patient history, clinical examination and imaging form the basis for correct decision-making in treating posterior unstable shoulder. Radiographic evaluation should include anteroposterior, axillary and scapular Y view. Computed tomography (CT) scans can be useful to evaluate bone loss, and Magnetic Resonance Imaging (MRI) is better to evaluate any soft tissue lesions and to define the quantity of bone damage.

During physical examination, active and passive range of motion should be carefully evaluated; a locked posterior dislocation should be suspected in patients that display a serious reduction of active and passive rotations, with recent traumatic history and "at-risk" upper limb behaviours (e.g., contact athletes, heavy workers and seizure patients). In case of recurrent posterior dislocation, patients report similar symptoms. Usually posterior subluxation can occur with internal rotation, flexion and adduction of the upper limb.

The following tests are useful to evaluate the posterior shoulder instability.

Jerk test: patient is seated with upper limb internally rotated and flexed at 90°, the examiner with one hand secures the shoulder, with the other hand applies a posterior force while adducing the limb; the test is considered positive if it causes pain or sense of apprehension, possibly a subluxation.

Load and shift test: patient in lateral decubitus with shoulder abducted at 90° and flexed elbow, the examiner applies a posterior force to the arm; the test is positive if the patient has pain of sense of apprehension, possibly a subluxation.

Posterior drawer test: the shoulder and elbow are flexed at 90°; the examiner applies a posterior force to the humerus while pulling the forearm anteriorly. The test is positive if it causes pain or a posterior dislocation of above 50%.

36.3 Reverse Hill–Sachs Treatment

36.3.1 Conservative Treatment

Lesions involving less than 25% of the articular surface can be treated in a conservative way with reduction in narcosis and immobilization with an arm sling at 30° of external rotation for 4–6 weeks. Surgical treatment must be considered in patients with larger bone defects, locked posterior dislocation (more than 3 weeks from trauma) and recurrent dislocation after a failed conservative treatment.

36.3.2 Surgical Treatment

Current surgical techniques can be divided in two groups: anatomical and non-anatomical reconstructions. The target of anatomical approach is to restore the original shape of humeral head. This can be obtained by different bone grafting techniques or by performing a filling of the bone defect with injection of bone graft [5–8]. The target of non-anatomical surgery is to restore stability by filling the defect with soft tissue [2, 9, 10].

36.4 McLaughlin Technique

McLaughlin reported good results in patients treated with transfer of the subscapularis tendon into the bone defect [2] (Fig. 36.2). According to

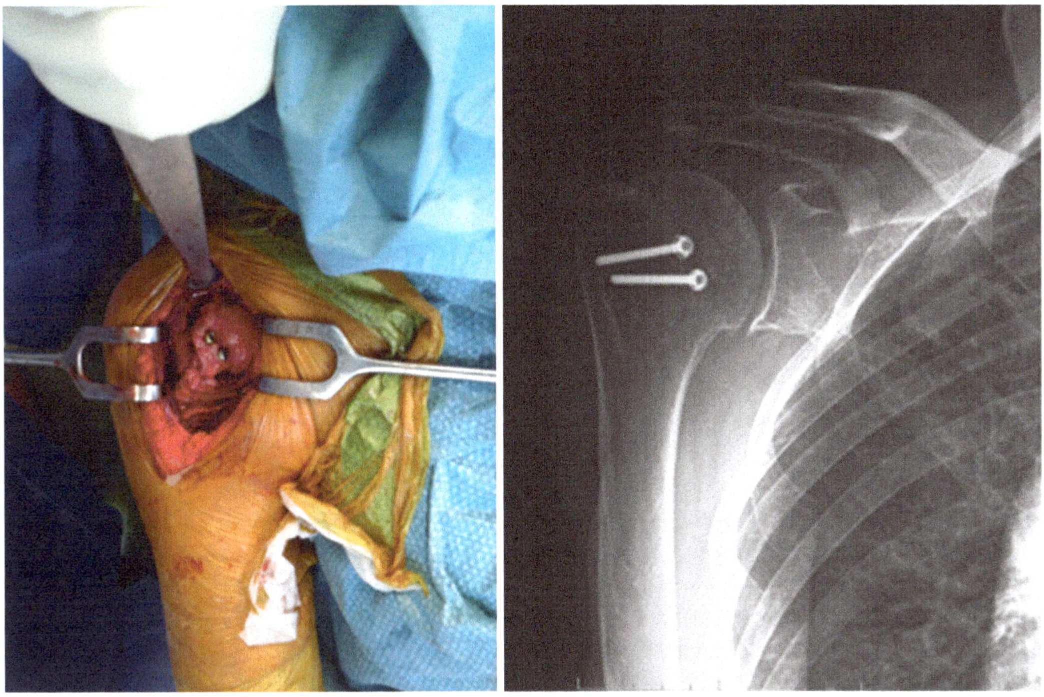

Fig. 36.2 Transfer of the subscapularis tendon into the bone defect and stabilization with two screws (McLaughlin technique): intraoperative image and post-operative X-ray

the literature, there is consensus that this procedure should be carried out when the following conditions are met: lesion up to 45% of the articular surface and surgery performed within 6 months from the dislocation.

The patient is secured in beach chair position; via a deltopectoral approach; the subscapularis tendon is exposed and sectioned at 1 cm from its insertion on the lesser tuberosity; the humeral head is then reduced and the bone defect exposed. At this point, external rotation to the limb is applied and two anchors are placed at the medial margin of the lesion: the medial surface of the tendon is then sutured using mattress stitches; the lateral margin of the tendon is then secured to the bone with transosseous suture. Stabilization is also possible using two screws. Following defect correction, the shoulder joint is immobilized in neutral rotation for 3 weeks, the limb is instead immobilized at 15° of external rotation for 6 weeks with dedicated arm sling.

This technique has been modified by Hughes and Neer in 1975 performing bone transfer into the reverse Hill–Sachs using the lesser tuberosity [11]. Charalambous et al. instead described a new technique that avoided tenotomy of the subscapularis tendon, which is instead mobilized and used to fill the bone defect [12].

Limits of these procedures are similar and include reduced internal rotation strength and increased difficulty in performing prosthetic surgery of the shoulder, if needed [7].

36.5 Arthroscopic Techniques

The patient is placed in lateral decubitus position with the affected shoulder at 20–30° of abduction. The joint is carefully examined with combination of 30° and 70° arthroscopes; if any capsular or posterior labrum lesion is found, a repair is performed by suture anchors. Posterior rim engagement is then evaluated in internal rotation of the humeral head. Via posterior portal access, the reverse Hill–Sachs lesion can be easily and clearly visualized with a 70° arthroscope. The lesion is debrided in order to evaluate its extension, size and location; using an arthroscopic burr, the lesion is prepared for repair. One or two anchors are placed in the lesion and the previously mobilized subscapularis tendon is secured with mattress stitches; double mattress stitches should be used in order to avoid tissue necrosis, described by Koo et al. as a potential pitfall of this technique [13]. This procedure, also known as "reverse remplissage", converts the reverse Hill–Sachs lesion into an extra-articular defect thereby reducing engagement and symptoms correlated to the defect.

Regarding arthroscopic techniques literature is limited: Krackhardt et al. first described this technique in 2006 [10], later Martetschläger et al. in 2013 reported a variation in which the suture anchors were placed, one superior and one inferior into the defect [14].

Arthroscopic reverse remplissage is a minimally invasive technique that provides better visualization of the lesion and thereby avoids surgical comorbidities compared to open techniques, like tenotomy of subscapularis tendon or lesser tuberosity osteotomy. Its main limit is alteration of the subscapularis' biomechanics thereby causing reduced internal rotation of the shoulder. To reduce this problem, Duey and Burkhart developed a variation of this procedure in which they filled the reverse Hill–Sachs lesion with the middle glenohumeral ligament [15]. This technique seems to provide a better internal rotation; authors advise the use of this technique in case of lesions involving less than one-third of the articular surface.

Post-operatively, the upper limb is immobilized in arm sling for 6 weeks before starting physical therapy. The patient should be instructed on elbow, wrist and shoulder movement. After sling removal, the patient begins passive physiotherapy with a progressive program of stretching and strengthening; after 12 weeks from the operation, a more advanced course of strengthening begins. Return to full activities should be expected between 6- and 9-months post-op depending on the characteristics of the repaired lesion.

36.6 Bone Grafting Techniques

Reconstruction of the humeral head defect by osteochondral allograft has been successfully used in posterior dislocations with a defect of the humeral head involving up to 40% of the articular surface [5–15]. This technique helps in the restoration of the spherical shape of the humeral head, and the bone defect can be corrected using both allograft and autograft [8] (Figs. 36.1, 36.3, and 36.4).

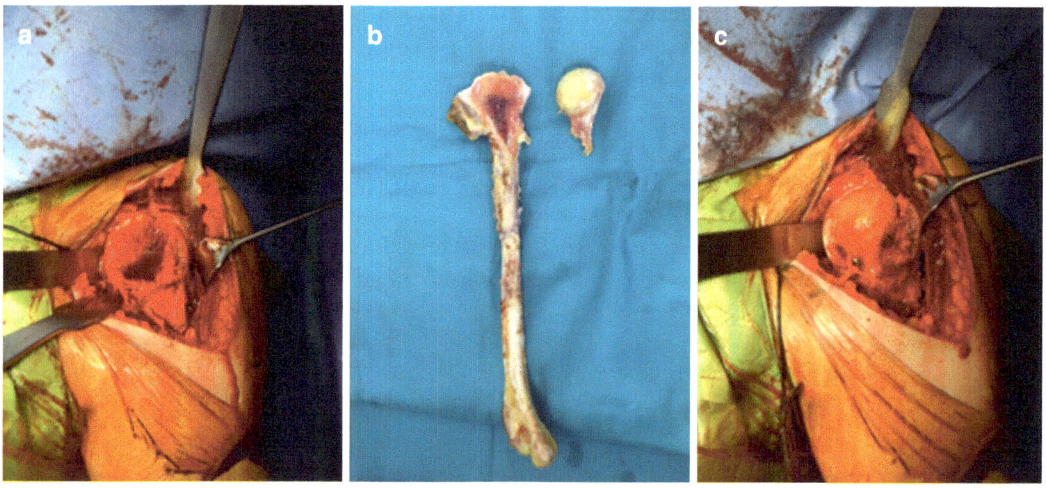

Fig. 36.3 Intraoperative images of allograft implant in severe bone loss of the proximal humeral head in posterior dislocation. (**a**) Image of proximal humerus after preparation of socket for allograft implant. (**b**) Humeral component taken from allograft for implant. (**c**) Final result after fixation with two 4.5 mm cannulated screws

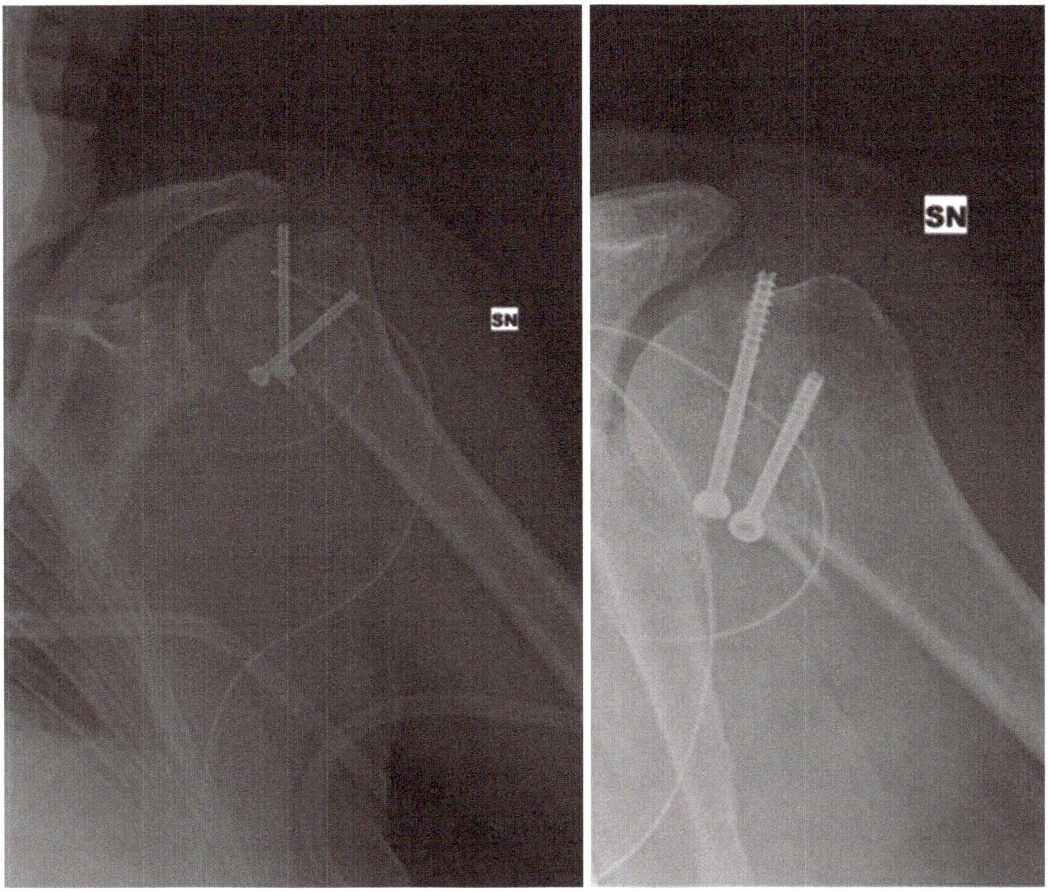

Fig. 36.4 Post-operative radiological evaluation after allograft implantation

Autograft shows better and faster integration, but its major limitation is the retrieval of enough bone material to fill the defect. On the other hand, allografts are easily available through bone bank, but they are associated with slow bone integration and likelihood of infectious disease transmission. All bone specimens admitted into the bone banks are frozen and stored at −80 °C, tested for bacterial contamination and serologically against HAV, HBV, HCV and HIV; this makes the infectious risk of allograft usage limited. Bone grafting allows for anatomical reconstruction of the humeral head, thereby avoiding rotational limitations, permitting a latter prosthetic treatment.

Regarding allograft choice and management, the most used and best suited grafts are proximal humerus or femoral head; during the operation, the defect is carefully measured and an oscillating bone saw is used to fulfil a wedge of the same size from the graft; it is then fixed into the lesion with two or three bone screws.

These techniques are best suited for young patients with good bone quality. Compressive forces can produce dislocation or collapse of the graft in patients with osteoporotic bone; for this reason, this technique should be considered with caution in these patients.

The upper limb is immobilized in an arm sling for 6 weeks after surgery. Passive physiotherapy should be started the first post-operative day with forward elevation and external rotation exercises; internal rotation is not permitted for 6 weeks. Active physiotherapy begins after sling removal and resisted exercises after 12 weeks.

Another possible option for treating these bone defects, in case of recent dislocations with impact fracture, is to a perform a plasty of the proximal humerus. This procedure utilizes an inflatable balloon, in an effort to reduce the impaction fracture and to create a space to theoretically allow safer injection of cement into the fractured humeral head. The most widely used cement product is polymethyl methacrylate, commonly used in spinal surgery for kyphoplasty (Figs. 36.5, 36.6, and 36.7).

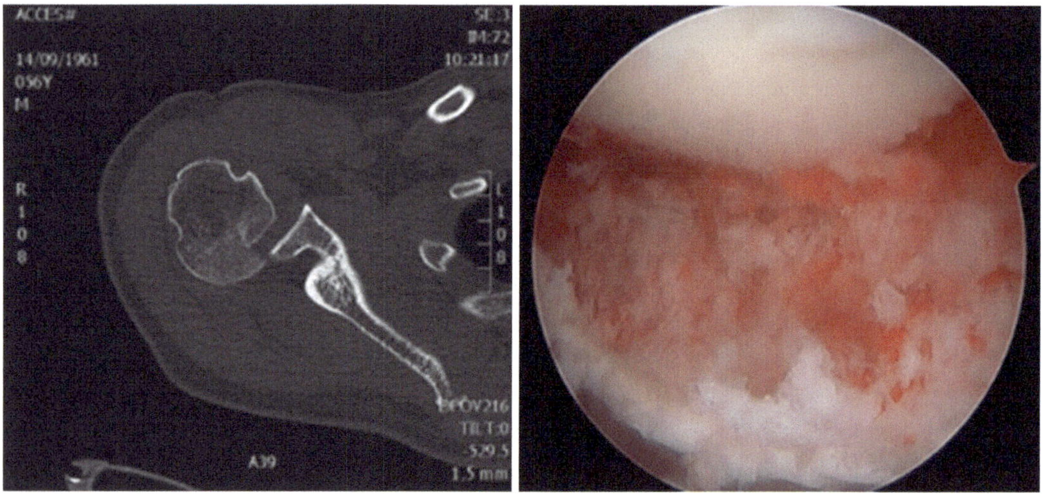

Fig. 36.5 Posterior dislocation of humeral head with impact fracture of anterior articular surface. Pre-operative MRI and intra-operative arthroscopic view

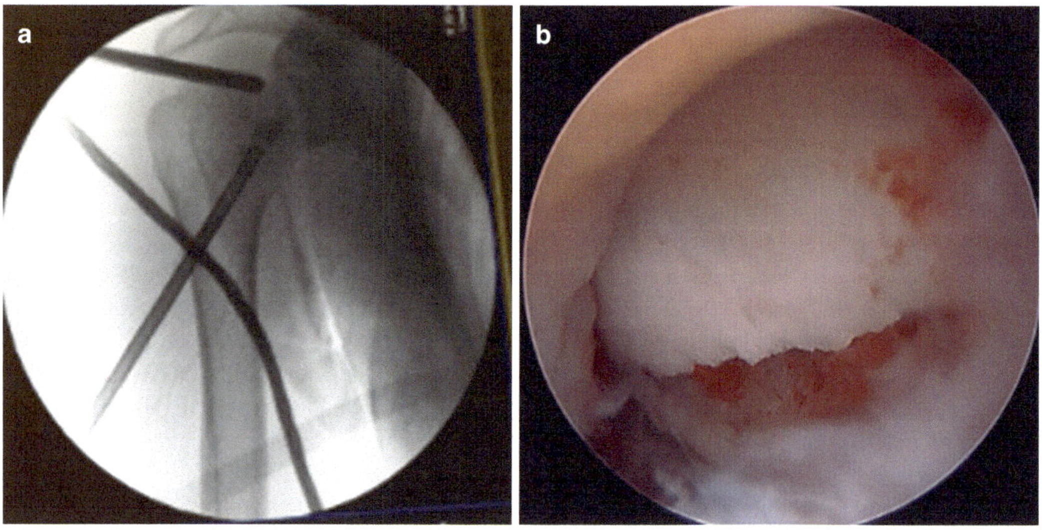

Fig. 36.6 (**a**) Intra-operative fluoroscopic image of percutaneous reduction and filling with polymethyl methacrylate of bone fracture consequence of a posterior dislocation. (**b**) Arthroscopic image of humeral head at the end of the procedure

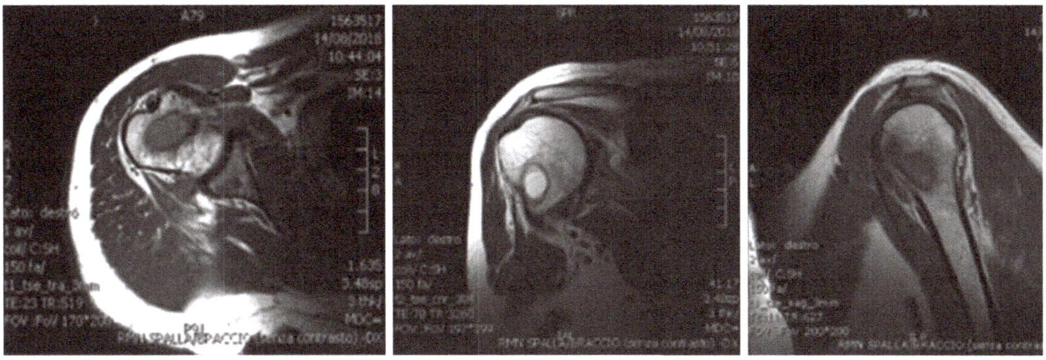

Fig. 36.7 MRI control: 1 month after surgery

36.7 Prosthetic Treatment

In case of lesion involving more than 50% of the articular surface or chronic dislocations, partial shoulder replacement or total shoulder arthroplasty can be considered. In case of associated degenerative lesions of the glenoid, a total anatomical prosthesis is indicated; but if concurrent rotator cuff lesions are present, an inverse prosthesis is recommended.

The operation is carried out with patient in beach chair position with deltopectoral approach. The long head of the biceps tendon is identified and a tenotomy/tenodesis is performed. The subscapularis tendon is then identified and stitches are places before performing a tenotomy at about 1 cm from its insertion in the lesser tuberosity. The joint is then gently reduced in case of chronic dislocation and displaced anteriorly with exposition of the humeral head. The head is removed with a cut at the level of the anatomical neck in order to facilitate glenoid preparation in case of total shoulder replacement. Following preparation of the humeral canal, the definitive prosthesis components are placed. As a general rule, the surgical technique follows the steps used in traditional prosthetic implants, but specific attention has to be focused on final implant stability.

36.8 Conclusions

Posterior shoulder instability is a rare and an often-misdiagnosed condition. In the absence of a clear clinical history, like an anterior trauma or repeated stresses of the posterior capsule linked to working or sport trauma, it is often hard to hypothesize a posterior instability. Usually symptoms are mild and insidious; therefore a good patient history and a careful clinical examination are mandatory along with proper imaging techniques. An early diagnosis and a proper treatment for the acute traumatic posterior dislocation is crucial, in order to prevent it from becoming a chronic affection. In cases with associated reverse Hill–Sachs lesion, it is useful to evaluate the engagement of the lesion into the posterior glenoid rim and the percentage of missing humeral articular surface with a CT or MRI study. Depending on the size of the articular surface and the patient's needs, the surgical technique is chosen. Massive bone loss or presence of associated tears, such as massive rotator cuff tear or glenohumeral arthritis, can be considered potential indications for a shoulder replacement.

References

1. Robinson CM, Seah M, Akhtar MA. The epidemiology, risk of recurrence, and functional outcome after an acute traumatic posterior dislocation of the shoulder. J Bone Joint Surg Am. 2011;93(17):1605–13.
2. McLaughlin HL. Posterior dislocation of the shoulder. J Bone Joint Surg Am. 1952;24 A(3):584–90.
3. Saupe N, White LM, Bleakney R, Schweitzer ME, Recht MP, Jost B, Zanetti M. Acute traumatic posterior shoulder dislocation: MR findings. Radiology. 2008;248(1):185–93.
4. Cicak N. Posterior dislocation of the shoulder. J Bone Joint Surg Br. 2004;86(3):324–32.

5. Gerber C, Lambert SM. Allograft reconstruction of segmental defects of the humeral head for the treatment of chronic locked posterior dislocation of the shoulder. J Bone Joint Surg Am. 1996;78(3):376–82.
6. Martinez AA, Navarro E, Iglesias D, Domingo J, Calvo A, Carbonel I. Long-term follow-up of allograft reconstruction of segmental defects of the humeral head associated with posterior dislocation of the shoulder. Injury. 2013;44(4):488–91.
7. Diklic ID, Ganic ZD, Blagojevic ZD, Nho SJ, Romeo AA. Treatment of locked chronic posterior dislocation of the shoulder by reconstruction of the defect in the humeral head with an allograft. J Bone Joint Surg Br. 2010;92(1):71–6.
8. Khayal T, Wild M, Windolf J. Reconstruction of the articular surface of the humeral head after locked posterior shoulder dislocation: a case report. Arch Orthop Trauma Surg. 2009;129(4):515–9.
9. Hawkins RJ, Neer CS II, Pianta RM, Mendoza FX. Locked posterior dislocation of the shoulder. J Bone Joint Surg Am. 1987;69(1):9–18.
10. Krackhardt T, Schewe B, Albrecht D, Weise K. Arthroscopic fixation of the subscapularis tendon in the reverse Hill-Sachs lesion for traumatic unidirectional posterior dislocation of the shoulder. Arthroscopy. 2006;22(2):227.e1–6.
11. Hughes M, Neer CS II. Glenohumeral joint replacement and postoperative rehabilitation. Phys Ther. 1975;55(8):850–8.
12. Charalambous CP, Gullett TK, Ravenscroft MJ. A modification of the McLaughlin procedure for persistent posterior shoulder instability: technical note. Arch Orthop Trauma Surg. 2009;129(6):753–5.
13. Koo SS, Burkhart SS, Ochoa E. Arthroscopic double-pulley remplissage technique for engaging Hill-Sachs lesions in anterior shoulder instability repairs. Arthroscopy. 2009;25(11):1343–8.
14. Martetschläger F, Padalecki JR, Millett PJ. Modified arthroscopic McLaughlin procedure for treatment of posterior instability of the shoulder with an associated reverse Hill-Sachs lesion. Knee Surg Sports Traumatol Arthrosc. 2013;21(7):1642–6.
15. Duey RE, Burkhart SS. Arthroscopic treatment of a reverse Hill–Sachs lesion. Arthrosc Tech. 2013;2(2):e155–9.

Glenoid Osteotomy

37

Bartłomiej Kordasiewicz, Michał Janyst, and Maciej Kiciński

37.1 Introduction

Glenohumeral instability is a common disease with the incidence rate of 56 per 100,000 people per year. There is a significant difference between prevalence of the condition in male patients: 82.2 per 100,000 and female patients: 30.9 per 100,000 [1]. On the other hand, posterior shoulder instability is less common than anterior and affects only 2–4% of patients suffering from glenohumeral instability [2]. Among population of athletes, posterior shoulder instability is a much more common cause of instability (17.9%) comparing to overall population [3].

Patients suffering from posterior shoulder instability (PSI) can be divided into three different groups. First group are the patients with acute shoulder dislocation, which usually is associated with violent trauma. Second group are the patients with missed acute posterior dislocation. In majority of cases missed acute posterior dislocation results in chronic fixed posterior dislocation. The last and the most common type of posterior shoulder instability is recurrent posterior subluxation [4].

As less than one-third of the humeral head is articulating in the glenoid fossa, glenohumeral joint tends to be instable [5]. Stability of glenohumeral joint is maintained due to both static and dynamic restraints. Main anatomic structures responsible for static stability are: proper joint congruency, glenoid labrum, joint capsule, and ligaments. Dynamic stability is maintained by three main groups of muscles: scapula stabilizers, scapulohumeral muscles, and rotator cuff [6].

37.2 Pathogenesis

Posterior shoulder instability may be caused by macrotrauma, microtrauma, or result from abnormalities of soft tissues, as well as glenohumeral dysplasia (atraumatic). Traumatic background is more frequent [7].

Macrotrauma is caused by a single event, in which load is applied axially and arm adducted internally rotated and flexed [8]. It may be also caused by a maximum muscle contraction during epileptic seizures or electrocution. This type of injury is also accompanied with high risk of other injuries, such as: reverse Hill-Sachs lesions, fractures of surgical neck, and injuries of rotator cuff or labrum.

B. Kordasiewicz (✉)
Trauma and Orthopaedics Department, SPSK im. A. Grucy, Otwock, Poland

Centre of Postgraduate Medical Education, Warsaw, Poland
e-mail: bartekko@tlen.pl

M. Janyst · M. Kiciński
Trauma and Orthopaedics Department, SPSK im. A. Grucy, Otwock, Poland
e-mail: m.kicinski@ideaortopedia.pl

R. Brzóska et al. (eds.), *360° Around Shoulder Instability*,
https://doi.org/10.1007/978-3-662-61074-9_37

Posterior shoulder instability caused by microtrauma may occur during repetitive injury, in which posterior capsule and labrum is damaged. Such type of instability may by provoked by overhead sport such as volleyball or swimming. Chronic microtrauma usually does not primarily lead to dislocation but results in instability and subluxation [9].

Atraumatic posterior shoulder instability may be result of innate collagen abnormality resulting in ligament and capsule laxity. Anatomical variations of glenoid or glenoid hypoplasia also can result in posterior shoulder instability. Possible cause of instability may be excessive retroversion of glenoid resulting in eccentric loading of glenohumeral joint [10]. It may lead to progression of arthritis; however, it was not confirmed by other authors [11, 12].

Walch et al. proposed to distinguish patients with posterior shoulder instability from patients with static posterior subluxation (PPSHH). This is a group of patients that do not have symptoms of instability in provocative tests. One of the risk factor leading to this condition is also excessive retroversion of the glenoid. Comparing to healthy population, patients with PPSHH have also excessive glenoid retroversion of 15° comparing to healthy population with 2° to 8°. They have a higher mean age (40 years) comparing to the mean age of patients with posterior shoulder instability (20–27 years). It was proposed that PPSHH can lead to development of arthritis; however, it remains a hypothesis [13].

37.3 Glenoid Types

Evaluation of glenoid version provides an important data that enables to distinguish the potential cause of posterior shoulder instability. There are currently many methods of glenoid type evaluation. The main controversy is determination of scapular axis. Currently two main types of glenoid type measurement can be described [14].

In the first method, described by Friedman, scapular axis is determined by a line set from the medial angle of scapula to the center of glenoid fossa [11]. To determine the glenoid version, perpendicular line to the axis is drawn (line of neutral version). Angle between the line of neutral version and anterior and posterior edges of the glenoid determines the glenoid version (Fig. 37.1). In the second method, axis is determined by the line drawn complementary to scapular body. Angle between the axis and the line between anterior and posterior glenoid rim determines the glenoid version.

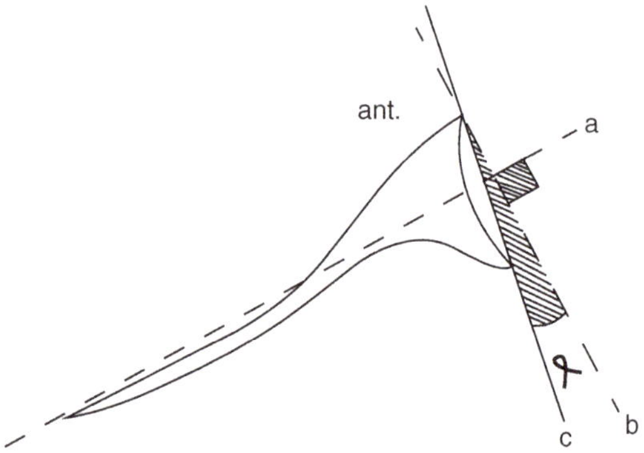

Fig. 37.1 To determine the glenoid version, perpendicular line to the axis is drawn (line of neutral version). Angle between the line of neutral version and anterior and posterior edges of the glenoid determines the glenoid version. Walch. (1999). Morphologic study of the glenoid in primary glenohumeral osteoarthritis. J Arthroplasty, 14(6):756-60. (With permission of Elsevier)

According to modified Walch classification of primary glenohumeral osteoarthritis, glenoid morphology can be divided into four different subsets (Fig. 37.2) [15, 16]. In type A, the humeral head is centered, that is why strengths in glenohumeral joint are equally distributed. The erosion may be minor (A1) or major (A2).

In type B, the humeral head is subluxated posteriorly. Type B may be further divided into subsets: B0—pre-osteoarthritic posterior subluxation; B1—posterior narrowing of joint, subchondral sclerosis, and osteophytes; B2—erosion of posterior rim, excessive retroversion of glenoid; and B3—monoconcave, posterior wear, subluxation of humeral head >70% or retroversion of glenoid >15°.

Type C is defined when retroversion is higher than 25° regardless of erosion (C1) and also when biconcave, posterior bone loss or posterior translation of humeral head occurs (C2). In type D, glenoid anteversion occurs or humeral head is subluxated less than 40%.

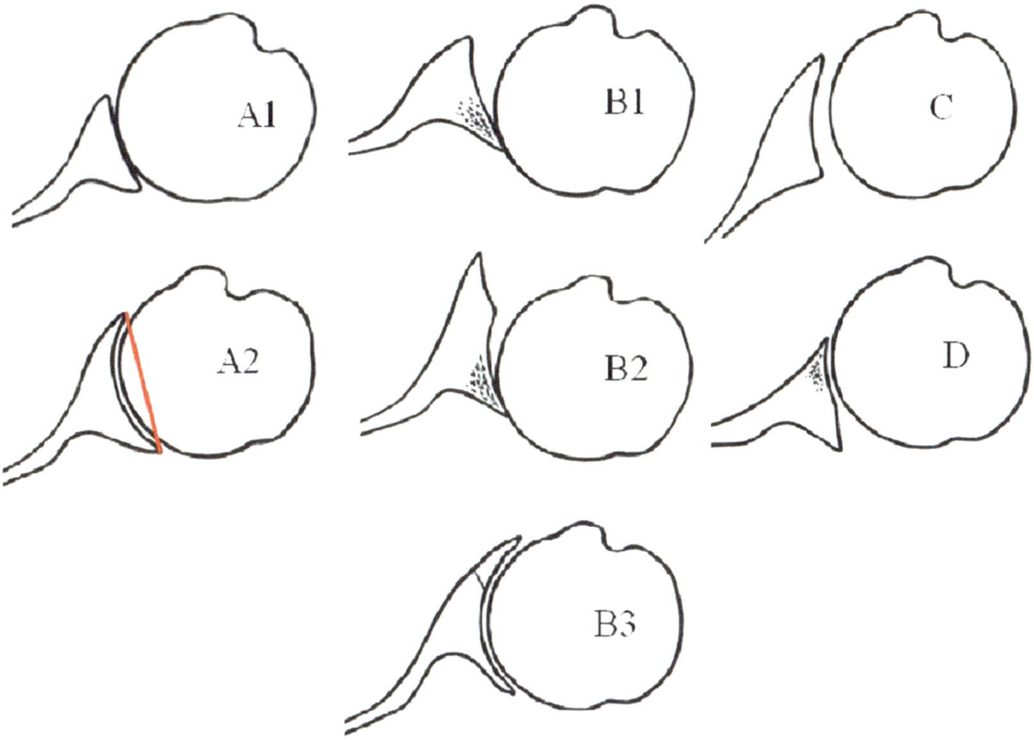

Fig. 37.2 Different types of the glenoid in primary glenohumeral osteoarthritis. Modified Walch classification. A line drawn from the anterior to posterior native glenoid rim transects the humeral head in the A2 glenoid but not in the A1 glenoid. Bercik MJ, et al. A modification to the Walch classification of the glenoid in primary glenohumeral osteoarthritis using three-dimensional imaging. J Shoulder Elbow Surg 2016;25:1601–6. (With permission of Elsevier)

The above classification describes glenoid deformity in osteoarthritis. It has never been proved it could be adapted to the posterior insta bility evaluation. Despite this fact, the methodology of bony architecture evaluation remains the same.

The influence of morphology of the glenoid on posterior shoulder instability is still debated. Patients suffering from posterior shoulder instability have an increased retroversion of glenoid, which was shown by Parada et al. On the other hand, they do not have increased posterior humeral subluxation, thus it is not a reliable indicator of the presence or absence of symptomatic posterior shoulder instability. This may incline that correction of the glenoid retroversion may be an interesting therapeutic approach for this group of patients [17]. Studies also suggest that patients with biconcave glenoid have higher rate of posterior shoulder instability [18].

37.4 Glenoid Osteotomy as a Therapeutic Option

Many therapeutic options have been proposed for treatment of posterior shoulder instability. As a first-line treatment in patients with atraumatic posterior shoulder instability without bony pathologies, usually conservative approach is chosen. There is no consensus concerning the optimal length of such approach; however, minimum 6 months of nonsurgical treatment should be performed [7]. The conservative approach is focused on strengthening both the rotator cuff muscles and scapular stabilizers. With 60–90% success rate, this method allows to successfully treat the majority of patients [19, 20].

Following unsuccessful conservative treatment, surgical management should be considered. Surgical options can be divided into two groups: soft tissue repair and osseous repair. Soft tissue repair includes reverse Bankart repair, capsular plication, posterior-inferior capsular shift, reverse Putti-Platt procedure, and thermal capsulorrhaphy. Osseous procedures include posterior glenoid osteotomy, McLaughlin's procedure, and total shoulder arthroplasty. In this publication, glenoid osteotomy will be further evaluated.

As increased glenoid retroversion could be a major factor resulting in posterior shoulder instability, patients with glenoid retroversion >20° that underwent unsuccessful capsular plication are one group that may benefit from glenoid osteotomy [7]. This hypothetical approach requires further evaluation – literature suggests that approximately 70% of patients following correction of glenoid retroversion show no signs of instability.

Other group of patients that can benefit from this procedure are patients with deficiency of the osseous socket or rim with associated soft-tissue abnormalities of the labrum and capsule, as well as malformation in the mechanical alignment or orientation of the socket identified as glenoid hypoplasia. However, the combination of bone deficiency and increased retroversion makes glenoid osteotomy very challenging.

37.5 Surgical Technique

Open glenoplasty for posterior shoulder instability was firstly employed by Kretzler and Blue [21]. In general, operation is indicated for patients with atraumatic and symptomatic instability with increased glenoid retroversion (>20°), or glenoid dysplasia following unsuccessful conservative or soft tissue repair [7].

The procedure is performed in prone or alternatively in a lateral decubitus position. Mobile image intensifier system (C-arm) is positioned to perform axillary radiographs. Lateral decubitus position also requires attachment of arm to the traction system, in contrary to prone position. Posterolateral corner of the acromion is marked.

A 6–7 cm long incision starting medially to the posterolateral corner of acromion extending toward the posterior axillary fold is made. Following division of skin and subcutaneous tissue, deltoid fascia is exposed, incised, and deltoid muscle is retracted. The tendons of the teres minor and infraspinatus are exposed. Attention must be taken to the suprascapular nerve, which is located 0.5–2 cm medially to the glenoid neck and axillary nerve in quadrilateral space. Next, the infraspinatus muscle is dissected and elevated. The posterior glenohumeral capsule is incised in a T-shaped manner. Osteotomy is performed intracapsularly, medially to the posterior rim of the glenoid, 7–8 mm from the articular surface. A K-wire may be placed laterally to the osteotomy, and it may serve as a guide pin (Fig. 37.3a, b). Attention must be given not to damage the anterior cortex. The depth of the incision may be monitored using fluoroscopy. Following osteotomy, structural autograft harvested from spina

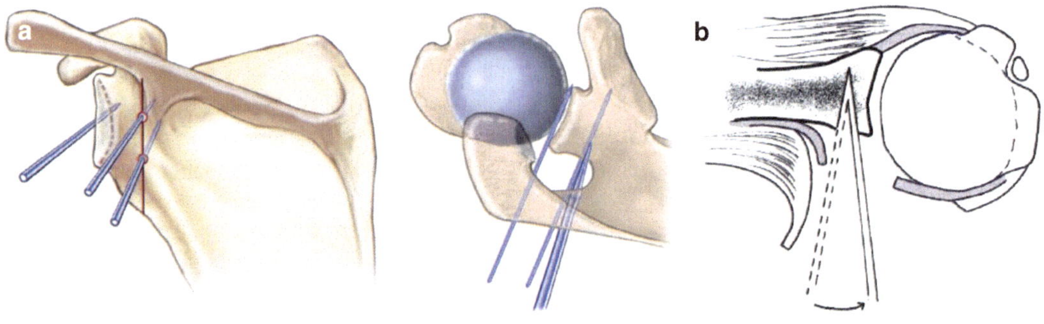

Fig. 37.3 Glenoid ostetomy. (**a**) A K-wire may be placed laterally to the osteotomy and serve as a guide pin. (**b**) Anterior cortex should not be damaged during osteotomy. Ortmaier R. et al. Posterior open wedge osteotomy of the scapula neck for the treatment of advanced shoulder osteoarthritis with posterior head migration in young patients. J Shoulder Elbow Surg, 2017. 26(7): 1278–1286 (with permission of Elsevier). Seebauer L et al. Posterior glenohumeral instability. Der Orthopäde. 1998;27:542–555. (With permission of Springer Nature)

scapulae or iliac spine is placed. The size of the graft is determined following both preoperative and intraoperative measurements. If the osteotomy is not stable or anterior cortex is damaged, posterior T-plate may be placed.

In order to reinforce the posterior capsule, plication of the posterior capsule should be performed. Subsequently all muscles are repaired, and wound closed.

37.6 Results and Potential Complications

Glenoid osteotomy is a rare method of posterior shoulder instability treatment. There are not many series of randomized studies investigating long-term outcome and potential complications. One of the biggest study investigating long-term results of such treatment was performed by Inui and Nobuhara [20]. The authors provided a series of 249 osteotomies performed on 211 patients. They included into the study patients suffering from atraumatic posteroinferior instability resulting from glenoid dysplasia. Mean follow-up was 7 years. Result of treatment was investigated using Rowe score and Japan Shoulder Society Shoulder Instability Score (JSS-SIS). Following the procedure, 205 (82.3%) shoulders were assessed as stable using JSS-SIS. The mean Rowe score was 36 preoperatively versus 88 postoperatively. As a complication, 12 patients required revision surgery because of anterior instability. Authors also describe seven cases of intra-articular fractures occurred during the procedure and one case requiring subacromial arthrolysis. Although the study does not include the control group, it provides a thorough perspective into the long-term outcome of the procedure.

Graichen et al. evaluated the glenoid osteotomy in both traumatic and atraumatic patients with posterior shoulder instability. Thirty-two patients were included into the study, 17 of them were atraumatic, while 15 cases of PSI was caused by micro- or macrotrauma [22]. Clinical result was measured in the Constant-Murley and Rowe scores. The mean glenoid retroversion improved from −9.35° preoperatively to −4.62° postoperatively. It was associated with good or excellent clinical outcome in 81% of cases evaluated in Constant score while in 72% of cases in Rowe score. Authors emphasize that there is a substantial difference in the recurrence rate following osteotomy in patients with traumatic (50%) and atraumatic (15.4%) PSI origin. Moreover, authors stated that patients undergoing osteotomy had a higher rate of arthrosis (30%) and had a complication rate of 20.8%. Reduction of range of motion was experienced in two cases and both infection and nerve damage in one case.

Other study comparing results of osteotomy in patients with either traumatic or atraumatic posterior shoulder instability was performed by Hawkins. The study included 12 osteotomies. The average follow-up was 61 months. Author obtained average correction rate of 10.8° (−1° to +24°). In 2 out of 12 patients, instability persisted. Author underlined that the procedure was associated with a high rate of complications. He reported one case of acromion fracture, one intra-articular fracture, one infection, one coracoid impingement, one loss of correction due to graft prolapse, and one osteoarthritis [23].

Pogorzelski et al. performed osteotomy in atraumatic patients with increased glenoid retroversion (>20°) following unsuccessful conservative treatment. Six osteotomies performed on five patients were enclosed to the study. Postoperative retroversion of glenoid was 11.2 ± 9.4° comparing to 26.0 ± 8.6° preoperatively. The mean follow-up was 26.8 months. Four patients reported complete recovery. One patient, in whom two osteotomies were performed, showed signs of persistent instability. No revision surgeries were performed [24].

Lacheta et al. have studied the long-term results of osteotomy in 13 shoulders (12 patients) with posterior shoulder instability concomitant with glenoid retroversion higher than 10°. Outcome of the procedure was evaluated both radiographically and clinically (using Rowe score and Oxford instability score). Retroversion of glenoid improved from 23° (12°–35°) preoperatively to 13° (range 1°–28°) postoperatively. Authors stated that in only one case, treatment was unsuccessful due to persistent instability [25].

37.7 Conclusions

Posterior shoulder instability is probably a multifactorial disorder, and hence treatment may be a difficult problem. In the group of atraumatic patients that bony pathologies are excluded, at first conservative treatment for at least 6 months should be implemented. Such approach is a sufficient treatment in 80% of cases. Following unsuccessful conservative treatment, the optimal group of patients for osteotomy should be elected. Glenoid osteotomy is a potential method of treatment particularly in young patients with glenoid morphology problems. In majority of studies, mean age of patients qualified for treatment varied from 20 to 27 years.

Glenoid osteotomy is a rarely performed procedure and can potentially lead to complications; therefore, it should be performed after meticulous preoperative planning by experienced surgeons.

Although further studies are required to evaluate potential indications for this procedure, glenoid osteotomy is a therapeutic option for patients with posterior shoulder instability associated with increased glenoid retroversion or glenoid dysplasia.

References

1. Liavaag S. The epidemiology of shoulder dislocations in Oslo. Scand J Med Sci Sports. 2011;21:e334–40.
2. Robinson CM. The epidemiology, risk of recurrence, and functional outcome after an acute traumatic posterior dislocation of the shoulder. J Bone Joint Surg Am. 2011;93(17):1605–13.
3. Lanzi JT. Epidemiology of posterior glenohumeral instability in a young athletic population. Am J Sports Med. 2017;45(14):3315–21.
4. Hawkins. Posterior shoulder instability. Orthopedics. 1988;11(1):101–7.
5. Warner JJP. Complex and revision problems in shoulder surgery. Philadelphia: Lippincott Williams & Wilkins; 2005.
6. Bäcker. Biomechanics of posterior shoulder instability—current knowledge and literature review. World J Orthop. 2018;9(11):245–54.
7. Tannenbaum E. Evaluation and management of posterior shoulder instability. Sports Health. 2011;3(3):253–63.
8. Fronek. Posterior subluxation of the glenohumeral joint. J Bone Joint Surg Am. 1989;71(2):205–16.
9. Millet PJ. Recurrent posterior shoulder instability. J Am Acad Orthop Surg. 2006;14(8):464–76.
10. Hurley. Posterior shoulder instability. Surgical versus conservative results with evaluation of glenoid version. Am J Sports Med. 1992;20(4):396–400.
11. Friedman. The use of computerized tomography in the measurement of glenoid version. J Bone Joint Surg Am. 1992;74(7):1032–7.
12. Randelli M. Glenohumeral osteometry by computed tomography in normal and unstable shoulders. Clin Orthop Relat Res. 1986;208:151–6.
13. Walch G. Static posterior subluxation of the humeral head: an unrecognized entity responsible for glenohumeral osteoarthritis in the young adult. J Shoulder Elbow Surg. 2002;11(4):309–14.
14. Roleau DM. Glenoid version: how to measure it? Validity of different methods in two-dimensional computed tomography scans. J Shoulder Elbow Surg. 2010;19(8):1230–7.
15. Bercik. A modification to the Walch classification of the glenoid in primary glenohumeral osteoarthritis using three-dimensional imaging. J Shoulder Elbow Surg. 2016;25(10):1601–6.
16. Walch G. Morphologic study of the glenoid in primary glenohumeral osteoarthritis. J Arthroplasty. 1999;14(6):756–60.
17. Parada SA. Comparison of glenoid version and posterior humeral subluxation in patients with and without posterior shoulder instability. Arthroscopy. 2017;33(2):254–60.
18. Denard. Current concepts in the surgical management of primary glenohumeral arthritis with a biconcave glenoid. J Shoulder Elbow Surg. 2013;22(11):1589–98.
19. Burkhead. Treatment of instability of the shoulder with an exercise program. J Bone Joint Surg Am. 1992;74(6):890–6.
20. Inui. Glenoid osteotomy for atraumatic posteroinferior shoulder instability associated with glenoid dysplasia. Bone Joint J. 2018;100-B(3):331–7.
21. Kretzler. Recurrent posterior dislocation of the shoulder in cerebral palsy. J Bone Joint Surg Am. 1966;48:1221.
22. Graichen. Effectiveness of glenoid osteotomy in atraumatic posterior instability of the shoulder associated with excessive retroversion and flatness of the glenoid. Int Orthop. 1999;23(2):95–9.
23. Hawkins. Glenoid osteotomy for recurrent posterior subluxation of the shoulder: assessment by computed axial tomography. J Shoulder Elbow Surg. 1996;5(5):393–400.
24. Pogorzelski J. Open-wedge-Glenoidosteotomie als Therapie bei posteriorer Schulterinstabilität aufgrund vermehrter Glenoidretroversion. Oper Orthop Traumatol. 2016;28:438–48.
25. Lacheta. Posterior open wedge glenoid osteotomy provides reliable results in young patients with increased glenoid retroversion and posterior shoulder instability. Knee Surg Sports Traumatol Arthrosc. 2019;27(1):299–304.

Part III

Multidirectional Instability: Anatomy and Etiology

Anatomy in Multidirectional Instability

38

Giuseppe Milano, Alessandro Colosio, and Davide Fattoretto

38.1 Introduction

Multidirectional shoulder instability (MDI) was initially described by Neer and Foster [1] as a condition in which dislocation occurs in more than one direction, with minimal or no causative trauma. Typical patients with MDI of the shoulder are adolescents and young adults, who may sometimes voluntarily subluxate their glenohumeral joints.

The main symptoms reported are pain, instability and disability of the shoulder, and they occur with an abnormal movement of the joint in two or more directions; in some cases, the abnormal movement causing dislocation may prevail in one direction.

MDI appears to be caused by several anatomical factors acting simultaneously. Neer and Foster attributed the disease to the redundancy of the capsule [1], while other authors [2–4] hypothesized that it was due to morphological changes of the glenoid, enlargement of the capsule, incompetence of the glenohumeral ligaments or an increase in the glenohumeral volume.

Joint laxity, a fundamental characteristic of the disease, may be congenital (in which case, often bilateral), or may be due to the microtrauma of repetitive movements, for example in athletes who overload the upper limbs.

There are different classifications of instability, introduced over the years. Initially they were distinguished based on the directions of instability, that is in two or three directions [5]. In 2002, Gerber and Nyffeler [6] introduced a new classification of dynamic instability: unidirectional or multidirectional, with or without hyperlaxity. The Stanmore classification [7] is an easy and complete classification that distinguishes three different groups according to the respective cause of instability: type I concerns patients that have suffered trauma resulting in structural damage to the glenohumeral joint, leading to shoulder instability; type II concerns patients that show a constitutional deficit such as capsular insufficiency or reduced concavity of the glenoid surface, which predisposes these patients to shoulder instability without the need for significant trauma; and type III describes a type of instability that is not generated by structural defects, but rather caused by an aberrant activation pattern of the rotator cuff and periscapular muscles (Fig. 38.1).

G. Milano (✉)
Department of Medical and Surgical Specialties, Radiological Sciences, and Public Health, University of Brescia, Brescia, Italy

Department of Bone and Joint Surgery, Spedali Civili, Brescia, Italy

A. Colosio · D. Fattoretto
Department of Medical and Surgical Specialties, Radiological Sciences, and Public Health, University of Brescia, Brescia, Italy

R. Brzóska et al. (eds.), *360° Around Shoulder Instability*,
https://doi.org/10.1007/978-3-662-61074-9_38

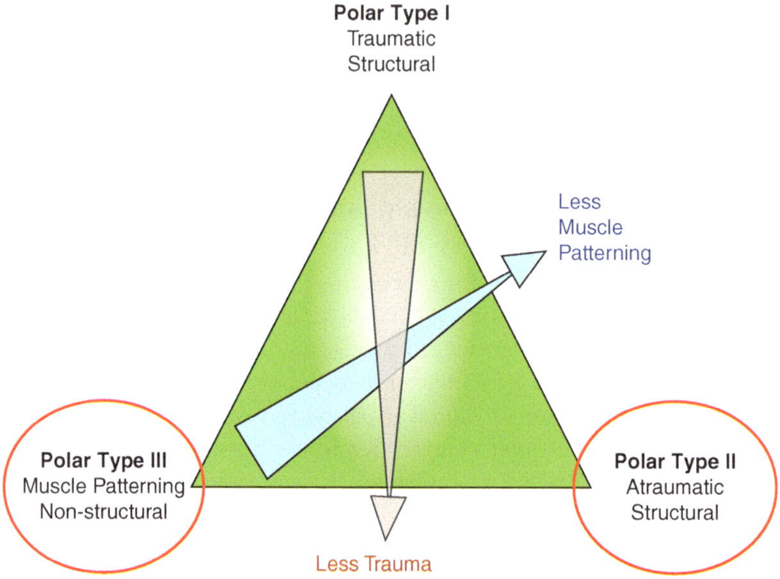

Fig. 38.1 The Stanmore classification is an easy and complete classification that distinguishes three different groups according to the respective cause of instability [7]

38.2 Clinical Evaluation

The clinical diagnosis of atraumatic MDI is based on a combination of typical clinical history and objective shoulder instability in two or more directions. A typical presentation is a general shoulder pain associated with involuntary and recurrent sensations of instability, subluxation or dislocation, during daily life movements or during sleep, without initial traumatic dislocation [8]. In subjects who practice an upper-limb sports, such as gymnastics, volleyball and swimming, it may present as a lower resistance or difficulty in athletic performance, in association with pain.

Bilateral onset of symptoms is considered typical, but not mandatory for the diagnosis of MDI. There are several clinical methods for measuring the translation of the humeral head beyond the edge of the glenoid in two or more directions. Tests indicate inferior, anterior and posterior laxity and not necessarily instability. When performing these tests, special attention should be paid to pain and apprehension. Generalized ligament laxity should also be assessed. Already through these tests, it is possible to make an initial distinction between the types of instability, especially in view of their direction. An inferior laxity is present if positive sulcus sign or Gagey test have been found (Fig. 38.2). Signs for anterior instability are defined as positive findings in the apprehension test, the relocation test or an increased anterior translation. Posterior instability is considered in case of positive findings in either the jerk test or the posterior apprehension test as well as with an increased posterior translation of the glenohumeral joint [9, 10].

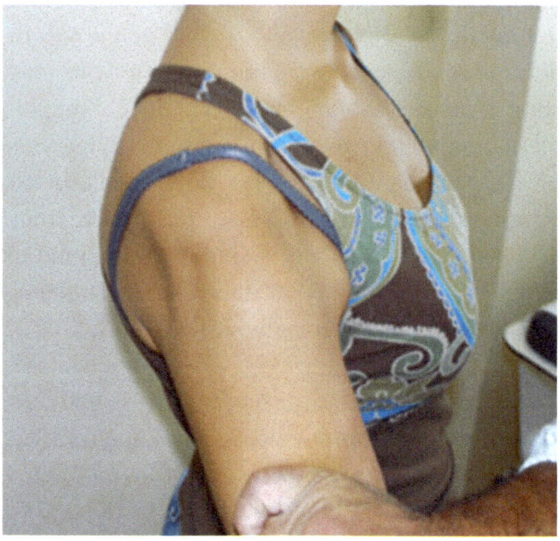

Fig. 38.2 An inferior laxity is present if sulcus sign is positive

38.3 Imaging

Imaging is a crucial step in the diagnosis of MDI. Radiographs and computed tomography (CT) scans are useful in case of bone abnormalities, while magnetic resonance (MR) analyzes the anatomy of soft tissues, which is fundamental in the study of MDI.

MR-arthrography (MRA) can detect the labrum, rotator interval and glenohumeral ligaments, through to the distension of the capsule. Diagnostic features and measurements can be acquired on standard MRA or using abduction and external rotation (ABER) position to better evaluate capsular redundancy [10].

Labral tears, due to micro-traumas or less commonly to macro-traumas, can be visualized, albeit the most common finding in MDI is a pathological capsule with an increase in glenohumeral joint volume and the size of the rotator interval. In ABER images, some typical signs have a good accuracy in the diagnosis of MDI. Examples are the "crescent sign", that is the combination of an improvement layer between the humeral head and the anterior–inferior glenohumeral ligament (AIGHL), and the "triangle sign", that is a triangular space between the humeral head, AIGHL and the glenoid, suggestive of a decentring humeral head [10].

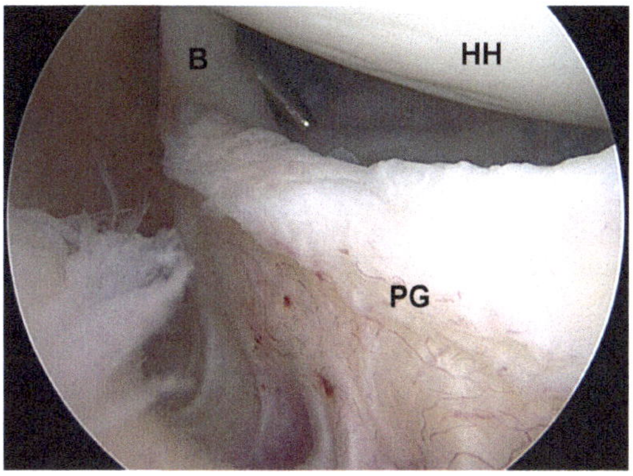

Fig. 38.3 Capsule redundancy is a key factor predisposing to multidirectional instability (MDI) (*PG* posterior glenoid, *B* biceps, *HH* humeral head)

38.4 Pathoanatomy

Among the causes of MDI, in addition to the presence of congenital generalized ligamentous laxity and the presence of repeated macro- and micro-traumas, there is a predisposition dictated by the specific anatomy of the shoulder. When instability occurs, especially in MDI, it means that one or more of the mechanisms for containing the shoulder is failing.

38.4.1 Capsular Laxity

Capsule redundancy is a key factor predisposing to MDI (Fig. 38.3). Dewing et al. [11] have demonstrated the presence of elongation of capsular cross-sectional areas in MDI patients compared to healthy subjects. Although some studies have highlighted the role of repetitive episodes of instability in the development of capsular laxity [12], authors such as Uhthoff and Piscopo [13] found the presence of a redundant capsule in 23% of foetal and embryonic shoulders, concluding that an enveloped and redundant anterior capsule may be a variant of development, as well as the consequence of trauma.

Several studies have demonstrated that the open anterior–inferior capsular shift effectively decreases capsular volume and laxity, preserving normal glenohumeral joint biomechanics [14–17], while cadaveric models have been used to demonstrate effective reduction in anterior, posterior and inferior glenohumeral translation after both anterior–inferior capsular shift and anterior capsulolabroplasty (with a decrease in capsular volume from 19% to 60%) [19].

38.4.2 Glenohumeral Ligaments and Rotator Interval

Another possible factor in MDI is the incompetence of the glenohumeral ligaments, which act as static stabilisers of the joint. The major static constraints against anterior instability are provided by the anteroinferior aspect of the capsule and the anterior band of the inferior glenohumeral ligament (i.e. AIGHL) [18], whereas major static constraint against posterior instability is provided by the posterior aspect of the capsule and the posterior band of the inferior glenohumeral ligament (PIGHL) [19]. The posterior glenoid, articular cartilage and periosteum are also important static stabilizers preventing posterior shoulder instability [20, 21].

The rotator interval (RI) is also being considered increasingly important in shoulder stability. The RI can be defined as a triangular space within the shoulder capsule, located between the supraspinatus and subscapularis tendons, the coracohumoral ligament and the superior glenohumeral ligament. It is thought to contribute to the humeral head stability, mainly during abduction, as well as to stability of the long head of the biceps tendon [22, 23]. Some reports found that sectioning of the RI results in marked posterior and inferior translation of the humeral head [24].

Rotator interval laxity, clinically demonstrated as a persistent positive inferior sulcus sign with the arm in external rotation, is associated with anterior–superior shoulder instability and found more often in patients who suffer shoulder dislocation and in those with systemic joint hyperlaxity [6, 22].

Lee et al. [21] hypothesized that the increased size of the RI and capsular dimension measured on MRA would be helpful for strengthening the clinical diagnosis of the MDI when MRA does not show any labral, rotator cuff or osseous structural abnormalities. They discovered that width and depth of the RI were statistically significantly larger in the MDI group compared to a control group. Similarly, the capsular dimensions at the inferior and posteroinferior regions were statistically significantly larger in the MDI group than in a control group [21].

Rotator interval closure, using open or arthroscopic techniques, was suggested to improve humeral head stability [25–27]. Chechik et al. [27] performed a retrospective study to compare the results of arthroscopic anterior shoulder instability repair (arthroscopic Bankart repair, ABR) with and without closure of the RI (arthroscopic rotator interval closure, ARIC). They observed that the patients in the ABR + ARIC group had a significantly higher prevalence of multidirectional shoulder laxity than those in the ABR group and a small or no Hill–Sachs lesion. However, the prevalence of systemic joint hyperlaxity did not differ significantly between the groups.

38.4.3 Glenoid Labrum

Although capsuligamentous structures play an important role in ensuring shoulder stability in healthy subjects compared to the glenoid labrum, when these structures are of poor quality and their biomechanical functioning is not optimal, like in hyperlax shoulders, the contribution of the glenoid labrum to shoulder stability seems to become crucial. An interesting concept in the evaluation of the glenoid labrum in MDI has been related to the loss of containment in the chondrolabral portion due to loss of posterior labral height and to posterior chondrolabral clefts as anatomical variations [28, 29]. Chondrolabral clefts are defined as a medium curved or triangular fissure with a high signal intensity between the glenoid labrum and the articular cartilage [29]. The labrum should have smooth and regular margins for the lesion to be diagnosed as a chondrolabral clefts. A large study by Campbell et al. [30] evaluated the presence of posterior chondrolabral fissures in more than 1000 shoulders through an MRI study. The results showed that posterior chondrolabral cleft is not a rare condition (9% of the sample) and that often, when present, it is a bilateral condition. More importantly, however, these lesions seem to be associated with a specific morphology of the glenoid, in particular a rounded and truncated posterior glenoid edge with respect to the healthy shoulders (21.9% vs. 1.5%) (Fig. 38.4). Furthermore, it was noted that the presence of chondrolabral clefts was more frequently associated with previous stories of shoulder instability than those who did not have them (14% vs. 8%) and the hazard ratio for the development of instability in the shoulders with a posterior chondrolabral crack was 3.5. Authors hypothesized that the morphological variations of the glenoid observed may

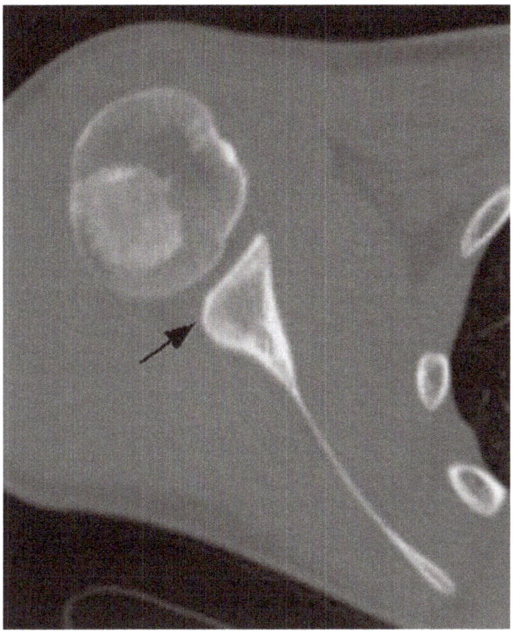

Fig. 38.4 Computed tomography scan (CT scan) of a right shoulder with multidirectional instability (MDI). A truncated posterior glenoid edge is evident (arrow)

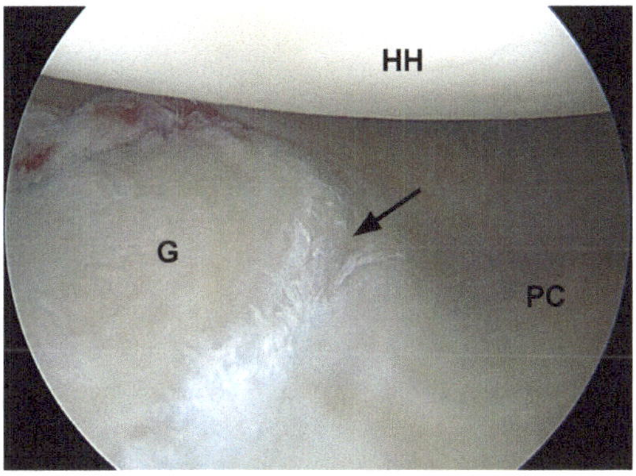

Fig. 38.5 Chondrolabral clefts (arrow) in a shoulder with multidirectional instability (MDI). This type of defect may decrease the degree of negative intra-articular pressure, resulting in a greater propensity to atraumatic joint instability (*HH* humeral head, *G* glenoid, *PC* posterior capsule)

decrease the concavity compression effect at the extremes of shoulder movement and that the presence of a chondrolabral clefts may decrease the degree of negative intra-articular pressure, resulting in a greater propensity to atraumatic joint instability (Fig. 38.5).

38.4.4 Glenoid Version

The relationship between glenoid version and glenohumeral instability has been explored in the past decades, with the early literature showing conflicting results, above all about the connection between glenoid version and anterior instability [31]. In contrast, growing evidence has suggested a relationship between glenoid version and posterior instability [32, 33].

On CT images, version can be measured using the glenoid vault method as discussed by Poon and Ting [34]. First, an isosceles triangle is drawn within the glenoid cavity. Then, a line bisecting the triangle is drawn and a line perpendicular to this bisector is drawn. Finally, a line paralleling the glenoid endosteal face is drawn, which is then compared with the perpendicular line of the bisector to give the glenoid version.

Using the Poon and Ting's method, Kikuchi et al. [35] found that posterior instability increased with a posterior tilt of more than 15° and anterior instability increased with an anterior tilt of more than 5°. However, Bokor et al. [36] found that the measured retroversion can vary by more than 10° with minor rotation of the scapula. Furthermore, retroversion depends to a great extent on the position of the transverse image section relative to the glenoid and three-dimensional analyses of the glenoid shape supported a spiral twist in the joint surface of the glenoid cavity with progressive decrease of glenoid retroversion from the upper to the lower part of the cavity [37].

In the study of Von Eisenhart Rothe et al. [37], in the healthy individuals, the mean retroversion average was 3.9° ± 1.3° (range, 0.82–5.6°) with no significant gender-related difference. In patients with atraumatic instability, a significantly ($P < 0.05$) increased retroversion (9.4° ± 4.8°) was observed with a range of 2.6–16.6°.

38.4.5 Glenoid Concavity

The shape of the glenoid is closely related to shoulder stability and its abnormality is believed to affect the position of the humeral head in the shoulders with atraumatic instability. However, it is not yet entirely clear how the shape of the glenoid in shoulders with atraumatic instability differs from that of normal shoulders.

One of the main mechanisms of shoulder stabilization is the compression of the rotator cuff, which pushes the humeral head into the concavity of the glenoid, stabilizing it against the translational forces of decentralization, especially in the medium range of motion [38, 39].

Several authors [40] described a correlation between the depth of the glenoid and the stability ratio (i.e. the ratio between the maximum translational force against which a shoulder can be stabilized by a given concavity compression force [38]) of a shoulder and how the lack of glenoid concavity is associated with MDI [41].

The effectiveness of the concavity–compression stabilization mechanism is determined by the concavity of the glenoid and the direction in which this concavity is pointed. It seems that the shoulders with posterior atraumatic instability showed loss of inclination angle and loss of concavity at the lower glenoid, compared to healthy shoulders [42].

To prove this, Howell et al. [43] found that the stabilization degree of compression varied along the circumference of the glenoid. This can be attributed to the greater effective depth of the concavity of the glenoid in the superior–inferior plane (4.8 mm) than in the anterior–posterior plane (2.2 mm) [40]. The result was that the stability ratio was higher in the superior–inferior direction (64%) than in the anterior–posterior direction (33–35%) [43].

These results become relevant for MDI, where the joint is typically unstable in the mid-range of motion. The flatness of the articular surface of the glenoid, therefore, can be defined as a factor predisposing to this type of instability, allowing a relatively easy translation in different directions due to the lack of effective depth of the glenoid (Fig. 38.6).

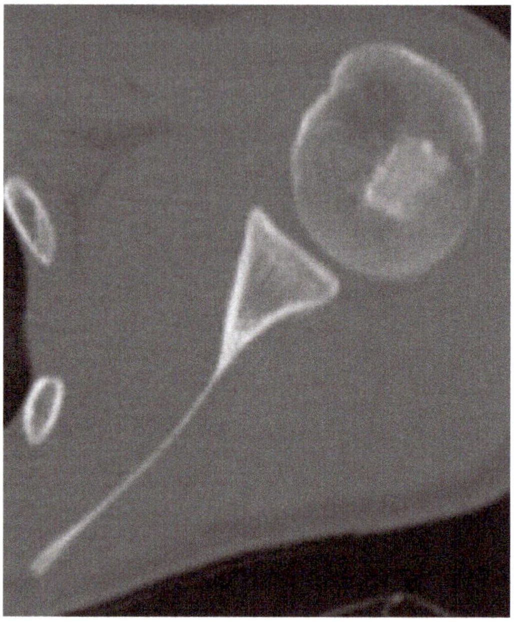

Fig. 38.6 Computed tomography (CT) scan of a left shoulder with multidirectional instability (MDI). Flatness of the articular surface is a factor predisposing to this type of instability, allowing a relatively easy translation in different directions due to the lack of effective depth of the glenoid

38.4.6 Glenoid Hypoplasia

Glenoid hypoplasia, also known as glenoid dysplasia or dysplasia of the scapular neck, is a failure of ossification of the posteroinferior two-thirds of the glenoid.

Once thought to be a rare condition, more recent studies have shown that the incidence of glenoid hypoplasia ranges from 18% to 35%, depending on the chosen diagnostic criteria [44, 45].

Although the natural course of glenoid hypoplasia is not well documented, chronic glenohumeral joint instability predisposes patients to develop accelerated degenerative joint disease and glenoid retroversion, increasing patient susceptibility to posterior labral tears, subluxation or dislocation [44–46].

During physical examination, patients with symptomatic posterior glenoid dysplasia usually present with signs of posterior shoulder instability. Variable presentation with a painful, diminished range of motion, resulting in a suggestion of weakness, can occur. As such, clinical examination for posterior shoulder instability does not allow for clear and simple distinction among traumatic causes, collagen disorder-related laxity and causes associated with glenoid dysplasia.

Axial and 3D CT shoulder imaging of the hypoplastic glenoid shows rounding of the posteroinferior glenoid rim, glenoid retroversion and widening of the inferior glenohumeral joint space due to the failure of ossification of the glenoid. A smooth concentric articular cartilaginous surface of the glenoid and a hypertrophied articular cartilage inferiorly may be better appreciated when intraarticular contrast is injected with CT-arthrography (CTA). An arthrogram provides information about the soft tissues of the shoulder including labral pathology and capsular abnormalities such as increased capsular area and capsular tears or avulsions.

Weishaupt et al. [47] characterized glenoid abnormalities in a series of patients with atraumatic, recurrent posterior instability and found both increased retroversion and posteroinferior osseous deficiency.

38.4.7 Scapular Dysfunction

Just as important as the soft tissue and bone anatomy is the scapular movement. For example, it is not uncommon to see individuals with MDI who have decreased upward rotation of the scapula during arm abduction [48]. Less upward rotation of the scapula results in less inclination of the glenoid in the scapula plane and therefore less stability in the lower direction [49].

The resting scapular position has an internal rotation that is around 35° and a much more variable front inclination. Reduced scapular inclination worsens inferior shoulder instability; in contrast, increased inclination prevents inferior displacement of the humeral head by tightening the superior capsule, thus increasing the slope of the glenoid fossa, and act as a bony cam, tightening the overlying structures and stabilizing the humeral head in the glenoid fossa.

In normal arm elevation, the scapula rotates upward and externally and tilts posteriorly during shoulder elevation [7]. Evidence exists that scapular and glenohumeral kinematics are altered in unstable shoulders. Using radiographic methods, Ozaki [48] reported decreased scapular abduction and excessive glenohumeral translation with shoulder elevation in subjects with MDI when compared with a control group.

Ruediger et al. [50] evaluated shoulders with unidirectional instability and MDI using MRI in static position with and without isometric muscle contraction. They found excessive translations in the MDI group compared with asymptomatic shoulders and a decentralization of the humeral head with isometric contraction compared with the asymptomatic and anterior instability groups.

Subsequently, Ogston et al. [50] confirmed that patients with MDI have a disruption in normal scapular kinematics when compared with a matched control group.

The lack of upward rotation and increased internal rotation in MDI suggests difficulty with scapular control, which can lead to injury of the subacromial structures and alteration of the functioning of shoulder musculature due to altered scapular kinematics. In fact, this kind of patients tend to place the shoulder in internal rotation, with a typical winging of the inferior medial tip of the scapula (type I dyskinesis) or of the entire medial border (type II dyskinesis) (Fig. 38.7).

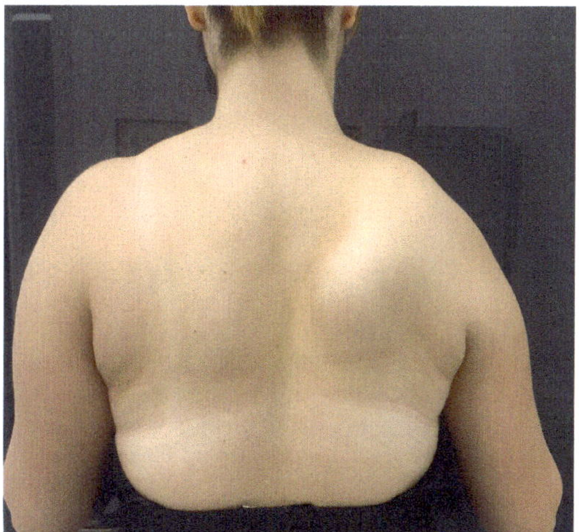

Fig. 38.7 Scapular dyskinesis in the right shoulder of a patient affected by multidirectional instability (MDI)

The reasons for abnormal scapular motion are the hyperactivity of the internal rotators of the shoulder, anterior deltoid, pectoralis major and latissimus dorsi, and a strongly reduced activity of the posterior deltoid and external rotators [7]. These findings provide objective evidence of abnormal scapular mechanics and supports the inclusion of scapular stability exercises in rehabilitative programs. In addition, rotator cuff strengthening and stabilization methods should be employed because these patients demonstrated rotator cuff weakness and activation of these muscles may improve the stability of the glenohumeral joint by recentring the humeral head [50, 51].

References

1. Neer CS II, Foster CR. Inferior capsular shift for involuntary inferior and multidirectional instability of the shoulder. A preliminary report. J Bone Joint Surg Am. 1980;62:897–908.
2. Ikeda H, Tsukanishi S, Nobuhara K. Shoulder in-stability: its relationship to glenoid dysplasia. Seikesaigaigeka. 1984;27:1757–65.
3. Jerosch J, Castro WH. Shoulder instability in Ehlers-Danlos syndrome. An indication for surgical treatment? Acta Orthop Belg. 1990;56:451–3.
4. Schenk TJ, Brems JJ. Multidirectional instability of the shoulder: pathophysiology, diagnosis, and management. J Am Acad Orthop Surg. 1998;6:65–72.
5. Neer CS II. Involuntary inferior and multidirectional instability of the shoulder: etiology, recognition, and treatment. Instr Course Lect. 1985;34:232–8.
6. Gerber C, Nyffeler RW. Classification of glenohumeral joint instability. Clin Orthop Relat Res. 2002;400:65–76.
7. Lewis A, Kitamura T, Bayley JIL. The classification of shoulder instability: new light through old windows! Curr Orthop. 2004;18:97–108.
8. Johnson SM, Robinson CM. Shoulder instability in patients with joint hyperlaxity. J Bone Joint Surg Am. 2010;92:1545–57.
9. Bahk M, Keyurapan E, Tasaki A, Sauers EL, McFarland EG. Laxity testing of the shoulder: a review. Am J Sports Med. 2007;35(1):131–44.
10. Schaeffeler C, Waldt S, Bauer JS, Kirchhoff C, Haller B, Schröder M, Rummeny EJ, Imhoff AB, Woertler K. MR arthrography including abduction and external rotation images in the assessment of atraumatic multidirectional instability of the shoulder. Eur Radiol. 2014;24:1376–85.
11. Dewing CB, McCormick F, Bell SJ, Solomon DJ, Stanley M, Rooney TB, Provencher MT. An analysis of capsular area in patients with anterior, posterior, and multidirectional shoulder instability. Am J Sports Med. 2008;36:515–22.
12. Ahmad CS, Freehill MQ, Blaine TA, Levine WN, Bigliani LU. Anteromedial capsular redundancy and labral deficiency in shoulder instability. Am J Sports Med. 2003;31:247–52.
13. Uhthoff HK, Piscopo M. Anterior capsular redundancy of the shoulder: congenital or traumatic? An embryological study. J Bone Joint Surg Br. 1985;67:363–6.
14. Ahmad CS, Wang VM, Sugalski MT, Levine WN, Bigliani LU. Biomechanics of shoulder capsulorrhaphy procedures. J Shoulder Elbow Surg. 2005;14(1 Suppl S):12S–8S.
15. Sugalski MT, Wiater JM, Levine WN, Bigliani LU. An anatomic study of the humeral insertion of the inferior glenohumeral capsule. J Shoulder Elb Surg. 2005;14(1):91–5.
16. Wang VM, Sugalski MT, Levine WN, Pawluk RJ, Mow VC, Bigliani LU. Comparison of glenohumeral mechanics following a capsular shift and anterior tightening. J Bone Joint Surg Am. 2005;87(6):1312–22.
17. Warner JJP, Johnson D, Miller M, Caborn DNM. Technique for selecting capsular tightness in repair of anterior-inferior shoulder instability. J Shoulder Elb Surg. 1995;4(5):352–64.
18. Ovesen J, Nielsen S. Stability of the shoulder joint. Cadaver study of stabilizing structures. Acta Orthop Scand. 1985;56:149–51.
19. Ovesen J, Nielsen S. Posterior instability of the shoulder. A cadaver study. Acta Orthop Scand. 1986;57:436–9.
20. Kim SH, Noh KC, Park JS, Ryu BD, Oh I. Loss of chondrolabral containment of the glenohumeral joint in atraumatic posteroinferior multidirectional instability. J Bone Joint Surg Am. 2005;87:92–8.
21. Lee HJ, Kim NR, Moon SG, Ko SM, Park JY. Multidirectional instability of the shoulder: rotator interval dimension and capsular laxity evaluation using MR arthrography. Skelet Radiol. 2013;42(2):231–8. https://doi.org/10.1007/s00256-012-1441-2.
22. Hunt SA, Kwon YW, Zuckerman JD. The rotator interval: anatomy, pathology, and strategies for treatment. J Am Acad Orthop Surg. 2007;15:218–27.
23. Stokes DA, Savoie FH, Field LD, Ramsey JR. Arthroscopic repair of anterior glenohumeral instability and rotator interval lesions. Orthop Clin N Am. 2003;34:529–38. https://doi.org/10.1016/S0030-5898(03)00091-9.
24. Hewitt M, Getelman MH, Snyder SJ. Arthroscopic management of multidirectional instability: pancapsular plication. Orthop Clin North Am. 2003;34:549–57. https://doi.org/10.1016/S0030-5898(03)00094-4.
25. Perthes G. Operationen bei habituelller Schulterluxation. Deutsch Ztschr Chir. 1906;85:199–207.
26. Mologne TS, Zhao K, Hongo M, Romeo AA, An KN, Provencher MT. The addition of rotator interval closure after arthroscopic repair of either ante-

rior or posterior shoulder instability: effect on glenohumeral translation and range of motion. Am J Sports Med. 2008;36:1123–31. https://doi.org/10.1177/0363546508314391.
27. Chechik O, Maman E, Dolkart O, Khashan M, Shabtai L, Mozes G. Arthroscopic rotator interval closure in shoulder instability repair: a retrospective study. J Shoulder Elb Surg. 2010;19(7):1056–62.
28. Cooper DE, Arnoczky SP, O'Brien SJ, Warren RF, DiCarlo E, Allen AA. Anatomy, histology, and vascularity of the glenoid labrum. J Bone Joint Surg Am. 1992;74A(1):46–52.
29. Tuite MJ, Currie JW, Orwin JF, Baer GS, Munoz del Rio A. Sublabral clefts and recesses in the anterior, inferior, and posterior glenoid labrum at MR arthrography. Skeletal Radiol. 2013;42(3):353–62.
30. Campbell SE, Dewitt RM, Cameron KL, Thompson AK, Owens BD. Posterior chondrolabral cleft: clinical significance and associations with shoulder instability. HSS J. 2014;10(3):208–12.
31. Privitera DM, Siegel EJ, Miller LR, Sinz NJ, Higgins LD. Glenoid version and its relationship to glenohumeral instability and labral tears. J Shoulder Elb Surg. 2016;25(7):1056–63.
32. Brewer BJ, Wubben RC, Carrera GF. Excessive retroversion of the glenoid cavity. A cause of non-traumatic posterior instability of the shoulder. J Bone Joint Surg Am. 1986;68:724–31.
33. Owens BD, Campbell SE, Cameron KL. Risk factors for posterior shoulder instability in young athletes. Am J Sports Med. 2013;41:2645–9.
34. Poon PC, Ting FS. A 2-dimensional glenoid vault method for measuring glenoid version on computed tomography. J Shoulder Elb Surg. 2012;21:329–35.
35. Kikuchi K, Itoi E, Yamamoto N, Seki N, Abe H, Minagawa H, Shimada Y. Scapular inclination and glenohumeral joint stability: a cadaveric study. J Orthop Sci. 2008;13(1):72–7.
36. Bokor DJ, O'Sullivan MD, Hazan GJ. Variability of measurement of glenoid version on computed tomography scan. J Shoulder Elb Surg. 1999;6:595–8.
37. Von Eisenhart Rothe R, Mayr HO, Hinterwimmer S, Graichen H. Simultaneous 3D assessment of glenohumeral shape, humeral head centering, and scapular positioning in atraumatic shoulder instability: a magnetic resonance-based in vivo analysis. Am J Sports Med. 2010;38(2):375–82.
38. Lazarus MD, Sidles JA, Harryman DT II, Matsen FA III. Effect of a chondral-labral defect on glenoid concavity and glenohumeral stability. J Bone Joint Surg. 1996;78A:94–102.
39. Matsen FA III, Thomas SC, Rockwood CA Jr, Wirth MA. Glenohumeral Instability. In: Rockwood Jr CA, Matsen III FA, editors. The shoulder. 2nd ed. Philadelphia: WB Saunders; 1998. p. 611–754.
40. Lippitt SB, Vanderhooft JE, Harris SL, Sidles JA, Harryman DT II, Matsen FA III. Glenohumeral stability from concavity-compression: a quantitative analysis. J Shoulder Elbow Surg. 1993;2(1):27–35.
41. Moroder P, Ernstbrunner L. Anterior shoulder instability is associated with an underlying deficiency of the bony glenoid concavity. Arthroscopy. 2015;31(7):1223–31.
42. Inui H, Sugamoto K, Miyamoto T, Yoshikawa H, Machida A, Hashimoto J, Nobuhara K. Glenoid shape in atraumatic posterior instability of the shoulder. Clin Orthop Relat Res. 2002;403:87–92.
43. Howell SM, Gallnat BJ. The glenold·labral socket a can strained articular surface. Clin Orthop. 1989;243:122–5.
44. Harper KW, Helms CA, Haystead CM, Higgins LD. Glenoid dysplasia: incidence and association with posterior labral tears as evaluated on MRI. Am J Roentgenol. 2005;184(3):984e8.
45. Baca MJ, King RW, Bancroft LW. Glenoid hypoplasia. Radiol Case Rep. 2016;11(4):386–90.
46. Jean K. Classifications of glenoid dysplasia, glenoid bone loss and glenoid loosening: a review of the literature. Eur J Orthop Surg Traumatol. 2013;23(3):301–10.
47. Weishaupt D, Zanetti M, Nyffeler RW, Gerber C, Hodler J. Posterior glenoid rim deficiency in recurrent (atraumatic) posterior shoulder instability. Skelet Radiol. 2000;29(4):204–10.
48. Ozaki J. Glenohumeral movements of the involuntary inferior and multidirectional instability. Clin Orthop Relat Res. 1989;(238):107–11.
49. Itoi E, Motzkin NE, Money BF, et al. Scapular inclination and inferior stability of the shoulder. J Shoulder Elb Surg. 1992;1:131–9.
50. Ogston JB, Ludewig PM. Differences in 3-dimensional shoulder kinematics between persons with multidirectional instability and asymptomatic controls. Am J Sports Med. 2007;35(8):1361–70.
51. Hsu H, Luo Z, Stone J, An K. Influence of rotator cuff tear on glenohumeral stability: the effect of size and location of the tear from a "created-defect" model. J Shoulder Elb Surg. 1997;6:413–22.

Hyperlaxity and Multidirectional Shoulder Instability

39

Wojciech Solecki, Adrian Błasiak, Hubert Laprus, and Roman Brzóska

39.1 Hyperlaxity

Generalized joint hypermobility is a physiological condition characterized with increased range of motion of various joints of an individual. This hyperlaxity can be congenital caused by disorders of connective tissue like Marfan syndrome, Ehlers-Danlos syndrome, or osteogenesis imperfecta. Another form of congenital disorder in which hyperlaxity is the only clinical sign is known as benign joint hypermobility syndrome (BJHS) [1].

Acquired joint hypermobility is often developed in athletes due to repetitive microtrauma and stretching of normal joint capsuloligamentous restraints. Acquired hypermobility is most commonly observed in gymnasts, swimmers, or throwing sportsmen [2, 3].

The prevalence of joint hyperlaxity not associated with a systemic disease ranges from 4 to 13% in general population and can reach up to 40% among school children and adolescents. Mean joint mobility is higher in females than in males and it decreases with age [4–7].

The diagnosis of joint hyperlaxity is based on several proposed criteria, yet still remains vague.

Table 39.1 Beighton score

1. Ability to touch palms flat to floor with knees straight	(one point)
2. Elbow extension >10°	(one point for each side)
3. Knee extension >10°	(one point for each side)
4. Ability to touch thumb to forearm	(one point for each side)
5. Fifth finger metocarpalphalageal joint extension >90°	(one point for each side)
Scores of 4 or above indicate **Generalised Joint Hypermobility**	

The most common is the Beighton score modified by Junge et al. [8, 9] (Table 39.1).

Less common, but extended in comparison to the mentioned above, is the Hospital del Mar score [10].

Beighton score is also considered as one of the major criteria in Brighton criteria designed to make diagnosis of the benign joint hypermobility syndrome [11].

Cameron et al. proved a correlation of Beighton score higher than 2 with a 2.5 higher risk of developing shoulder instability [12]. Chahal et al. showed that external rotation of the shoulder above 85° is a predisposing factor for traumatic shoulder dislocation [13].

A high prevalence of hyperlaxity has been reported in recurrent instability after both open and arthroscopic stabilization procedures [3, 14, 15].

W. Solecki (✉) · A. Błasiak · H. Laprus · R. Brzóska
Shoulder and Upper Limb Department,
St. Luke's Hospital, Bielsko-Biala, Poland
e-mail: wsolecki@lukasza.pl

R. Brzóska et al. (eds.), *360° Around Shoulder Instability*,
https://doi.org/10.1007/978-3-662-61074-9_39

39.2 Multidirectional Shoulder Instability

Unlike hyperlaxity, instability refers to a pathological symptomatic luxation or subluxation of the joints. Multidirectional instability of the shoulder (MDI) is defined as symptomatic instability in two or more directions. Two main types of MDI are recognized: with hyperlaxity (congenital or acquired) and without hyperlaxity. MDI with hyperlaxity is classified by Gerber and Nyffeler as type B6 [16] (Table 39.2). It usually has an insidious onset without trauma. MDI without hyperlaxity is usually associated with a traumatic onset and concomitant capsulolabral lesions. It is classified as a B5 group in Gerber and Nyffeler's classification of dynamic shoulder instability and is less common [16].

Table 39.2 Gerber and Nyffeler Classification of glenohumeral joint instability

Classification	Description
B1: Chronic Locked Dislocation	Locked instability caused by major trauma
B2: Unidirectional Instability without hyperlaxity	Symptoms elicited in a single direction Traumatic capsulolabral lesions frequently present
B3: Unidirectional Instability with hyperlaxity	Symptoms elicited in a single direction Patulous capsular tissue frequently present Presence of capsulolabral lesion less likely
B4: Multidirectional Instability without hyperlaxity	Symptoms elicited in two or more directions Anterior and posterior capsulolabral lesions frequently present
B5: Multidirectional Instability with hyperlaxity	Symptoms elicited in rem or more directions Patulous capsular tissue frequently present Signs of generalized hyperlaxity frequently present Frequent recurrent subluxation
B6: Uni or Multidirectional Instability with voluntary reduction	At first dislocation is not noticed and voluntary reduction is symptomatic. With time they learn to put the shoulder in dislocation position and reduce it

MDI can also be classified according to the dominant direction of instability into anteroinferior with a posterior subluxation, posteroinferior with an anterior subluxation, or global instability [17].

39.3 Biomechanics

Stability of the shoulder is provided by static and dynamic stabilizers. The static restraints include joint capsule, glenohumeral ligaments, labrum, and glenoid cavity. The dynamic stabilizers consist of rotator cuff and shoulder girdle muscles. Due to abnormalities in elastic fibers observed in patients with hyperlaxity and MDI, inferior capsular structures are patulous and redundant resulting in increased glenohumeral volume [18, 19]. Furthermore, subjects with MDI exhibit altered movement pattern, neuromotor control, and stabilizing muscles activation of the shoulder girdle complex comparing to healthy population [20–22]. MDI with hyperlaxity should also be distinguished from functional shoulder instability—a term proposed by Moroder [23] for atraumatic instability without structural abnormalities, caused only by abnormal muscle activation patterns.

39.4 Treatment

The goal of treatment in MDI is to remove pain and restore balance between maintaining acceptable range of motion while preventing the recurrence of instability.

In case of MDI, it is important to define dominant direction of instability by thorough clinical examination. MRI, MR arthrography, or CT scan can be helpful in finding concomitant soft tissue and bony lesions. If no lesions are present, a physiotherapy program is the first line of treatment and should be continued for at least 6–12 months. The rehabilitation should be performed in a specialized center under the guidance of the same team, and sport level or discipline should be modified. If the conservative treatment is successful, stabilizing exercises should be continued further on in order to maintain the stability.

Surgical treatment is applied when pain [24] and structural lesions of glenohumeral joint are present or when conservative treatment fails. The lesions in MDI include lesions of capsulo-ligamento-labral complex, humeral avulsion of glenohumeral ligament, or bony lesions of glenoid and humeral head.

It is important that surgical treatment is also followed by physiotherapy to achieve or maintain proper kinematics of shoulder girdle muscles [25].

Open surgical techniques include inferior capsular shift or anterior-inferior capsular shift [26, 27] With the development of the arthroscopy, more techniques were developed such as capsule plication, capsular shift, labral augmentation, reconstruction of capsuloligamentous complex, rotator interval closure, and thermal capsulorrhaphy.

According to Longo [28], surgical treatment of MDI is associated with 10% of recurrence rate, comparing with 21% after conservative treatment. Both open and arthroscopic techniques provide comparable rate of success in terms of recurrence, but arthroscopy provides less postoperative restriction of range of motion [24].

Arthroscopic techniques based on thermal shrinkage of the capsule are proven to be unreliable with recurrence rate between 24.5 and 59%, which provides more outcome than conservative treatment [24, 28–30].

There is also no clear evidence for isolated rotator interval closure effectiveness [31, 32].

Among arthroscopic procedures, capsule plication seems to be the most efficient to address patulous and redundant inferior capsule. Ponce proved that each 1 cm plication of the capsule decreases volume of the glenohumeral joint by around 10%. This means that use of five sutures decreases the volume by 50% which is an equivalent to the open capsular shift [33].

Using suture anchors in the glenoid is more reliable than simple sutures placed in the capsule or the labrum. Anchors should be introduced starting from the inferior part of the capsule as they are the most challenging and accessible only before capsule plication.

39.5 Conclusion

It is crucial that the first-line treatment of MDI with hyperlaxity without any structural lesions should be a proper rehabilitation program in a specialized center for at least 12 months, optimally with the same team of physiotherapists. Surgical treatment should be advocated only after physiotherapy fails and symptoms like pain or instability persist.

Precautions should be taken when performing capsule plication in patients with hyperlaxity. Patients with a very gentle, parchment capsule are prone to develop capsule lesions. Excessively shrunken capsule leads to an overconstrained humeral head at one of the glenoid borders, limitation of range of motion, crepitation and pain. Excessive plication can also result in HAGL or HAGL-like lesions or can lead to the development instability in the opposite direction.

In patients with hyperlaxity and glenoid hypoplasia, it is extremely difficult to obtain stability with surgical means. In these cases, arthroscopy should be only considered when the pain persists despite the conservative treatment.

References

1. Kirk JA, Ansell BM, Bywaters EL. The hypermobility syndrome. Ann Rheum Dis. 1967;26:419.
2. Perry J. Anatomy and biomechanics of the shoulder in throwing, swimming, gymnastics, and tennis. Clin Sports Med. 1983;2:247–70.
3. Saccomanno MF, Fodale M, Capasso L, Cazzato G, Milano G. Generalized joint laxity and multidirectional instability of the shoulder. Joints. 2014;1(4):171–9.
4. Everman DB, Robin NH. Hypermobility syndrome. Pediatr Rev. 1998;19:111–7.
5. Hakim AJ, Grahame R. Joint hypermobility. Best Pract Res Clin Rheumatol. 2003;17:989–1004.
6. Larsson LG, Baum J, Mudholkar GS, Srivastava DK. Hypermobility: PREVALENCE and features in a Swedish population. Br J Rheumatol. 1993;32:116–9.
7. Remvig L, Jensen DV, Ward RC. Epidemiology of general joint hypermobility and basis for the proposed criteria for benign joint hypermobility syndrome: review of the literature. J Rheumatol. 2007;34:804–9.
8. Beighton P, Solomon L, Soskolne CL. Articular mobility in an African population. Ann Rheum Dis. 1973;32:413–8.

9. Junge T, Jespersen E, Wedderkopp N, Juul-Kristensen B. Inter-tester reproducibility and inter-method agreement of two variations of the Beighton test for determining generalized joint hypermobility in primary school children. BMC Pediatr. 2013;13:214.
10. Bulbena A, Duró JC, Porta M, et al. Clinical assessment of hypermobility of joints: assembling criteria. J Rheumatol. 1992;19(1):115–22.
11. Grahame R, Bird HA, Child A, et al. The revised (Brighton 1998) criteria for the diagnosis of benign joint hypermobility syndrome (BJHS). J Rheumatol. 2000;27:1777–9.
12. Cameron KL, Duffey ML, DeBerardino TM, et al. Association of generalized joint hypermobility with a history of glenohumeral joint instability. J Athl Train. 2010;45:253–8.
13. Chahal J, Leiter J, McKee MD, Whelan DB. Generalized ligamentous laxity as a predisposing factor for primary traumatic anterior shoulder dislocation. J Shoulder Elbow Surg. 2010;19(8):1238–42.
14. Meehan RE, Petersen SA. Results and factors affecting outcome of revision surgery for shoulder instability. J Shoulder Elbow Surg. 2005;14(1):31–7.
15. Zabinski SJ, Callaway GH, Cohen S, et al. Revision shoulder stabilization: 2- to 10-year results. J Shoulder Elbow Surg. 1999;8:58–65.
16. Gerber C, Nyffeler RW. Classification of glenohumeral joint instability. Clin Orthop Relat Res. 2002;400:65–76.
17. Merolla G, Cerciello S, Chillemi C, Paolo P, De Santis E, Porcelli G. Multidirectional instability of the shoulder: biomechanics, clinical presentation, and treatment strategies. Eur J Orhop Surg Traumatol. 2015;25(6):975–85.
18. Castagna A, Cesari E, Gigante A, Di Matteo B, Garofalo R, Porcellini G. Age-related changes of elastic fibers in shoulder capsule of patients with glenohumeral instability: a pilot study. BioMed Res Int. 2018;2018:8961805, 7 pages.
19. Lee HJ, Kim NR, Moon SG, Ko SM, Park JY. Multidirectional instability of the shoulder: rotator interval dimension and capsular laxity evaluation using MR arthrography. Skeletal Radiol. 2013;42(2):231–8.
20. Beasley L, Faryniarz DA, Hannafin JA. Multidirectional instability of the shoulder in the female athlete. Clin Sports Med. 2000;19:331–49.
21. Guerrero P, Busconi B, Deangelis N, Powers G. Congenital instability of the shoulder joint: assessment and treatment options. J Orthop Sports Phys Ther. 2009;39:124–34.
22. Morris AD, Kemp GJ, Frostick SP. Shoulder electromyography in multidirectional instability. J Shoulder Elbow Surg. 2004;13:24–9.
23. Moroder P, Danzinger V, Maziak N, et al. Characteristics of functional shoulder instability. J Shoulder Elbow Surg. 2020;29(1):68–78, ISSN 1058-2746
24. Chen D, Goldberg J, Herald J, Critchley I, Barmare A. Effects of surgical management on multidirectional instability of the shoulder: a meta-analysis. Knee Surg Sports Traumatol Arthrosc. 2016;24(2):630–9.
25. Illyes A, Kiss J, Kiss RM. Electromyographic analysis during pull, forward punch, elevation and overhead throw after conservative treatment or capsular shift at patient with multidirectional shoulder joint instability. J Electromyogr Kinesiol. 2009;19:e438–47.
26. Levine WN, Arroyo JS, Pollock RG, et al. Open revision stabilization surgery for recurrent anterior glenohumeral instability. Am J Sports Med. 2000;28:156–60.
27. Neer CS II, Foster CR. Inferior capsular shift for involuntary inferior and multidirectional instability of the shoulder. A preliminary report. J Bone Joint Surg Am. 1980;62(6):897–908.
28. Longo UG, Rizzello G, Loppini M, et al. Multidirectional instability of the shoulder: a systematic review. Arthroscopy. 2015;31(12):2431–43.
29. Hawkins RJ, Krishnan SG, Karas SG, Noonan TJ, Horan MP. Electrothermal arthroscopic shoulder capsulorrhaphy: a minimum 2-year follow-up. Am J Sports Med. 2007;35(9):1484–8.
30. Toth AP, Warren RF, Petrigliano FA, Doward DA, et al. Thermal shrinkage for shoulder instability. HSS J. 2011;7(2):108–14.
31. Cicak N, Klobucar H, Bicanic G, Trsek D. Arthroscopic extracapsular plication to treat multidirectional instability of the shoulder. Arthroscopy. 2005;21:1278.
32. Snyder SJ. Shoulder arthroscopy. New York: Lippincott Williams and Wilkins; 2003. p. 22–8.
33. Ponce BA, Rosenzweig SD, Thompson KJ, et al. Sequential volume reduction with capsular plications: relationship between cumulative size of plications and volumetric reduction for multidirectional instability of the shoulder. Am J Sports Med. 2011;39:526–31.

Conservative Treatment of Multidirectional Instability of the Shoulder

40

Wojciech Solecki, Patryk Kłaptocz, Adrian Blasiak, and Roman Brzóska

40.1 Introduction

Shoulder joint provides the biggest range of motion among all joints in human body, but at the same time it is the least stable and most commonly dislocated joint [1].

Static restraints of glenohumeral (GH) joint include glenoid concavity, negative intraarticular pressure, labrum, GH ligaments and capsule [2]; other important factors include humeral head retro-torsion and joint congruence [3].

Multifold periscapular muscles and especially rotator cuff muscles contribute as dynamic stabilizers of the GH joint [4, 5]. Cooperation between those muscles provides good stabilization to this extremely mobile joint [6]. Proper motor control and proprioception is crucial for correct functioning of the mentioned mechanisms [7–9].

40.2 Multidirectional Instability of the Shoulder

Multi-directional instability (MDI) of GH joint is a symptomatic instability with either subluxations or luxations in more than one direction. In majority of cases, MDI is atraumatic and results from coexistence of repetitive stretching exercises or microtrauma and congenital joint laxity and capsule redundancy [10–12].

Frequently the main complaint is pain during specific movements, sensation of instability or apprehension in the GH joint.

Patients with generalized laxity represent poorer proprioception than those without laxity [13]. Subjects with MDI exhibit altered movement pattern, neuromotor control and stabilizing muscles activation of the shoulder girdle complex comparing to healthy population [14–16]. In those patient's, scapula is usually set in downward rotation and its upward rotation is significantly restricted [5, 17]. As a result, contact between humeral head and glenoid is unsettled due to larger translation of the humeral head [5, 18].

Natural history of MDI shows that spontaneous recovery or increase of instability occur in only 22.9% cases of atraumatic shoulder instability after at least 3 years [19].

The most recommended initial treatment of MDI is rehabilitation based mainly on kinesiotherapy [10, 12, 20, 21].

Rehabilitation programs focus on stabilization and positioning of the scapula, improvement of muscle control and activation, proprioception and modification of activity to tolerable level. This is based on the rationale, that strengthening of rotator cuff and periscapular muscles compensates deficiency of static stabilizers.

W. Solecki (✉) · P. Kłaptocz · A. Blasiak · R. Brzóska
Shoulder and Upper Limb Department,
St. Luke's Hospital, Bielsko-Biala, Poland
e-mail: wsolecki@lukasza.pl

R. Brzóska et al. (eds.), *360° Around Shoulder Instability*,
https://doi.org/10.1007/978-3-662-61074-9_40

Active stabilization is obtained by achieving better co-contraction balance of agonist–antagonist muscles resulting in improved humeral head position within acceptable range of motion. Proprioception is also affected by shoulder fatigue, therefore proprioception drills and strengthening of the muscles are crucial in treatment of MDI [13, 22].

Long follow-up after surgery suggests that plicated capsule becomes redundant over time [23], that is why it seems reasonable to compensate passive stabilizers of GH joint by strengthening exercises of rotator cuff and periscapular muscles.

40.3 Evidence-Based Results of Conservative Rehabilitation in MDI

40.3.1 Rehabilitation and Surgical Treatment

Several authors compared conservative and surgical treatment of MDI in order to establish proper treatment guidelines. Tillander et al. [24] compared effect of rehabilitation to open inferior capsule shift in patients with MDI. Rehab protocol consisted of 4 phases, lasted for at least 21 weeks and included strengthening of rotator cuff and stabilization of scapula.

Results showed poor effect of conservative treatment: 55% patients were unsatisfied, 44% of them decided to undergo surgery. Authors concluded that patients with MDI and clinical instability respond only moderately to the exercise program. Illyes et al. [25] examined 130 shoulders with MDI. Subjects were divided into two groups: first underwent conservative treatment and second, arthroscopic capsular shift plus conservative rehabilitation. Healthy individuals served as a control group. Rehabilitation protocol included proprioceptive exercises, neuromotor control reeducation and training of correct movement patterns. Scapula and GH joint strengthening exercises in close and open kinetic chain were performed. Mirrors and biofeedback were used in order to maximize the effect of rehabilitation. Measurement of muscle activation was performed with the Electromyography (EMG) examination.

Conservative treatment lasted over 24 weeks and included strengthening of the rotator cuff, pectoralis major, biceps brachii, triceps brachii and deltoid muscles. Increased normalization of muscle activity was observed in this group but not in such extent as in the group with preceding surgery. Normal muscle activation was obtained in the control group. Unfortunately, authors did not share details regarding type, frequency and dosage of exercises.

The same group of authors [26] measured scapulothoracic rhythm and relative displacement between the rotation centres of the humerus and scapula on the same research groups. Results proved improvement of scapula kinematics and humeral head centralization in MDI group, but in order to receive full physiological function surgery and rehabilitation was necessary.

Ide et al. [27] tested rehabilitation training for MDI with use if the orthosis to maintain the scapula in upward rotation. Program lasted for 8 weeks. Isometric exercises of rotator cuff and stabilization of scapula were performed. Later on, isotonic exercises with theraband and in the end wall push-ups were implemented. Outcomes demonstrated significant change in Rowe score, increased external and internal rotation strength and decreased Internal Rotation/Exteranal Rotation (IR/ER) ratio.

40.4 Effects of Rehabilitation Programs

Few studies report outcomes of rehabilitation in atraumatic MDI and the results vary among authors. Warby et al. [21] stated that this might be due to heterogeneity of patients and different methods of evaluation. There is low-quality evidence of improvement of Rowe score, periscapular strength and kinematics proving the impact of rehabilitation in MDI patients.

Burkhead and Rockwood [20] described a rehab protocol for posterior instability and MDI. The 3–4 months program was based on the principle of progressive resistance and consisted of two phases. In the first phase, exercises were performed using six types of rubber Therabands with increasing resistance. Second phase included similar exercises but with increasing weights instead of Therabands. Authors noted good and excellent result of Rowe score in 88% of participants with atraumatic MDI and involuntary subluxations and in 100% of participants with MDI and voluntary subluxations provided they didn't have any psychological problems.

Misamore et al. [28] tested the results of a home exercise program on a group of 64 patients with MDI. Program consisted of four phases but specific details of the drills were not provided. The goal of phase I was to limit pain by rest from provocative activities, analgesics and gentle exercises. Phase II included progressive strengthening exercises performed for 15–20 min three times daily in a pain-free manner.

Strengthening exercises of rotator cuff included internal and external rotation, forward flexion, abduction and extension. Strength of periscapular muscles was improved by exercises for retraction, elevation and depression of the scapula. Increasing resistance was implied by elastic tubing and weights. In phase III, functional exercises tailored for specific sport were implemented. During phase IV, patients returned to their work or sport. Patients were instructed to continue program in order to maintain the effects.

Study showed poor or fair outcome of exercises or decision about surgical intervention in 66% participants at 2 years follow-up and 70% at 8 years follow-up.

In 2016 Watson et al. [29, 30] published a detailed description of a new rehabilitation program for MDI. It was the first published program that provided enough details to replicate in clinical practice since the program by Burkhead and Rockwood in 1992 [20]. Program focuses on scapula stabilization exercises in the first place followed by strengthening of rotator cuff muscles and sport specific exercises. Program consists of six stages. Stage 1: "Scapula control and coronal plane control at 0–30° abduction" begins with scapula setting, which is the foundation whole program according to the authors. Scapula stabilization is achieved by scapula upward rotation, elevation and posterior tilt exercises with gradually increasing resistance. Next phase focuses on gaining control within increasing arc of abduction in coronal plane. Then drills for strengthening of internal and external rotation are implemented. During stage 2 posterior musculature is strengthened to prevent posterior humeral head translation. In stage 3, forward flexion control is achieved in range 0–45°. Range of abduction and flexion is increased to 90° in stage 4. Stage 5 consists of isolated deltoid drills in order to specifically strengthen and gain control of anterior, middle and posterior part of this muscle. Stage 6 consists of sport-specific and functional-specific drills. After finishing all the stages, patients are encouraged to continue with a maintenance program to preserve the effect of rehabilitation [29].

Watson rehabilitation program was compared to the program proposed by Burkhead and Rockwood in a randomized clinical trial published in 2018 by Warby et al. [31]. Forty-one patients were randomly allocated in one of the programs and outcomes were measured after 12 and 24 weekly sessions of therapy. The study revealed that Watson program was superior in terms of the Western Ontario Shoulder Index (WOSI) and limitation of abduction at 12 weeks and in WOSI, Melbourne Instability Shoulder Score (MISS) and pain at 24 weeks follow-up.

40.5 Conclusions

Kinesiotherapy plays an important role in treatment in all kinds of MDI. It is beneficial especially in cases of atraumatic instability and should be considered as the main treatment. Duration and dosage and load during the drills are described in the mentioned programs and should be individually modified according to the patient's response. Burkhead stated that the patients' maximized their stability after 3–4 months of therapy. Misamore et al. observed that most of the patients who did not respond to the therapy after 3 months, did not improve in further follow-up [20, 28].

Illyes states that 6 months of therapy is usually attempted before considering surgery [25].

Watson proposed a 24-week exercise program [29]. It is recommended to continue exercises after finishing the program to maintain the result. In authors' opinion, rehabilitation should be carried out for at least 12 months with control visits every 3 months before considering surgical intervention. When rehabilitation fails, surgical procedures such as arthroscopic capsular shift or capsulorrhaphy are performed. Surgery should also be followed by proper rehabilitation to obtain proper position of scapula, proprioception and neuromotor function of rotator cuff and periscapular muscles.

Results of rehabilitation vary among authors, from very promising to poor. This is probably caused by differences among study groups in terms of age and sports activity [20, 24, 28]. Compliance in performing home exercises was also questioned [28]. Furthermore in some studies, patients with traumatic history were included in the statistics [16, 32].

MDI patients have different movement patterns and changed muscle activation [11, 16] and these disorders should be addressed during rehabilitation. At present, the protocol proposed by Watson et al. [29, 30] besides being precisely described is proven to be the most efficient in treatment of MDI.

References

1. Kibler WB. The role of the scapular in athletic shoulder function. Am J Sports Med. 1998;26:325–37.
2. Wang VM, Flatow EL. Pathomechanics of acquired shoulder instability: a basic science perspective. J Shoulder Elbow Surg. 2005;14(1 Suppl S):2S–11S.
3. Tannenbaum E, Sekiya JK. Evaluation and management of posterior shoulder instability. Sport Health. 2011;3(3):253–63.
4. Debski RE, Sakone M, Woo SL, Wong EK, Fu FH, Warner JJ. Contribution of the passive properties of the rotator cuff to glenohumeral stability during anterior-posterior loading. J Shoulder Elbow Surg. 1999;8(4):324–9.
5. Ogston JB, Ludewig PM. Differences in 3-dimensional shoulder kinematics between persons with multidirectional instability and asymptomatic controls. Am J Sports Med. 2007;35:1361–70.
6. Provencher MT, LeClere LE, King S, McDonald LS, Frank RM, Mologne TS, et al. Posterior instability of the shoulder: diagnosis and management. Am J Sports Med. 2011;39(4):874–86.
7. Allegrucci M, Whitney SL, Lephart SM, Irrgang JJ, Fu FH. Shoulder kinesthesia in healthy unilateral athletes participating in upper extremity sports. J Orthop Sports Phys Ther. 1995;21(4):220–6.
8. Herrington L, Horsley I, Rofl C. Evaluation of shoulder joint position sense in both asymptomatic and rehabilitated professional rugby players and matched controls. Phys Ther Sport. 2010;11(1):18–22.
9. Myers JB, Lephart SM. The role of the sensorimotor system in the athletic shoulder. J Athl Train. 2000;35(3):351–63.
10. Bahu MJ, Trentacosta N, Vorys GC, Covey AS, Ahmad CS. Multidirectional instability: evaluation and treatment options. Clin Sports Med. 2008;27:671–89.
11. Barden JM, Balyk R, Raso VJ, Moreau M, Bagnall K. Atypical shoulder muscle activation in multidirectional instability. Clin Neurophysiol. 2005;116:1846–57.
12. Saccomanno MF, Fodale M, Capasso L, Cazzato G, Milano G. Generalized joint laxity and multidirectional instability of the shoulder. Joints. 2013;1(4):171–9.
13. Blasier RB, Carpenter JE, Huston LJ. Shoulder proprioception. Effect of joint laxity, joint position, and direction of motion. Orthop Rev. 1994;23(1):45–50.
14. Beasley L, Faryniarz DA, Hannafin JA. Multidirectional instability of the shoulder in the female athlete. Clin Sports Med. 2000;19:331–49.
15. Guerrero P, Busconi B, Deangelis N, Powers G. Congenital instability of the shoulder joint: assessment and treatment options. J Orthop Sports Phys Ther. 2009;39:124–34.
16. Morris AD, Kemp GJ, Frostick SP. Shoulder electromyography in multidirectional instability. J Shoulder Elbow Surg. 2004;13:24–9.
17. Illyes A, Kiss RM. Kinematic and muscle activity characteristics of multidirectional shoulder joint instability during elevation. Knee Surg Sports Traumatol Arthrosc. 2006;14:673–85.
18. Basmajian JV, Bazant FJ. Factors preventing downward dislocation of the adducted shoulder joint. J Bone Joint Surg. 1959;41:1182–6.
19. Kuroda S, Sumiyoshi T, Moriishi J, et al. The natural course of atraumatic shoulder instability. J Shoulder Elbow Surg. 2001;10(2):100–4.
20. Burkhead WZ Jr, Rockwood CA Jr. Treatment of instability of the shoulder with an exercise program. J Bone Joint Surg Am. 1992;74:890–6.
21. Warby SA, Pizzari T, Ford JJ, Hahne AJ, Watson L. The effect of exercise-based management for multidirectional instability of the glenohumeral joint: a systematic review. J Shoulder Elbow Surg. 2014;23:128–42.
22. Voight ML, Hardin JA, Blackburn TA, et al. The effects of muscle fatigue on and the relationship of arm dominance to shoulder proprioception. J Orthop Sports Phys Ther. 1996;23(6):348–52.

23. Mallon WJ, Speer KP. Multidirectional instability: current concepts. J Shoulder Elbow Surg. 1995;4(Pt 1):54–64.
24. Tillander B, Lysholm M, Norlin R. Multidirectional hyperlaxity of the shoulder: results of treatment. Scand J Med Sci Sports. 1998;8:421–5.
25. Illyes A, Kiss J, Kiss RM. Electromyographic analysis during pull, forward punch, elevation and overhead throw after conservative treatment or capsular shift at patient with multidirectional shoulder joint instability. J Electromyogr Kinesiol. 2009;19:e438–47.
26. Kiss RM, Illyes A, Kiss J. Physiotherapy vs. capsular shift and physiotherapy in multidirectional shoulder joint instability. J Electromyogr Kinesiol. 2010;20:489–501.
27. Ide J, Maeda S, Yamaga M, Morisawa K, Takagi K. Shoulder strengthening exercise with an orthosis for multidirectional shoulder instability: quantitative evaluation of rotational shoulder strength before and after the exercise program. J Shoulder Elbow Surg. 2003;12:342–5.
28. Misamore GW, Sallay PI, Didelot W. A longitudinal study of patients with multidirectional instability of the shoulder with seven- to ten-year follow-up. J Shoulder Elbow Surg. 2005;14:466–70.
29. Watson L, Warby S, Balster S, Lenssen R, Pizzari T. The treatment of multidirectional instability of the shoulder with a rehabilitation program: Part 1. Shoulder Elbow. 2016;8(4):271–8.
30. Watson L, Warby S, Balster S, Lenssen R, Pizzari T. The treatment of multidirectional instability of the shoulder with a rehabilitation programme: part 2. Shoulder Elbow. 2016;9(1):46–53.
31. Warby SA, Ford JJ, Hahne AJ, Watson L, Balster S, Lenssen R, Pizzari T. Comparison of 2 exercise rehabilitation programs for multidirectional instability of the glenohumeral joint: a randomized controlled trial. Am J Sports Med. 2018;46(1):87–97.
32. Kiss J, Damrel D, Mackie A, Neumann L, Wallace WA. Non-operative treatment of multidirectional shoulder instability. Int Orthop. 2001;24:354–7.

Multidirectional Shoulder Instability–Operative Treatment

41

Przemysław Lubiatowski, Joanna Wałecka, and Hubert Laprus

41.1 Introduction

There has been a lot of confusion about how to define multidirectional shoulder instability (MDI), and it is well known that multidirectional dislocations of the glenohumeral joint are less common than anterior instability. The prevalence of multidirectional shoulder instability (MDI) is highest in young men (twice that in women). Different clinical and pathophysiological aspects put emphasis on either direction of instability, contributing factors, laxity or presence of intra-articular lesions [1–3] (Table 41.1). MDI can be identified if symptomatic subluxations or dislocations occur in more than two directions. It has been understood classically to occur with the presence of congenital laxity and redundant joint capsule but often proved by repetitive microtrauma.

Gerber has classified the MDI types as dynamic ones occurring without hyperlaxity (B4), with hyperlaxity (B5) or with voluntary reduction (B6) [4]. B4 seems to be rare. It is traumatic, typically with complex capsulolabral lesions (e.g. 360°). Patients have both anterior and posterior apprehensions with no joint laxity. This group of patients usually needs early surgery to repair torn tissue. B5 is typical MDI occurring mostly in very young patients with shoulder and generalized joint laxity. There is usually no major trauma, but multiple minor traumas (e.g. due to sports). Patients lose control over shoulder stabilization. It is usually presented as subluxations, also. Usually no major lesions can be identified; however, typical radiological or arthroscopic findings include widening of rotator interval, pathologist capsule and stretched ligaments. Type B5 would mostly correspond to polar type 2 in the Stanmore classification [5]. The Stanmore system attempts to find a place for all patients. The concept is that patients can be at one of three poles, in which case they will exhibit a defined set of features placing them there. Polar type 1 patients will have a defined history of a significant trauma, display unidirectional instability and have a Bankart lesion. At the second pole, patients have a less-defined history of trauma but are likely to have a structural lesion. At the third pole, patients have no structural abnormality and may be habitual dislocators or have a significant muscle patterning abnormality and may be habitual dislocators or have a significant muscle patterning abnormality system that allows patients to move around the triangle over time. This system allows patients to move around the triangle over time.

The following chapter summarizes both the indications and contraindications for surgery in

P. Lubiatowski · J. Wałecka (✉)
Rehasport Clinic, Poznań, Poland
e-mail: p.lubiatowski@rehasport.pl

H. Laprus
St Luke's Hospital, Bielsko-Biała, Poland

R. Brzóska et al. (eds.), *360° Around Shoulder Instability*,
https://doi.org/10.1007/978-3-662-61074-9_41

Table 41.1 Surgical scenario for laxity treatment

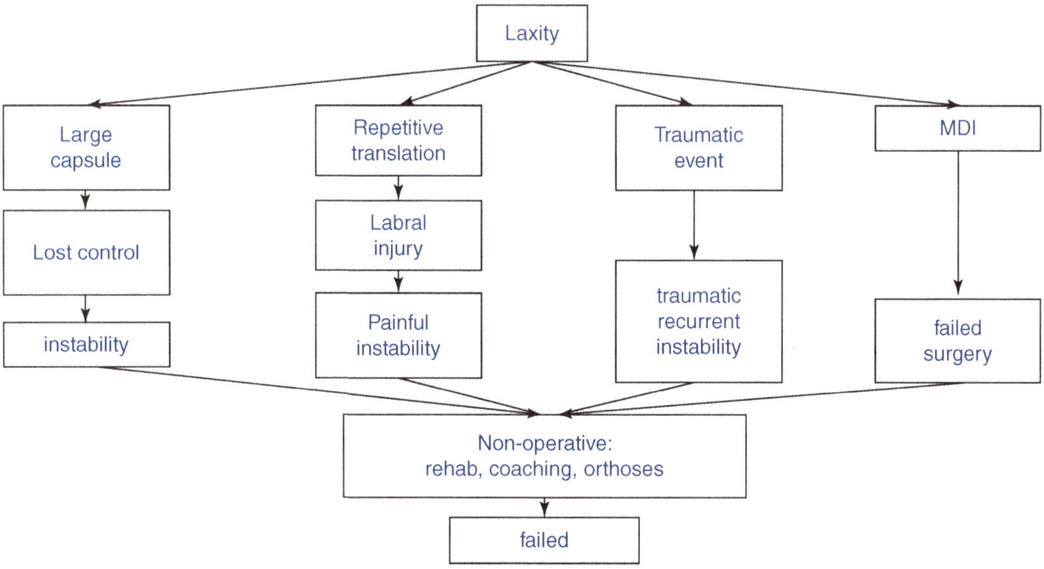

MDI. The purpose of this chapter is to present the most common surgical treatment techniques in MDI and to discuss the results of such treatment based on the author's experience and current literature, comparing it with conservative treatment.

41.2 Conservative Treatment

For atraumatic MDI (B5 and B6), conservative treatment seems to be beneficial [6–8]. Studies reveal that with long-term observation (over 24 weeks) conservative treatment focused on extending strength of the rotator cuff muscles, pectoralis major, biceps brachii, triceps brachii and deltoid muscles increases muscle activity but not as much as rehabilitation as a second step after arthroscopic capsular shift.

MDI patients have different movement patterns and changed muscle activation [9, 10]. Whether this is a cause or an effect, or perhaps just an adaptation process allowing function in this kind of disorder, is not clearly known. Scapular control and proper active positioning seem to be the foundation of the rehabilitation process. On this basis, glenohumeral stability and controlled movement may be regained. Part of the process is to support patients' efforts and decrease pain and anxiety. Often it may require team work with a specialized physiotherapist, shoulder surgeon and psychologist.

Conservative treatments have also been reported to yield poor results. In some studies, up to 50% of patients remain unstable and dissatisfied with the therapy [1, 2].

41.3 Surgical Treatment

Surgical treatments in many studies have shown superior results to non-operative treatments; however, direct comparison cannot be made since all surgeries were performed in cases where rehabilitation had failed. In Longo's systematic review, surgery was performed in 21% with MDI [11]. Arthroscopic plication for MDI showed a high rate of success with a recurrence rate of 6% and slightly more common for open plication, with a rate of 10% [3]. Only 5% of patients needed revision surgery. Patients after open shift had a more limited range of shoulder movement at follow-up compared to those treated arthroscopically. Indications for surgery for MDI have to be based on a thorough clinical assessment. Several factors should be taken into consideration. Acute traumatic onset may indicate a tear in the tissues which possibly did not heal and may need to be addressed with repair, as opposed to atraumatic and gradual onset which typically would respond well to a rehabilitation programme. Other factors also have been evaluated—such as presence of accompanying pain, loss of control, participation in sports, the volitional component, psychological status and genetic disorders. Many of these need be addressed with non-operative measures first, before surgery is considered. Eliminating pain or overuse could restore the stability and function. The degree of instability (dislocations vs. subluxations) has to be addressed. True dislocations are far more disabling and sometimes associated with organic lesions, which will make non-operative measures less effective. Prior treatment needs to be explored—rehabilitation or surgery. Thorough orthopaedic examination has to be performed to identify signs and direction of instability. A variety of provocative tests—anterior apprehension, posterior apprehension, Kim's, jerk—have been described to detect anterior or posterior instability. Another set of tests aims to modify (or relieve) symptoms, mostly by co-contracture of cuff muscles, scapular assistance or postural correction.

Hyperlaxity might be a substantial ground for operative failure. Generalized joint and tissue laxity have to be examined in patients with MDI and PI symptoms. The Beighton score is simple, reliable and repeatable to assess laxity, and a score of 4 or more (out of 9 points) supports a clinical diagnosis of hyperlaxity. Imaging studies are necessary to identify the underlying glenohumeral pathology. Conventional radiography usually shows a normal appearance, but osseous pathologies—glenoid dysplasia or retroversion—may be easily diagnosed. More advanced imaging may be necessary in chronic cases which fail to respond to therapy or which include a traumatic component. We mostly rely on magnetic resonance arthrography. The range of soft tissues lesions occurring in MDI includes increased joint volume, plastic deformation of the capsule and a "family" of labral lesions—Kim's, GLAD, Bankart, posterior Bankart, HAGL, RHAGL and chondrolabral erosion of the glenoid rim. Bone pathology may be congenital (increased glenoid retroversion, glenoid hypoplasia) or secondary attrition (posterior or anterior glenoid erosions, engaging humeral head defects).

A basic indication for surgical treatment of MDI is clinically disabling instability and pain, showing no improvement with a rehabilitation programme in an otherwise psychologically stable patient. A 6-month period of non-operative treatment has been widely accepted in the literature, although this has not been scientifically proven. In the case of patients with typical labral tears or attritional bone defects, a long delay may not be necessary. Special consideration is required for patients with recurrent or persistent instability following surgical treatment. Thorough evaluation of failure is essential to establish the reason—wrong qualification, inferior technique, failure to heal, stretching, or non-compliant patient [12, 13]. Specific factors have to be considered, including hardware failures, infection, nerve lesions, secondary arthritis or stiffness. If surgery is planned again all risks have to be evaluated and explained to the patient. A decision needs to be taken as to whether repeating the procedure has a chance of success. In some cases salvage procedures—bone block, overtensioning and arthrodesis—may be advisable.

41.4 Surgical Techniques

Various techniques, mostly arthroscopic, may need to be used depending on intra-articular pathology. Capsular laxity is addressed with capsular shift. Labral tears may need to be treated using suture anchors. Bone deficiency of the glenoid may need bone block (anterior or posterior) or coracoid transfer. For some patients, a combination of surgical procedures is used, e.g. labral repair with capsular shift.

41.4.1 Arthroscopic Capsular Shift: Author's Technique [14]

Shoulder arthroscopy is performed in a standard way. Three arthroscopic portals are used. Before starting the procedure, a standard arthroscopic evaluation is performed and joint volume is measured. The most important part is to manage the anteroinferior capsule and inferior glenohumeral ligament. The surface of the displaced capsule is rasped or gently shaved to cause superficial bleeding. An anteroinferior anchor is introduced at position 5.30 of the glenoid rim for the right shoulder, or at 6.30 for the left. The capsular shift is then performed (Fig. 41.1). We use both the anterior portals simultaneously. A precise portion of the capsule is gripped with a suture manipulator or grasper via the anterosuperior portal and shifted upwards towards the anchor site (Fig. 41.2). We can repeat this manoeuvre if too little or too much tissue has been engaged. A flap of the capsule is then pierced with a penetrating grasper, and the suture is retrieved. A standard sliding knot is tightened over the shifted capsule

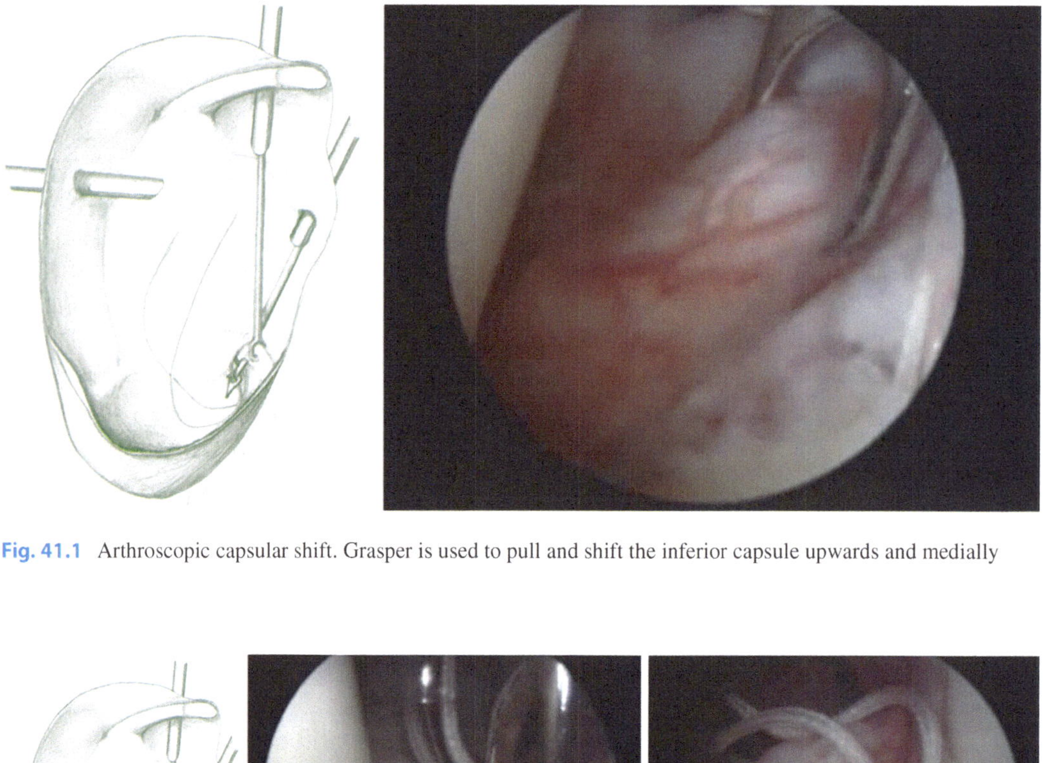

Fig. 41.1 Arthroscopic capsular shift. Grasper is used to pull and shift the inferior capsule upwards and medially

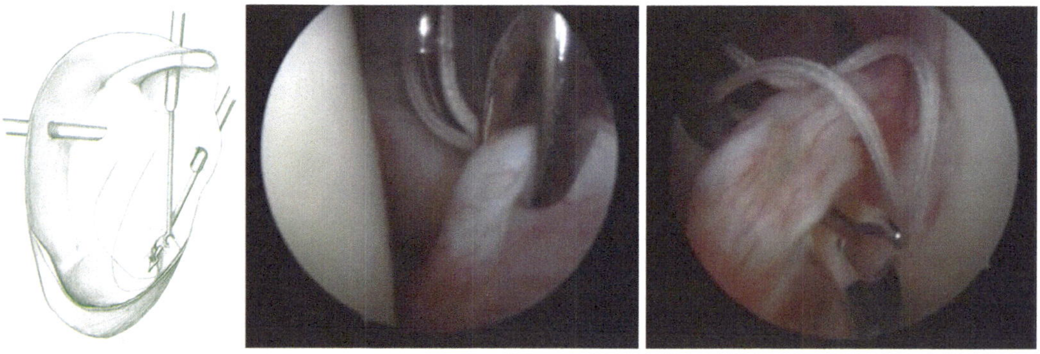

Fig. 41.2 Arthroscopic capsular shift. Shifted capsule is pierced through mid-glenoid portal

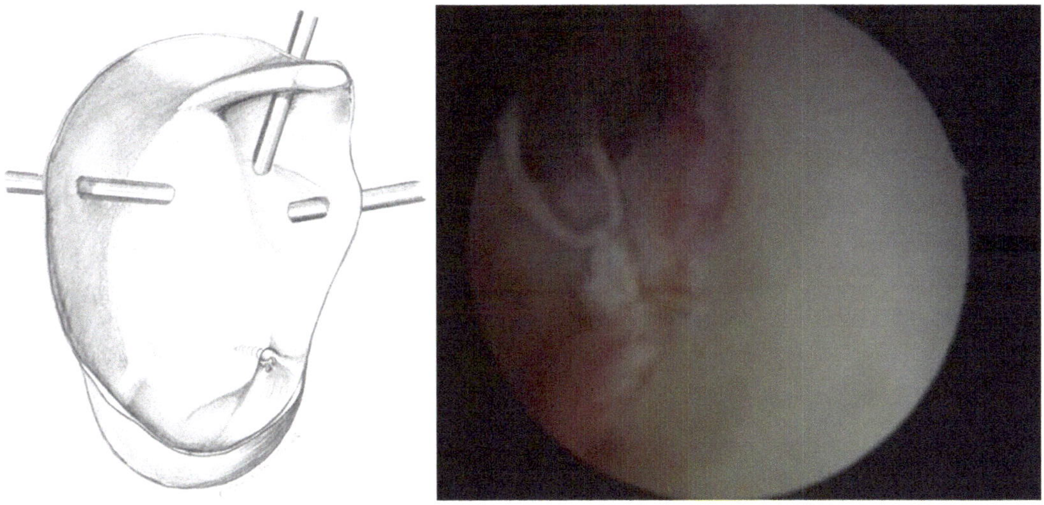

Fig. 41.3 Arthroscopic capsular shift. Shifted capsule is sutured to labrum or glenoid anchor

(Fig. 41.3). Next, an additional capsular shift is performed with more superior capsule middle glenohumeral ligament (MGHL). If necessary, the posteroinferior capsule can be shifted using the same technique. In cases of massive instability with spacious joints, the authors perform rotator interval closure (Fig. 41.4).

Arthroscopic clinical and cadaver studies have shown that after arthroscopic capsular shift the surgeon is able to achieve 61% of joint volume reduction, which is greater than classic arthroscopic Bankart repair with 37% of reduction [15]. However, volume reduction can also be anticipated when labral repair is performed. Tissue management always involves some degree of capsular plication. For this kind of capsular plication pendant f.e posterior Bankart repair, labrum mobilization allows lift the capsule towards the glenoid. Fixing implants secured with mattress stitches are usually used in its reconstruction. Stitches surrounding the labrum should be avoided, as they can lead to ischaemia, labral reinjury and damage to the cartilage. Mattress stitches, apart from their proven effectiveness, prevent contact between the hard stitch material and the humeral head's cartilage (Fig. 41.5).

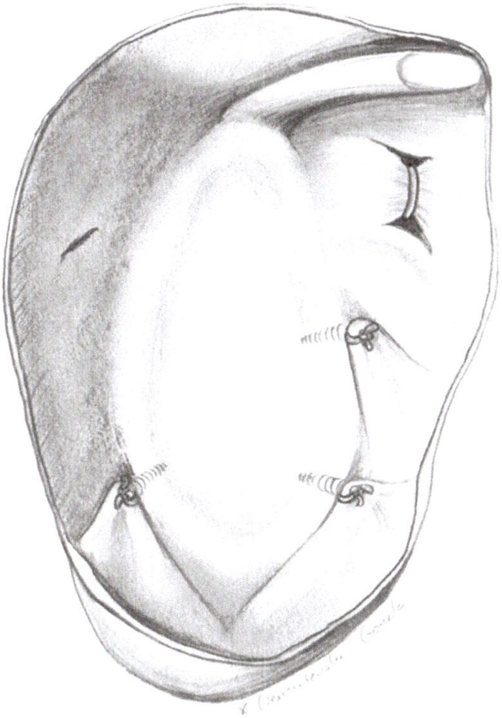

Fig. 41.4 Arthroscopic capsular shift. Final picture with anterior and posterior shift and rotator interval closure

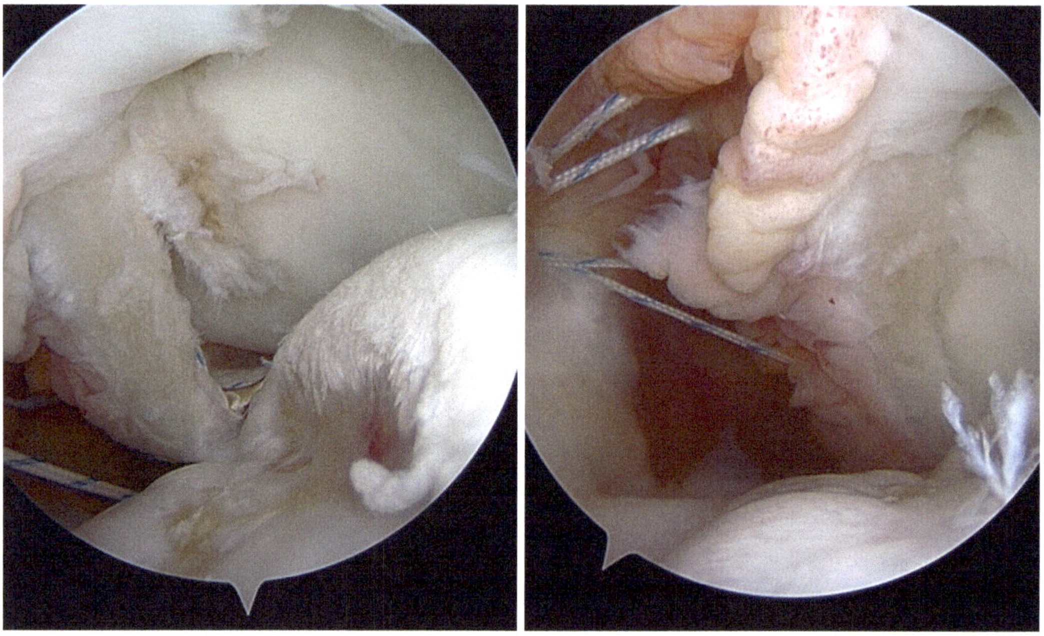

Fig. 41.5 Posterior labrum injury repair with capsular plication using mattress sutures

41.5 Contraindications for Surgery

Not all patients with MDI may or should be operated on. One contraindication for surgery is the volitional component of instability, meaning willful subluxation due to psychological disorder, medico-legal issues or secondary gains. Other contraindications include neurological disorders affecting muscular control (miastenia, ataxia, uncontrolled epilepsy). Surgical treatment should be proposed with caution in cases of genetic disorders causing laxity (e.g. Ehlers–Danlos syndrome). The patient's compliance is an important issue. Thorough explanation of the whole process is necessary, as well as careful planning of both the surgical procedure and the postoperative regimen with a specialist rehabilitation programme. Patients with MDI unwilling to cooperate or with no access to rehabilitation should not be operated on.

41.6 Salvage Procedures

41.6.1 Bone Block Procedure

Bone deficiency is not a common problem in MDI. However, both anterior and posterior glenoid defects may occur and need to be addressed. Coracoid transfer has been shown to be a successful procedure for anterior defects over many years. Both open and arthroscopic techniques have been developed. A classic open procedure can be combined with anterior capsular shift. In such cases, the released coraco-acromial ligament can be used to reinforce the anterior capsule. Arthroscopic coracoid transfer is a relatively new technique and some technical aspects are still developing. Suter button fixation of the coracoid is combined with capsular and labral repair. If needed the posterior capsule and posterior band of the inferior glenohumeral ligament can also be shifted and tensioned. Posterior bone block stabilization is usually recommended in cases of posterior glenoid erosion or hypoplasia [16, 17]. Both open and arthroscopic approaches have been proposed with various methods of fixation (screws, anchors and suture buttons). For both the approaches, soft tissue tensioning is also possible.

41.7 Fusion

This salvage procedure introduced by Diaz [18] is a viable treatment option for patients with refractory shoulder instability. In his study, Diaz proved that the average time to bony union after arthrodesis was 3.5 months (the range was 2.5–5 months). The patients reported significant overall subjective improvement, and none complained of instability postoperatively. However, it should be understood that this procedure, because of extreme limitation of function and the possibility of residual pain, should only be considered as a last step in surgery.

41.8 Capsular Release

Adhesive capsulitis is a complication caused by scarring between shoulder tissue layers and requires an individualized treatment protocol. Restriction of passive internal and external rotation caused by contractured coracohumeral ligament and rotator interval is typically observed. Forsythe et al. suggest that capsulitis might be a result of too aggressive rotator interval closure [13]. During rotator interval closure by shifting the middle glenohumeral ligament (MGHL) to the superior glenohumeral ligament (SGHL), loss of external rotation is often observed. This is especially the case in P-MDI revision surgery when excessive rotator interval closure might be the result of imbrication in an adduct arm. In these cases, for successful adhesion treatment, arthroscopic rotator interval release is required [12]. Biceps inflammation and biceps adhesions might also produce capsulitis. Tonino et al. suggest that intra-articular biceps adhesions should be treated by arthroscopic excision of the biceps tendon. Biceps tenodesis with capsular release seems too aggressive for a short postoperative period [19].

41.9 Conclusion

Multidirectional shoulder instability is a complex disorder and always needs careful and thorough evaluation. Typically it is effectively treated with non-operative measures, and surgical treatment of MDI is not the primary approach, though in case of failed rehabilitation and especially in post-traumatic cases, it has shown very good results. In every case possible limitations and contraindications to surgery have be taken into consideration.

References

1. Misamore GW, Sallay PI, Didelot W. A longitudinal study of patients with multidirectional instability of the shoulder with seven- to ten-year follow-up. J Shoulder Elbow Surg. 2005;14:466–70.
2. Tillander B, Lysholm M, Norlin R. Multidirectional hyperlaxity of the shoulder: results of treatment. Scand J Med Sci Sports. 1998;8:421–5.
3. Chen D, Goldberg J, Herald J, Critchley I, Barmare A. Effects of surgical management on multidirectional instability of the shoulder: a meta-analysis. Knee Surg Sports Traumatol Arthrosc. 2016;24(2):630–9.
4. Gerber C, Nyffeler RW. Classification of glenohumeral joint instability. Clin Orthop Relat Res. 2002;400:65–76.
5. Lewis A, Kitamura T, Bayley JIL. The classification of shoulder instability: new light through old windows! Curr Orthop. 2004;18:97–108.
6. Burkhead WZ Jr, Rockwood CA Jr. Treatment of instability of the shoulder with an exercise program. J Bone Joint Surg Am. 1992;74:890–6.
7. Kiss J, Damrel D, Mackie A, Neumann L, Wallace WA. Non-operative treatment of multidirectional shoulder instability. Int Orthop. 2001;24:354–7.
8. Warby SA, Pizzari T, Ford JJ, Hahne AJ, Watson L. The effect of exercise-based management for multidirectional instability of the glenohumeral joint: a systematic review. J Shoulder Elbow Surg. 2014;23:128–42.
9. Barden JM, Balyk R, Raso VJ, Moreau M, Bagnall K. Atypical shoulder muscle activation in multidirectional instability. Clin Neurophysiol. 2005;116:1846–57.

10. Illyes A, Kiss RM. Kinematic and muscle activity characteristics of multidirectional shoulder joint instability during elevation. Knee Surg Sports Traumatol Arthrosc. 2006;14:673–85.
11. Longo UG, Rizzello G, Loppini M, Locher J, Buchmanna S, Maffulli N, Denaro V. Multidirectional instability of the shoulder: a systematic review. Arthroscopy. 2015;31(12):2431–43.
12. Brzoska R, Laprus H, Ranosz P, Kłaprocz P, Rynkiewicz T. Management of failed posterior and multidirectional instability repair. In: Milano G, Grasso A, Calvo A, Brzóska R, editors. Management of failed shoulder surgery. Berlin: Springer; 2018. https://doi.org/10.1007/978-3-662-56504-9_4.
13. Forsythe B, Ghodadra N, Romeo AA, Provencher MT. Management of the failed posterior/multidirectional instability patient. Sports Med Arthrosc. 2010;18(3):149–61.
14. Lubiatowski P, Ogrodowicz P, Wojtaszek M, Breborowicz M, Długosz J, Romanowski L. Arthroscopic capsular shift technique and volume reduction. Eur J Orthop Surg Traumatol. 2012;22(6):437–41.
15. Lubiatowski P, Długosz J, Ślęzak M, Ogrodowicz P, Stefaniak J, Walecka J, Romanowski L. Effect of arthroscopic techniques on joint volume in shoulder instability: Bankart repair versus capsular shift. Int Orthop. 2017;41(1):149–55. https://doi.org/10.1007/s00264-016-3275-3.
16. Schwartz DG, Goebel S, Piper K, Kordasiewicz B, Boyle S, Lafosse L. Arthroscopic posterior bone block augmentation in posterior shoulder instability. J Shoulder Elbow Surg. 2013;22(8):1092–101.
17. Boileau P, Hardy MB, McClelland WB Jr, Thélu CE, Schwartz DG. Arthroscopic posterior bone block procedure: a new technique using suture anchor fixation. Arthrosc Tech. 2013;2(4):e473–7.
18. Diaz JA, Cohen SB, Warren RF, Craig EV, Allen AA. Arthrodesis as a salvage procedure for recurrent instability of the shoulder. J Shoulder Elbow Surg. 2003;12(3):237–41. https://doi.org/10.1016/S1058-2746(02)86883-5.
19. Tonino PM, Gerber C, Itoi E. Complex shoulder disorders: evaluation and treatment. J Am Acad Orthop Surg. 2009;17:125–36.

Part IV

Future Perspectives in the Instability Treatment

New Directions in Grafting Technologies: Up to Date

42

A. Marmotti, I. Zorzolo, E. Bellato, G. Agati, and F. Castoldi

42.1 Introduction

The shoulder is the most mobile joint, thus the most inherently unstable. The incidence for first-time dislocations is 21.9 per 100,000 population of which up to 6.1% will develop further symptomatic instability [1].

Recurrent anterior posttraumatic instability is commonly associated with osseous defects on both the glenoid and humeral side. The prevalence of anteroinferior glenoid erosion or rim fracture has been reported with a range from 8% to 95%, whereas the occurrence of a Hill–Sachs lesion ranges from 84% to 93% [2]. Glenoid bone defects are caused by dislocation episodes and they impair the stability of the joint, hence predisposing to recurrence.

In the mid-range arc of motion, the joint stability is achieved by negative intraarticular pressure and by the concavity-compression effect resulting from muscle contractions that center the humeral head in the glenoid concavity [3]. A large bony defect of the glenoid causes an insufficient concavity-compression effect, while the increase of joint volume, combined with the capsule thinning, makes the joint unable to maintain a negative intraarticular pressure. In addition, muscle imbalances also may lead to a humeral head that is not centered in the glenoid socket. Joint capsule and glenohumeral ligaments, in particular the anterior band of the inferior glenohumeral ligament (AIGHL), play a role in the end-range stability in abduction and external rotation. Bankart lesion causes a functional impairment of the AIGHL, and the surgical repair is a successful treatment for end-range instability. However, in presence of glenoid bone loss, surgical repair becomes ineffective for the concomitant mid-range instability [2].

Glenoid bone loss is the most important risk factor for complications after a primary arthroscopic Bankart procedure, increasing the morbidity and the costs [4]. Several authors have tried to establish the "critical" limit beyond of which the arthroscopic repair is prone to failure. The amount of bone loss, which demands conversion to an open procedure with bony augmentation, has been reported to range from 20% to 27% [5–15]. Burkhart et al. [7, 13, 16] reported that an inverted pear-shaped glenoid, equivalent to at least 27% of bone loss, predicted failure after arthroscopic stabilization, and they recommended bone-blocking procedures in presence of this specific glenoid shape. The arthroscopic failure rate reported with critical bone loss was as high as 67% compared to 4% of that reported in subjects without significant bone loss. These results have been confirmed by numerous authors

A. Marmotti (✉) · I. Zorzolo · E. Bellato · G. Agati · F. Castoldi
Department of Orthopaedics and Traumatology, University of Turin, Torin, Italy
e-mail: enrico.bellato@unito.it

R. Brzóska et al. (eds.), *360° Around Shoulder Instability*,
https://doi.org/10.1007/978-3-662-61074-9_42

[5, 9, 11, 14, 17–20]. However, the critical bone loss identifies the risk of instability recurrence or re-operation, and it does not take in account functional results. Sahaha et al. [18] placed the "subcritical" glenoid bone loss at 13.5%: above this threshold, high demand patients would experience a clinically unacceptable result even without recurrent instability.

The Hill-Sachs lesion is the compression fracture generated when the posterolateral humeral head impinges against the anterior rim of the glenoid [21]. It has been described by Burkhart and De Beer [16] as "engaging" when, arthroscopically, it comes in contact with the glenoid anterior margin with the arm abducted and maximally externally rotated, creating a risk of joint displacement. The depth [22], size [23], and volume [22] of the Hill-Sachs lesions have been wrongfully thought to be parameters to estimate the risk of engagement. On the other hand, the relative location of the Hill-Sachs lesion and the glenoid width are the most important parameters.

In a cadaver study, Yamamoto et al. [24] demonstrated that the contact area between the humeral head and the anterior glenoid rim with the arm abducted at 90° spans from the medial margin of the footprint of the rotator cuff for 18.4 mm ± 2.5 mm, which is equivalent to 84% ± 14% of the glenoid width. This contact zone is defined the "glenoid track" and can be used to evaluate whether or not there is a risk of engagement. If the Hill-Sachs lesion remains within the glenoid track, there is no risk of engagement, but if the Hill-Sachs lesion extends medially over the glenoid track, it might engage. In another study, it was later demonstrated that the width of the glenoid track was 83% of the glenoid width [25]. Di Giacomo et al. [2, 26] not only have developed a TC method that uses the concept of the glenoid track to determine the engagement risk, but they highlighted how the bone loss in recurrent instability is bipolar, affecting both the anterior glenoid and the posterolateral humeral head, and how these defects interplay. Restoring the glenoid width with bone-blocking surgery widens significantly the glenoid track, so that some preoperative off-track lesion could fell on-track after the bone-blocking, not requiring additional treatment. The on-track versus off-track concept has been demonstrated to be a better predictor of failed arthroscopic stabilization than solely quantifying glenoid osseous defect [27].

42.2 Glenoid Grafting

Glenoid bone grafting surgery is necessary in order to restore the glenoid width and to prevent instability recurrence. Several autograft and allograft techniques have been tested without one being clearly superior to the others. The ideal graft should anatomically reconstruct the defect, redistributing the contact pressure and preventing the progression of osteoarthritis secondary to instability. The graft should have a high rate of integration, a low resorption rate, and a low risk of hardware fixation complications. When a 30% glenoid bone defect is present, the glenohumeral contact pressures increase by up to 390% in the anteroinferior quadrant of the glenoid [28].

42.2.1 Coracoid Transfer Procedures

Helfet [29] described a procedure known as the Bristow's procedure, whereby 1 cm of the distal coracoid and the conjoined tendon were transferred, by means of a slit through the subscapularis tendon, on the anterior neck of the scapula. The graft was fixed with suture through the conjoined and subscapular tendons. A dynamic buttress was created across the anterior aspect of the glenoid to enhance shoulder stability in abduction and external rotation. However, isolated Bristow procedure have been only 50% successful at preventing shoulder instability [30].

In the coracoid transfer described by Latarjet [31], the coracoid is harvested between the insertions of the coracobrachialis and pectoralis minor tendon using a chisel, laid flat with its posterior surface against the glenoid neck and its lateral surface towards the joint, after a preferably vertical split of the subscapularis muscle, and then stabilized by one screw. The subscapularis muscle and the capsule are repaired by suture over the bone graft and reinforced with the coracoacromial ligament (CAL).

Latarjet's original procedure resulted in an extraarticular, nonanatomic repair that may stabilize the shoulder through three principles [32, 33]:

1. Bony stabilization by the transfer of the coracoid segment. It is effective especially in the mid-range motion by the glenoidplasty effect. The reconstruction of the glenoid concavity prevents anterior translation of the humeral head by means of positioning the coracoid process flush to the glenoid margin.
2. Sling effect through the transfer of the conjoined tendon. The interaction between conjoint tendons and the inferior part of the subscapularis tendon is the most important stabilizing mechanism at the end-range motion with the arm in abduction and external rotation and it contributes to mid-range stability.
3. Capsule strengthening through the transferred CAL contributes to stabilize the arm in the end range with the arm in abduction and neutral rotation.

The surgical technique for the Latarjet procedure evolved and several modifications have been proposed [34]: splitting the subscapularis horizontally L-shape or in a shape of an "L", positioning the graft flush to the articular surface, effectively performing a glenoidplasty, using two screws or a specific plate for the fixation, repairing the capsule over the graft (thus making it "intraarticular"), performing capsular shifts and even performing the surgery arthroscopically [35]. These technical differences make a direct comparison between studies difficult.

A highly debated surgical aspect is the orientation of the coracoid graft: either with the lateral aspect of the coracoid toward the joint line as described by Latarjet [31, 36, 37] or by rotating the graft by 90°, with the inferior face of the coracoid toward the articular surface, exploiting the coracoid natural curvature that resembles the glenoid in the so-called "congruent-arc Latarjet" [38–40].

The Latarjet procedure is fairly successful in preventing instability recurrence, with a dislocation rate from 2.94% to 10% [34]. A drawback of this surgery is that it can cause neurological injuries, especially to the musculocutaneous and axillary nerves, approximately at 1% rate in large reviews [34], although it has been reported as high as 20% in some series [41, 42]. There are several complication related to the graft: (1) bone block nonunion can occur in 1.5–9% of cases and is usually related to unicortical or single screw fixation; (2) graft fracture occurs in 1.5% of cases and usually happens for an intraoperative overtightening of the screws [43]; (3) bone block partial lysis is frequent but only rarely leads to unsatisfactory outcomes and, apparently, the resorption is more pronounced in patients with less glenoid bone loss [44]. The screws used for the fixation may cause anterior pain if the head of the screw is protruding toward the subscapularis muscle or it may produce posterior pain if the length of screw is excessive causing protrusion of the tip beyond the posterior border of the glenoid. Implant breakage is often secondary to graft nonunion [43]. Stiffness and loss of external rotation is an important concern for young and active patients; however, if the subscapularis is respected during the graft placement, only an average of 5° of external rotation is lost [43].

Osteoarthritis after the Latarjet procedure is a long-term complication. Fourteen years after surgery, Allain et al. [45] reported that 37% of patients had glenohumeral arthritis. It can be partially explained by technical mistakes as the lateral overhang of the graft or the malposition of the implant. Furthermore, considering how much the glenohumeral contact pressure increases in case of bone loss [28], a nonanatomical graft is not capable to redistribute the pressure, thus predisposing to "instability osteoarthritis." Bouju et al. [46] suggested that maintaining the coracoid in an extraarticular position may prevent the graft from "rubbing" on the glenoid surface, thus reducing the progression of osteoarthritis.

42.2.2 Autograft

Anterior glenoid bone grafting is sometimes referred as the Eden-Hybinette procedure. This surgery was firstly performed using tibial autograft, secured by placing it between the glenoid and detached labrum [12]. As for the Latarjet procedure, there is not a single technique described in literature. Usually a corticocancellous iliac crest bone graft is harvested, the inner table is placed flush to the glenoid surface and then it is fixed with screws and contoured to replicate the anatomic profile of the native glenoid [12]. This anatomic approach is followed by soft tissue repair that makes the graft either intraarticular [47] or extraarticular [48]. Studies have reported good to excellent outcomes; however, these studies are limited by small population groups and short follow-up period [47–49]. Recently arthroscopic-assisted techniques for iliac crest autograft have been described [50, 51].

In a long-term follow-up study, Rahme et al. [52] reported a prevalence of glenohumeral arthritis of 47%. However, conclusive evidence was not available to suggest whether this was the result of the trauma from recurrent instability prior to repair or a consequence of the surgical treatment. As for the Latarjet procedure, loss of external rotation is a common complication [47, 52].

In order to prevent complications related to the use of fixing devices and in order to obtain a more anatomic stabilization, Auffarath et al. [53, 54] developed an implant-free technique: the J-grafting. After assessing the glenoid bone loss, a bicortical iliac crest graft is harvested and then the cancellous bone is removed, obtaining a roughly J-shaped graft with a keel of cortical bone that is thinned using the high-speed burr. After a partial glenoid osteotomy, the graft keel is securely impacted to the anterior aspect of the glenoid and its surface is milled down to the level of the adjacent intact glenoid cartilage surface. In laboratory studies, the J-grafting restored near-native glenohumeral contact areas and pressures, provided secure initial graft fixation, and demonstrated excellent osseous glenohumeral stability at time zero [55]. In a long-term follow-up study, J-grafting showed to be a reliable procedure for preventing instability recurrence, with only 3% of relapses, with good functional results. Nevertheless, 32% of patient showed signs of osteoarthritis [56]. So the initial hope that the J-bone grafting may hamper the progression of "instability arthropathy" (due to the anatomic graft remodeling and the formation of cartilage-like soft tissue on the graft) still remains unfulfilled [57]. As for other techniques, an arthroscopic-assisted version of J-grafting has been described [58].

A common concern in using iliac crest bone autograft is the donor-site morbidity. Major complications include neurologic and vascular injury, deep infection, large hematoma, bowel herniation, fracture, or pelvic instability with impaired gait. Minor complications include superficial infection, seroma, unacceptable cosmesis, and temporary paresthesia. Major complications are rare and typically require treatment, while minor complications may linger for months to years [59].

An unusual and rarely used osteochondral autograft for glenoid reconstruction is the distal clavicle [60]. The distal part of the clavicle (6 to 8 mm) is harvested by a section perpendicular to the acromio-clavicular joint surface obtaining a bone segment with a width as large as to match the glenoid bone loss. The graft can be fixed either with screw or suture anchor, and the soft tissue are reinserted to create and intra-articular position of the graft. As the clinical experiences are very limited, so are the biomechanical studies [61, 62]. However, it appears that the distal clavicle may viably restore the glenoid anatomy, even better than a glenoid allograft [62].

42.2.3 Allograft

Several sources of allografts have been used to address glenoid bone loss, including glenoid bone [63], iliac crest [64], distal tibia [65], femoral head [66], and humeral head [67]. Preshaped osseous allograft are also available for implant [68]. These allografts are supposed to be more anatomic than the coracoid transfer, and they do not produce donor-site morbidity, unlike iliac crest bone autograft. Moreover, osseocartilaginous allograft could theoretically allow for reestablishing both the bone geometry and the joint surface, decreasing the risk of future "instability arthropathy."

Multiple surgical techniques have been described. Most of the reconstructions are described as intraarticular [58, 63–67], and graft fixation can be achieved by either screws [65–67], suture anchors [64], or J-grafting [58]. Allograft reconstruction of the glenoid has shown good to excellent clinical outcomes, despite a small loss of external rotation, a low rate of recurrent instability, high rates of graft union, and very low rates of graft resorption [69]. Nevertheless, these results are based on small, short follow-up studies, so no conclusive data could be drafted on the late osteoarthropathy onset.

Biomechanical studies performed on either anatomic specimens or computer models compared how coracoid transfer and different grafts can restore articular geometry and normalize contact pressure, in the hope to prevent further articular damage. Willemot et al. [70] found that glenoid allografts most accurately restored articular geometry, classic Latarjet performed well on average but exhibited large variability, tibial allograft restored only the coronal arc, and congruent arc Latarjet was the worst option for anatomic reconstruction. However, these findings have not been widely confirmed by other biomechanical works. Another study found the tibial plafond and iliac crest allografts to better match the axial arc and restore the depth of the glenoid, while the congruent arc Latarjet reconstruction was able to better restore the native glenoid coronal radius [71]. According to Bhatia et al. [72], distal tibia allograft is better in reducing joint contact pressure compared to the Latarjet procedure, but the articular geometry was not considered in the study.

Nonetheless, there are innate disadvantages in using the allografts. Despite proper precautions, there is a small risk of disease transmission [73]. Osteochondral grafts can potentially reconstruct the articular surface, but this potentiality is considerably reduced if the graft has been cryopreserved, as the availability of chondrocytes is reduced both in vitro [74] and in vivo [75]. Fresh allografts are not widely available and their use is logistically challenging because they must be implanted within 14–28 days to avoid biological decline of the tissue [76].

42.3 Humeral Grafting

Symptomatic engaging Hill-Sachs lesions have been addressed with several surgical strategies including humeroplasty, disimpaction with elevation and bone grafting, remplissage, arthroplasty, and humeral head augmentation using either prosthetic cap or allograft matched to defect size [77].

The use of osteochondral allografts has been proposed to address moderate to large humeral-side defects (>40% of the articular surface) [78]. However, since it is a fairly recent technique with limited indications, only case reports or studies with a small cohort and short follow-up are available in literature. Furthermore, most of them are focused on the treatment of reverse Hill-Sachs for posterior recurrent instability.

The Fresh-frozen femoral [79–82] or humeral head [83–85] osteochondral allografts are shaped to fit into the humeral defect and seated flush with the surrounding articular surface, allowing for reproducing the native articular contour, as well as filling the subchondral bony defect. As for glenoid allograft, fresh-frozen allograft are essentially acellular [75], reducing the advantage of a chondral surface. For this reason, some authors [86–88] suggested the use of fresh allograft, despite the reduced availability and the short time window period of implantation [76]. Instead of side-matched fresh humeral allograft, Provencher et al. [89] have proposed the use of a talus allograft, considering its highly congruent radius of curvature, the strong weight-bearing properties, and the presence of a thick cartilage layer. The concept of using this type of graft is related to the fact that the humeral head is located closely to the central portion of the body, and this aspect increases the risk of graft harvest contamination from the donor, because of greater potential for exposure to pathogens. Indeed it seems that the talus may offer a lower risk of contamination, being located far from major organs.

Bulk allograft can be press-fit into the bone deficit [80, 83, 90] or fixed with screws [81, 82, 84–86, 88, 91, 92]. Some studies [90–92] suggested the use of osteochondral bone plugs, similarly to mosaicplasty technique, to fill up the humeral bone deficit. As for other reconstructive surgeries, humeral head plug allograft procedure has been performed arthroscopically [90].

A recent review [93] outlined that humeral head augmentation with an osteochondral allograft may improve shoulder range of motion and functional scores, and these aspects may lead to a low subsequent dislocation rate. However, the procedure is burdened by a 20–30% complication rate including minor intra-operatory complications as capsular avulsion and damages to the long head of the biceps. Finally, there is a high rate of allograft reabsorption up to 36% of cases and, most importantly, 50% of patients required conversion to a total shoulder arthroplasty after 5 years or more of follow up.

42.4 New Perspectives

A new perspective in the concept of bone grafting comes from the field of the basic science. Indeed, from a "basic" view point, some of the current limitations in the use of bone graft are linked to the occurrence of bone resorption. In order to prevent such a complication, a possible solution may be represented by the use of a cellular bone graft that allows for obtaining a bone structure of optimal quality. At present, two speculative alternatives are suggested from the literature.

The first option may be represented by the concept of infusing bioscaffolds with growth factors that facilitate the homing of mesenchymal stem cells. This fascinating opportunity may lead to the repopulation of the bone scaffold by means of stem cells originating directly from the host reservoir and, thus, perfectly biocompatible. Migrating cells may theoretically be engaged in the scaffold incorporation by means of local osteogenic differentiation and bone matrix production, obtaining a stable cellularized bone graft. This idea has been already exploited in a promising preclinical rabbit model in 2010 [94]. Lee et al. [94] have realized an anatomically correct bioscaffold mimicking the rabbit proximal humeral joint made of a composite of poly-e-caprolactone and hydroxyapatite, and they spatially infused the scaffold with transforming growth factor beta 3-adsorbed collagen hydrogel. The hydrogel carrying the growth factor allowed for a progressive release of the bioactive molecule, and the end term result at 4 months after implantation was astonishing: tgf-beta 3-infused samples presented a greater number of chondrocytes and a better quality of the matrix compared to that of tgf-beta-free samples. A cartilage surface was recapitulated and the neo-cartilage was avascular, and it was also integrated with a neo-subchondral bone that showed the presence of blood vessels. This result represented a proof of concept of a new and totally different basic science approach to regenerate complex tissues and a possible alternative to the more common cell delivery methods.

The second option seems no less appealing than the previous one. Indeed, the use of bone grafting may be further improved by the concept of recapitulating the endochondral ossification inside the bone graft. An ideal bone graft should be similar to natural bone, thus obtaining a functional bone organ by means of tissue engineering may be a possible alternative to reach an optimal quality of the graft and, hopefully, to reduce the bone resorption process of the graft itself. Scotti et al. have introduced this concept in 2013 [95]. In their experiment, human mesenchymal stem cells from bone marrow were firstly seeded into scaffold made by collagen and cultivated in a chondrogenic hypertrophic medium in order to obtain a construct with neo-tissue resembling hypertrophic cartilage. Then, they implanted the constructs in the dorsal subcutaneous pooches of nude mice, and after 12 week they observed a subtotal remodeling of the constructs with the presence of bone marrow, vessel, and bone. In the central core, they described the appearance of bone matrix along with trabecular bone structure while at the periphery of the construct they observed the presence of compact, cortical bone. The histologic result obtained by the authors is greatly different from the common process of bone remodeling and scaffold incorporation and may represent a future attractive strategy for improving bone grafting technology. In line with

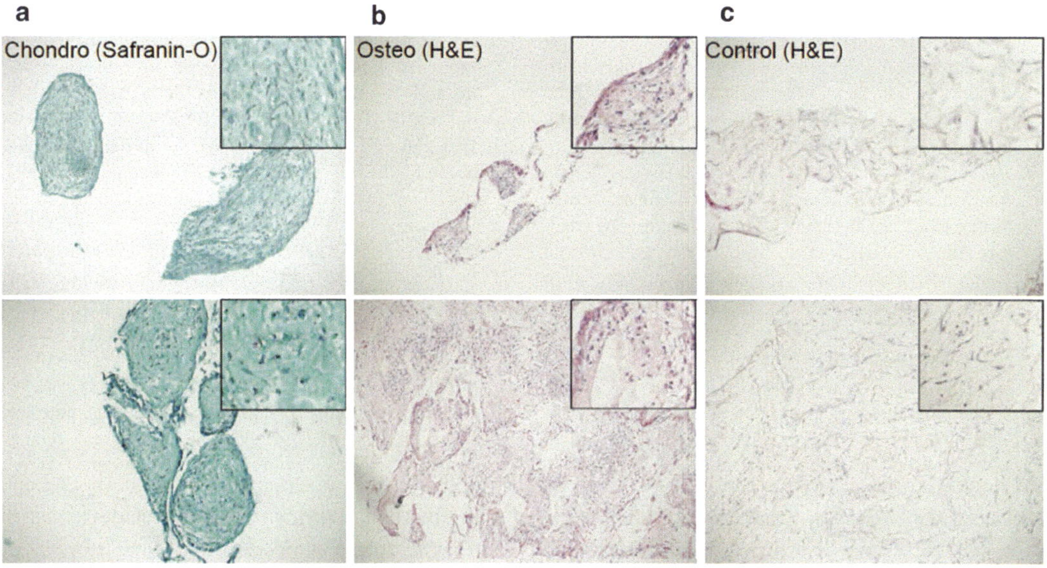

Fig. 42.1 Hypertrophic differentiation of UC-MSCs seeded onto Orthoss granules. Safranin O staining (**a**) and H&E staining (**b**, **c**); UC-MSCs seeded onto Orthoss granules and cultured for 5 weeks in the hypertrophic medium (**a**), osteogenic medium (**b**), or basal medium (**c**). Cartilage matrix production is visible in (**a**). Runt-related transcription factor 2 (RUNX2) also known as core-binding factor subunit alpha-1 (CBF-alpha-1) is a protein that in humans is encoded by the RUNX2 gene. RUNX2 is a key transcription factor associated with osteoblast differentiation

these theories, a recent work of Marmotti et al. suggested also the possibility to use an allogeneic source of cells to realize osteochondral scaffold [96]. An allogeneic source may allow for optimizing the osteochondral strategy by means of eliminating the need of tissue harvest and thus hypothesizing an “off-the-shelf” cellular product that could be readily available, providing a stem cell factory to manufacturing the technology. The authors selected a stem cells line from the umbilical cord stroma by means of a minimal manipulation process, and they seeded the cells into a commonly used commercial bioderived bone substitute made from highly purified bovine bone mineral. In vitro, in presence of hypertrophic chondrogenic medium, they observed chondral matrix production (Fig. 42.1) along with a strong expression of the osteogenic factor RUNX2 (Runt-related transcription factor 2 or core-binding factor subunit alpha-1) that characterizes the osteogenic traits of the hypertrophic phase of endochondral development. This result anticipates the possibility to develop endochondral ossification combining umbilical cord mesenchymal stem cells with commercially available bone substitute in order to theorize a possible future use of the off-the-shelf endochondral allografts to improve bone grafting technologies.

References

1. Shields DW, Jefferies JG, Brooksbank AJ, et al. Epidemiology of glenohumeral dislocation and subsequent instability in an urban population. J Shoulder Elb Surg. 2018;27:189–95. https://doi.org/10.1016/j.jse.2017.09.006.
2. Di Giacomo G, de Gasperis N, Scarso P. Bipolar bone defect in the shoulder anterior dislocation. Knee Surg Sport Traumatol Arthrosc. 2016;24:479–88. https://doi.org/10.1007/s00167-015-3927-7.
3. Itoi E. Pathophysiology and treatment of atraumatic instability of the shoulder. J Orthop Sci. 2004;9(2):208–13.
4. Wiesel BB, Gartsman GM, Press CM, et al. What went wrong and what was done about it: pitfalls in the treatment of common shoulder surgery. J Bone Joint Surg Ser A. 2013;95:2061–70.
5. Boileau P, Villalba M, Héry JY, et al. Risk factors for recurrence of shoulder instability after arthroscopic Bankart repair. J Bone Joint Surg Am. 2006;88:1755–63. https://doi.org/10.2106/JBJS.E.00817.

6. Ahmed I, Ashton F, Robinson CM. Arthroscopic Bankart repair and capsular shift for recurrent anterior shoulder instability: functional outcomes and identification of risk factors for recurrence. J Bone Joint Surg Am. 2012;94:1308–15. https://doi.org/10.2106/JBJS.J.01983.
7. Burkhart SS, Danaceau SM. Articular arc length mismatch as a cause of failed Bankart repair. Arthroscopy. 2000;16:740–4. https://doi.org/10.1053/jars.2000.7794.
8. Beran MC, Donaldson CT, Bishop JY. Treatment of chronic glenoid defects in the setting of recurrent anterior shoulder instability: a systematic review. J Shoulder Elb Surg. 2010;19:769–80.
9. Bigliani LU, Newton PM, Steinmann SP, et al. Glenoid rim lesions associated with recurrent anterior dislocation of the shoulder. Am J Sports Med. 1998;26:41–5. https://doi.org/10.1177/03635465980260012301.
10. Chen AL, Hunt SA, Hawkins RJ, Zuckerman JD. Management of bone loss associated with recurrent anterior glenohumeral instability. Am J Sports Med. 2005;33:912–25.
11. Ochoa E, Burkhart SS. Glenohumeral bone defects in the treatment of anterior shoulder instability. Instr Course Lect. 2009;58:323–36.
12. Lynch JR, Clinton JM, Dewing CB, et al. Treatment of osseous defects associated with anterior shoulder instability. J Shoulder Elb Surg. 2009;18:317–28.
13. Lo IKY, Parten PM, Burkhart SS. The inverted pear glenoid: an indicator of significant glenoid bone loss. Arthrosc J Arthrosc Relat Surg. 2004;20:169–74. https://doi.org/10.1016/j.arthro.2003.11.036.
14. Itoi E, Lee SB, Berglund LJ, et al. The effect of a glenoid defect on anteroinferior stability of the shoulder after Bankart repair: a cadaveric study. J Bone Joint Surg Am. 2000;82:35–46. https://doi.org/10.2106/00004623-200001000-00005.
15. Yamamoto N, Itoi E, Abe H, et al. Effect of an anterior glenoid defect on anterior shoulder stability: a cadaveric study. Am J Sports Med. 2009;37:949–54. https://doi.org/10.1177/0363546508330139.
16. Burkhart SS, De Beer JF. Traumatic glenohumeral bone defects and their relationship to failure of arthroscopic Bankart repairs: significance of the inverted-pear glenoid and the humeral engaging Hill-Sachs lesion. Arthroscopy. 2000;16(7):677–94. https://doi.org/10.1053/jars.2000.17715.
17. Yamamoto N, Muraki T, Sperling JW, et al. Stabilizing mechanism in bone-grafting of a large glenoid defect. J Bone Joint Surg Am. 2010;92:2059–66. https://doi.org/10.2106/JBJS.I.00261.
18. Shaha JS, Cook JB, Song DJ, et al. Redefining "critical" bone loss in shoulder instability. Am J Sports Med. 2015;43:1719–25. https://doi.org/10.1177/0363546515578250.
19. Milano G, Grasso A, Russo A, et al. Analysis of risk factors for glenoid bone defect in anterior shoulder instability. Am J Sports Med. 2011;39(9):1870–6. https://doi.org/10.1177/0363546511411699.
20. Chuang TY, Adams CR, Burkhart SS. Use of preoperative three-dimensional computed tomography to quantify glenoid bone loss in shoulder instability. Arthroscopy. 2008;4(4):376–82. https://doi.org/10.1016/j.arthro.2007.10.008.
21. Hill HA, Sachs MD. The grooved defect of the humeral head: a frequently unrecognized complication of dislocations of the shoulder joint. Radiology. 1940;35(6):690–700. https://doi.org/10.1148/35.6.690.
22. Sommaire C, Penz C, Clavert P, et al. Recurrence after arthroscopic Bankart repair: is quantitative radiological analysis of bone loss of any predictive value? Orthop Traumatol Surg Res. 2012;98(5):514–9. https://doi.org/10.1016/j.otsr.2012.03.015.
23. Rowe CR, Zarins B, Ciullo JV. Recurrent anterior dislocation of the shoulder after surgical repair. Apparent causes of failure and treatment. J Bone Joint Surg Am. 1984;66(2):159–68. https://doi.org/10.2106/00004623-198466020-00001.
24. Yamamoto N, Itoi E, Abe H, et al. Contact between the glenoid and the humeral head in abduction, external rotation, and horizontal extension: a new concept of glenoid track. J Shoulder Elb Surg. 2007;16(5):649–56. https://doi.org/10.1016/j.jse.2006.12.012.
25. Omori Y, Yamamoto N, Koishi H, et al. Measurement of the glenoid track in vivo as investigated by 3-dimensional motion analysis using open MRI. Am J Sports Med. 2014;42(6):1290–5. https://doi.org/10.1177/0363546514527406.
26. Di Giacomo G, Itoi E, Burkhart SS. Evolving concept of bipolar bone loss and the Hill-Sachs lesion: from "engaging/non-engaging" lesion to "on-track/off-track" lesion. Arthroscopy. 2014;30:90–8. https://doi.org/10.1016/j.arthro.2013.10.004.
27. Shaha JS, Cook JB, Rowles DJ, et al. Clinical validation of the glenoid track concept in anterior glenohumeral instability. J Bone Joint Surg Am. 2016;98(22):1918–23. https://doi.org/10.2106/JBJS.15.01099.
28. Ghodadra N, Gupta A, Romeo AA, et al. Normalization of glenohumeral articular contact pressures after Latarjet or iliac crest bone-grafting. J Bone Joint Surg Am. 2010;92(6):1478–89. https://doi.org/10.2106/JBJS.I.00220.
29. Helefet AJ. Coracoid transplantation for recurring dislocation of the shoulder. J Bone Joint Surg Br. 1958;40-B(2):198–202. https://doi.org/10.1302/0301-620X.40B2.198.
30. Schauder KS, Tullos HS. Role of the coracoid bone block in the modified Bristow procedure. Am J Sports Med. 1992;20(1):31–4. https://doi.org/10.1177/036354659202000109.
31. Latarjet M. [Treatment of recurrent dislocation of the shoulder]. Lyon Chir. 1954;49:994–7.
32. Wellmann M, De Ferrari H, Smith T, et al. Biomechanical investigation of the stabilization principle of the Latarjet procedure. Arch Orthop Trauma Surg. 2012;132:377–86. https://doi.org/10.1007/s00402-011-1425-z.

33. Yamamoto N, Muraki T, An KN, et al. The stabilizing mechanism of the Latarjet procedure: a cadaveric study. J Bone Joint Surg Am. 2013;95:1390–7. https://doi.org/10.2106/JBJS.L.00777.
34. Cowling PD, Akhtar MA, Liow RYL. What is a Bristow-Latarjet procedure? A review of the described operative techniques and outcomes. Bone Joint J. 2016;98-B:1208–14. https://doi.org/10.1302/0301-620X.98B9.37948.
35. Lafosse L, Lejeune E, Bouchard A, et al. The Arthroscopic Latarjet procedure for the treatment of anterior shoulder instability. Arthroscopy. 2007;23(11):1242.e1–5. https://doi.org/10.1016/j.arthro.2007.06.008.
36. Hovelius L, Korner L, Lundberg B, et al. The coracoid transfer for recurrent dislocation of the shoulder. Technical aspects of the Bristow-Latarjet procedure. J Bone Joint Surg Am. 1983;65(7):926–34. https://doi.org/10.2106/00004623-198365070-00007.
37. Lafosse L, Bongiorno V, Schwartz DG. Arthroscopic Latarjet procedure. In: Shoulder arthroscopy: principles and practice. Milano G and Grasso A (Eds.). London: Springer-Verlag. 2014;451–59. https://doi.org/10.1007/978-1-4471-5427-3.
38. de Beer JF, Roberts C. Glenoid bone defects-open Latarjet with congruent arc modification. Orthop Clin North Am. 2010;41:407–15.
39. Boileau P, Mercier N, Roussanne Y, et al. Arthroscopic Bankart-Bristow-Latarjet procedure: the development and early results of a safe and reproducible technique. Arthroscopy. 2010;26(11):1434–50.
40. Doursounian L, Debet-Mejean A, Chetboun A, Nourissat G. Bristow-Latarjet procedure with specific instrumentation: study of 34 cases. Int Orthop. 2009;33(4):1031–6. https://doi.org/10.1007/s00264-008-0606-z.
41. Metais P, Clavert P, Barth J, et al. Preliminary clinical outcomes of Latarjet-Patte coracoid transfer by arthroscopy vs. open surgery: prospective multicentre study of 390 cases. Orthop Traumatol Surg Res. 2016;102(8S):S271 6. https://doi.org/10.1016/j.otsr.2016.08.003.
42. Griesser MJ, Harris JD, McCoy BW, et al. Complications and re-operations after Bristow-Latarjet shoulder stabilization: a systematic review. J Shoulder Elb Surg. 2013;22(2):286–92.
43. Domos P, Lunini E, Walch G. Contraindications and complications of the Latarjet procedure. Shoulder Elbow. 2018;10(1):15–24. https://doi.org/10.1177/1758573217728716.
44. Di Giacomo G, de Gasperis N, Costantini A, et al. Does the presence of glenoid bone loss influence coracoid bone graft osteolysis after the Latarjet procedure? A computed tomography scan study in 2 groups of patients with and without glenoid bone loss. J Shoulder Elb Surg. 2014;23(4):514–8. https://doi.org/10.1016/j.jse.2013.10.005.
45. Allain J, Goutallier D, Glorion C. Long-term results of the Latarjet procedure for the treatment of anterior instability of the shoulder. J Bone Joint Surg Am. 1998;80(6):841–52. https://doi.org/10.1002/bjs.18002610104.
46. Bouju Y, Gadéa F, Stanovici J, et al. Shoulder stabilization by modified Latarjet-Patte procedure: results at a minimum 10 years' follow-up, and role in the prevention of osteoarthritis. Orthop Traumatol Surg Res. 2014;100:S213–8. https://doi.org/10.1016/j.otsr.2014.03.010.
47. Warner JJP, Gill TJ, O'Hollerhan JD, et al. Anatomical glenoid reconstruction for recurrent anterior glenohumeral instability with glenoid deficiency using an autogenous tricortical iliac crest bone graft. Am J Sports Med. 2006;34(2):205–12. https://doi.org/10.1177/0363546505281798.
48. Churchill RS, Moskal MJ, Lippitt SB, Matsen FA. Extracapsular anatomically contoured anterior glenoid bone grafting for complex glenohumeral instability. Tech Shoulder Elb. 2001;2:210–8.
49. Scheibel M, Nikulka C, Dick A, et al. Autogenous bone grafting for chronic anteroinferior glenoid defects via a complete subscapularis tenotomy approach. Arch Orthop Trauma Surg. 2008;128(11):1317–25. https://doi.org/10.1007/s00402-007-0560-z.
50. Kalogrianitis S, Tsouparopoulos V. Arthroscopic iliac crest bone block for reconstruction of the glenoid: a fixation technique using an adjustable-length loop cortical suspensory fixation device. Arthrosc Tech. 2016;5(6):e1197–202. https://doi.org/10.1016/j.eats.2016.07.007.
51. Boehm E, Gerhardt C, Kraus N, Scheibel M. Arthroscopic glenoid reconstruction for chronic anteroinferior shoulder instability using a tricortical iliac crest bone graft. JBJS Essent Surg Tech. 2016;6(4):e39. https://doi.org/10.2106/JBJS.ST.16.00080.
52. Rahme H, Wikblad L, Nowak J, Larsson S. Long-term clinical and radiologic results after Eden-Hybbinette operation for anterior instability of the shoulder. J Shoulder Elb Surg. 2003;12(1):15–9. https://doi.org/10.1067/mse.2002.128138.
53. Auffarth A, Schauer J, Matis N, et al. The J-bone graft for anatomical glenoid reconstruction in recurrent posttraumatic anterior shoulder dislocation. Am J Sports Med. 2008;36(4):638–47. https://doi.org/10.1177/0363546507309672.
54. Auffarth A, Kralinger F, Resch H. Anatomical glenoid reconstruction via a J-bone graft for recurrent posttraumatic anterior shoulder dislocation. Oper Orthop Traumatol. 2011;23(5):453–61. https://doi.org/10.1007/s00064-011-0055-5.
55. Pauzenberger L, Dyrna F, Obopilwe E, et al. Biomechanical evaluation of glenoid reconstruction with an implant-free J-bone graft for anterior glenoid bone loss. Am J Sports Med. 2017;45(12):2849–57. https://doi.org/10.1177/0363546517716927.
56. Moroder P, Plachel F, Becker J, et al. Clinical and radiological long-term results after implant-free, autologous, iliac crest bone graft procedure for the treatment of anterior shoulder

instability. Am J Sports Med. 2018;46:2975–80. https://doi.org/10.1177/0363546518795165.
57. Auffarth A, Resch H, Matis N, et al. Cartilage morphological and histological findings after reconstruction of the glenoid with an iliac crest bone graft. Am J Sports Med. 2018;46:1039–45. https://doi.org/10.1177/0363546517749813.
58. Anderl W, Kriegleder B, Heuberer PR. All-arthroscopic implant-free iliac crest bone grafting: new technique and case report. Arthroscopy. 2012;28:131–7. https://doi.org/10.1016/j.arthro.2011.10.027.
59. Shin SR, Tornetta P. Donor site morbidity after anterior iliac bone graft harvesting. J Orthop Trauma. 2016;30:340–3. https://doi.org/10.1097/BOT.0000000000000551.
60. Tokish JM, Fitzpatrick K, Cook JB, Mallon WJ. Arthroscopic distal clavicular autograft for treating shoulder instability with glenoid bone loss. Arthrosc Tech. 2014;3:e475–81. https://doi.org/10.1016/j.eats.2014.05.006.
61. Kwapisz A, Fitzpatrick K, Cook JB, et al. Distal clavicular osteochondral autograft augmentation for glenoid bone loss: a comparison of radius of restoration versus latarjet graft. Am J Sports Med. 2018;46:1046–52. https://doi.org/10.1177/0363546517749915.
62. Petersen SA, Bernard JA, Langdale ER, Belkoff SM. Autologous distal clavicle versus autologous coracoid bone grafts for restoration of anterior-inferior glenoid bone loss: a biomechanical comparison. J Shoulder Elb Surg. 2016;25:960–6. https://doi.org/10.1016/j.jse.2015.10.023.
63. Petrera M, Veillette CJ, Taylor DW, et al. Use of fresh osteochondral glenoid allograft to treat posteroinferior bone loss in chronic posterior shoulder instability. Am J Orthop. 2013;42(2):78–82.
64. Zhao J, Huangfu X, Yang X, et al. Arthroscopic glenoid bone grafting with nonrigid fixation for anterior shoulder instability: 52 patients with 2- to 5-year follow-up. Am J Sports Med. 2014;42(4):831–9. https://doi.org/10.1177/0363546513519227.
65. Provencher MT, Ghodadra N, LeClere L, et al. Anatomic osteochondral glenoid reconstruction for recurrent glenohumeral instability with glenoid deficiency using a distal tibia allograft. Arthroscopy. 2009;25(4):446–52. https://doi.org/10.1016/j.arthro.2008.10.017.
66. Weng PW, Shen HC, Lee HH, et al. Open reconstruction of large bony glenoid erosion with allogeneic bone graft for recurrent anterior shoulder dislocation. Am J Sports Med. 2009;37(9):1792–7. https://doi.org/10.1177/0363546509334590.
67. Tjoumakaris FP, Sekiya JK. Combined glenoid and humeral head allograft reconstruction for recurrent anterior glenohumeral instability. Orthopedics. 2008;31(5):497. https://doi.org/10.3928/01477447-20080501-28.
68. Smucny M, Miniaci A. A new option for glenoid reconstruction in recurrent anterior shoulder instability. Am J Orthop (Belle Mead NJ). 2017;46(4):199–202.
69. Sayegh ET, Mascarenhas R, Chalmers PN, et al. Allograft reconstruction for glenoid bone loss in glenohumeral instability: a systematic review. Arthroscopy. 2014;30(12):1642–9. https://doi.org/10.1016/j.arthro.2014.05.007.
70. Willemot LB, Akbari-Shandiz M, Sanchez-Sotelo J, et al. Restoration of articular geometry using current graft options for large glenoid bone defects in anterior shoulder instability. Arthroscopy. 2017;33:1661–9. https://doi.org/10.1016/j.arthro.2017.04.002.
71. Noonan B, Hollister SJ, Sekiya JK, Bedi A. Comparison of reconstructive procedures for glenoid bone loss associated with recurrent anterior shoulder instability. J Shoulder Elb Surg. 2014;23:1113–9. https://doi.org/10.1016/j.jse.2013.11.011.
72. Bhatia S, Van Thiel GS, Gupta D, et al. Comparison of glenohumeral contact pressures and contact areas after glenoid reconstruction with latarjet or distal tibial osteochondral allografts. Am J Sports Med. 2013;41:1900–8. https://doi.org/10.1177/0363546513490646.
73. Buck BE, Malinin TI, Brown MD. Bone transplantation and human immunodeficiency virus: an estimate of risk of acquired immunodeficiency syndrome (AIDS). Clin Orthop Relat Res. 1989;(240):129–36.
74. Rodrigo JJ, Thompson E, Travis C. Deep-freezing versus 4 degrees preservation of avascular osteocartilaginous shell allografts in rats. Clin Orthop Relat Res. 1987;(218):268–75.
75. Oakeshott RD, Farine I, Pritzker KPH, et al. A clinical and histologic analysis of failed fresh osteochondral allografts. Clin Orthop Relat Res. 1988;(233):283–94.
76. Williams SK, Amiel D, Ball ST, et al. Prolonged storage effects on the articular cartilage of fresh human osteochondral allografts. J Bone Joint Surg Am. 2003;85(11):2111–20. https://doi.org/10.2106/00004623-200311000-00008.
77. Patel RM, Amin NH, Lynch TS, Miniaci A. Management of bone loss in glenohumeral instability. Orthop Clin North Am. 2014;45:523–39. https://doi.org/10.1016/j.ocl.2014.06.005.
78. Snir N, Wolfson TS, Hamula MJ, et al. Arthroscopic anatomic humeral head reconstruction with osteochondral allograft transplantation for large Hill-Sachs lesions. Arthrosc Tech. 2013;2(3):e289–93. https://doi.org/10.1016/j.eats.2013.04.002.
79. Gerber C, Lambert SM. Allograft reconstruction of segmental defects of the humeral head for the treatment of chronic locked posterior dislocation of the shoulder. J Bone Joint Surg Am. 1996;78(3):376–82. https://doi.org/10.1016/j.jse.2014.03.017.
80. Yagishita K, Thomas BJ. Use of allograft for large Hill-Sachs lesion associated with anterior glenohumeral dislocation—a case report. Injury. 2002;33(9):791–4. https://doi.org/10.1016/S0020-1383(02)00043-8.
81. Diklic ID, Ganic ZD, Blagojevic ZD, et al. Treatment of locked chronic posterior dislocation of the shoulder by reconstruction of the defect in the humeral head with an allograft. J

Bone Joint Surg Br. 2010;92(1):71–6. https://doi.org/10.1302/0301-620X.92B1.22142.
82. Patrizio L, Sabetta E. Acute posterior shoulder dislocation with reverse Hill-Sachs lesion of the epiphyseal humeral head. ISRN Surg. 2011;2011:851051. https://doi.org/10.5402/2011/851051.
83. Johnson DL, Warner JJP. Osteochondritis dissecans of the humeral head: treatment with a matched osteochondral allograft. J Shoulder Elb Surg. 1997;6(2):160–3. https://doi.org/10.1016/S1058-2746(97)90038-0.
84. McCarty LP, Cole BJ. Reconstruction of the glenohumeral joint using a lateral meniscal allograft to the glenoid and osteoarticular humeral head allograft after bipolar chondrolysis. J Shoulder Elb Surg. 2007;16(6):e20–4. https://doi.org/10.1016/j.jse.2006.10.018.
85. Martinez AA, Navarro E, Iglesias D, et al. Long-term follow-up of allograft reconstruction of segmental defects of the humeral head associated with posterior dislocation of the shoulder. Injury. 2013;44(4):488–91. https://doi.org/10.1016/j.injury.2012.10.027.
86. Provencher MT, LeClere LE, Ghodadra N, Solomon DJ. Postsurgical glenohumeral anchor arthropathy treated with a fresh distal tibia allograft to the glenoid and a fresh allograft to the humeral head. J Shoulder Elb Surg. 2010;19(6):e6–e11. https://doi.org/10.1016/j.jse.2010.03.006.
87. Black LO, Ko J-WK, Quilici SM, Crawford DC. Fresh osteochondral allograft to the humeral head for treatment of an engaging reverse Hill-Sachs lesion. Orthop J Sport Med. 2016;4:2325967116670376. https://doi.org/10.1177/2325967116670376.
88. Nathan ST, Parikh SN. Osteoarticular allograft reconstruction for Hill-Sachs lesion in an adolescent. Orthopedics. 2012;35(5):e744–7. https://doi.org/10.3928/01477447-20120426-33.
89. Provencher MT, Sanchez G, Schantz K, et al. Anatomic humeral head reconstruction with fresh osteochondral talus allograft for recurrent glenohumeral instability with reverse Hill-Sachs lesion. Arthrosc Tech. 2017;6:e255–61. https://doi.org/10.1016/j.eats.2016.10.017.
90. Chapovsky F, Kelly JD IV. Osteochondral allograft transplantation for treatment of glenohumeral instability. Arthroscopy. 2005;21(8):1007. https://doi.org/10.1016/j.arthro.2005.04.005.
91. DiPaola MJ, Jazrawi LM, Rokito AS, et al. Management of humeral and glenoid bone loss--associated with glenohumeral instability. Bull NYU Hosp Jt Dis. 2010;68(4):245–50.
92. Trajkovski T, Mayne IP, Deheshi BM, Ferguson PC. Synovial chondromatosis of the shoulder: open synovectomy and insertion of osteoarticular allograft with internal fixation to repair intraoperative glenohumeral joint instability. Am J Orthop (Belle Mead NJ). 2011;40(8):E154–8.
93. Saltzman BM, Riboh JC, Cole BJ, Yanke AB. Humeral head reconstruction with osteochondral allograft transplantation. Arthroscopy. 2015;31(9):1827–34.
94. Lee CH, Cook JL, Mendelson A, Moioli EK, Yao H, Mao JJ. Regeneration of the articular surface of the rabbit synovial joint by cell homing: a proof of concept study. Lancet. 2010;376(9739):440–8. https://doi.org/10.1016/S0140-6736(10)60668-X.
95. Scotti C, Piccinini E, Takizawa H, Todorov A, Bourgine P, Papadimitropoulos A, Barbero A, Manz MG, Martin I. Engineering of a functional bone organ through endochondral ossification. Proc Natl Acad Sci U S A. 2013;110(10):3997–4002. https://doi.org/10.1073/pnas.1220108110. Epub 2013 Feb 11
96. Marmotti A, Mattia S, Castoldi F, Barbero A, Mangiavini L, Bonasia DE, Bruzzone M, Dettoni F, Scurati R, Peretti GM. Allogeneic umbilical cord-derived mesenchymal stem cells as a potential source for cartilage and bone regeneration: an in vitro study. Stem Cells Int. 2017;2017:1732094. https://doi.org/10.1155/2017/1732094.

Glenohumeral Joint Instability: Basic Science and Potential Treatment Options

43

Lukas Ernstbrunner, David Ackland, and Laura de Girolamo

43.1 Introduction

The glenohumeral joint facilitates the large range of upper limb motion that is essential for undertaking most activities of daily living. The shallow concavity of the bony glenoid and fibrocartilaginous labrum, together with the humeral head, comprises an inherently unstable joint that is dependent on the integrity and morphology of the articular surfaces, as well as the simultaneous activity of the rotator cuff for glenohumeral joint compression and stability. The scapulothoracic joint provides an additional stabilization by increasing upper limb range of motion and providing a moving "seat" for the humeral head, while the bony glenoid concavity, joint capsule and ligaments generate passive support to the glenohumeral joint, particularly in the mid-range and end range of joint motion. Disease or trauma to any of these bony or soft-tissue stabilizers may result in glenohumeral instability.

This chapter will review biomechanics of the normal and unstable shoulder, grafting techniques for the restoration of shoulder stability, and possible future directions in shoulder instability treatment.

43.2 Shoulder Structure and Function

43.2.1 Bony Stability

Normal shoulder function is a compromise between mobility and stability, with the large upper limb range of motion made possible by the shallow glenoid anatomy and mismatch with humeral articular geometry: a maximum 30% of the humeral articular cartilage is in contact with the glenoid at a given time, with contact pressure and area varying significantly with joint position [1]. The osseous and cartilaginous radii vary across the articular surfaces and are strongly dependent on plane of motion, influencing the degree of joint conformity [2]. The degree of mismatch in glenoid and humeral head radii has been shown to vary between 0.1 and 13.6 mm, with one study indicating that degree of mismatch had a significant influence on scores for glenoid radiolucent lines, which were best when the radial mismatch was between 6 and 10 mm

L. Ernstbrunner (✉)
Department of Orthopaedics, Balgrist University Hospital, University of Zurich, Zurich, Switzerland
e-mail: lukas.ernstbrunner@alumni.pmu.ac.at

D. Ackland
Department of Biomedical Engineering, University of Melbourne, Parkville, VIC, Australia
e-mail: dackland@unimelb.edu.au

L. de Girolamo
IRCCS Istituto Ortopedico Galeazzi, Milano, Italy
e-mail: laura.degirolamo@grupposandonato.it

R. Brzóska et al. (eds.), *360° Around Shoulder Instability*,
https://doi.org/10.1007/978-3-662-61074-9_43

[3]. However, incongruence of contacting joint surfaces is an essential feature of a healthy diarthrodial joint, since this allows articular contact areas to change during motion so cartilage can be flushed with synovial fluid during humeral motion [4]. More recent studies showed that recurrent anterior shoulder instability is associated with an inherited glenoid concavitiy deficiency and that the depth of the concavity is a main factor of the bony shoulder stability [5, 6].

43.2.2 Muscular Stability

Stability of the glenohumeral joint is dependent on a balance of the net forces and moments produced by the surrounding musculature to generate a net joint force that passes within the circumference of the glenoid fossa [7]. The simultaneous activation of the rotator cuff muscles, and other muscules spanning the glenohumeral joint, compresses the head of the humerus into the glenoid fossa, stabilizing the joint by concavity compression and preventing anterior–posterior and superior–inferior translations. The force produced by an individual shoulder muscle, and the direction of the muscle's force or its "line of action," determines the extent to which a muscle generates shear or compression at the glenohumeral joint, and therefore, whether it has destabilizing or stabilizing capacity, respectively. The rotator cuff muscles are oriented to provide significant compressive force at the glenohumeral joint, resisting the shear force transmitted via external upper limb forces, or imparted by muscles that are steeply inclined and have destabilizing capacity, such as the deltoid, latissimus dorsi and pectoralis major [8]. Whether or not these destabilizing muscles forces play a role in dynamic (atraumatic) instability is currently under investigation.

In addition to an individual muscle's line of action as a determinate of its stabilizing or destabilizing capacity, two simultaneously activated muscles that produce opposing joint moments may interact to produce a stabilizing "force couple" that results in glenohumeral joint compression. For example, during humeral abduction, the deltoid generates an agonist elevation moment and superior-directed force, which when combined with the antagonist moment and inferior-directed force of the inferior rotator cuff muscles, results in a scapular-plane force couple that compresses the glenohumeral joint (Fig. 43.1) [8, 9]. In a similar manner, humeral flexion and extension requires simultaneous activation of the anterior and posterior rotator cuff muscles to produce joint compression via a transverse-plane force couple [10]. The co-contraction of agonistic and anatonistic muscles during humeral movement, and the humeral compression from the resulting muscle force couple, is an essential mechanism required for glenohumeral joint stability during active upper limb motion.

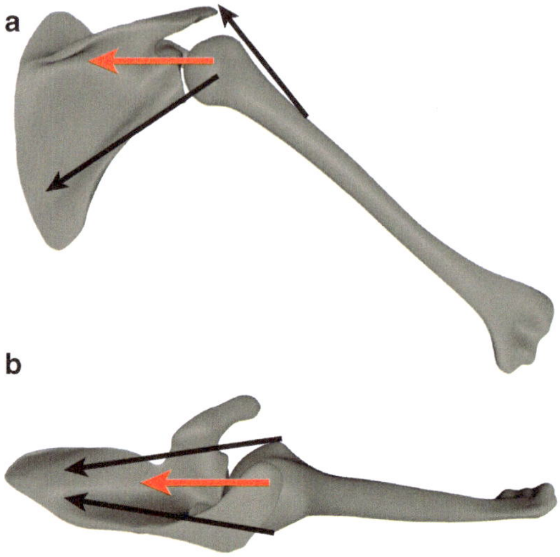

Fig. 43.1 Illustration of muscle force couples that provide glenohumeral joint stability by concavity compression, including the scapular-plane force couple formed between the middle deltoid and the inferior rotator cuff muscles (**a**) and the transverse-plane force couple formed between the anterior and posterior rotator cuff muscles (**b**). Black arrows indicate muscle lines of action, while the resultant glenohumeral joint compressive force direction is illustrated with red arrows

43.2.3 Labral and Ligamentous Stability

The glenoid labrum, a triangular section ring that resides on the periphery of the glenoid, functions to deepen the glenoid, increase joint congruency, and improve the stability of the glenohumeral joint. While the labrum constitutes up to 50% of the concavity depth [11], its function is dependent on its stiffness and structural integrity, as well as glenohumeral joint compressive forces generated by the shoulder musculature. Higher compressive joint forces increase the resistance of the joint to dislocation and help to maintain the humeral head centred in the glenoid during shoulder motion. There is an ongoing debate about the stabilizing role of the glenoid labrum, and biomechanical studies suggest that repair of a detached labrum by creating a "bump" does not provide any stabilizing effect [12].

The capsuloligamentous complex comprises a series of glenohumeral ligaments that are lax through the mid-range of movement but become progressively taut and provide glenohumeral joint stability toward the end-range of motion. For instance, the inferior glenohumeral ligament resists anteroinferior humeral head translation, especially with the arm externally rotated and abducted, while the superior glenohumeral ligament resists inferior translation of the adducted arm. The concept of ligamentous laxity during the mid-ranges of motion allows for dynamic muscle loading to be the primary joint stabilizing mechanism.

The ligament wrap length determines when a ligament provides passive restraint from translation. For example, long wrapping lengths of the inferior glenohumeral ligament during external rotation has been associated with passive posterior rotation [13]. This facilitates positioning of the humeral head in the glenoid fossa and prevention of anterior translation of the humeral head. Deficiency of this ligament reduces anterior translation restraint and may result in anterior subluxation. Ligaments may also provide stability to the glenohumeral joint by providing neurological feedback that directly mediates joint position and stabilizing muscle reflexes. It has been shown that proprioception of the symptomatic shoulder is disrupted in shoulders with joint instability compared to asymptomatic shoulders, with shoulder reconstruction having an important role in restoration of proprioceptive function [14].

43.2.4 Other Stabilizing Factors

Shoulder stability is also provided by a relatively constant capsular volume and ligament tension, which helps to maintain a negative intra-articular pressure and prevent excessive glenohumeral joint translation [15]. In addition, the long head of biceps tendon showed at least in biomechanical studies a humeral head depressor function [16]. For example, when the long head of biceps tendon is ruptured, the humeral head is known to translate superiorly during abduction [17]. Biomechanical studies have also shown that tension in the long head of biceps reduces superior–inferior and anterior–posterior translations, with anterior and posterior stabilizing function when the arm is internally and externally rotated, respectively [18]. However, the physiological role of the long biceps tendon is unknown. Finally, scapulothoracic motion, which allows increased humeral elevation beyond the 90° provided by the glenohumeral joint, provides a stabilizing "seat" for the head of the humerus at high elevation angles. The ratio of scapular to humeral motion has been reported as 1:2 beyond 30° of humeral elevation; however, shoulders with multidirectional instability (MDI) have an increased ratio, while shoulders with full-thickness rotator cuff tears or impingement have a lower ratio [19].

43.3 Glenohumeral Instability and Pathology

Glenohumeral instability may be defined by the inability of the humeral head to maintain congruency with the glenoid fossa during active humeral motion, and this may be associated with a range of pathological conditions affecting the active stabilizers (muscle-tendon units) and passive stabilizers (bony glenoid concavity, glenohumeral ligaments and glenoid labrum), or a combination. In the majority of patients with recurrent anterior instability, the primary dislocation is traumatic. Interestingly, posterior instability, which only accounts for about 5% of all patients with shoulder instabilities, is often non-traumatic. In patients with traumatic instability, symptoms are typically encountered in specific upper limb positions, while patient with atraumatic instability are affected in various upper limb configurations. Inherited or post-traumatic changes in the passive stabilizers of the glenohumeral joint are thought to be the primary factor associated with instability [5, 6, 20]; however, changes in the active stabilizers, muscle-tendon function and force/moment balance and neuromuscular control strategies may also contribute to increased translation and incidence of joint dislocation [11].

Gerber and Nyffeler introduced classification of dynamic instability as either unidirectional or multidirectional and with or without hyperlaxity [21]; however, providing a comprehensive classification of glenohumeral instability is made challenging by the many interacting biomechanical features of the pathology and the functional signs. For example, multidirectional instability (MDI), the condition where dislocation occurs in more than one direction with minimal or no causative trauma [22], has been identified based on the direction of dislocation: anterior-inferior with posterior subluxation, posterior-inferior with anterior subluxation, and global dislocation, with additional classifications based on combinations of instability directions. The pathoanatomy of MDI due to ligamentous laxity is associated with a redundant capsule resulting in increased glenohumeral joint volume and greater joint translations caused by excessive elastin in the capsular tissue; however, these quantities are difficult to measure clinically, and are ultimately influenced by loading of the active force-generating structures.

Glenohumeral joint dislocation occurs in 11.2 per 100,000 individuals annually [23], with initial and recurrent dislocations causing injury to the capsulolabral complex and the bony glenoid rim. Factors such as hyperlaxity or age under 18 years at the time of the first dislocation are associated with a high recurrency rate. There is an ongoing debate about surgical stabilization procedures in recurrent shoulder instability to prefer and specific surgical procedures include soft-tissue-based or glenoid reconstruction/grafting techniques. Large glenoid bone loss is known to diminish shoulder stability and lead to high failure rate of soft-tissue stabilization procedures [24]. This is because glenohumeral joint function is dependent on the entire glenoid articular surface to distribute contact forces and maintain joint congruency under the active muscle contraction conditions. Therefore, at least in situations with glenoid bone loss, glenoid grafting techniques have been shown to be superior to capsulolabral repairs [25].

It is established that even one-time shoulder dislocation can be associated with glenohumeral arthropathy and risk factors of ultimate arthropathy include traumatic dislocation, alcohol abuse, smoking, recurrence, contralateral instability or older age at primary dislocation and stabilization procedure [26–30]. The probably most crucial factor is the preoperative stage of dislocation arthropathy as suggested by Hovelius et al. in their landmark study [29]: The process of dislocation arthropathy, independently of the method of obtained stabilization (conservatively or surgically), cannot be reversed. They showed that 25 years after primary dislocation the rate of moderate or severe arthropathy in patients who had only one dislocation without surgery was 18%, 34% in those patients with recurrent dislocation without surgery, and 26% in those with successful surgery. Notwithstanding, there is also a certain percentage of patients developing a so-called iatrogenic arthropathy due to graft malpositioning, which results in increased glenohumeral contact pressure and posterior humeral head displacement [31, 32].

Besides the aforementioned soft-tissue-based or glenoid reconstruction/grafting techniques, no established treatment option has found its way to clinical application.

43.4 Future Directions in the Treatment of Glenohumeral Instability

Two surgical options for anterior shoulder instability are currently proposed, based on the extent of glenoid bone loss. When the glenoid defects are substantial, bony reconstruction techniques, such as an iliac crest bone grafting or a coracoid transfer procedure, are preferred [33].

Alternatively, for patients with a reduced or without an osseous lesion, soft-tissue stabilization procedures are the gold standard [33]. Nevertheless, the glenoid bone defect size remains small to intermediate in almost 90% of all cases [11]. Therefore, this vast majority does not require, as for ongoing treatment recommendations, a bony reconstruction but, on the other hand, this condition may constitute a biomechanically relevant defect able to threat the results of conventional soft-tissue stabilization procedures [34]. In fact, even "subcritical" glenoid bone lesions may negatively affect the functional outcome after soft-tissue stabilization procedures, with this problem emphasized in active patients [34]. To avoid these difficulties, a more liberal use of bone-grafting techniques (like the commonly used Latarjet procedure or iliac crest bone graft transfer) has been suggested, although more prone to complications (screw problems, pseudarthrosis, graft migration, nerve injury, and donor-site morbidity), together with an unnatural augmentation of the glenoid is produced with extensive bone graft resorption [35, 36].

Due to these premises, new approaches have been developed to address small to intermediate glenoid defects. In this perspective, the arthroscopic Bankart-Plus procedure has been proposed for patients with anterior shoulder instability and small to intermediate glenoid defects [37]. The technique is easy to perform because many steps are similar to the conventional arthroscopic Bankart repair. In this procedure, an allogeneic demineralized spongy bone matrix is inserted between the labrum and the glenoid neck, to compensate for the glenoid bone loss and increase the volume and stabilizing effect of the labrum. This enhanced stabilization, due to increased volume of the capsulolabral complex and concavity of the glenoid, may be due to either allograft development into bony apposition because of its osteoconductive properties or its transformation into scar tissue [38]. This procedure might be indicated also in other patients with compromised stability of the shoulder, as lack of sufficient labral tissue or constitutional flattened concavity [6, 39]. In the recent years, a growing interest in biological treatments, as alternative approaches to favour integration of graft, graft substitutes, or implants with bone and soft tissues, has gained attention. Indeed, biologics are able to stimulate the healing of the injured area through different mechanisms of actions. Among them, blood derivatives such as Platelet Rich Plasma (PRP), a low-cost way to obtain many growth factors [40] is a product enriched in platelets that contain an undifferentiated cocktail of anti-inflammatory, pro-inflammatory, anabolic, and catabolic mediators able to elicit the body's natural healing response are the most used. Likewise, cell concentrates such as those isolated from bone marrow and adipose tissue contain mesenchymal stem cells (MSCs), which are known for their ability to both differentiates into tissue-specific cells and interact with the tissue resident cells by secreting a plethora of different molecules, have recently increased their popularity.

The PRP therapeutic potential mainly relies on the platelets alpha granules which are rich in alluring growth factors. These include transforming growth factor-beta (TGF ß), epidermal growth factor (EGF), platelet derived growth factor (PDGF), fibroblast growth factor (bFGF), insulin like growth factor (IGF-1), stromal derived factor 1 alpha, bone morphogenic protein (BMP-2) and many other factors which mediate all the biological actions of PRP. Indeed, cumulative array of these growth factors possess unique multitasking abilities which include promotion of cellular chemotaxis, proliferation and differentiation, removal of tissue debris, angiogenesis and the laying down of extracellular matrix. The relative feasibility of PRP preparation is complemented by its alluring clinical safety profile: being a completely autologous product, PRP negates the chances of disease transmission and plausible immunogenic reactions. Several different PRP preparations are currently used, mainly varying in platelet and leukocyte concentration. There is no general consensus on the optimal PRP preparation. However, the findings collected so far seem to indicate that PRP with elevated leukocyte content, that is, leukocyte (neutrophil)-rich PRP (LRPRP), is associated with pro-inflammatory effects and elevated catabolic cytokines, such as interleukin-1β, tumor necrosis factor-α, and metalloproteinases [41]. Nevertheless, the clinical significance of these different PRP preparations is still being elucidated. As a striking PRP, which can be used alone or as a surgical augmentation, has given favourable results to enhance bone healing, although there is no clinical consensus to support the routine use of PRP to enhance bone healing [42, 43]. However, PRP was successful in the treatment of tibial fracture or osteotomy, posterior lumbar interbody fusion and calcaneal fractures [44].

PRP was also demonstrated to provide both short-term and long-term pain reliefs for tendon and ligament injuries, especially in the treatment of lateral epicondylitis and rotator cuff injuries [42]. For the latter application, the few studies that have been published about the use of PRP injection have compared clinical outcomes of subacromial injection of PRP to placebo and corticosteroids, with no studies evaluating direct injection into the tendon itself [45]. Although studies to date have demonstrated equivocal improvement in patient-reported outcomes from subacromial injections of PRP for rotator cuff tendinopathy, additional studies with longer follow-up are needed. When PRP was used a surgical augmentation in rotator cuff repair, the majority of individual studies have shown little difference in these outcome measures for PRP as an augment in arthroscopic rotator cuff repair compared to repair alone [46, 47]. However, given the significant heterogeneity of the PRP preparations large meta-analyses demonstrate a lack of evidence for the use of PRP as augmentation for rotator cuff repair. Some subgroup analyses seem to show that there may be some benefits in small or medium tears, treated with double-row repair, as well as a positive effect of PRP in immediate postoperative pain reduction.

Cell concentrate from bone marrow or adipose tissue are under extensive investigation given their properties to restore the tissue homeostasis. This is due to the presence of MSCs that is cells with a perivascular origin that are able to respond to trauma or tissue impairment by activating a pro-regenerative potential. MSCs have been shown to interact with resident cells through the release of several molecule families with different actions including, but not limited to anti-apoptotic, anti-scarring, pro-angiogenic and immunomodulatory.

Similar to PRP, cell concentrates greatly vary in composition and thus biological properties and there are not conclusive evidences about their efficacy in the musculoskeletal system yet.

However, bone marrow aspirate concentrate (BMAC) showed potential benefits for the repair of cartilage lesions, bony defects, and tendon injuries [48]. Also stromal vascular fraction (SVF) isolated from adipose tissue or microfragmented adipose tissue (micro-fat) was reported to be effective and safe in the field of orthopedic disorders, with documented results at joint level (osteoarthritis, meniscus tear), bone (osteonecrosis of the femoral head, bone and non-union fracture), and tendon/ligament (Achilles tendinopathy, lateral epicondylosis) regeneration [49]. BMAC and SVF/micro-fat rely on both mesenchymal stem cells and growth factors able to direct local cells to stimulate regeneration, repair and potentially graft repopulation, specific to each treated tissue as bone, cartilage or tendons. Compared to bone marrow, adipose tissue is considered a preferred source due to its ease of accessibility and the availability of a large number of mesenchymal stem cells per gram of tissue and a supposed higher immunomodulatory effect. To date, no data are available for the treatment of shoulder instability with any of these biologic products, but since regenerative approaches have been demonstrated an useful tool in similar tissues and disorders, in the future the combination of innovative regenerative-based products and ongoing surgical procedures might be a useful strategy to merge biological and biomechanical approaches as leading route for future biotechnological applications.

43.5 Conclusion

The glenohumeral joint is the most mobile joint of the body, but also an inherently unstable articulation. Stabilization of the joint is linked to a complex balance between static and dynamic tissue stabilizers. To date, consolidated surgical procedures are available for anterior shoulder instabilities with substantial bony glenoid defects, for patients without osseous lesions and, recently, for cases with small to intermediate glenoid defects. This new option sheds light on the possibility of using allogeneic demineralized spongy bone matrix, with the aim of compensating for the glenoid bone loss by increasing the volume of the labrum and thus its stabilizing effect, in a wide cohort of patients. Due to the possible allograft development into bony apposition because of either its osteoconductive properties or its transformation into scar tissue, the idea of biological-based regeneration and its enhancement has gained interest and the use of regenerative-based products in combination with classical procedures aimed at supporting biomechanics may be the key of future and improved techniques.

References

1. Warner JJ, et al. Articular contact patterns of the normal glenohumeral joint. J Shoulder Elbow Surg. 1998;7(4):381–8.
2. Zumstein V, et al. The glenohumeral joint—a mismatching system? A morphological analysis of the cartilaginous and osseous curvature of the humeral head and the glenoid cavity. J Orthop Surg Res. 2014;9:34.
3. Doyle AJ, Burks RT. Comparison of humeral head retroversion with the humeral axis/biceps groove relationship: a study in live subjects and cadavers. J Shoulder Elbow Surg. 1998;7(5):453–7.
4. Zumstein V, Kraljevic M, Muller-Gerbl M. Glenohumeral relationships: subchondral mineralization patterns, thickness of cartilage, and radii of curvature. J Orthop Res. 2013;31(11):1704–7.
5. Ernstbrunner L, et al. Biomechanical analysis of the effect of congruence, depth and radius on the stability ratio of a simplistic 'ball-and-socket' joint model. Bone Joint Res. 2016;5(10):453–60.
6. Moroder P, et al. Anterior shoulder instability is associated with an underlying deficiency of the bony glenoid concavity. Arthroscopy. 2015;31(7):1223–31.
7. Wu W, et al. Subject-specific musculoskeletal modeling in the evaluation of shoulder muscle and joint function. J Biomech. 2016;49(15):3626–34.
8. Ackland DC, Pandy MG. Lines of action and stabilizing potential of the shoulder musculature. J Anat. 2009;215:184–97.
9. Lucas DB. Biomechanics of the shoulder joint. Arch Surg. 1973;107(3):425–32.
10. Wattanaprakornkul D, et al. The rotator cuff muscles have a direction specific recruitment pattern during shoulder flexion and extension exercises. J Sci Med Sport. 2011;14(5):376–82.
11. Griffith JF, et al. Prevalence, pattern, and spectrum of glenoid bone loss in anterior shoulder dislocation: CT analysis of 218 patients. AJR Am J Roentgenol. 2008;190(5):1247–54.
12. Yamamoto N, et al. Does the "bumper" created during Bankart repair contribute to shoulder stability? J Shoulder Elbow Surg. 2013;22(6):828–34.
13. Karduna AR, et al. Kinematics of the glenohumeral joint: influences of muscle forces, ligamentous constraints, and articular geometry. J Orthop Res. 1996;14(6):986–93.
14. Lephart SM, et al. Proprioception of the shoulder joint in healthy, unstable, and surgically repaired shoulders. J Shoulder Elbow Surg. 1994;3(6):371–80.
15. Lugo R, Kung P, Ma CB. Shoulder biomechanics. Eur J Radiol. 2008;68(1):16–24.
16. Warner JJ, McMahon PJ. The role of the long head of the biceps brachii in superior stability of the glenohumeral joint. J Bone Joint Surg Am. 1995;77(3):366–72.
17. Abboud JA, Soslowsky LJ. Interplay of the static and dynamic restraints in glenohumeral instability. Clin Orthop Relat Res. 2002;400:48–57.
18. Pagnani MJ, et al. Role of the long head of the biceps brachii in glenohumeral stability: a biomechanical study in cadavera. J Shoulder Elbow Surg. 1996;5(4):255–62.
19. Halder AM, Itoi E, An KN. Anatomy and biomechanics of the shoulder. Orthop Clin North Am. 2000;31(2):159–76.
20. Gottschalk MB, et al. Posterior shoulder instability: does glenoid retroversion predict recurrence and contralateral instability? Arthroscopy. 2015;31(3):488–93.
21. Gerber C, Nyffeler RW. Classification of glenohumeral joint instability. Clin Orthop Relat Res. 2002;400:65–76.
22. Merolla G, et al. Multidirectional instability of the shoulder: biomechanics, clinical presentation, and treatment strategies. Eur J Orthop Surg Traumatol. 2015;25(6):975–85.
23. Dodson CC, Cordasco FA. Anterior glenohumeral joint dislocations. Orthop Clin North Am. 2008;39(4):507–18, vii
24. Burkhart SS, De Beer JF. Traumatic glenohumeral bone defects and their relationship to failure of arthroscopic Bankart repairs: significance of the inverted-pear glenoid and the humeral engaging Hill-Sachs lesion. Arthroscopy. 2000;16(7):677–94.
25. Zimmermann SM, et al. Long-term restoration of anterior shoulder stability: a retrospective analysis of arthroscopic bankart repair versus open latarjet procedure. J Bone Joint Surg Am. 2016;98(23):1954–61.

26. Allain J, Goutallier D, Glorion C. Long-term results of the Latarjet procedure for the treatment of anterior instability of the shoulder. J Bone Joint Surg Am. 1998;80(6):841–52.
27. Ernstbrunner L, Gerber C. Editorial commentary: computed tomography-based analysis of the arthroscopic latarjet procedure suggests graft positioning is more variable than expected. Arthroscopy. 2018;34(7):2041–4.
28. Ernstbrunner L, et al. Arthroscopic versus open iliac crest bone grafting in recurrent anterior shoulder instability with glenoid bone loss: a computed tomography-based quantitative assessment. Arthroscopy. 2018;34(2):352–9.
29. Hovelius L, Saeboe M. Neer Award 2008: arthropathy after primary anterior shoulder dislocation—223 shoulders prospectively followed up for twenty-five years. J Shoulder Elbow Surg. 2009;18(3):339–47.
30. Ladermann A, et al. Risk factors for dislocation arthropathy after Latarjet procedure: a long-term study. Int Orthop. 2013;37(6):1093–8.
31. Ghodadra N, et al. Normalization of glenohumeral articular contact pressures after Latarjet or iliac crest bone-grafting. J Bone Joint Surg Am. 2010;92(6):1478–89.
32. Montgomery WH Jr, et al. Anteroinferior bone-grafting can restore stability in osseous glenoid defects. J Bone Joint Surg Am. 2005;87(9):1972–7.
33. Bushnell BD, et al. Bony instability of the shoulder. Arthroscopy. 2008;24(9):1061–73.
34. Shaha JS, et al. Redefining "critical" bone loss in shoulder instability: functional outcomes worsen with "subcritical" bone loss. Am J Sports Med. 2015;43(7):1719–25.
35. Butt U, et al. Complications associated with open coracoid transfer procedures for shoulder instability. J Shoulder Elbow Surg. 2012;21(8):1110–9.
36. Di Giacomo G, et al. Does the presence of glenoid bone loss influence coracoid bone graft osteolysis after the Latarjet procedure? A computed tomography scan study in 2 groups of patients with and without glenoid bone loss. J Shoulder Elbow Surg. 2014;23(4):514–8.
37. Moroder P, et al. The Arthroscopic Bankart-Plus Procedure for treatment of anterior shoulder instability with small to intermediate glenoid defects. Arthrosc Tech. 2018;7(4):e379–84.
38. Yamamoto N, et al. Stabilizing mechanism in bone-grafting of a large glenoid defect. J Bone Joint Surg Am. 2010;92(11):2059–66.
39. Kim JY, et al. Morphological characteristics of the repaired labrum according to glenoid location and its clinical relevance after arthroscopic bankart repair: postoperative evaluation with computed tomography arthrography. Am J Sports Med. 2014;42(6):1304–14.
40. Kon E, et al. Platelet-rich plasma (PRP) to treat sports injuries: evidence to support its use. Knee Surg Sports Traumatol Arthrosc. 2011;19(4):516–27.
41. Dragoo JL, et al. Comparison of the acute inflammatory response of two commercial platelet-rich plasma systems in healthy rabbit tendons. Am J Sports Med. 2012;40:1274–81.
42. Marcazzan S, et al. Efficacy of platelet concentrates in bone healing: a systematic review on animal studies—part B: large-size animal models. Platelets. 2018;29(4):338–46.
43. Guzel Y, et al. The biomechanical and histological effects of platelet-rich plasma on fracture healing. Knee Surg Sports Traumatol Arthrosc. 2015;23:1378–83.
44. Roffi A, et al. Does PRP enhance bone integration with grafts, graft substitutes, or implants? A systematic review. BMC Musculoskelet Disord. 2013;14:330.
45. Le ADK, et al. Current clinical recommendations for use of platelet-rich plasma. Curr Rev Musculoskelet Med. 2018;11(4):624–34.
46. Holtby R, et al. Impact of platelet-rich plasma on arthroscopic repair of small- to medium-sized rotator cuff tears: a randomized controlled trial. Orthop J Sports Med. 2016;4:2325967116665559.
47. Cai Y, et al. Efficacy of platelet-rich plasma in arthroscopic repair of full-thickness rotator cuff tears: a meta-analysis. J Shoulder Elbow Surg. 2015;24:1852–9.
48. Gianakos AL, et al. Clinical application of concentrated bone marrow aspirate in orthopaedics: a systematic review. World J Orthop. 2017;8(6):491–506.
49. Pak J, et al. Current use of autologous adipose tissue-derived stromal vascular fraction cells for orthopedic applications. J Biomed Sci. 2017;24(1):9.

The manufacturer's authorised representative in the EU is Springer Nature Customer Service Centre GmbH, Europaplatz 3, 69115 Heidelberg, Germany. If you have any concerns regarding our products, please contact ProductSafety@springernature.com

Printed and bound by CPI Group (UK) Ltd, Croydon, CR0 4YY
30/09/2026
02225240-0019